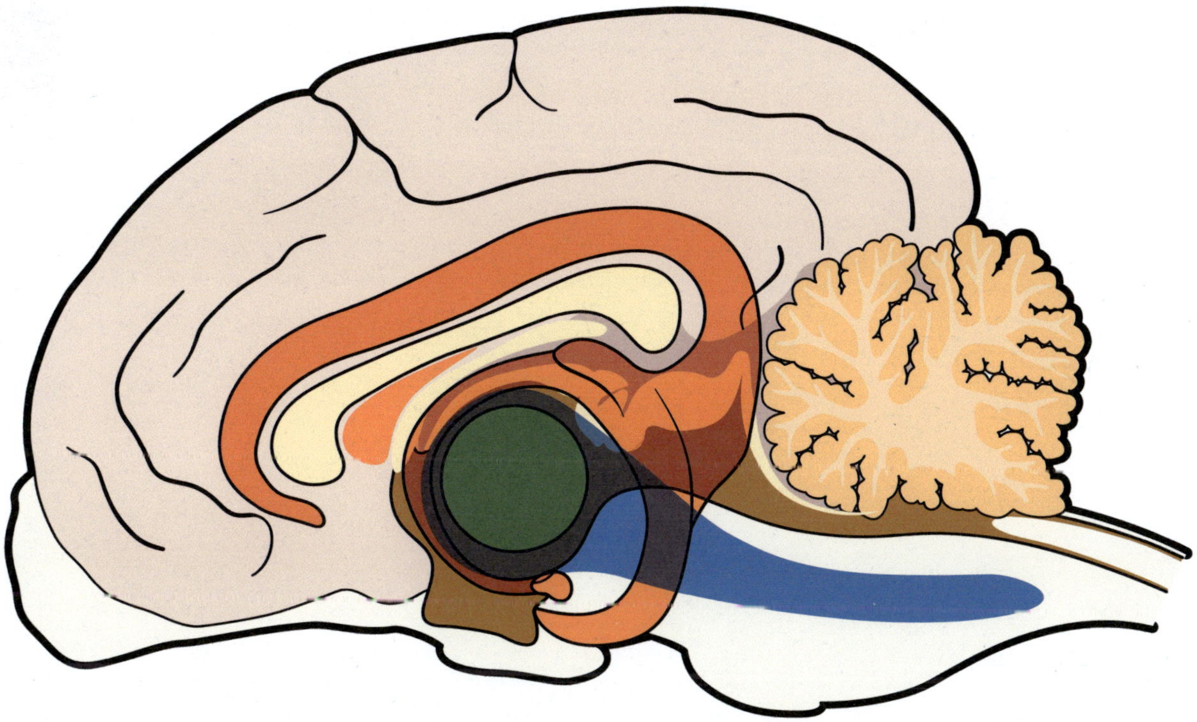

VETERINARY INTERNAL MEDICINE

EDITORS-IN-CHIEF
EDWARD FELDMAN
FEDERICO FRACASSI

CANINE NEUROLOGY

EDITORS
Luisa De Risio
Gualtiero Gandini

edra PUBLISHING

VETERINARY INTERNAL MEDICINE SERIES - Edward Feldman, Federico Fracassi. Editors-in-chief.
Luisa De Risio, Gualtiero Gandini - Canine neurology

ISBN: 978-1-957260-50-1
eISBN: 978-1-957260-80-8

Book Publishing Manager: Costanza Smeraldi

Cover: Laura Barzacca

Layout: T&T studio s.a.s, Milano

Copyediting: Melissa Testa, Grupo Asìs

edra
PUBLISHING

Edra Publishing US LLC
3309 Northlake Boulevard
Suite 203, Palm Beach Gardens
FL, 33403
EIN: 844113980
info@edrapublishing.com
www.edrapublishing.com

Printed in Italy by "Kosmoprint" S.r.l. Rimini (RN)

Series editors

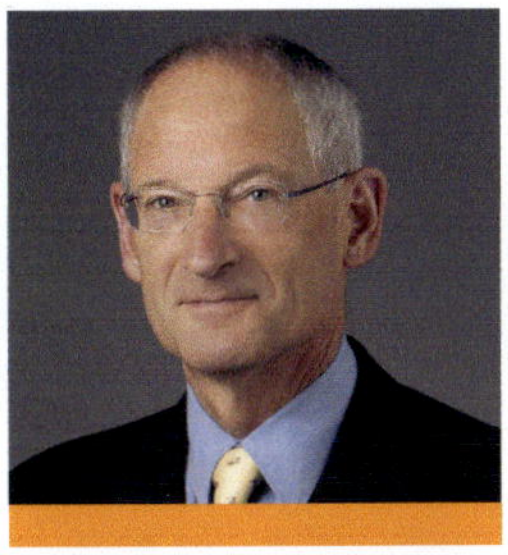

Edward C. Feldman
DVM, ACVIM Diplomate (SAIM), Emeritus Professor of Small Animal Internal Medicine, University of California, Davis, USA

Dr. Feldman earned his DVM from the University of California in 1973. He joined the Davis faculty in 1979 after an internship at the Animal Medical Center in New York City, a Residency with Dr. Stephen Ettinger in the world's first referral only private veterinary practice in Berkeley California, a year in general practice and another on faculty at the University of Saskatchewan, in Canada. He has authored more than 160 peer-reviewed scientific publications, 110 scientific abstracts, and 75 book chapters.

Dr. Feldman has coedited the last six editions of The Textbook of Veterinary Internal Medicine with Dr. Stephen Ettinger and the last two also with Dr. Etienne Côté. He coauthored the four editions of Canine and Feline Endocrinology with Dr. Richard Nelson and the 4th edition also with Drs. Claudia Reusch, Catharine Scott-Moncrieff, and Ellen Behrend. He coedited Feline Endocrinology with Dr. Fracassi and Dr. Peterson.

Dr. Feldman has lectured in more than 45 of the 50 United States and 43 countries.

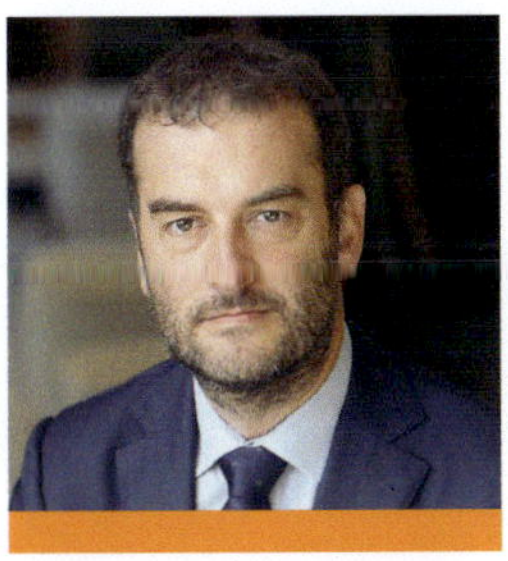

Federico Fracassi
DVM, ECVIM Diplomate (SAIM) Professor of Small Animal Internal Medicine University of Bologna, Italy

Dr. Fracassi graduated in Veterinary Medicine (DVM) at the University of Bologna, Italy. In 2005 he defended his PhD thesis and then completed a Residency in Internal Medicine at the University of Zurich, Switzerland.

He is now an Associate Professor of Veterinary Internal Medicine at the University of Bologna. His publication list consists of more than 100 journal articles.

He is the editor of "Veterinaria", a peer-reviewed journal and associate editor of JSAP. He coedited Feline Endocrinology with Dr. Feldman and Dr. Peterson. He has edited the book "Diagnostic and therapeutic algorithms in internal medicine for dogs and cats".

Dr. Fracassi has lectured in 22 countries.

Book editors

Luisa De Risio

DVM (Hons), PhD, PGCert Vet Ed, PGCert IAWEL, FHEA, DECVN, FRCVS, RCVS and EBVS® European Specialist in Veterinary Neurology

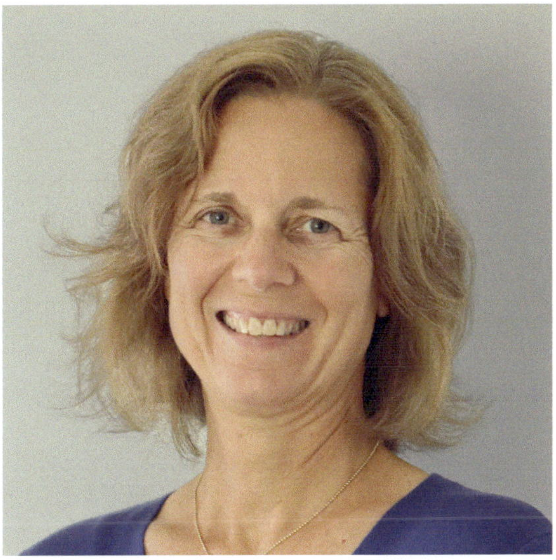

Dr. Luisa De Risio is a boarded veterinary neurologist with experience in conducting and leading research in academia, nonprofit organisations and industry. She earned her degree in Veterinary Medicine and her PhD from the University of Parma (Italy) in 1996 and 2000, respectively. She also completed an internship at a small animal referral hospital in Paris (France) and trained as a neurologist and neurosurgeon at North Carolina State University (USA). She became a Diplomate of the European College of Veterinary Neurology in 2004. Luisa was Faculty at the University of Parma until 2005 when she moved to the UK to become the Head of Neurology and subsequently Head of Research at the Animal Health Trust. Luisa joined Mars as a Clinical Research Director for Linnaeus in January 2020 and built a comprehensive program of clinical research support for Linnaeus Associates, fostering mutuality and productive scientific collaborations with other divisions in Mars Petcare. Luisa has been appointed as MVH global Director, Associate Research and joined the MVH Medical Affairs Science Team on 1 January 2025.

Luisa has worked with and led teams of people with different backgrounds, nationalities, and cultures. She achieved the Level 5 Certificate in Leadership and Management from the Institute of Leadership and Management in 2017, the Fellowship by Meritorious Contributions to Clinical Practice by the Royal College of Veterinary Surgeons in 2018, the Postgraduate Certificate in Veterinary Education at the Royal Veterinary College in 2020, and the Postgraduate Certificate in International Animal Welfare, Ethics and Law at the University of Edinburgh in 2025. She has been Honorary Professor of Veterinary Neurology at Nottingham Trent University (2021–2024) and vice president of the European College of Veterinary Neurology (2022–2024). Luisa has lectured at numerous continuing education and scientific meetings, published more than 100 papers in peer-reviewed journals, written numerous book chapters, and edited two textbooks on canine and feline seizure disorders.

Gualtiero Gandini

DVM, PhD, PGCert Vet Ed, FHEA, DECVN and EBVS® European Specialist in Veterinary Neurology

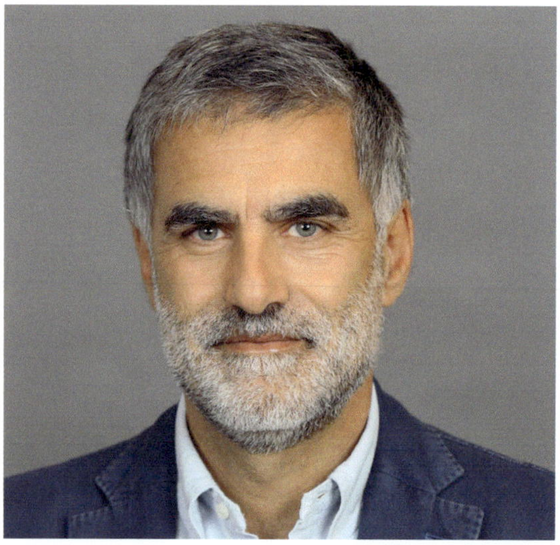

Dr. Gualtiero Gandini is full professor at the Department of Veterinary Medical Sciences of the University of Bologna (Italy). He graduated cum laude from the Faculty of Veterinary Medicine of Bologna and completed a PhD in Internal Medicine. In 2003, he achieved board certification in neurology by the European College of Veterinary Neurology (ECVN). In 2008 elected President of the European Society and College of Veterinary Neurology (ESVN/ECVN) and he has served in the Executive Committee for 12 years (2000–2012). In 2022 he was elected for the second time President of the European Society and College of Veterinary Neurology (ESVN/ECVN). He also served as president of the Italian Society of Veterinary Neurology (SINVet) (2021–2024), of which he has been a member since 1998.
He is an expert of the European System of Evaluation of Veterinary Training (ESEVT) within the European Association of Establishments for Veterinary Education (EAEVE). From 2015 to 2021, he directed the degree programme in veterinary medicine of the University of Bologna. From 2017 to 2021, he was the National Representative of the European Board of Veterinary Specialization (EBVS) for Italy. Dr. Gandini has lectured in more than 150 national and international courses and has been an invited speaker at over 35 national and international congresses. He has also organized the four European editions of the international neurology *"Brain Camp" - Veterinary Neuroscience Course* for residents in neurology. He is an author/coauthor of more than 100 scientific publications, 71 in peer-reviewed international journals.

Contributors

Federica Balducci, DVM, DECVN
Veterinary Hospital AniCura, I Portoni Rossi
Bologna, Italy

Renee Barber, DVM, PhD, DACVIM (Neurology)
Small Animal Medicine & Surgery
College of Veterinary Medicine
University of Georgia
Athens, GA (USA)

Elsa Beltrán, Lda. Vet., DECVN, PGDipVetEd, FHEA, MRCVS
Department of Clinical Science & Services
The Royal Veterinary College, University of London
Hatfield, UK

Sofie F.M. Bhatti, DVM, PhD
Department of Small Animals, Faculty of Veterinary Medicine
Ghent University
Ghent, Belgium

Ezio Bianchi, DVM, DECVN
Department of Veterinary Science
University of Parma
Parma, Italy

Giulia Cagnotti, DVM, MRCVS, PhD, DECVN
Department of Veterinary Science
University of Turin
Turin, Italy

Marios Charalambous, DVM, PhD, DACVIM (Neurology), DECVN, FHEA, MRCVS
Clinic for Small Animals, Department of Neurology
University of Veterinary Medicine Hannover
Hannover, Germany

Louise Clark, BVMS, CertVA, DECVAA, MSc, FRCVS
Davies Veterinary Specialists
Hitchin, UK

Joan R. Coates, DVM, MS, DACVIM (Neurology)
Department of Veterinary Medicine and Surgery,
College of Veterinary Medicine
University of Missouri
Columbia, MO (USA)

Ronaldo Casimiro da Costa, DMV, MSc, PhD, DACVIM (Neurology)
Department of Veterinary Clinical Sciences, College of Veterinary Medicine
The Ohio State University
Columbus, OH (USA)

Steven De Decker, DVM, PhD, MvetMed, DECVN, FHEA, PGCert VetEd, MRCVS
Queen Mother Hospital for Animals
The Royal Veterinary College, University of London
Hatfield, UK

Alberta de Stefani, DVM, MRCVS, PhD, DECVN, PGDipVetEd, FHEA
Queen Mother Hospital for Animals
The Royal Veterinary College, University of London
Hatfield, UK

Cristian Falzone, DVM, DECVN
Diagnostica Piccoli Animali
Zugliano (VI), Italy

Joe Fenn, BVetMed, MVetMed, DECVN, FHEA, MRCVS
Queen Mother Hospital for Animals
The Royal Veterinary College, University of London
Hatfield, UK

Rodrigo Gutierrez Quintana, MVZ, MVM, DECVN, MRCVS
School Of Biodiversity, One Health & Veterinary Medicine
University of Glasgow
Glasgow, UK

Silke Hecht, Dr. med. vet., DACVR, DECVDI
Department of Small Animal Clinical Sciences
College of Veterinary Medicine
University of Tennessee
Knoxville, TN (USA)

Mark Lowrie, MA, VetMB, MVM, DECVN, MRCVS, RCVS & EBVS®
European Recognized Specialist in Veterinary Neurology
Movement Referrals
Runcorn, UK

Oliver Marsh, BVM BVS, DECVN, MRCVS
DWR Veterinary Specialists
Six Mile Bottom, Cambridgeshire, UK

Lara Matiasek, DVM, DECVN
Centre for Clinical Veterinary Medicine
LMU Munich, Germany

Marika Menchetti, DVM, PhD, DECVN
San Marco Veterinary Clinic and Laboratory
Veggiano (PD), Italy

Diane Messum, MCSP, HCPC, BSc(Hons), MSc, ACPAT Cat A, RAMP
Davies Veterinary Specialists
Hitchin, UK

Sarah A. Moore, DVM, DACVIM (Neurology)
BluePearl Pet Hospitals
Tampa, FL (USA)

Dennis O'Brien, DVM, PhD, DACVIM (Neurology)
College of Veterinary Medicine
University of Missouri
Columbia, MO (USA)

Natasha Olby, DVM, PhD, MRCVS, DACVIM (Neurology)
Department of Clinical Sciences, College of Veterinary Medicine
NC State University
Raleigh, NC (USA)

John H. Rossmeisl, DVM, MS, DACVIM (SAIM and Neurology)
Department of Small Animal Clinical Sciences,
College of Veterinary Medicine
Virginia Tech
Blacksburg, VA (USA)

Clare Rusbridge, BVMS, PhD, DECVN, FRCVS
The School of Veterinary Medicine
University of Surrey
Guildford, UK
Wear Referrals Veterinary Specialist & Emergency Hospital
Bradbury, UK

Lluís Sánchez, Ldo. Vet., DECVN, MRCVS
Willows Veterinary Centre & Referral Service
West Midlands, UK

Fabio Stabile, DVM, MRCVS, PhD, DECVN
Wear Referrals
Bradbury, UK

Catherine Stalin, MA, VetMB, DECVIN, MRCVS
School Of Biodiversity, One Health & Veterinary Medicine
University of Glasgow
Glasgow, UK

Frank Steffen, DVM, DECVN
Vetsuisse Faculty
University of Zurich
Zurich, Switzerland

Series preface

"Oh! You are a veterinarian? I (or my brother, my sister, my son, my daughter...) always wanted to be a veterinarian." All of us, as veterinary students and later as veterinarians, have often heard comments like this. Becoming a veterinarian seems to be such a wonderful career to nonveterinarians: helping helpless dogs and cats. Veterinarians should be happy and satisfied in their *chosen* profession because they are able to earn a living by caring for loved pets. The journey to satisfaction and happiness for veterinarians, however, never seems to follow an obvious, straight, or level path.

The 1950s witnessed a dramatic growth in the popularity of pet dogs and in the number of veterinarians who cared exclusively for pets. The popularity of cats soon followed. Today, more dogs and cats are considered "members of the family" than ever before in human history, and their owners want to protect their family members from illness or to resolve any illness. There are more veterinarians who care for dogs and cats currently than ever before in human history. Veterinary medicine has evolved remarkably to meet the ever-growing medical care expectations and demands of dog and cat owners.

When learning of a diagnosis, prognosis, treatment, and/or the cost of care for their ill pet, some owners become distressed. These emotions are often directed at the "messenger" of the bad news: the veterinarian. The veterinarian, in turn, may not respect their own knowledge and feel inadequate. One reason that a veterinarian may feel inadequate is the realization that it is impossible for anyone in general practice to be expert and current on all the canine and feline conditions encountered in a day, week, or month: everything from orthopedics to oncology, from vaccinology to dermatology, from ophthalmology to cardiology. Nor is it possible for an internal medicine specialist to be expert and current in each condition they encounter, from endocrinology to gastroenterology or from respiratory conditions to chronic kidney disease. Further, it is clear that cats are not small dogs. Perceived "knowledge deficiencies" can cause veterinarians to feel they are failing to meet their clients' expectations.

The internal medicine textbooks in this new series offer one approach for enjoying veterinary practice. We encourage colleagues to embrace developing expertise in one area. By focusing on and studying one organ system in either the dog or cat, one can achieve greater knowledge and skills and, in turn, greater confidence. Each book in this series offers a clear path to learning current opinions on pathophysiology, diagnosis, treatment, prognosis, and costs associated with illnesses involving one system in one species. Confidence gained in a focused area can be sensed by devoted owners. Further, confidence in one area of internal medicine also creates confidence in sharing limitations: "I am extremely confident in diagnosing and managing some conditions but I lack that level of expertise in all other conditions".

The books in this series have been constructed to help build expertise in one organ system in either the dog or the cat. Each book is edited by one or two specialists with outstanding international credentials. Each editor was tasked with building a text that contains all the information found in general internal medicine textbooks, but with much more in-depth discussions on each condition. Each book has early chapters focusing on differential diagnoses of owner concerns, physical examination findings, and laboratory and/or imaging results. These are excellent for students as they begin to apply their basic knowledge to clinical cases. These chapters also provide a quick review for experienced general practitioners and specialists. Each chapter provides at least one algorithm designed to take the reader from a vague owner concern, physical examination finding, or laboratory abnormality to a specific diagnosis with step-by-step instructions. The "techniques section" in each text teaches currently employed procedures, most with videos. In-depth chapters on known illnesses comprise 70 to 80% of each book's content. The editors have provided a larger number of chapters, a larger number of expert contributors, and greater depth on each organ system than any general textbook can supply. The material has a level of credibility that no internet site can claim. Each book can guide the reader through a more complete journey of understanding than is available in any other veterinary resource.

Edward Feldman
Federico Fracassi

Preface

It has been an honour and a privilege to contribute the Canine neurology textbook to the novel Veterinary Internal Medicine Series led by Prof. Ed Feldman and Prof. Federico Fracassi.

Neurology is a rapidly evolving and advancing field, often perceived as challenging and intimidating. This new textbook, entirely dedicated to canine neurology, provides up-to-date, evidence-based, clinically applicable information to support veterinary practitioners both in primary and secondary care. The aim is to improve knowledge and confidence in dealing with the neurology canine patient and promote contextualized care to benefit the patients, their owners, and the veterinary team. This book is also a precious resource for house officers and residents studying for board examination and for veterinary interns and students wishing to deepen their knowledge of neurology.

The book comprises four sections and includes figures, videos, tables, and algorithms to provide both quick access to key practical information and more in-depth knowledge. The first section includes short chapters focused on common neurologic presentations based on the owner's presenting concerns and/or physical examination findings. Each chapter includes an algorithm to provide visually engaging and easily accessible information on clinical approach, differential diagnoses, diagnostic investigations, and treatment. The second section focuses on the foundations of clinical neurology: an accurate approach to the neurology patient, a well-conducted neurologic examination, and correct interpretation of the findings to establish a robust neuroanatomic localization and a differential diagnosis list. The third section provides insights into diagnostic procedures, including laboratory investigations, neuroimaging, and electrodiagnostics. The fourth section of the book provides comprehensive yet accessible evidence-based and clinically relevant information on numerous neurologic disorders. Each chapter includes details on pathophysiology, diagnosis, treatment, and prognosis; helpful illustrations and videos; and a key points box to highlight essential information.

This textbook is the result of the dedication and expertise of a global team of authors with the excellent support of EDRA's Costanza Smeraldi and Melissa Testa, overseen by Prof. Ed Feldman and Prof. Federico Fracassi. It has been wonderful to work with you all, an absolute dream team!

We hope that this textbook will equip the readers with the knowledge, skills, and confidence to optimize the care they provide to their neurology patients and bring joy in their clinical practice. Equally, we hope it will spark their interest in further advancing clinical neurology and engaging in lifelong learning.

Luisa De Risio
Gualtiero Gandini

The Editors endorse the WSAVA position statement on cosmetic alterations in companion animals.
Please see the whole WSAVA statement at the following webpage:
https://wsava.org/wp-content/uploads/2024/02/WSAVA-Position-Statement-on-Cosmetic-Alterations-in-Companion-Animals.pdf

Abbreviations

Ab antibody
ABC airway, breathing, circulation
ABR auditory brainstem response
ACP acute canine polyradiculoneuritis
ACVIM American College of Veterinary Internal Medicine
AD Alzheimer's disease
ADC apparent diffusion coefficient
AE adverse effect
AF annulus fibrosus
AILP acquired idiopathic laryngeal paralysis
ALP alkaline phosphatase
ALS amyotrophic lateral sclerosis
ALT alanine aminotransferase
Angio SNAP serum antigen test for Angiostrongylus vasorum
ANNPE acute noncompressive nucleus pulposus extrusion
APPs acute-phase proteins
aPTT activated partial thromboplastin time
ARAS ascending reticular activating system
ASD antiseizure drug
ASM antiseizure medication
AST aspartate aminotransferase
Aβ amyloid beta
BAEPs brainstem auditory evoked potentials
BAER brainstem auditory evoked response
BAST bile acid stimulation test
BBB blood–brain barrier
BD bladder dysfunction
BDNF brain-derived neurotrophic factor
BID twice a day
BUN blood urea nitrogen
BVA British Veterinary Association
BWST body weight supported treadmill
CBC complete blood count
CBD cannabidiol
CBF cerebral blood flow
CCDS canine cognitive dysfunction syndrome
CCG cranial cervical ganglion
CCSM caudal cervical spondylomyelopathy
CDPs cord dorsum potentials
CE clinical examination
CISS constructive interference in steady state
CK creatine kinase
CKCS Cavalier King Charles Spaniel
CM Chiari malformation
CMAP compound muscle action potential
CMG caudal mesenteric ganglia
CM-N Chiari malformation – normal
CM-P Chiari malformation – pain
CN cranial nerve
CNS central nervous system
CO client-owned
CPSP central poststroke pain
CPTs choroid plexus tumors
CRDs complex repetitive discharges
CRI constant rate infusion
CRP C-reactive protein
CS cluster seizures
CSF cerebrospinal fluid
CSM cervical spondylomyelopathy
CT computed tomography
CVA cerebrovascular accident
DA-CSM disc-associated cervical spondylomyelopathy
DEEH disc-associated extensive epidural hemorrhage
DISH diffuse idiopathic spinal hyperostosis
DISHAAL disorientation, changes in social interactions, disturbances in the sleep/wake cycle, house soiling, activity changes, anxiety, loss of learning
DLSS degenerative lumbosacral stenosis
DM degenerative myelopathy
DPMS descending pain modulatory system
DWI diffusion-weighted imaging
DZP diazepam
ECG electrocardiogram
ED extradurally
EDX electrodiagnostic
EEG electroencephalography
EFS episodic falling syndrome
EMG electromyography
EPS endplate spikes
ERG electroretinography
ESP erector spinae plane
EUS external urethral sphincter
FC fecal continence
FCEM fibrocartilaginous embolic myelopathy
FINFUN Finnish neurological functional testing battery
FLAIR fluid-attenuated inversion recovery
fT4 free thyroxin
FVNUO facial and vestibular neuropathy of unknown origin
GABA gamma-aminobutyric acid
GE gradient echo
GFAP glial fibrillary acidic protein
GGT gamma-glutamyl transferase
GME granulomatous meningoencephalomyelitis
GP general proprioceptive
HNPE hydrated nucleus pulposus extrusion
HPA hypothalamic–pituitary–adrenal
HRQoL health-related quality of life
IASP International Association for the Study of Pain
iCa ionized calcium
ICH intracranial hypertension
ICP intracranial pressure
ID intradural
IE idiopathic epilepsy
IFN Idiopathic facial neuropathy
IHTS idiopathic head tremor syndrome
IIVDE intradural intraparenchymal disc extrusion
IM intramedullary
IM intramuscular, intramuscularly

IMP imepitoin
IN intranasal
IPVD idiopathic peripheral vestibular disease
ITN Idiopathic trigeminal neuropathy/trigeminal neuritis
IUS internal urethral sphincter
IV intravenous, intravenously
IVD intervertebral disc
IVDD intervertebral disc disease
IVDE Hansen type I intervertebral disc extrusion
IVDH intervertebral disc herniation
IVDP Hansen type II intervertebral disc protrusion
IVETF International Veterinary Epilepsy Task Force
IVS idiopathic vestibular syndrome
KBr potassium bromide
LASER light amplification by stimulated emission of radiation
LEV levetiracetam
LFB Luxol fast blue
LMN lower motor neuron
LUT lower urinary tract
LUTI lower urinary tract infection
MAO-B monoamine oxidase
MCT medium-chain triglyceride
MDZ midazolam
MEPPs miniature endplate potentials
MEPs motor evoked potentials
MFS modified Frankel score
MG myasthenia gravis
MGBA microbiota–gut–brain axis
MLF medial longitudinal fasciculus
MNCS motor nerve conduction studies
MRI magnetic resonance imaging
MST median survival times
MUAP motor unit action potential
MUO meningoencephalomyelitis of unknown origin
NAD nicotinamide adenine dinucleotide
NBD neurogenic bladder dysfunction
NDP negative deep pain
NE necrotizing encephalitis
NeuPSIG Neuropathic Pain Special Interest group
NION Noninfectious, idiopathic optic neuritis
NLE necrotizing leukoencephalitis
NM neuromuscular
NMDA N-methyl-D-aspartate
NMDA–R N-methyl-D-aspartate receptor
NME necrotizing meningoencephalitis
NMES neuromuscular electrical stimulation
NMJ neuromuscular junction
NP nucleus pulposus
NSAID nonsteroidal anti-inflammatory drug
NST Nerve sheath tumor
OA-CSM osseous-associated cervical spondylomyelopathy
OMI otitis media/interna
PARR polymerase chain reaction for antigen receptor rearrangements
PAS periodic acid–Schiff
PB phenobarbital
PBMT photobiomodulation therapy
PCR polymerase chain reaction
PG pelvic ganglia
PGE prostaglandin E
PGSD paroxismal gluten-sensitive dyskinesia
PKD paroxysmal kinesigenic dyskinesia
PLR pupillary light reflex
PLs pelvic limbs
PLT platelet
PMC pontine micturition center
PMM progressive myelomalacia
PMMA polymethyl methacrylate
PN polyneuropathy
PNH peripheral nerve hyperexcitability
PNKD paroxysmal nonkinesigenic dyskinesia
PNS peripheral nervous system
PNST peripheral nerve sheath tumor
PO per os, orally
PRN pro re nata (when required)
PROM passive range of motion
PSRF pedicle-screw rod fixation
PT prothrombin time
PTs primary tumors
PU/PD polyuria/polydipsia
PVD peripheral vestibular disease
QID 4 times a day
QoL quality of life
QST Quantitative Sensory Testing
R rectal
RBC red blood cells
RCT randomized controlled trial
RGC retinal ganglion cell
RNS repetitive nerve stimulation
RT radiation therapy/treatment
SAA serum amyloid A
SAD spinal arachnoid diverticula
SAMe S-adenosyl-L-methionine
SAMS spinocerebellar ataxia with myokymia and/or seizures
SB serum biochemistry
SBA serum bile acid
SC subcutaneously
SC subcutaneous injection
SC spinal cord
SCM serum concentration monitoring
SCWT Soft Coated Wheaten Terrier
SE status epilepticus
SM syringomyelia
SM-M syringomyelia – mild
SM-S syringomyelia – severe
SNAPs sensory nerve action potentials
SNCS sensory nerve conduction studies
SNPs single nucleotide polymorphisms
SPA spontaneous pathological activity
SPE serum protein eletrophoresis
SPFs seizure-precipitating factors
SRMA steroid-responsive meningitis-arteritis
SSEPs somatosensory evoked potentials
STIR short tau inversion recovery
STs secondary tumors
SW susceptibility weighted
T1W T1-weighted
T2W T2-weighted
tCa total calcium
TCA tricyclic antidepressants
TENS transcutaneous electrical nerve stimulation
TIA transient ischemic attack
TID 3 times a day
TLs thoracic limbs
TNCC total nucleated cell count
TOF time-of-flight
TPM topiramate
TSH thyroid-stimulating hormone
TT4 total thyroxin
UA urinalysis
UAR utricle asymmetricity ratio
UC urinary continence
UMN upper motor neuron
VD vestibular disease
VEPs visual evoked potentials
VGKC voltage-gated potassium channel
WBC white blood cell
WC window center
WGS whole genome sequence
WSAVA World Small Animal Veterinary Association
WW window width
ZNS zonisamide

Table of contents

SECTION III Techniques and procedures

SECTION IV Neurological diseases

Abnormal mentation and behavior

Rodrigo Gutiérrez Quintana
MVZ, MVM, DECVN, MRCVS

Definition and pathophysiology

Mentation and behavior are important factors that need to be assessed by the clinician in every patient as part of the physical examination or complete neurological examination. Normal mentation and behavior are characterized by appropriate interactions with the external environment and suitable responses to external stimuli.[1] *Mentation* or *mental status* is a general term that encompasses a combination of the level of consciousness (awareness and wakefulness) and cognition (mental processing).[2] *Behavior* is the observable response of an animal to a given situation or stimulus.[3]

The neural basis for maintaining normal mentation and behavior involves a dynamic interplay of various regions within the cerebrum and brainstem, with the following areas playing a critical role (Fig. 1.1):[3,4,5]

- **Ascending reticular activating system (ARAS):** The ARAS is a set of connected nuclei in the reticular formation of the brainstem, which are responsible for stimulating the cerebral cortex via the diencephalon to maintain consciousness and wakefulness. It is formed by ill-defined areas in the central portion of the brainstem, from the medulla oblongata to the diencephalon. It projects to the thalamus, and from there it stimulates the entire cerebral cortex. The main function of the ARAS is to adjust the level of activity in the cortex. It filters incoming sensory information and modulates consciousness levels.
- **Diencephalon:** The thalamus acts as a relay station for sensory information, directing sensory inputs to different parts of the cerebral cortex. It plays a crucial role in integrating sensory experiences and contributing to awareness.
- **Limbic system:** The limbic system refers to brain structures that border the diencephalon forming two incomplete ring-like structures. Its most important structures include the amygdala, hippocampus, hypothalamus, basal nuclei, and cingulate gyrus. It supports many different functions, including emotion, behavior, memory, and olfaction.
- **Cerebral cortex:** The cerebral cortex is where decision making, problem solving, and planning occurs, and it could be said that it is the true seat of consciousness.

Abnormal mentation usually indicates a disease process that is causing dysfunction of the brainstem and/or forebrain. Neurological disorders affecting the forebrain can also lead to abnormal behavior that can be reported by the owners or observed in the consult room.[1,3]

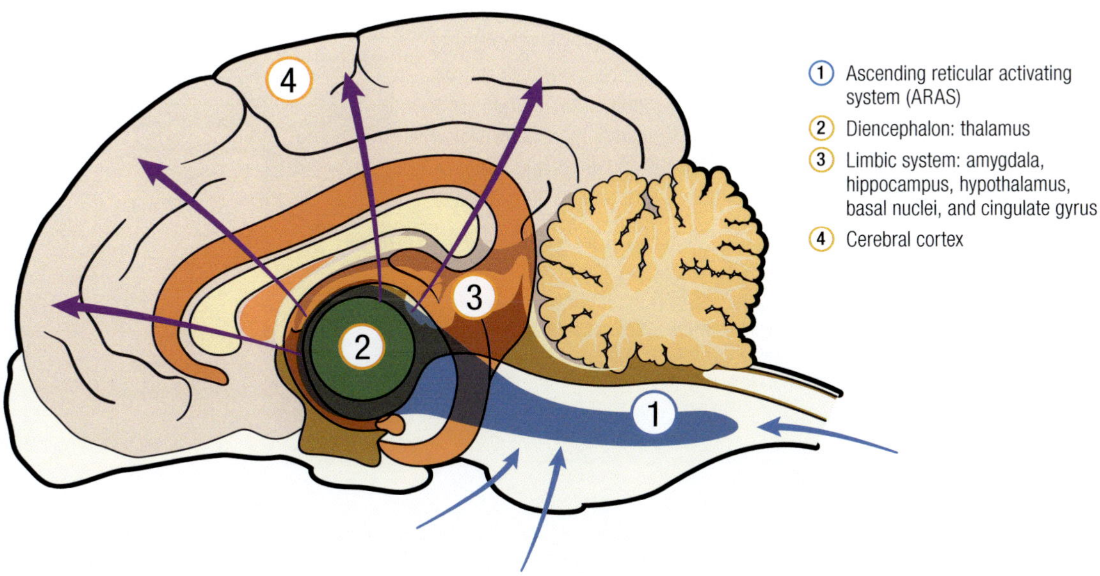

FIG. 1.1 Anatomical regions playing a critical role in mentation and behavior.

Clinical signs

Clinical signs of abnormal mentation encompass a broad spectrum of alterations in cognitive function, awareness, wakefulness, and behavior. These changes can be episodic or constant, subtle or severe, acute or chronic, progressive or nonprogressive.

Mental status is assessed through questioning the owner and by evaluating how the dog interacts with its environment in the consult room and ideally outdoors. Being observant is particularly important. It is useful to create a stress-free environment for the dog, and it is often better to assess mentation and behavior before performing any examination, for example while taking the medical history, so the dog is more relaxed. In some cases, asking the owner to record videos at home can be beneficial. Patients are classified as alert if they respond in a predictable fashion to external stimuli (visual, auditory, and tactile).

In order of increasing severity, the level of consciousness may be classified as (Video 1.1):[1]

- **Drowsiness:** The animal has a reduced ability to sustain consciousness without the application of external stimuli; slow arousal to auditory or tactile stimuli.
- **Stupor:** The animal is unconscious and remains unresponsive to environmental stimuli but responsive to noxious stimulation.
- **Coma:** The animal is unconscious and remains unresponsive to both environmental and noxious stimulation.

Another term that has been used to describe mental status in dogs is confusion. It describes an inability to think with appropriate speed and clarity, and in veterinary medicine this interpretation remains subjective. Some terms used in a nonstandardized fashion in the veterinary literature to describe mental status include depressed, delirium, obtundation and lethargy; these terms are difficult to apply to animals and the author recommends avoiding them.[1]

Changes in behavior can be variable and may include anxiety, aggression, fear, excessive vocalization, house soiling, and repetitive behaviors. Animals with focal, lateralized forebrain lesions may be unaware of sensory information coming from the contralateral side of the body and tend to walk in circles (towards the side of the lesion); this is known as hemi-inattention or hemi-neglect syndrome (see Video 1.1).[3]

It is very important to perform a complete neurological examination in patients with altered mentation and behavior, as it may be possible to identify other clinical signs that can help to further localize the lesion affecting the central nervous system. Using the modified Glasgow Coma Scoring System is recommended in patients with more severe alterations of consciousness, particularly secondary to traumatic brain injuries. This scoring system enables grading of the initial neurological status and serial monitoring of the patient with impaired consciousness and can provide an idea of prognosis. The three categories that should be evaluated include level of consciousness, motor activity, and brainstem reflexes.[6,7,8] Decerebrate rigidity can be observed in stuporous or comatose animals. It is characterized by opisthotonos and extension of all limbs, which is due to loss of descending input from the supratentorial structures to the brainstem centers responsible for flexion of the limbs.[3,4]

Video 1.1

Examples of altered mentation and behavior in dogs. Some of the videos are courtesy of Adriana Kaczmarska and Alfonso Cabral Naranjo.

Diagnostic approach

Algorithm 1.1 shows the approach to the patient with altered mentation and behavior and Tables 1.1 and 1.2 summarize the list of differential diagnoses.

Algorithm 1.1 Note 1 Severe alterations in the level of consciousness such as stupor or coma are acute and life-threatening situations in which the initial approach should aim to stabilize (airway, breathing, circulation [ABC]) the patient.[1,3,9] Excluding undetermined causes, the most common causes of stupor and coma in dogs in a recent study included traumatic brain injury, hypoglycemia, shock, seizures, and renal or hepatic dysfunction.[9]

Algorithm 1.1 Note 2 The diagnostic approach should always include a complete clinical history, with a good description of mental status and behavior by the owner and, if possible, videos of what they are observing at home. Identifying any triggers to the abnormal behavior can be useful. A complete physical and neurological examinations are essential.

Algorithm 1.1 Note 3 Diagnostic testing should start by ruling out extracranial causes with hematology and biochemistry profiles, a urinalysis, and blood pressure measurement. Depending on the results, further endocrine testing could be considered. Thoracic radiographs are recommended in older animals.

Algorithm 1.1 Note 4 Once extracranial causes have been excluded, advanced imaging (magnetic resonance imaging or computed tomography) of the brain and cerebrospinal fluid examination should be performed.

TABLE 1.1 Extracranial causes for altered mentation and behavior in dogs.

Mechanism of disease	*Metabolic*	*Nutritional*	*Toxic*
Specific diseases	■ Hypoglycemia* ■ Hepatic encephalopathy* ■ Shock* ■ Uremia* ■ Syncope ■ Electrolyte disturbances ■ Hyperthermia ■ Hypothyroidism	■ Thiamine deficiency	■ Lead ■ Avermectins ■ Milbemycin ■ Barbiturates ■ Ethylene glycol ■ Opioids ■ Anticonvulsants ■ Recreational drugs ■ Metaldehyde

* Most common causes of stupor and coma in dogs.[9]

ALGORITHM 1.1

Approach to the patient with altered mentation and behavior.

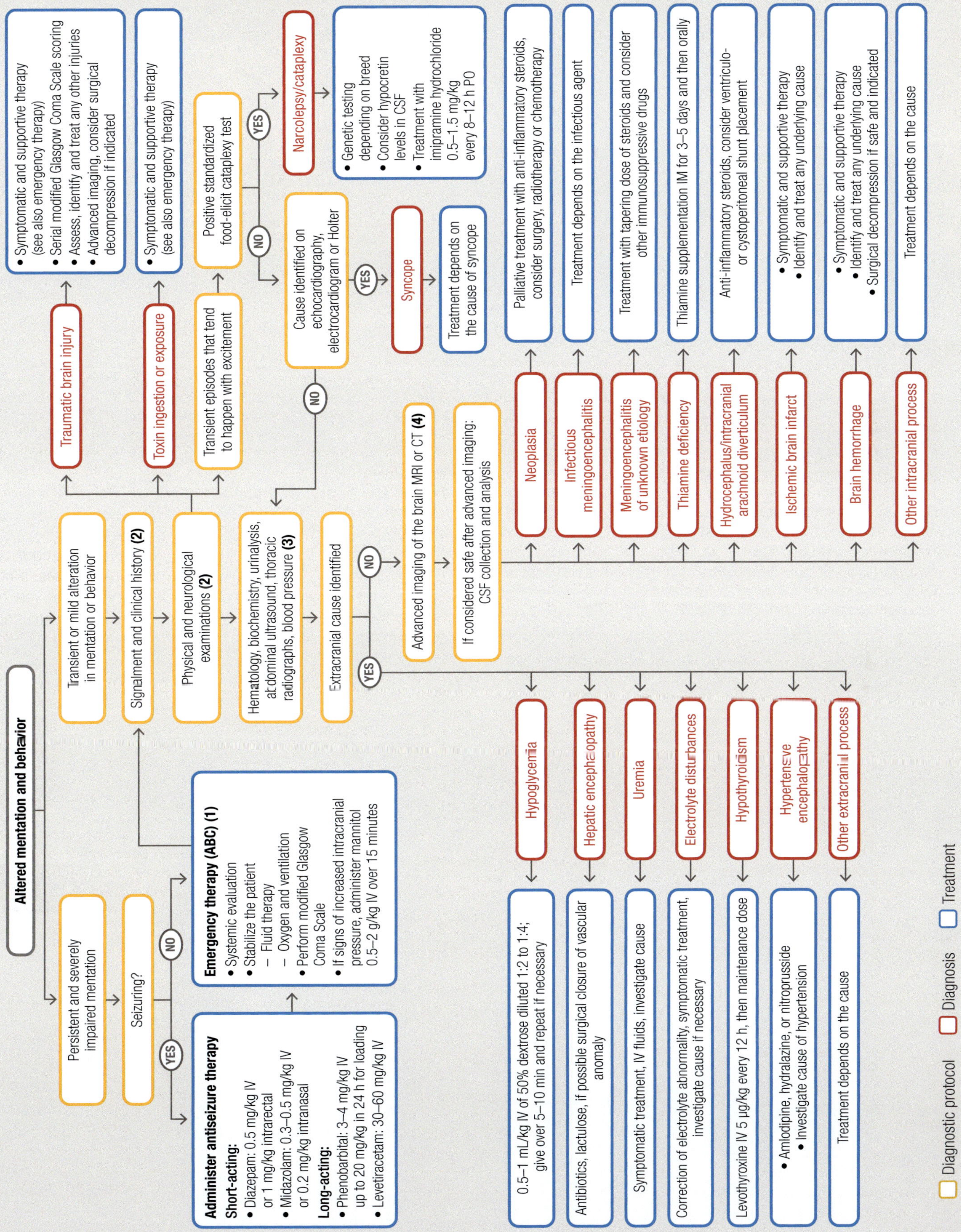

TABLE 1.2 Intracranial causes for altered mentation and behavior in dogs.

Mechanism of disease	Degenerative	Congenital anomaly	Neoplasia	Idiopathic	Inflammatory Infectious	Trauma	Vascular
Specific diseases	■ Inherited neuro-degenerative diseases	■ Hydrocephalus ■ Intracranial arachnoid diverticulum	■ Primary or secondary brain tumor ■ Local extension to the brain of head tumors	■ Narcolepsy ■ Idiopathic epilepsy (cluster seizures, status epilepticus, postictal)*	■ Infectious encephalitis (viral, bacterial, protozoal, fungal or parasitic) ■ Meningo-encephalitis of unknown etiology	■ Traumatic brain injury*	■ Ischemic brain infarct ■ Brain hemorrhage ■ Hypertensive encephalopathy

* Most common causes of stupor and coma in dogs.[9]

References

1. Platt S. Altered stated of consciousness in small animals. *Vet Clin North Am Small Anim Pract.* 2014 Nov;44(6):1039–1058.
2. Wilber ST, Ondrejka JE. Altered Mental Status and Delirium. *Emerg Med Clin North Am.* 2016 Aug;34(3):649-665.
3. Bagley RS, Platt S. Coma stupor and mentation changes. In: Platt S, Olby N. (eds.) *BSAVA manual of canine and feline neurology.* 4th ed. United Kingdom, BSAVA; 2013. p.136–166.
4. De Lahunta A, Glass EN, Kent M. *De Lahunta's Veterinary Neuroanatomy and Clinical Neurology.* 5th ed. United States of America: Elsevier; 2021.
5. Bodien YG, Chatelle C, Edlow BL. Functional networks in disorders of consciousness. *Semin Neurol.* 2017 Oct;37(5):485–502.
6. Platt SR, Radaelli ST, McDonnell JJ. The prognostic value of the modified Glasgow Coma Scale in head trauma in dogs. *J Vet Intern Med.* 2001 Nov-Dec;15(6):581–584.
7. Cameron S, Weltman JG, Fletcher DJ. The prognostic value of admission point-of-care testing and modified Glasgow Coma Scale score in dogs and cats with traumatic brain injuries (2007-2010): 212 cases. *J Vet Emerg Crit Care (San Antonio).* 2022 Jan;32(1):75–82.
8. Her J, Yanke AB, Gerken K, et al. Retrospective evaluation of the relationship between admission variables and brain herniation in dogs (2010-2019): 54 cases. *J Vet Emerg Crit Care (San Antonio).* 2022 Jan;32(1):50–55.
9. Parratt CA, Firth AM, Boag AK, et al. Retrospective characterization of coma and stupor in dogs and cats presenting to a multicenter out-of-hours service (2012-2015): 386 animals. *J Vet Emerg Crit Care (San Antonio).* 2018 Nov;28(6):559–565.

CHAPTER 2

Seizures

Fabio Stabile
DVM, MRCVS, PhD, DECVN

Definition of seizure

The term *seizure* is used to describe any sudden, short-lasting, and transient event experienced by a patient. As such, the term *seizure* does not imply that the event is epileptic in origin, and it can be used to describe any event of abnormal behavior, abnormal mental state, abnormal muscle tone, and abnormal posture and/or movement.[1]

Epileptic seizures

Characteristics of epileptic seizures

Epileptic seizures are defined as the transient manifestations of motor/behavioral/autonomic signs due to excessive, synchronous, usually self-limiting epileptic neuronal activity in the brain.[1,2] They can be caused by a variety of etiologies including structural epilepsy and idiopathic epilepsy. Epileptic seizures tend to manifest in three distinct sequential phases: a prodrome (or preictal phase), an ictus (or ictal phase), and a postictal phase. Their definition and characteristics, as described by the International Veterinary Epilepsy Task Force (IVETF) in 2015, are provided in Box 2.1.[1]

If epileptic seizures are consistently and objectively evoked by a specific stimulus or by a specific activity of the patient, these are defined as reflex epileptic seizures. Reported stimuli/provocative factors include light flashes, a startle, a monotone sound, or a specific movement or action such as eating.[5,6] The term *provocative factor* refers to any transient/sporadic factor associated with the ability to induce seizures in patients with chronic epilepsy or in nonepileptic patients.[1]

Epileptic seizures can occur as isolated seizures, cluster seizures, or status epilepticus:[1]

- Cluster seizures are defined clinically as two or more epileptic seizures within a 24-hour period, with complete recovery of consciousness between the epileptic seizures.
- Status epilepticus is defined as a single epileptic seizure lasting longer than 5 minutes, or two or more epileptic seizures without complete recovery of consciousness in between the epileptic seizures.[1]

Box 2.1 Phases associated with epileptic seizures according to the IVETF.[1]

Prodrome or preictal phase

Period of variable duration (hours to days) during which caregivers may notice changes in their dog's disposition/behavior that might indicate a forthcoming epileptic seizure.[1] The most common prodromal signs reported by caregivers of epileptic dogs are long-lasting restlessness, clinginess, and anxiousness/fearful behaviors.[3] Identification of the prodrome offers an opportunity for pulse administration of fast-acting antiseizure drugs to prevent the occurrence of epileptic seizures.[4]

Ictus or ictal phase

The ictus is the manifestation of a focal or generalized epileptic seizure, or of a focal epileptic seizure evolving into a generalized epileptic seizure.[1]

Postictal phase

Period of variable duration (seconds to several hours or days) that follows the ictal phase of an epileptic seizure. It is typically characterized by disorientation, tiredness, ataxia, and failure to avoid stationary obstacles. Abnormal behaviors such as vocalization, a sudden urge to urinate or defecate, increased hunger or thirst, and excessive sleeping are also observed. Postictal blindness or aggression are also frequently reported.[1]

Epileptic seizure classification

The semiology of epileptic seizures is the description of the clinical signs witnessed during the different types of epileptic seizures and has been used to classify these as focal epileptic seizures, generalized epileptic seizures, and focal epileptic seizures with secondary generalization (Box 2.2).[1–4] Focal epileptic seizures are the manifestation of abnormal electrical activity originating in a localized group of neurons or network of neurons within one hemisphere. Therefore, the associated clinical signs reflect the functions of the cerebral region from which the abnormal electrical discharges originate. The clinical signs are typically lateralized and/or the manifestation of a specific function (i.e., motor, autonomic/behavioral signs, alone or in combination).

Generalized epileptic seizures result from abnormal electrical discharges involving both cerebral hemispheres. All motor manifestations are symmetrical from the onset of the seizure and often accompanied by a loss of consciousness and autonomic signs. Impairment or loss of consciousness and autonomic signs are not associated with myoclonic epileptic seizures. Focal epileptic seizures may evolve into generalized epileptic seizures when abnormal electrical discharges spread from an initially localized brain region to both cerebral hemispheres. This is the most common type of seizure observed in dogs. The onset of focal epileptic seizures often only lasts seconds to minutes, after which secondary generalization with convulsions is observed. The onset of a focal epileptic seizure may be difficult to detect by the dog's caregivers due to its brief nature.[1–4]

Reactive seizures

Reactive seizures (also called provoked seizures) are seizures occurring in response to a transient disturbance in function caused by a metabolic or nutritional disorder or exposure to an exogenous toxin in an otherwise normal/healthy brain. Treatment of the underlying cause of reactive seizures can result in seizure remission.[1]

Epilepsy

Epilepsy is defined as a disease of the brain characterized by an enduring predisposition to generate epileptic seizures. This definition applies to any patient experiencing at least two (or more) unprovoked epileptic seizures, >24 hours apart from each other.[1]

Structural epilepsy

Structural epilepsy refers to epilepsy caused by cerebral pathology such as vascular (ischemic/hemorrhagic), inflammatory/infectious, or traumatic lesions; developmental abnormalities; or a neoplastic or degenerative disease. The diagnosis of an underlying structural pathology by advanced diagnostic imaging (magnetic resonance imaging [MRI] or computed tomography [CT]), cerebrospinal fluid examination (when indicated), DNA testing (when possible) or postmortem examination is required to reach a diagnosis of structural epilepsy.[1]

Idiopathic epilepsy

Idiopathic epilepsy refers to epilepsy of known or presumed genetic origin. Idiopathic epilepsy is a disease in its own right, with an age of onset reported between 6 months and 6 years of age. Dogs with idiopathic epilepsy have a normal interictal general physical and neurological examination, and a normal blood analysis and urinalysis. The IVETF recommends it as a bridging term, with three subclassifications:

1. Genetic epilepsy: when a causative genetic mutation has been identified.
2. Suspected genetic epilepsy: when a genetic influence is strongly suspected and supported by a high breed prevalence (>2%), pedigree analysis, and/or familial accumulation of epileptic individuals.
3. Epilepsy of unknown cause: when the underlying etiology is unknown, and there is no indication of structural epilepsy based on the results of advanced diagnostic investigations (including blood tests, MRI of the brain, and CSF analysis).[1]

Further details on idiopathic epilepsy can be found in Chapter 16.

Box 2.2 Classification of epileptic seizures based on semiology according to the International Veterinary Epilepsy Task Force.[1]

Focal epileptic seizures

- Motor: focal motor phenomena such as facial twitches, repeated jerking movements of the head, rhythmic blinking, repeated rhythmic jerking movements of one extremity.
- Autonomic: parasympathetic and epigastric phenomena such as pupil dilation, hypersalivation, vomiting, defecation.
- Behavioral: short-lasting episodes of changes in behavior such as anxiousness, attention seeking/"clinging" to the caregiver, restlessness, unexplainable fear reactions.

Generalized epileptic seizures

- Convulsive generalized epileptic seizures
  - Tonic: sustained muscle contraction lasting for the duration of the epileptic seizure.
  - Clonic: regularly repetitive myoclonus of a muscle group, appearing as repetitive jerking movements due to repetitive contraction and relaxation of the muscle group involved.
  - Tonic-clonic: repetitive alternation of a tonic phase and a clonic phase (Video 2.1).
  - Myoclonic: sudden, brief jerking movements usually affecting both sides of the body, caused by involuntary muscular/muscle group contraction (Video 2.2).
- Nonconvulsive generalized epileptic seizures
  - Atonic (also called drop attacks): characterized by a sudden and generalized loss of muscle tone, which usually causes a collapsing episode.

Focal epileptic seizures evolving into generalized epileptic seizures

The epileptic seizure will start with regional/lateralized motor, autonomic, and/or behavioral signs only to progress rapidly into a convulsive stage with bilateral tonic, clonic, or tonic-clonic convulsions and loss of consciousness.

Video 2.1

Three-year-old spayed female Dalmatian diagnosed with idiopathic epilepsy experiencing a generalized epileptic seizure. The patient is unconscious, shows autonomic signs (hypersalivation) and tonic-clonic contractions of all four limbs. The episode cannot be interrupted by the owner. In the postictal phase, the dog recovers and appears confused and ataxic on all four limbs.

Video 2.2

Nine-year-old spayed female Weimaraner experiencing myoclonic epileptic seizures. Note the sudden, brief jerking movements usually affecting both sides of the body, caused by involuntary muscular/muscle group contraction. The patient was affected by insulinoma. In this condition, myoclonic epileptic seizures are caused by severe hypoglycemia. Video courtesy of Dr. Bruno Lopes.

Disorders mimicking epileptic seizures

Movement disorders

Movement disorders are neurological conditions characterized by abnormal, involuntary muscular contraction/relaxation caused by abnormalities in the central or peripheral nervous system.[2] These involuntary movements appear to be painless and may be episodic or may occur continuously (i.e., myoclonus caused by canine distemper virus infection). They are not associated with impairment of consciousness or autonomic clinical signs. Movement disorders include:

- Tremors, which are rhythmic bursts of motor neuron activity occurring in opposing muscle groups creating a biphasic character with a range of frequencies varying from 1 to 2 Hz up to 12 Hz or higher. Tremors can be focal (i.e., affecting one limb or the head) or generalized (i.e., affecting all body). See Chapter 18 for further reading on tremors.[2]
- Peripheral nerve hyperexcitability (such as fasciculations, myokymia, neuromyotonia, myotonia, cramps, tetanus/tetany), which is due to a dysfunction of the motor nerve causing hyperexcitability caused by ion channel dysfunction, which presents with a wide variety of muscle contractions. Motor nerve hyperexcitability can be caused by a wide variety of central and peripheral nervous system diseases.[2]
- Myoclonus, which is defined as sudden, brief (<100 ms), involuntary contractions of a single muscle or a muscle group in variable locations (axial, proximal, or distal part of a limb).[1] Myoclonus manifests as "shock-like" movements of the body.[2]
- Paroxysmal dyskinesia, which is characterized by recurrent self-limiting episodes of abnormal and involuntary muscle contractions and movements.[2,7] Clinical signs associated with canine paroxysmal dyskinesias include, but are not limited to, dyskinesia, dystonic movements, and tremors.[2] Unlike epileptic seizures, episodes of paroxysmal dyskinesia may be prolonged (minutes to hours); in addition, consciousness is not impaired and autonomic signs are absent. The abnormal behavior reported in the postictal phase of epileptic seizures is typically not observed in patients experiencing episodes of paroxysmal dyskinesia.[2,7] See Chapter 19 for further details on paroxysmal dyskinesia.

Compulsive behavior disorders

Compulsive behavior disorder is characterized by a constant, time-consuming repetition of behaviors serving no obvious purposes, which are therefore referred to as stereotypies.[8,9] These behaviors include circling, fly biting, barking, chewing/licking, or self-mutilation. An increased state of anxiety, a conflict, frustration, or an inability to cope with stressful situations might all be a cause for these behavioral manifestations.[8] Consciousness is not affected, and the episodes may be interrupted by distracting the patient. No autonomic manifestations, prodrome, or postictal signs are observed.

Sleep disorders

The most commonly reported forms of sleep disorders are narcolepsy-cataplexy and rapid eye movement (REM) sleep disorder.

- Narcolepsy-cataplexy. Narcolepsy is a chronic sleep disorder characterized by excessive daytime sleepiness and sleep paralysis. Narcolepsy might progress to cataplexy, which is defined as a sudden loss of muscle tone elicited by an exciting stimulus (such as presentation of food or playing).[10] In dogs, the condition might be sporadic or occur in a familial form.[11] Cataplectic attacks are frequently characterized by initial weakness and collapse due to decreased muscle tone in the pelvic limbs progressing to involve the thoracic limbs, the cervical region, and the head. Dogs may collapse to the floor and remain motionless for a variable period of time ranging from a few seconds to several minutes. Dogs may first appear ataxic, often with sagging of the pelvic limbs, before finally collapsing. Autonomic signs (salivation, urination, or defecation) are not observed during cataplectic attacks. Muscle tone is always flaccid and never increased/spastic.[10,11] Sporadic or acquired narcolepsy is associated with a loss of production of the hypocretin peptides (suspected postnatal death of hypocretin neurons).[12] The underlying etiology for narcolepsy in dogs is likely variable; however, it has been demonstrated that familial narcolepsy in dogs is caused by mutations in the hypocretin receptor 2.[10]
- Rapid eye movement (REM) sleep disorder manifests as muscle twitching and/or slow to violent repetitive movements of all limbs, teeth grinding, and chewing movements during the active phase of REM sleep, with no autonomic manifestations.[10,13] The episodes can happen anytime during sleep and not only at night. Patients can be easily woken up from the episodes and manifest normal mentation immediately when awake. REM sleep disorder has been documented as a possible sequel to tetanus in dogs.[13]

Episodic pain

Episodic pain can present as self-limiting paroxysmal episodes mimicking epileptic seizures (Video 2.3, Fig. 2.1).[14] During these episodes, consciousness is preserved, although the animal may be less keen to interact due to the pain. Autonomic signs are generally not observed. The length of the episodes can vary from seconds to hours. Episodic pain can be caused by a variety of diseases. If the source of pain is not removed/addressed, then the patient may continue experiencing episodes, often multiple times a day.[14]

Vestibular disease

Vestibular disease causes transient and episodic vestibular signs such as vestibular ataxia (leaning to falling to a side), head tilt, and nystagmus, often associated with disorientation and occasionally with vomiting and/or salivation. Episodes can last for a variable period of time (seconds

Video 2.3

Four-year-old neutered male French Bulldog presented for suspected epileptic seizure activity due to recurrent episodes of sudden falls to the floor. The dog seemed anxious, before rolling into lateral recumbency and screaming. During the episodes, the patient assumed a tonic extension on all four limbs. The patient was reported to be normal between episodes by the caregiver. Despite a normal neurological examination, the patient manifested significant discomfort on palpation and lateral flexion of the cervical spine. Based on neurological assessment and magnetic resonance imaging of the cervical region, the dog was diagnosed with an extrusion of the C4–C5 intervertebral disc.

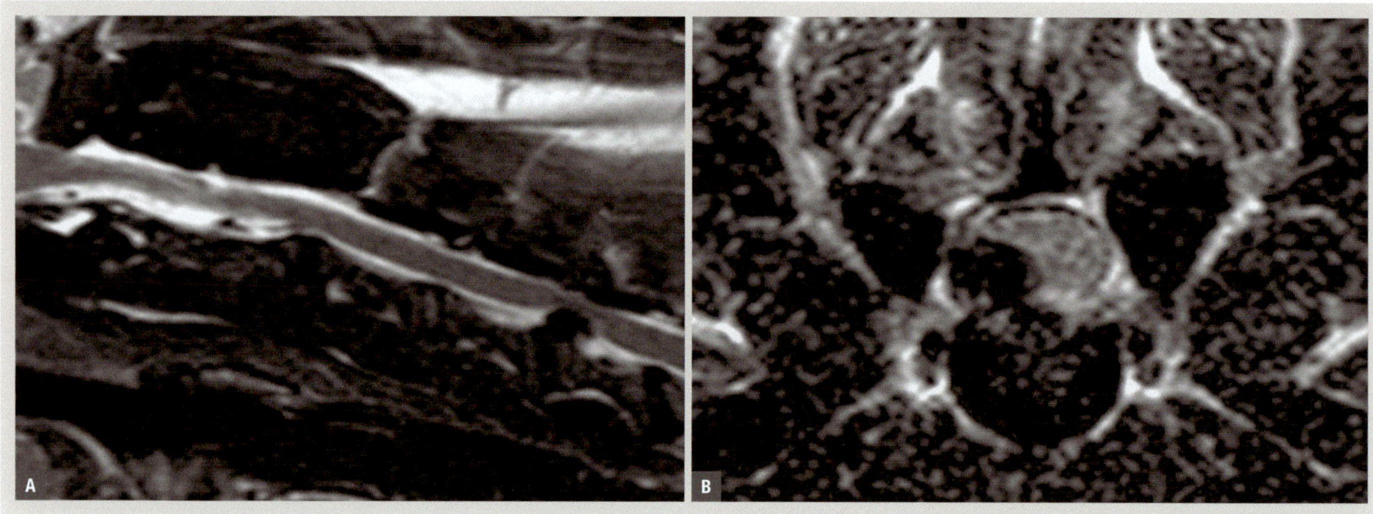

FIG. 2.1 Magnetic resonance images of the patient in Video 2.3. Right parasagittal T2-weighted image (left) of the cervical column showing a C4–C5 intervertebral disc extrusion compressing the spinal cord and spinal nerve. On the transverse T2-weighted image, through the C4–C5 intervertebral disc space (right), the extruded intervertebral disc material, visible as a large hypointense compressive lesion lateralized to the right, is moderately compressing the spinal cord and obliterating the foramen causing spinal nerve compression, likely causing the episodes of severe pain.

to hours). Normal mentation, apart from disorientation, is maintained throughout the episodes, which frequently occur in association with exercise. No pre- and postictal phases are recognized. Transient ischemic attacks, which are due to a brief period of inadequate perfusion in a territory of the carotid or vertebra-basilar arteries, have been reported as a possible underlying etiology in dogs.[15] See Chapter 23 for more information on idiopathic vestibular disease.

Neuromuscular disease

Neuromuscular disease is a disorder of the neuromuscular system frequently manifesting as collapsing episodes following exercise. Typically, consciousness is preserved, and no autonomic signs occur. Dogs tend to be intolerant to exercise. Gait analysis shows a short-strided and stilted gait, with a decreased ability of the affected dogs to support their weight. Patients may have a recent history of regurgitation, which should be differentiated from vomiting potentially associated with epileptic seizures.[16]

Syncope

Syncope is defined as a sudden loss of consciousness with a loss of postural tone, always associated with a spontaneous recovery, caused by a short-lasting interruption of cerebral blood perfusion, oxygen supply, or supply of essential nutrients.[17,18] Cyanosis of the mucous membranes and heart rate and rhythm abnormalities may be observed during the syncopal collapse. Cardiac disease is the most common cause of syncope in small animals, and arrhythmias represent one of the most frequently reported etiologies.[18] Atrial fibrillation, ventricular premature complexes, and ventricular tachycardia are commonly diagnosed arrhythmias associated with syncope in dogs. However, arrhythmias are not the only underlying etiology of syncope, and efforts to document or exclude arrythmias are essential.[17,18]

Diagnostic approach to seizures

Algorithm 2.1 reflects the possible differential diagnoses for seizures/paroxysmal disorders and the process that can be followed to narrow down the possibilities.

Algorithm 2.1 Note 1 For any patient presenting with a history of paroxysmal episodes, the patient's medical history and video footage of the paroxysmal episodes should be reviewed and a full description of the episodes obtained, including any information on suspected triggers and any abnormalities preceding and/or following the episodes.

Algorithm 2.1 Note 2 If the patient remains conscious during the episodes, consider the possibility that the patient is experiencing a form of paroxysmal dyskinesia (typically, autonomic signs and a postictal phase are not present) or vestibular attacks (in the presence of vestibular ataxia, head tilt, nystagmus, possible disorientation with or without vomiting and/or salivation).

Algorithm 2.1 Note 3 Consider full investigations into the underlying etiology of epileptic seizures including a full general and neurological examination, hematology, serum biochemistry, urinalysis, bile acid stimulation test with or without an MRI of the brain, and cerebrospinal fluid collection and analysis.

Algorithm 2.1 Note 4 To confirm syncope, check mucous membranes during an event and investigate if the episode is characterized by a flaccid muscle tone. Cardiological investigations might be required.

Algorithm 2.1 Note 5 Status epilepticus is a neurological emergency needing urgent investigations into the underlying etiology of epileptic seizures and urgent treatment.

Algorithm 2.1 Note 6 Cataplectic attacks should be suspected if the episodes are characterized by a loss of muscle tone. Investigations into narcolepsy-cataplexy might be indicated based on history and clinical assessment. Note episodes might last from seconds to several minutes.

ALGORITHM 2.1

Algorithm for the differential diagnosis of seizures.

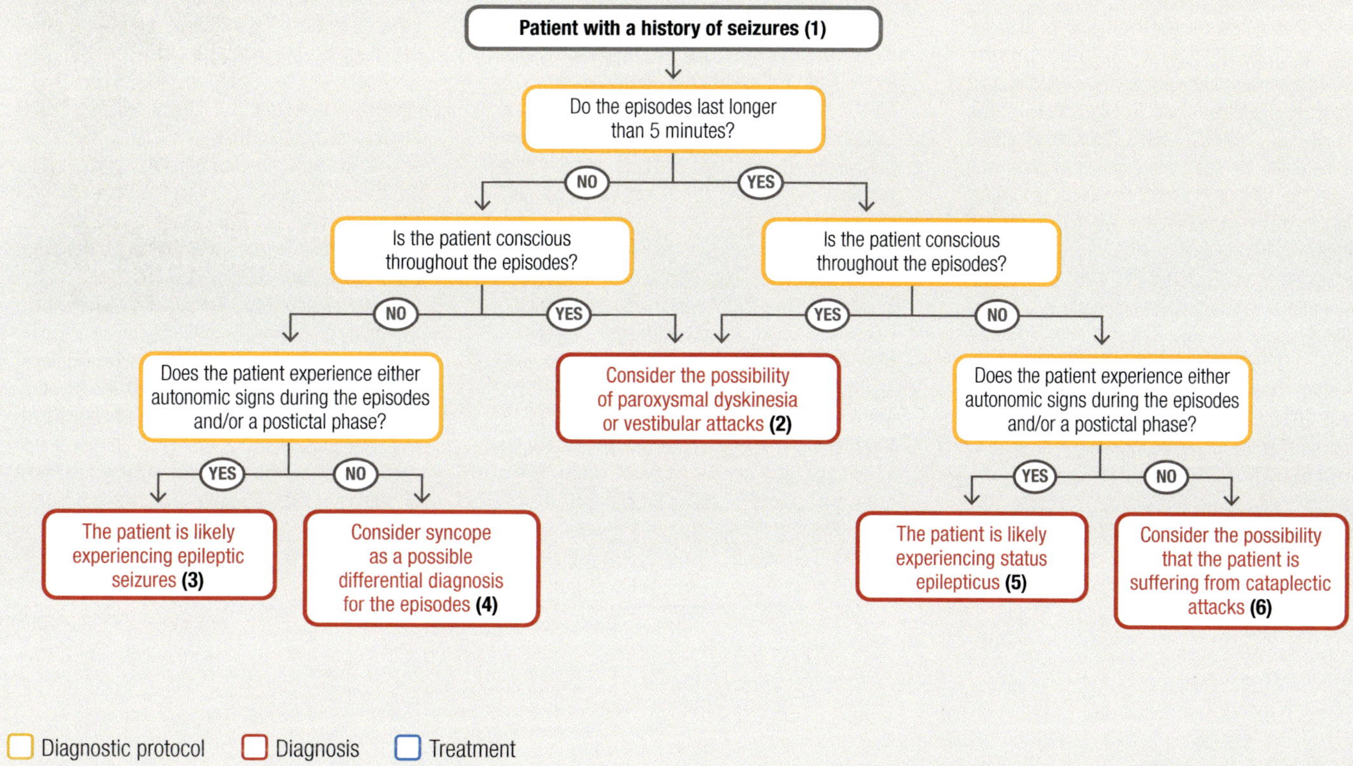

References

4. Berendt M, Farquhar RG, Mandigers PJ, et al. International veterinary epilepsy task force consensus report on epilepsy definition, classification and terminology in companion animals. *BMC Vet Res.* 2015 Aug 28;11:182.
5. Cerda-Gonzalez S, Packer RA, Garosi L, et al. International veterinary canine dyskinesia task force ECVN consensus statement: Terminology and classification. *J Vet Intern Med.* 2021;35:1218–1230.
6. Finnegan SL, Volk HA, Asher L, et al. Investigating the potential for seizure prediction in dogs with idiopathic epilepsy: owner-reported prodromal changes and seizure triggers. *Vet Rec.* 2020 Aug 22;187(4):152.
7. Packer RM, Nye G, Porter SE, Volk HA. Assessment into the usage of levetiracetam in a canine epilepsy clinic. *BMC Vet Res.* 2015 Feb 7;11:25.
8. Brocal J, Lowrie M, Wamsley G, et al. Epileptic seizures triggered by eating in dogs. *J Vet Intern Med.* 2020 May;34(3):1231–1238. [Erratum for Epileptic seizures triggered by eating in dogs. *J Vet Intern Med.* 2020 Sep;34(5):2175]
9. Forsgård JA, Metsähonkala L, Kiviranta AM, et al. Seizure-precipitating factors in dogs with idiopathic epilepsy. *J Vet Intern Med.* 2019 Mar;33(2):701–707.
10. Lowrie M, Garosi L. Classification of involuntary movements in dogs: paroxysmal dyskinesias. *Vet J.* 2017;220:65–71.
11. d'Angelo D, Sacchettino L, Carpentieri R, et al. An Interdisciplinary Approach for Compulsive Behavior in Dogs: A Case Report. *Front Vet Sci.* 2022 Mar 24;9:801636.
12. Luescher AU. Diagnosis and management of compulsive disorders in dogs and cats. *Vet Clin North Am Small Anim Pract.* 2003 Mar;33(2):253–267, vi.
13. Tonokura M, Fujita K, Nishino S. Review of pathophysiology and clinical management of narcolepsy in dogs. *Vet Rec.* 2007 Sep 15;161(11):375–380.
14. Baker TL, Foutz AS, McNerney V, et al. Canine model of narcolepsy: genetic and developmental determinants. *Exp Neurol.* 1982 Mar;75(3):729–742.
15. Ripley B, Fujiki N, Okura M, et al. Hypocretin levels in sporadic and familial cases of canine narcolepsy. *Neurobiol Dis.* 2001 Jun;8(3):525–534.
16. Shea A, Hatch A, De Risio L, Beltran E. Association between clinically probable REM sleep behavior disorder and tetanus in dogs. *J Vet Intern Med.* 2018 Nov;32(6):2029–2036.
17. De Bonis A, Marsh O, Stabile F. Mimicking focal epileptic seizures-episodic pain due to a facial foreign body in a puppy: Imaging characteristics and treatment. *Vet Rec Case Rep.* 2022 March;10(1).
18. Bentley RT, March PA. Recurrent vestibular paroxysms associated with systemic hypertension in a dog. *J Am Vet Med Assoc.* 2011 Sep 1;239(5):652–655.
19. Glass EN, Kent M. The clinical examination for neuromuscular disease. *Vet Clin North Am Small Anim Pract.* 2002 Jan;32(1):1–29, v.
20. Barnett L, Martin MW, Todd J, et al. A retrospective study of 153 cases of undiagnosed collapse, syncope or exercise intolerance: the outcomes. *J Small Anim Pract.* 2011 Jan;52(1):26–31.
21. Billen F, Van Israël N. Syncope secondary to transient atrioventricular block in a German shepherd dog with dilated cardiomyopathy and atrial fibrillation. *J Vet Cardiol.* 2006 May;8(1):63–68.

CHAPTER 3

Loss of balance, head tilt, and nystagmus

Catherine Stalin
MA, VetMB,
DECVN, MRCVS

Pathophysiology

Loss of balance, head tilt, and nystagmus are neurological signs exhibited when there is a lesion in the vestibular system. The vestibular system is key to maintaining an animal's posture and balance in relation to gravity, by ensuring the eyes, trunk, and limbs are correctly positioned in reference to head position or movement. In order to understand why these signs occur, it is important to first understand the functional anatomy of the vestibular system.

The system can be divided into peripheral and central components. The vestibular apparatus is situated peripherally within the bony labyrinth of the petrosal bone, suspended within this bony structure. It is a membranous labyrinth consisting of the utricle, the saccule, and three semicircular canals situated perpendicular to one another. Mechanoreceptor "hair cells" within the macula of the utricle and saccule and the crista ampullaris of the semicircular canals generate signals when they are bent by movement of the endolymph fluid within the labyrinth. The utricle and saccule sense gravitational movement in a horizontal and vertical plane, and the semicircular canals sense angular and rotational movement of the head. Sensory input from the hair cells is received by the vestibular ganglion, and afferent axons join to form the vestibular nerve and more proximally the vestibulocochlear nerve (cranial nerve VIII).

Centrally, the vestibular neurons mostly terminate in the vestibular nuclei, while a minority terminate in the cerebellum. There are four vestibular nuclei on either side of the brainstem networking with various parts of the body caudally and rostrally. It is these interconnections that help maintain posture and eye movement when the animal moves. Lateral and medial vestibulospinal tracts affect head position and activity of the limbs and trunk. The medial longitudinal fasciculus carries axons to the nuclei of cranial nerves III, IV, and VI, and thus affects eye position. Tracts to the cerebrum via the thalamus allow for conscious perception and, as with all systems, there is control through input and output from the cerebellum. In addition, some axons project to the reticular formation and vomiting center located within the brainstem (Fig. 3.1).

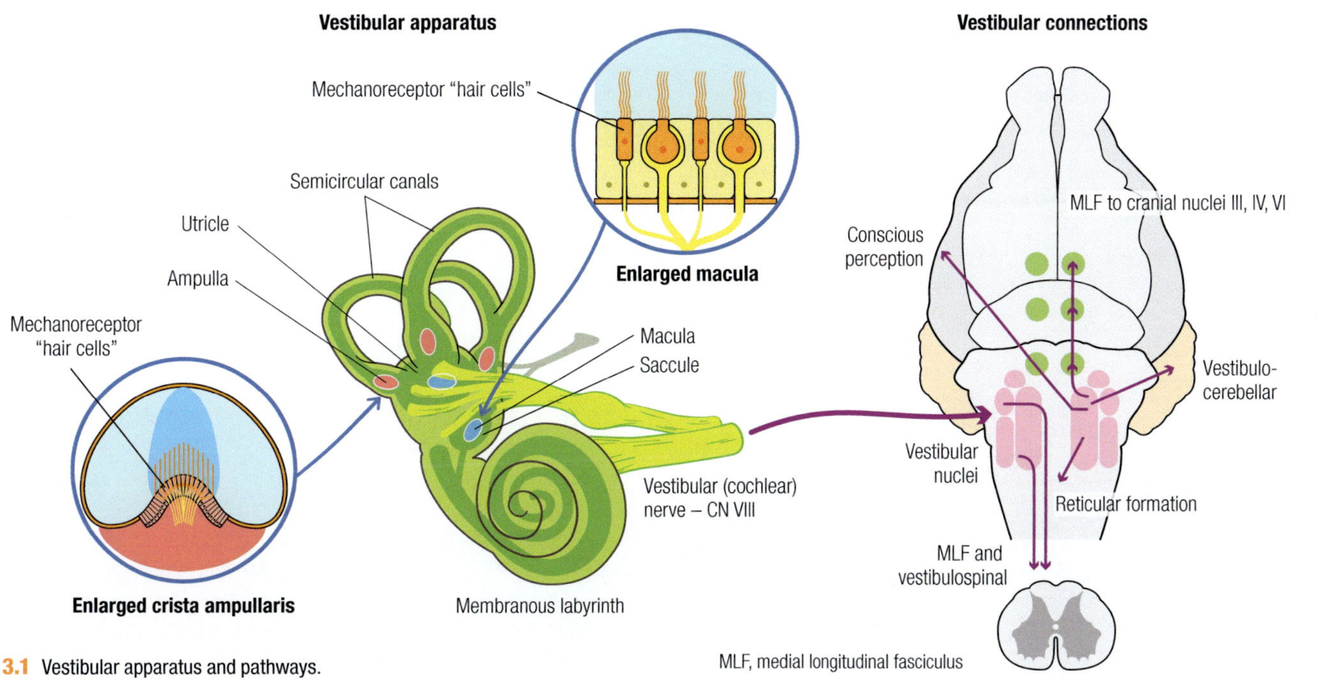

FIG. 3.1 Vestibular apparatus and pathways.

The vestibular neurons are tonically active, further excited or inhibited by deflection of the hair cells depending on the direction of head movement. Lesions in any part of the vestibular system reduce the signals received from that side, which is perceived as the contralateral side being more active. Hence, the system acts as though the animal's head is moving while it is stationary; the usual eye movements and change in limb and trunk tonicity seen when the animal normally moves are therefore witnessed as the abnormal loss of balance, head tilt, and nystagmus seen with vestibular disease when the animal is static.

Clinical signs

The clinical signs associated with vestibular disease include strabismus, nystagmus, head tilt, ataxia, rolling, and vomiting. However, not all these signs are obvious in all cases. Because of the close association of the system with other parts of the nervous system, it is not unusual to see other concurrent clinical signs, which can assist with the neuroanatomical localization of the lesion (Table 3.1). For example, the facial and sympathetic nerves course through the middle ear close to the vestibular nerve, and it is not uncommon to see facial paresis and Horner's syndrome associated with peripheral vestibular disease depending on the underlying etiology. Similarly, within the brainstem, the proximity of the nuclei with the descending upper motor neuron and ascending spinocerebellar pathways means paresis and general proprioceptive ataxia can be observed with central vestibular lesions. In addition, if a cerebellar lesion is the cause of the vestibular signs, there may be other concurrent cerebellar signs such as hypermetria.

Clinical signs are typically ipsilateral to the lesion, with a left-sided head tilt indicating a left-sided lesion. With nystagmus, the direction of the slow phase of eye movement indicates the side of the lesion. The only converse to this is when the lesion affects the vestibulocerebellar tracts, then the head tilt and slow phase eye movement is contralateral to the lesion. This is because the cerebellum normally has a negative effect on the vestibular system and when this is hampered, the affected side is perceived as being more active, the opposite of when there is dysfunction of the vestibular nuclei or nerve. This is referred to as paradoxical vestibular disease and can only be appreciated if accompanied by other cerebellar signs (such as hypermetria) that are ipsilateral to the lesion.

TABLE 3.1 Differentiating between central and peripheral vestibular disease.

	Peripheral vestibular disease	Central vestibular disease
Anatomical region	Vestibular apparatus and vestibular nerve	Vestibular nuclei and associated pathways
Head tilt	Towards lesion	To either side
Nystagmus	Horizontal or rotatory Slow phase towards lesion	Horizontal, rotatory, **or vertical**. Direction may change with head position
Absent conscious proprioception	Normal	Ipsilateral deficits – due to association with adjacent pathways in brainstem
Hypermetria	Normal	Ipsilateral – if vestibulocerebellar pathway affected. Seen with a contralateral head tilt
Cranial nerve deficits	Ipsilateral CN VII due to proximity with CN VIII	Ipsilateral CNs V–XII if extensive brainstem lesion
Horner's syndrome	Ipsilateral. CN VIII and sympathetic nerve can be affected with otitis media due to common pathway through middle ear	No – unless extensive lesion affecting sympathetic pathway in brainstem

CN, cranial nerve

Head tilt

Normal stimulation of the vestibulospinal tract leads to ipsilateral extensor tone and inhibition on the contralateral side of the body. When there is a lesion in any part of this pathway from the vestibular apparatus to the limbs, there is loss of this extensor tone reflected by a head tilt or collapse to the side of the lesion.

Strabismus

Normally, the eyeballs should remain central in the palpebral fissure when the head is elevated. When there is a lesion in the vestibular system, signaling to the nuclei of cranial nerves III, IV, and VI is affected and the eyeball does not move accordingly, frequently remaining ventrally deviated on the side of the lesion. This differs from a lesion in the extraocular muscles, nerves, or nuclei, which would prevent the eyeball from moving. In these cases, the strabismus is present when the head is in a neutral position and continues to have the same deviation when the head is moved.

Nystagmus

Physiological nystagmus occurs when an animal's head is rotated, and this is a useful test to assess normal function. This involuntary movement of the eyes is initiated by movement of the endolymph in the semicircular canals and signaling through the vestibular nerve and nuclei to innervate the extraocular eye muscles via the medial longitudinal fasciculus, which results in a slow phase of eye movement opposite to the direction of rotation. The fast return phase of the eye to a neutral position is initiated through stretch receptors in the muscles. An absence of this "vestibulo ocular reflex" is indicative of a lesion. Likewise, spontaneous nystagmus occurring when the animal's head is stationary also signifies a lesion and can be described as horizontal, rotatory, or vertical (Video 3.1), with the latter indicating central vestibular disease and the former a lesion in any part of the vestibular system. Typically, the direction of the slow phase indicates the side of the lesion but in central vestibular disease the direction of nystagmus can change with changes in head position.

Diagnostic approach

Algorithm 3.1 reflects the decision-making process when presented with a dog with vestibular disease.

Algorithm 3.1 Note 1 Most dogs presenting with vestibular signs will have peripheral disease, which in most cases will be idiopathic, especially if it presents at an older age. However, it is important to be aware of the key signs that immediately suggest central disease, such as vertical nystagmus, reduced conscious proprioception, involvement of multiple cranial nerves, or altered mentation.

ALGORITHM 3.1

Clinical approach to the patient with vestibular disease.

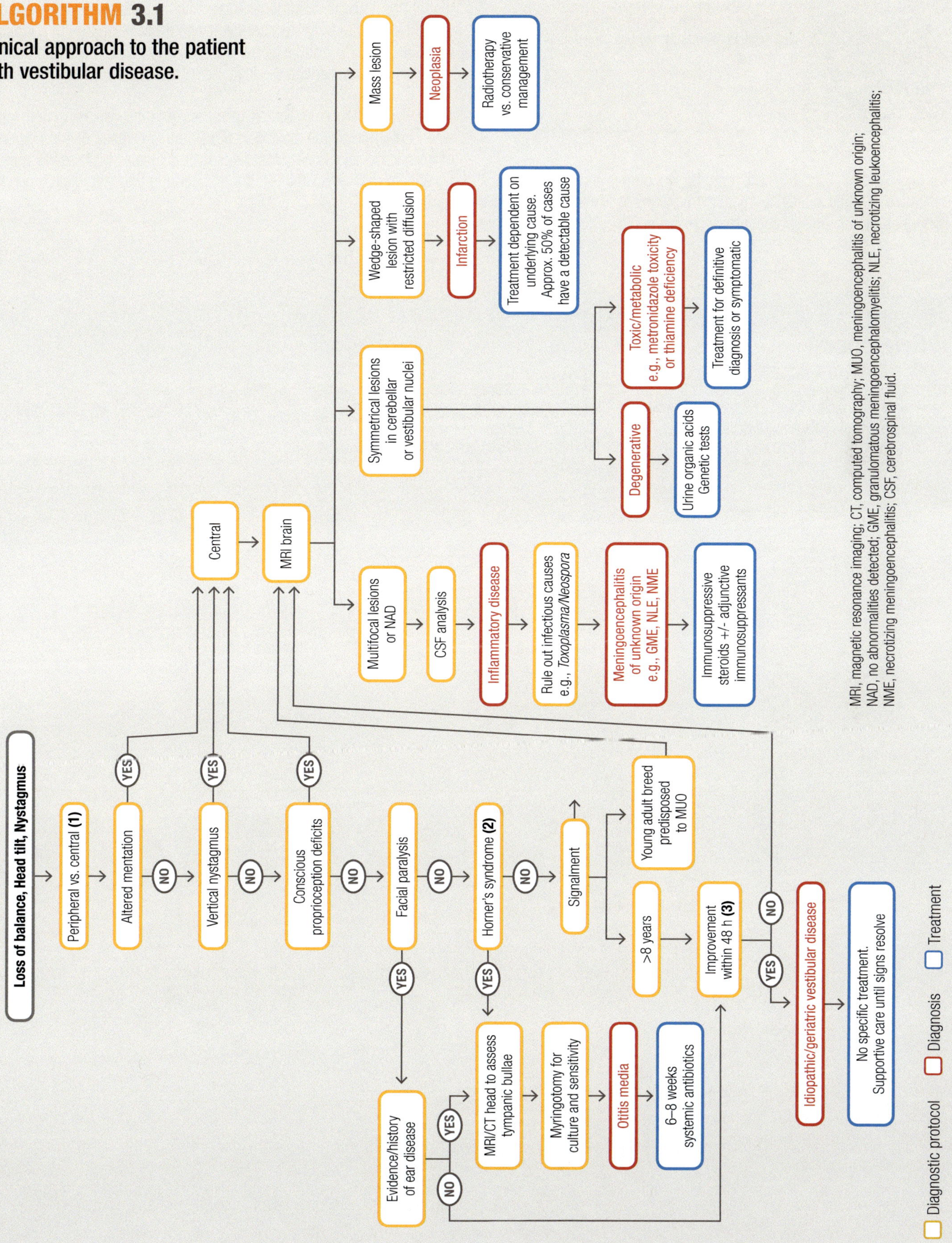

MRI, magnetic resonance imaging; CT, computed tomography; MUO, meningoencephalitis of unknown origin; NAD, no abnormalities detected; GME, granulomatous meningoencephalomyelitis; NLE, necrotizing leukoencephalitis; NME, necrotizing meningoencephalitis; CSF, cerebrospinal fluid.

Video 3.1

Dog with horizontal nystagmus and dog with vertical nystagmus.

Algorithm 3.1 Note 2 There can be accompanying clinical signs indicative of otitis media, particularly concurrent Horner's syndrome. Historically, a concurrent vestibular and facial nerve dysfunction was also thought to be more commonly suggestive of middle ear disease; however, in a recent study, approximately two thirds of dogs with peripheral vestibular disease and facial paralysis had no middle ear abnormalities and were diagnosed with the idiopathic form of the disease.

Algorithm 3.1 Note 3 Speed of recovery is also an important factor when determining the likelihood of idiopathic disease or the necessity of further investigations. Most dogs with idiopathic disease will make a significant recovery within 48 hours, although they will retain a head tilt for longer.

References

1. Orlandi R, Gutierrez-Quintana R, Carletti B et al. Clinical signs, MRI findings and outcome in dogs with peripheral vestibular disease: a retrospective study. *BMC Vet Res*. 2020 May 25; 16(1):159.
2. de Lahunta A, Glass E. Vestibular System: Special Proprioception. In: de Lahunta A, Glass E (eds.). *Veterinary Neuroanatomy and Clinical Neurology*, 3rd ed. Philadelphia, USA: W.B. Saunders; 2009. pp. 319–347.
3. Miller ME, Christensen GC, Evans HE. *Miller's Anatomy of the Dog*, 2nd ed. Philadelphia: W.B. Saunders; 1979.

CHAPTER 4

Anisocoria

Elsa Beltrán
Lda. Vet., DECVN, PGDipVetEd, FHEA, MRCVS

Pathophysiology

Anisocoria is a condition characterized by unequal pupil size. The resting pupil size and possible asymmetry should be assessed (by distant direct ophthalmoscopy) in normal light and then in a darkened room. Anisocoria results from a neurological dysfunction unless it is caused by a mechanical dysfunction of the iris dilator or sphincter muscles. The neurological causes of anisocoria with normal vision involve dysfunction of the parasympathetic pathway to the iris constrictor muscles (mydriatic pupil) or dysfunction of the sympathetic pathway to the iris dilator muscles (miotic pupil).

The parasympathetic innervation to the eye regulates the pupil response to the amount of environmental light (Fig. 4.1), while the sympathetic innervation to the eye regulates the pupil response to emotional factors (Fig. 4.2).

The afferent pathways that contribute to the parasympathetic innervation to the eye arise from the retina, where nerve impulses originate after light stimulation of the photoreceptors. These impulses travel within the retinal ganglion cell (RGC) axons (optic nerve) and reach the optic chiasm. The majority (around 75% in dogs) of the RGC axons decussate at the optic chiasm and continue as part of the optic tract. Around 80% of the axons from the RGC reach the lateral geniculate nucleus and finally the occipital lobe for conscious perception of vision. However, for parasympathetic innervation to the eye, around 10–20% of these RGC axons bypass the lateral geniculate nucleus and course ventrally to synapse in the pretectal nucleus, which is located in the rostral midbrain. From the pretectal nucleus, most axons (around 75% in dogs) cross over to the contralateral side and reach the parasympathetic nucleus of the oculomotor nerve (Edinger–Westphal nucleus in human anatomy), which is also located in the rostral part of the midbrain and very close to the midline. The remaining axons from the pretectal nucleus (around 35% in cats and 25% in dogs) reach the ipsilateral parasympathetic nucleus of the oculomotor nerve.

The efferent parasympathetic fibers (preganglionic fibers) from the oculomotor nucleus travel with the motor fibers of the oculomotor nerve, coursing ventrally and emerging on the medial side of the crus cerebri. The parasympathetic fibers are located medial to the motor fibers of the oculomotor nerve at the middle cranial fossa; they are therefore the first to be affected when a structural lesion (such as a pituitary mass) arises and extends laterally from the midline. The parasympathetic fibers leave the skull through the orbital fissure and synapse in the ciliary ganglion caudal to the eye. The postganglionic parasympathetic fibers (short ciliary nerves) innervate the iridal sphincter muscle and induce reciprocal cholinergic inhibition to the iridal dilator muscle, causing iridal sphincter contraction and dilator muscle relaxation (pupillary constriction).

The sympathetic innervation to the eye is also described as a three-order neuron pathway. The afferent pathways (first-order neurons) arise from the caudal nuclei of the hypothalamus, which is activated by emotional factors or noxious stimuli. These first-order neurons project caudally and ipsilaterally via the hypothalamic spinal tract (also known as lateral tectotegmental spinal tract) at the level of the spinal cord to the preganglionic cell bodies (second-order neurons), which are located in the lateral grey column, at the level of the T1–T3 spinal cord segments. The axons from the preganglionic neurons join the ventral roots of the segmental spinal nerves at this level and join the thoracic sympathetic trunk through the ramus communicans. The preganglionic fibers continue cranially as part of the cervical vagosympathetic trunk and terminate in the cranial cervical ganglion (CCG), located ventromedial to the tympanic bulla. There, the preganglionic fibers synapse with the postganglionic neurons (third-order neurons). The postganglionic fibers then project cranially through the tympano-occipital fissure, enter the cranial cavity, and exit through the orbital fissure. The postganglionic sympathetic fibers innervate the smooth muscles of the periorbita, Müller's muscle of the upper and lower eyelids, and the dilator muscles of the iris. The adrenergic (sympathetic) excitatory input to the dilator muscle causes contraction of this muscle and therefore mydriasis. Sympathetic stimulation also causes a reciprocal adrenergic inhibition of the other antagonist muscle and thus further relaxation of the iris sphincter muscle.

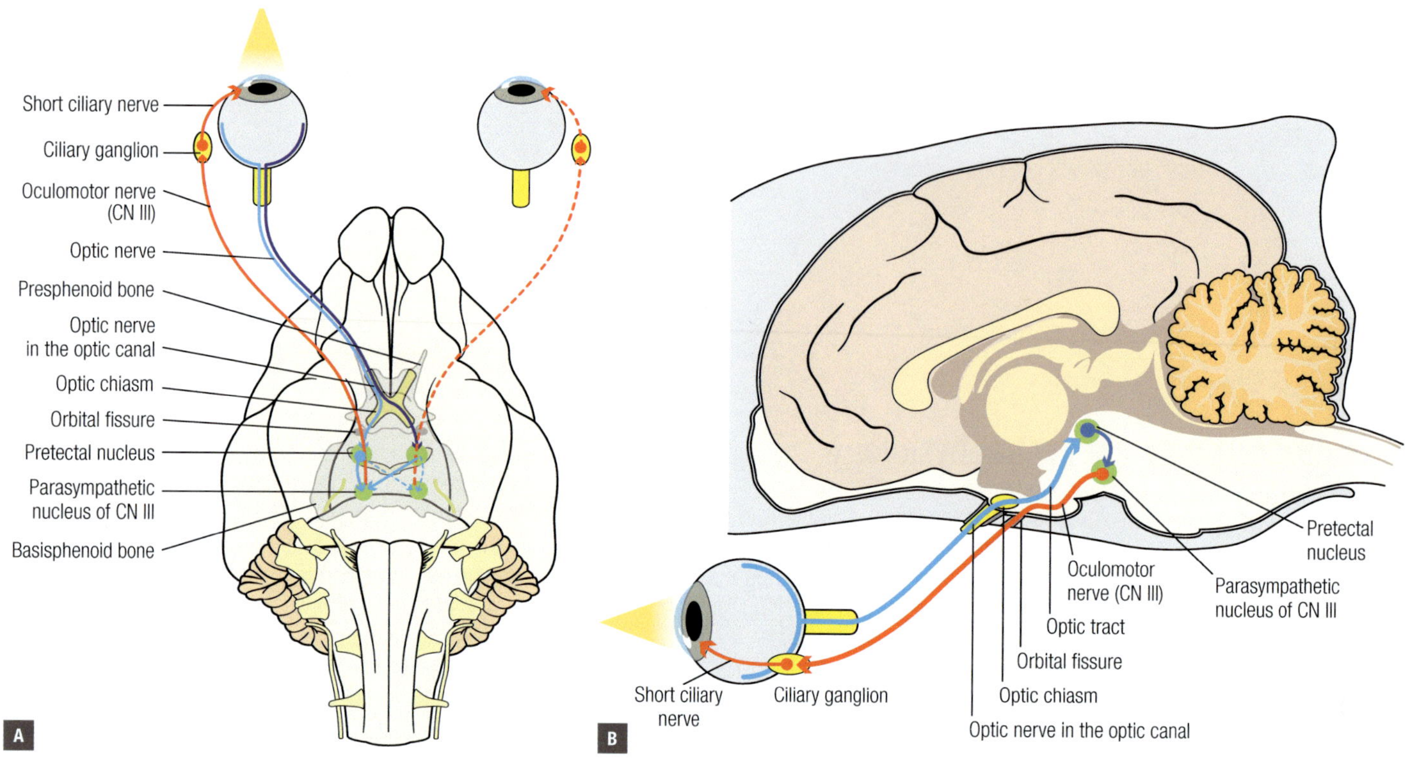

FIG. 4.1 Neuroanatomical pathway for the (direct and indirect) pupillary light reflex (PLR). The axons that contribute to the indirect PLR are represented with dotted lines. CN, cranial nerve.

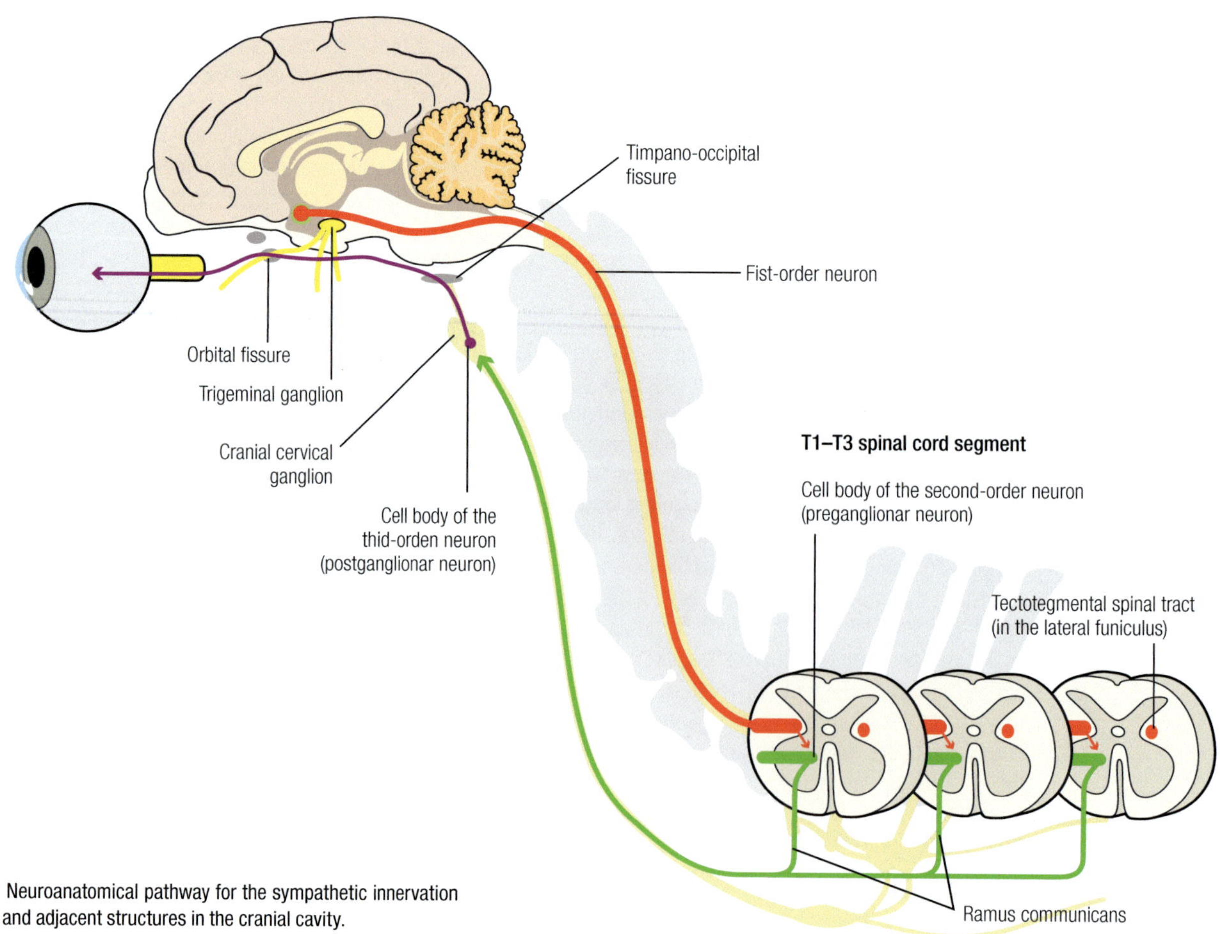

FIG. 4.2 Neuroanatomical pathway for the sympathetic innervation to the eye and adjacent structures in the cranial cavity.

Clinical signs

When the problem is in the mydriatic pupil

Internal ophthalmoparesis/-plegia is characterized by decreased (ophthalmoparesis) or absent (ophthalmoplegia) motor function of the iris sphincter and ciliary body muscle. This is due to a loss of parasympathetic innervation from the oculomotor nerve [cranial nerve (CN) III] or short ciliary nerves, observed clinically as areflexive mydriasis.

Most of the literature on dogs with internal ophthalmoparesis/-plegia are case reports with middle cranial fossa syndrome (also known as cavernous sinus syndrome).

Middle cranial fossa syndrome is a clinical disorder characterized by ipsilateral internal ophthalmoparesis/-plegia, paresis or plegia of the extraocular muscles (also known as external ophthalmoparesis /-plegia), and decreased to absent facial and corneal sensation. These clinical signs are due to a dysfunction of several cranial nerves that course at the level of the middle cranial fossa. These cranial nerves include CN III (motor and parasympathetic components), CN IV (trochlear nerve), CN VI (abducens nerve), the ophthalmic branch of CN V (trigeminal nerve), and postganglionic sympathetic nerve fibers. The maxillary branch of CN V, which passes through the round foramen, can also be affected. This is usually due to an intracranial or retrobulbar mass invading the orbital fissure or middle cranial fossa. Case reports in dogs have included chondrosarcoma, lymphoma, meningioma (Video 4.1), primitive neuroectodermal tumors, metastatic invasion of thyroid carcinomas, neuroendocrine carcinoma, and an aneurysm as the underlying cause.[1–3]

Lesions affecting the CN III alone and causing internal ophthalmoparesis/-plegia as the sole clinical signs are more rarely reported. Dysautonomia and pharmacological blockage with mydriatic agents such as atropine have to be considered. In dogs, oculomotor neuropathy has been reported to be secondary to intracranial meningiomas, intracranial suprasellar germ cell tumors, toxic contact (e.g., with *Datura stramonium*), or as an idiopathic cause.[4–6]

When the problem is in the miotic pupil

Horner's syndrome is a clinical disorder caused by a lack of sympathetic innervation to the head. Besides the miotic pupil, the clinical signs include ptosis of the upper eyelid, decreased tone of the lower eyelid, protrusion of the nictitating membrane, enophthalmos, and conjunctival hyperemia; crusts may also be observed inside the nares. The miotic pupil in patients with Horner's syndrome is most noticeable in the dark because the normal pupil dilates and the affected pupil remains miotic. Horner's syndrome results from lesions affecting first-, second- (preganglionic), or third-order (postganglionic) neurons. The presence of other clinical signs in association with Horner's syndrome can help to localize the lesion and formulate a differential diagnosis. Table 4.1 summarizes the most common differentials in dogs presented with Horner's syndrome.

Diagnostic approach

Algorithm 4.1 shows the diagnostic approach to patients with anisocoria. For the purposes of this chapter, the algorithm is focused mainly on the neurological causes.

When anisocoria is not considered mechanical (e.g., due to posterior synechiae, surgical injury), iatrogenic (pharmacologically induced) or physiological, then the diagnostic algorithm can be followed.

Algorithm 4.1 Note 1 A pharmacological test may be used to try to determine whether the underlying cause of the mydriatic pupil dysfunction is in the preganglionic neurons (oculomotor neuropathy) or the ganglionic neurons (short ciliary nerves). This test relies on denervation hypersensitivity, which usually takes 5 to 7 days to occur. It involves exposing the eye to direct-acting and indirect-acting parasympathomimetic eye drops. The direct-acting drugs elicit a more rapid and more complete miosis if the dysfunction is in the short ciliary nerves (postganglionic), whereas the indirect-acting drugs require the short ciliary nerves to be intact, and the lesion is therefore considered preganglionic. However, these tests are not consistently reliable, and investigations including advanced imaging might be needed in some patients.

Algorithm 4.1 Note 2 The occurrence of anisocoria with ipsilateral mydriasis associated with a naturally occurring cerebellar ischemic infarct in the region of the interposital nucleus has been described in dogs.[7]

Algorithm 4.1 Note 3 The concept behind this pharmacological test is similar to that described for the parasympathetic system (Algorithm Note 1), but in this case it involves exposing the eye to direct-acting and indirect-acting sympathomimetic drugs. The time to pupillary dilation following topical administration of 1% phenylephrine (direct-acting sympathomimetic agent) to both eyes should be determined. A time interval of less than 20 minutes suggests third-order Horner's syndrome, 20–45 minutes suggests second-order Horner's syndrome, and 60–90 minutes suggests first-order Horner's syndrome or no sympathetic denervation of the eye. If 10% phenylephrine is used, mydriasis occurs in 5–8 minutes with postganglionic (third-order neuron) lesions.

Pharmacological testing should only be used to guide the diagnosis, but it should not be used as the sole diagnostic test to localize the lesion.

Video 4.1

Nine-year-old male neutered Boxer with anisocoria. The abnormal pupil is the left (mydriatic) pupil. The neurological examination revealed a normal mental status, posture, and gait. The menace response was present in both eyes, with an absent direct/consensual pupillary light reflex (PLR) in the left eye and a normal PLR in the right eye. The vestibulo-ocular reflex was decreased in the left eye. The neurolocalization was the left oculomotor nerve. The main differential diagnoses included idiopathic oculomotor nerve neuropathy and neoplasia or inflammatory granuloma at the middle cranial fossa. The final diagnosis was a meningioma at the level of the middle cranial fossa.

TABLE 4.1 Horner's syndrome: possible neuroanatomical localizations and clinical signs and main differential diagnoses.

Neurons affected (order)	Localization	Possible signs of dysfunction that could be present ipsilateral to the affected eye	Diseases
1st order neurons	Brainstem	■ Altered level of consciousness ■ Cranial nerve deficits ■ General proprioceptive ataxia ■ Central vestibular dysfunction ■ Ipsilateral paresis or plegia	■ Meningioma ■ Glial tumor ■ Medulloblastoma ■ Lymphoma ■ Cerebrovascular accident ■ GME, NE, MUO ■ Infectious ■ Head trauma
1st order neurons	Lateral tectotegmental spinal tract (C1–C5 spinal cord segments)	■ General proprioceptive ataxia ■ Paresis or plegia on all four limbs/ipsilateral ■ Cervical hyperalgesia ■ Cervical muscle spasm/rigidity	■ Glial tumors ■ Lymphoma ■ Ischemic myelopathy ■ Acute nucleus pulposus extrusion ■ Spinal cord trauma
1st/2nd order neurons	C6–T2 spinal cord segments	■ General proprioceptive ataxia ■ Paresis or plegia on all four limbs or ipsilateral ■ Decreased spinal reflexes in thoracic limb(s) ■ Increased/normal spinal reflexes in pelvic limb(s) ■ Lameness (nerve root signature) ■ Cervicothoracic hyperalgesia ■ Cutaneous trunci muscle reflex decreased or absent ipsilateral	■ Same as C1–C5 spinal cord segments
2nd order neurons	T3–L3 spinal cord segments	■ General proprioceptive ataxia ■ Paresis or plegia on pelvic limb(s) ■ Increased spinal reflexes in the pelvic limb/s ■ Cranial thoracic spinal hyperalgesia ■ Cutaneous trunci muscle decreased or absent ■ Dysfunction of micturition (upper motor neuron bladder) and defecation	■ Same as C1–C5 spinal cord segments
2nd order neurons	T1–T3 ventral nerve roots	■ Lameness (nerve root signature) ■ Cutaneous trunci muscle reflex decreased or absent	■ Nerve sheath tumor ■ Sarcoma ■ Lymphoma ■ Trauma
2nd order neurons	Vagosympathetic trunk	■ Laryngeal paralysis ■ Dysphagia ■ Cough ■ Regurgitation	■ Thymoma ■ Lymphoma ■ Thyroid tumor ■ Trauma
3rd order neurons	Middle ear	■ Peripheral vestibular dysfunction ■ Facial paresis/paralysis	■ Otitis media/interna ■ Squamous cell carcinoma ■ Adenocarcinoma ■ Fibrosarcoma ■ Osteosarcoma
3rd order neurons	Middle cranial fossa	■ Internal/external ophthalmoparesis/-plegia	■ Pituitary tumors ■ Meningioma ■ Lymphoma ■ Inflammatory/infectious
3rd order neurons	Retrobulbar area	■ Exophthalmos ■ Hyperesthesia on palpation ■ CN deficits II, III, IV, V, VI	■ Orbital tumors ■ Inflammatory/infectious ■ Trauma
2nd/3rd order neurons		■ No other clinical signs	■ Idiopathic

CN, cranial nerves; GME, granulomatous meningoencephalomyelitis; NE, necrotizing encephalitis; MUO, meningoencephalomyelitis of unknown origin.

ALGORITHM 4.1

Diagnostic approach to patients with anisocoria.

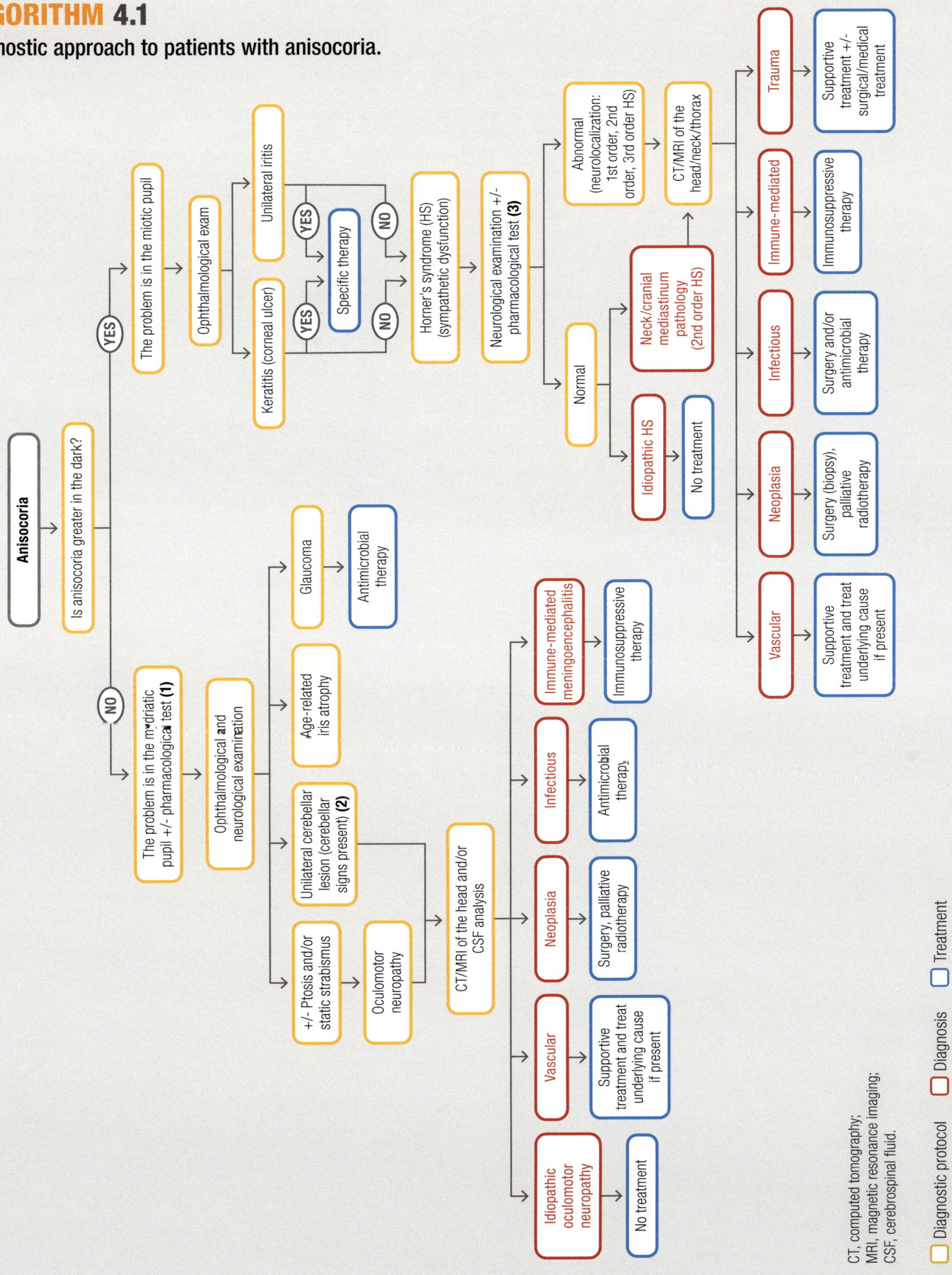

CT, computed tomography;
MRI, magnetic resonance imaging;
CSF, cerebrospinal fluid.

References

1. Theisen SK, Podell M, Schneider T, et al. A retrospective study of cavernous sinus syndrome in 4 dogs and 8 cats. *J Vet Intern Med.* 1996 Mar-Apr;10(2):65–71.
2. Rossmeisl JH Jr, Higgins MA, Inzana KD, et al. Bilateral cavernous sinus syndrome in dogs: 6 cases (1999-2004). *J Am Vet Med Assoc.* 2005 Apr 1;226(7):1105–1111.
3. Jones AM, Bentley E, Rylander H. Cavernous sinus syndrome in dogs and cats: case series (2002-2015). *Open Vet J.* 2018;8(2):186–192.
4. Webb AA, Cullen CL, Rose P, et al. Intracranial meningioma causing internal ophthalmoparesis in a dog. *Vet Ophthalmol.* 2005 Nov-Dec;8(6):421–425.
5. Hansen P, Clerc B. Anisocoria in the dog provoked by a toxic contact with an ornamental plant: Datura stramonium. *Vet Ophthalmol.* 2002 Dec;5(4):277–279.
6. Tetas Pont R, Freeman C, Dennis R, et al. Clinical and magnetic resonance imaging features of idiopathic oculomotor neuropathy in 14 dogs. *Vet Radiol Ultrasound.* 2017 May;58(3):334–343.
7. Danciu CD, Fenn J, Beltran E. Mydriasis associated with ischemic cerebrovascular infarct affecting the ipsilateral cerebellar interposital nucleus in two dogs. *J Vet Intern Med.* 2024 Aug 28. doi: 10.1111/jvim.17176. Epub ahead of print.
8. Glass E, DeLahunta A. Chapter 7. Lower motor neuron: general visceral efferent system. In: DeLahunta A, Glass E (eds.). *Veterinary Neuroanatomy and Clinical Neurology*, 3rd ed. St Louis, Missouri: Elsevier Saunders; 2015. pp. 197–221.
9. Webb AW, Cullen CL. Chapter 34. Neuro-ophthalmology. In: Gelatt KN, Gilger BC, Kern TJ (eds). *Veterinary Ophthalmology*, 5th ed. Iowa, USA: Wiley-Blackwell; 2013. pp. 1820–1897.

CHAPTER 5

Spinal pain

Joe Fenn
BVetMed, MVetMed, DECVN, FHEA, MRCVS

Pathophysiology

Pain has been defined as "an unpleasant sensory and emotional experience associated with, or resembling that associated with, actual or potential tissue damage".[1] This describes the conscious experience produced by the complex central processing of signals received by the brain following a noxious (potentially harmful) stimulus. Noxious stimuli are detected by nociceptors found in various tissues in the body, such as those comprising the structures of and surrounding the vertebral column in the case of spinal pain. Activation of nociceptors by mechanical or chemical stimuli generates action potentials that are transmitted by a combination of thinly myelinated A (fast pain) or unmyelinated C (slow pain) axons via spinal or cranial nerves, followed by central sensory tracts, the thalamus, and ultimately the cerebral cortex, for conscious perception. Increased sensitivity to normal levels of stimulus is referred to as hyperesthesia, such as that detected by spinal palpation on examination.

It is important to recognize that there are no nociceptors within the central nervous system tissue, such as the spinal cord itself. As a result, whilst innervated structures (e.g., paraspinal muscles, ligaments, or joints; intervertebral discs, specifically the annulus fibrosus; vertebral periosteum; meninges; or nerve roots) can all be sources of spinal pain, lesions affecting spinal cord grey or white matter alone (e.g., intramedullary neoplasia or fibrocartilaginous embolic myelopathy) often do not cause pain. The pathophysiology of spinal pain can therefore be variable and multifactorial, with multiple sources of potential discomfort present in the structures of the vertebral column and surrounding tissues.

Spinal pain or hyperesthesia can be caused by several pathological processes, provided that nociceptive pathways are stimulated. Spinal pain in dogs can be associated with diseases of traumatic, inflammatory, degenerative, congenital, neoplastic, or vascular origin (Table 5.1). These conditions can result in mechanical, chemical, or neuropathic pain. For example, traumatic injuries such as vertebral fractures/luxations can cause direct mechanical stimulation of nociceptors in the muscles, vertebrae, and joints as well as inflammation, which can lead to severe signs of spinal pain. Immune-mediated or infectious inflammatory diseases affecting tissues such as the meninges, joints, and muscles of the vertebral column lead to chemical stimulation of nociceptive pathways by inflammatory mediators, resulting in pain that can be diffuse and marked depending on the underlying disease. Some conditions in dogs, such as Chiari-like malformation and syringomyelia, may cause spinal hyperesthesia through abnormal central or peripheral somatosensory processing of nociceptive pathways, known as neuropathic pain. Although challenging to define or confirm clinically in animals, neuropathic pain in humans may be associated with specific signs such as dysesthesia (unpleasant abnormal sensation, e.g., a "burning" sensation) or paresthesia (abnormal sensation, e.g., tingling or "pins

TABLE 5.1 Differential diagnoses that can be associated with spinal pain in dogs according to their etiological classification.

	Diagnoses
Degenerative	■ Hansen type I intervertebral disc extrusion (IVDE) ■ Degenerative lumbosacral stenosis ■ Caudal cervical spondylomyelopathy ■ *Acute noncompressive nucleus pulposus extrusion (ANNPE)* ■ *Hydrated nucleus pulposus extrusion (HNPE)* ■ *Hansen type II intervertebral disc protrusion (IVDP)*
Anomalous	■ Atlantoaxial instability ■ Chiari-like malformation and syringomyelia ■ *Vertebral malformation/kyphosis*
Neoplasia	■ Extradural (vertebral - sarcoma, multiple myeloma, plasma cell tumor) ■ Extramedullary-intradural (peripheral nerve sheath tumor, meningioma, lymphoma) ■ *Intramedullary neoplasia (glioma, ependymoma, metastatic)*
Inflammatory	■ Discospondylitis ■ Steroid-responsive meningitis-arteritis (SRMA) ■ Spinal epidural empyema ■ Meningomyelitis of unknown origin (MUO) ■ Infectious meningomyelitis (bacterial, fungal, viral, protozoal) ■ Immune-mediated polymyositis ■ Immune-mediated polyarthritis ■ Paraspinal abscess
Traumatic	■ Vertebral fracture/luxation
Vascular	■ Spinal epidural hemorrhage

Conditions in italics are typically non painful but can be associated with mild spinal pain.

and needles"). It is also possible to see cervical spinal pain associated with increases in intracranial pressure due to lesions in the brain.

In the case of degenerative intervertebral disc disease, particularly Hansen type I intervertebral disc extrusions, dogs can demonstrate quite marked pain and focal spinal hyperesthesia associated with a multifactorial pain stimulus. The pathophysiology in this case is unclear but likely involves mechanical stimulation of nociceptors in the dorsal annulus fibrosus and dorsal longitudinal ligament as well as inflammatory mediator release (chemical stimulation) and neuropathic pain related to compression of the associated nerve roots.[2,3] Other conditions, such as compressive neoplasms and congenital anomalies associated with either vertebral instability or compression of soft tissues, can also result in spinal pain through variations of this pathophysiology.

Clinical signs

A suspicion of spinal pain in dogs is typically first raised by their behavior and demeanor; signs often include a reluctance to exercise, a stiff gait, increased sensitivity to touch, a low head carriage, or spontaneous vocalization. As a result, it is essential to obtain a thorough clinical history and pay particular attention to the owner's description of their dog's behavior and activity at home and when exercising. Some complaints or clinical signs can also be more suggestive of spinal pain in a specific region of the vertebral column. For example, a low head carriage or reluctance to raise the head suggests cervical spinal pain, whereas a reluctance to jump or climb stairs with a low tail carriage and difficulty posturing to defecate is more suggestive of caudal lumbar or lumbosacral spinal pain. The highly mobile nature of the cervical vertebral column also means that clinical signs of pain in this region can be characteristically intermittent, such as spontaneous yelping when moving the head. It is important to remember, however, that assessment of pain in animals is somewhat subjective, and responses will vary between individual animals. In addition, evidence of pain may sometimes be subtle, and spinal pain should always be considered as a possible contributor to more nonspecific primary complaints, such as lethargy or inappetence.

In addition to a comprehensive clinical history, a careful and thorough general physical and neurological examination is essential when evaluating for the presence of spinal pain or hyperesthesia in dogs. Rectal temperature is of particular importance, as the presence of pyrexia in a dog with spinal pain will guide the diagnostic approach by greatly increasing the index of suspicion for immune-mediated or infectious inflammatory differential diagnoses, particularly when combined with a young age and inflammatory leukogram in the case of cervical spinal pain.[4,5] On general physical examination, care should be taken to ensure that there are no potential causes of discomfort that could be misinterpreted as spinal pain, such as abdominal pain, painful soft tissue masses/swellings, or joint pain on orthopedic examination. Any history of gastrointestinal signs such as persistent vomiting or diarrhea should raise the index of suspicion for abdominal pain as a possible contributing factor to the clinical picture. It is therefore important to differentiate true thoracolumbar spinal pain from referred abdominal pain, through separate careful and gentle palpation of the abdominal structures alongside the neurological examination.

The neurological examination can be divided into "hands-off" and "hands-on" components, all of which provide important information in dogs with a suspicion of spinal pain (see Chapter 9 for a more detailed description of the neurological examination). The initial "hands-off" assessment of behavior, posture, and gait in the consultation room can offer some vital clues of spinal discomfort. Alongside the behavioral changes described above, particularly suggestive findings for spinal pain include a kyphotic posture (thoracolumbar pain; Fig. 5.1A), low head carriage with a reluctance to turn (cervical spinal pain; Fig. 5.1B), or a stiff gait and reluctance to walk. Another observation that may be supportive of neuropathic pain in the cervical region is the presence of spontaneous focal cervical myoclonus (cervical muscle "jerks"; Video 5.1). This may be related to the mechanical stimulation of compressed nerve roots in the cervical vertebral column, with a recent study speculating that it might be suggestive of a diagnosis of cervical Hansen type I intervertebral disc extrusion.[6]

The initial "hands-on" components of the neurological examination include the assessment of postural reactions, spinal reflexes, and cranial

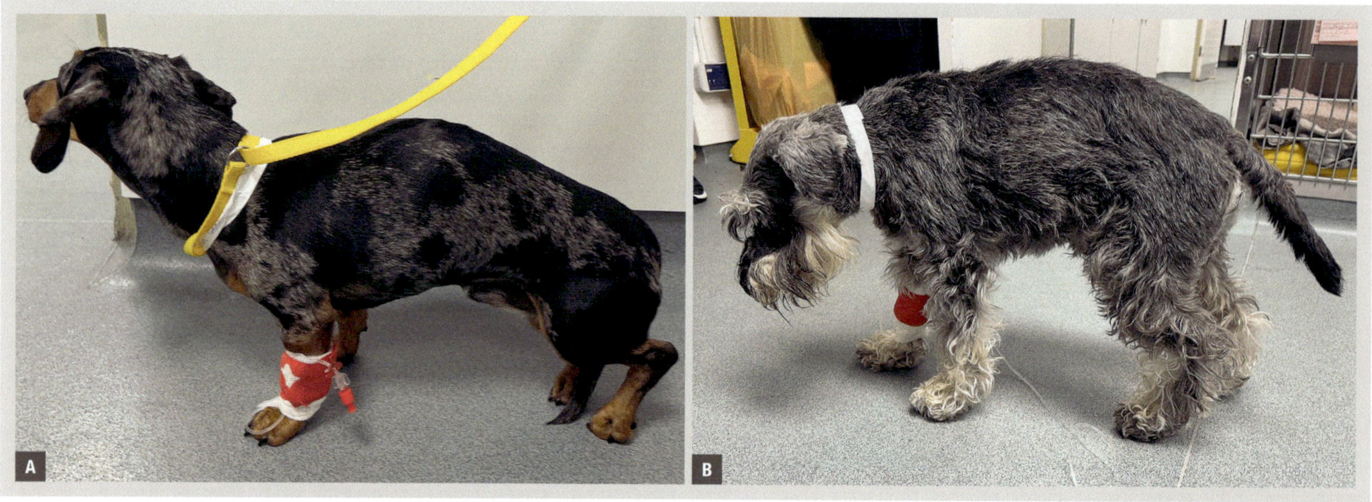

FIG. 5.1 Examples of postures suggestive of spinal pain: a kyphotic posture in a Miniature Dachshund with thoracolumbar spinal pain (A) and a low head carriage in a Miniature Schnauzer with marked cervical spinal pain (B).

ALGORITHM 5.1

Diagnostic approach to spinal pain.

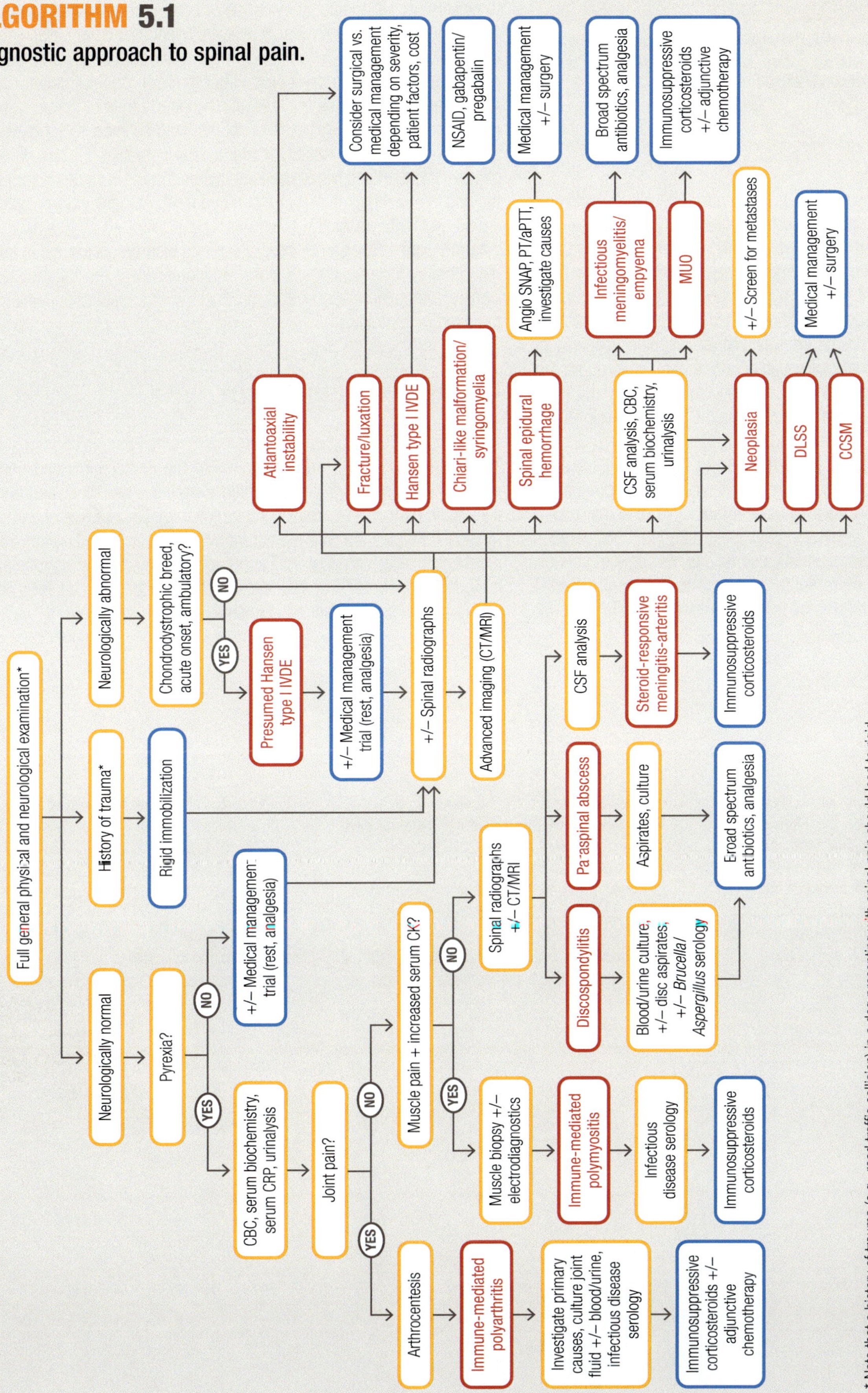

* Note that a history of trauma (e.g., road traffic collision) in a dog presenting with spinal pain should lead to rigid immobilization, ideally restrained on a spinal board, until fracture/luxation are excluded through diagnostic imaging.

CBC, complete blood count; CRP, C-reactive protein; CK, creatine kinase; CT, computed tomography; MRI, magnetic resonance imaging; IVDE, intervertebral disc extrusion; CSF, cerebrospinal fluid; NSAID, nonsteroidal anti-inflammatory drug; Angio SNAP, serum antigen test for *Angiostrongylus vasorum*; PT/aPTT, prothrombin time/activated partial thromboplastin time; MUO, meningoencephalitis of unknown origin; DLSS, degenerative lumbosacral stenosis; CCSM, caudal cervical spondylomyelopathy.

Diagnostic protocol · Diagnosis · Treatment

Video 5.1

Typical cervical muscle "jerks" in two French Bulldogs with cervical spinal pain associated with presumed cervical intervertebral disc extrusion.

nerve function. These steps are of great importance when evaluating dogs with signs of spinal pain, as certain differential diagnoses will be more relevant in dogs that are neurologically abnormal than in those presenting with spinal pain alone and no neurological deficits. Tests for the presence of spinal pain or hyperesthesia (e.g., palpation and manipulation of the neck, thoracolumbar vertebral column, and muscles) should be performed last in the neurological examination, followed by testing of deep and superficial pain perception in paraplegic dogs. Any distress caused by performing these potentially painful tests early in the examination could have a detrimental effect on the ability to perform and interpret the remainder of the neurological exam.

Vertebral column palpation is performed using firm digital pressure applied to either side of the spinous processes, with a conscious painful response (e.g., vocalization, turning to bite) indicative of spinal hyperesthesia. Interpretation of any response should take into consideration the breed and behavioral characteristics of the dog, as some more stoic dogs may demonstrate a more subtle response to discomfort. Gentle handling of the abdomen at the same time can detect tension in response to discomfort for additional evidence of pain. Firm palpation of the epaxial muscles laterally may also reveal evidence of pain, particularly in the cervical region in dogs with syringomyelia or lateralized nerve root compression due to Hansen type I intervertebral disc extrusion. Gentle manipulation of the neck may reveal a reduced range of dorsal, ventral, and lateral flexion, but extreme caution should be exercised if there is a suspicion of fracture, luxation, or atlantoaxial instability. It is also useful to observe for restricted head movement when turning in circles or tempting the dog to move their head with food or a treat. Alongside firm palpation, stress on the lumbosacral region can be maximized by extending the patient's hips at the same time, which can also be performed in lateral recumbency in large dogs. Finally, manipulation of the tail can reveal signs of lumbosacral discomfort, particularly in dorsal flexion, which tilts the sacrum ventrally.

Diagnostic approach

An example of the diagnostic approach to spinal pain is dogs in shown in Algorithm 5.1. Note the importance of the neurological and general physical examination findings, which determine the most appropriate diagnostic path. There are also scenarios in which a period of empirical medical management with a presumptive diagnosis based on the signalment and clinical signs is a valid approach, as long as clinical progression is closely monitored.[7] The reader can also refer to Table 5.1 for a list of differential diagnoses that can cause spinal pain.

References

1. Raja SN, Carr DB, Cohen M, et al. The revised International Association for the Study of Pain definition of pain: concepts, challenges, and compromises. *Pain.* 2020;161(9):1976–1982.
2. Fadda A, Oevermann A, Vandevelde M, et al. Clinical and pathological analysis of epidural inflammation in intervertebral disk extrusion in dogs. *J Vet Intern Med.* 2013;27(4):924–934.
3. Willems N, Tellegen AR, Bergknut N, et al. Inflammatory profiles in canine intervertebral disc degeneration. *BMC Vet Res.* 2016:1–12.
4. Grapes NJ, Packer RMA, De Decker S. Clinical reasoning in canine cervical hyperaesthesia: which presenting features are important? *Vet Rec.* 2020;187(11):448.
5. De Strobel F, Palus V, Vettorato E, Cherubini GB. Cervical hyperaesthesia in dogs: an epidemiological retrospective study of 185 cases. *J Small Anim Pract.* 2019;129:343–347.
6. Olender M, Couturier J, Gatel L, Cauvin E. Cervical jerks as a sign of cervical pain or myelopathy in dogs. *J Am Vet Med Assoc.* 2023;261(4):510–516.
7. Khan S, Freeman P. Bayesian clinical reasoning in the first opinion approach to a dog with suspected thoracolumbar pain. *J Small Anim Pract.* 2022:1–5.

CHAPTER 6

Gait abnormalities: ataxia, paresis, and paralysis

Gualtiero Gandini
DVM, PhD, DECVN

Pathophysiology

Gait abnormalities most often result from a dysfunction of the nervous or locomotor system. Correct identification of the system involved is critical to developing a list of differential diagnoses and selecting the most appropriate diagnostic investigations. Gait examination is of paramount importance and is a relevant part of the neurological and orthopedic examination. For the purpose of this book, this chapter will focus mainly on neurological gait abnormalities.

Functional anatomy of gait

In dogs, normal gait depends on the functional integrity of the cerebral cortex, brainstem, cerebellum, spinal cord (ascending and descending pathways), peripheral nerves (sensory and motor), neuromuscular junction, and muscles (Fig. 6.1).[1] Voluntary movement is initiated by nerve impulses generated in the cerebral cortex or brainstem. The cerebellum coordinates voluntary movements, and the vestibular system maintains balance during movement. Nerve impulses from the brain travel along the descending tracts of the spinal cord to the peripheral nerves and then to the muscles. Information about limb position during movement reaches the cerebellum and forebrain from the periphery via the proprioceptive ascending tracts of the spinal cord.[1,2] Voluntary movement is the result of the synergistic action of motor (descending) and sensory (ascending) functions with integration by the cerebellum.

Motor function

Two types of motor neurons form the descending motor pathways. The *upper motor neurons* (UMNs), whose cell bodies are located in the brain, initiate voluntary movements: their axons run down the central nervous system forming the descending tracts of the spinal cord and synapse with the *lower motor neurons* (LMNs), which are large neurons located in the ventral horn of the spinal cord. The axons of the LMNs exit the spinal cord and, together with other motor fibers, eventually form the efferent part of the peripheral nerves. These axons connect to striated muscle at the neuromuscular junction.[1]

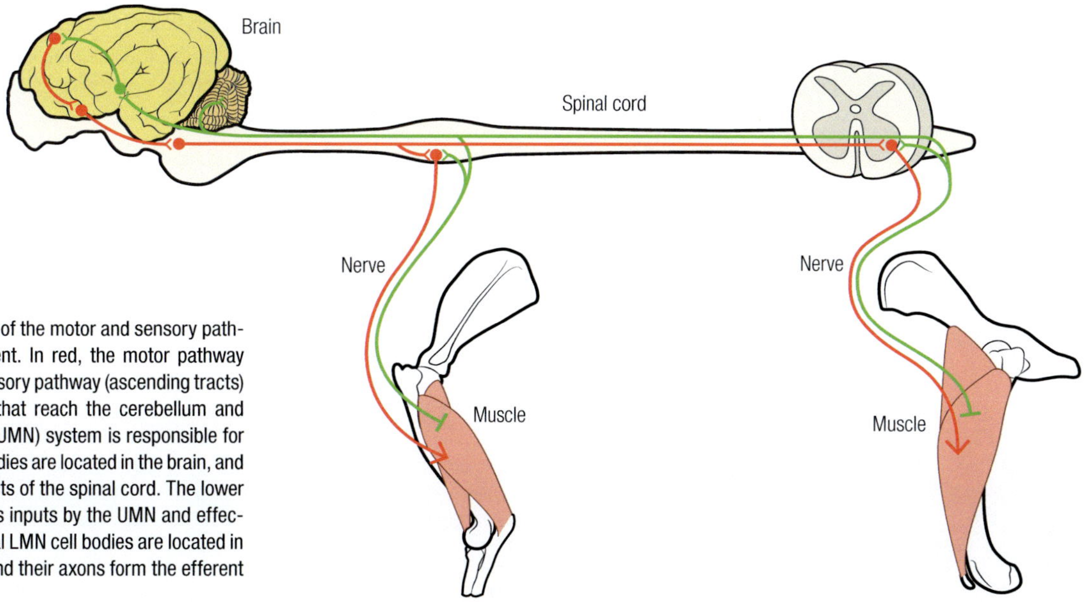

FIG. 6.1 Schematic representation of the motor and sensory pathways involved in voluntary movement. In red, the motor pathway (descending tracts). In green, the sensory pathway (ascending tracts) including the proprioceptive fibers that reach the cerebellum and forebrain. The upper motor neuron (UMN) system is responsible for initiating movement. The UMN cell bodies are located in the brain, and their axons form the descending tracts of the spinal cord. The lower motor neuron (LMN) system receives inputs by the UMN and effectively produces movement. The spinal LMN cell bodies are located in the ventral horn of the spinal cord, and their axons form the efferent part of the peripheral nerves.

Sensory function

Kinesthesia is the awareness of the position and movement of one's own body, especially the limbs. Kinesthetic information is detected and transmitted by general proprioceptive neurons. The general proprioceptive system schematically consists of a peripheral receptor (part of the sensory component of the peripheral nerves), the centripetal sensory fibers of the peripheral nerve, and the ascending spinal tracts carrying information to the cerebellum or cerebral cortex.[1] General proprioception, by providing continuous information about the position of the limbs during movement, is essential for the coordination of movement itself. Other sensory inputs necessary for movement coordination come from the *vestibular system* ("special proprioception") and the *visual system.*

Clinical features of gait abnormalities

Gait abnormalities can be classified into three broad categories*: ataxia, paresis*, and *lameness*. Ataxia and paresis represent neurological deficits, whereas lameness is more commonly caused by orthopedic disorders. In some cases, lameness may also be due to neurological disorders, especially those affecting the nerve roots, spinal nerves, or peripheral nerves supplying the limbs. Ataxia is associated with dysfunction of the sensory system. Paresis is a sign of dysfunction of the motor system.

Ataxia

Ataxia defines the inability to perform normal coordinated movements that is not caused by paresis or musculoskeletal disorders.[2,3]

Ataxia can be classified as *proprioceptive, cerebellar,* or *vestibular*.[1,2,3] Typically, cerebellar and vestibular ataxia affect all four limbs. Proprioceptive ataxia, depending on the site of the lesion, can involve the pelvic or all four limbs.

Proprioceptive ataxia results from lesions of nervous structures involved in the control of general proprioception (peripheral receptors and sensory nerve fibers, dorsal nerve roots, spinal cord, brainstem, cerebellum, and forebrain). In clinical practice, proprioceptive ataxia is often associated with disorders of the spinal cord. This type of ataxia is characterized by a loss of awareness of the spatial position of the body, particularly of the limbs (kinesthesia).[2]

The severity of proprioceptive ataxia depends on the extent of the lesion and can range from barely perceptible changes to obvious deficits. In the latter cases, the limbs are excessively abducted and/or adducted, hypo- and/or hypermetric during walking; they may cross, touch the other limb, and it is sometimes possible to observe a tendency to stand on the dorsum of the paw (*knuckling*).[2,3]

It is important to remember that the proprioceptive and motor pathways throughout the spinal cord and caudal brainstem are intimately connected, and proprioceptive ataxia is therefore often associated with paresis.[2]

Proprioceptive ataxia can be appreciated in ambulatory patients when paresis is mild to moderate. Severe, nonambulatory paresis does not permit objective appreciation of the ataxia.

Cerebellar ataxia is caused by disorders of the cerebellum or, more rarely, by lesions selectively affecting the spinocerebellar tracts. This type of ataxia is characterized by an inability to regulate the strength and range of movements, resulting in dysmetria, most commonly seen as hypermetria, an exaggerated elevation and protraction of the limb.[1,2,3] This type of ataxia may be associated with other cerebellar signs, such as a wide-base stance and intention tremor. Unlike proprioceptive ataxia, cerebellar ataxia is never associated with paresis.

Vestibular ataxia associated with unilateral vestibular lesions is characterized by a tendency to drift, fall, or roll to one side (usually ipsilateral to the lesion). This type of ataxia is associated with vestibular signs, such as head tilt, resting nystagmus, positional strabismus, and sometimes a tendency to circle.[1,2,3]

Paresis and paralysis

Paresis is the partial loss of voluntary motor function. *Paralysis (*or *plegia)* defines the complete loss of this function. Paresis and paralysis are two terms that define the same type of defect and differ only quantitatively. Paresis has varying degrees of severity and can be divided into ambulatory paresis (i.e., when the animal can stand and walk unassisted) and nonambulatory paresis (i.e., when the patient requires assistance to stand and walk) (Fig. 6.2).

Paresis/paralysis can affect one limb (monoparesis/monoplegia), the pelvic limbs (paraparesis/paraplegia), the thoracic and pelvic limbs on the same side (hemiparesis/hemiplegia), or all four limbs (tetraparesis/tetraplegia).[3] The keyword to understand paresis is weakness.[1] Depending on the severity, paresis is observed as hypometria, dragging of the toes (with abnormal nail wear in chronic cases), shorter strides, and an inability to support body weight.[2]

Paresis/paralysis can be the consequence of a UMN or a LMN lesion. Spastic paresis/paralysis occurs in lesions of the UMN, due to the lack

Video 6.1

Ten-year-old male Beagle showing mild lameness of the left thoracic limb. Note the elevation of the head when the affected limb touches the ground to reduce weight bearing (easily seen with the video in slow motion). At this stage of the examination, it is not possible to distinguish between an orthopedic and neurological origin of the lameness. The dog suffered from a lateralized cervicothoracic (C5–C6) disc extrusion, and the neurological examination showed neck rigidity during manipulation.

Video 6.2

Mixed-breed dog affected by mild thoracolumbar disc herniation showing marked proprioceptive ataxia of the pelvic limbs. Note the crossing and excessive abduction and adduction of the pelvic limbs, including spontaneous knuckling of the left pelvic limb especially when turning and changing pace. As in many spinal cord disorders, a very mild degree of concurrent paraparesis may be observed. The thoracic limbs are normal. The patient's tail had been docked for medical reasons.

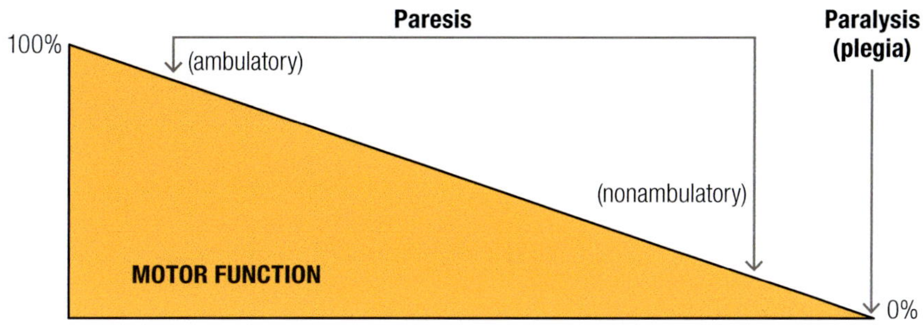

FIG. 6.2 Schematic representation of the concept of paresis and paralysis. Paresis is the partial loss of the ability to perform a voluntary movement. Paresis covers a wide range of motor changes depending on the severity of the lesion. At the mildest levels, ambulatory paresis is observed, while at the most severe levels, the paresis is so severe that, although some residual voluntary movement remains, walking is no longer possible. Paralysis is the complete loss of the ability to make voluntary movements.

of modulating effect by the UMN on the LMN, which, among other functions, maintains muscle tone. For the same reason, paresis/paralysis resulting from LMN damage is flaccid, due to the inability to maintain a normal muscle tone.[1,2]

Diagnostic approach

Algorithm 6.1 reflects the diagnostic approach that should be followed when presented with a dog with gait abnormalities. The dog's gait must be evaluated by observing the animal from the side, front, and back while walking in a straight line and turning on a nonslippery surface and, if appropriate, while walking up and down stairs. Gait assessment in an environment where the animal is psychologically and physically comfortable and, if required, part of the body weight is supported, should be encouraged as best practice.

Algorithm 6.1 Note 1 Proprioceptive ataxia is the only type of ataxia that, depending on the location of the lesion, may selectively affect the pelvic limbs. The presence of a head tilt is typically associated with vestibular ataxia. Intention tremors of the head are associated with hypermetria and spasticity, typical of cerebellar disorders.

Algorithm 6.1 Note 2 Some neurological disorders may only present with lameness. This is particularly true for lateralized disc herniations causing nerve root compression/inflammation or in the early stages of peripheral nerve sheath tumors (PNSTs).

Algorithm 6.1 Note 3 Both spinal cord and brainstem diseases can result in ataxia and paresis. Diseases affecting the brainstem also commonly result in impaired mentation and cranial nerve deficits.

Algorithm 6.1 Note 4 Proprioceptive ataxia is frequently associated with a degree of paresis, due to the proximity of the ascending proprioceptive fibers with the descending UMN fibers. Superficial lesions of the spinal cord may result in proprioceptive ataxia without concomitant paresis. On the contrary, more severe and deeper spinal cord lesions result in more prominent paresis (e.g., nonambulatory paresis) or, in the most severe cases, paralysis.

Algorithm 6.1 Note 5 Magnetic resonance imaging (MRI) is the gold standard in the investigation of central nervous system disorders. It is preferred to computed tomography due to its superior soft-tissue resolution. Cerebrospinal fluid (CSF) examination is recommended, especially when the differential diagnoses include inflammatory diseases.

Algorithm 6.1 Note 6 Inflammatory central nervous system disorders in dogs are mainly due to noninfectious disorders; most of them are grouped under the umbrella term of meningoencephalomyelitis of unknown origin (MUO). The diagnostic investigation of an inflammatory disorder includes MRI, CSF examination, and serology and polymerase chain reaction (PCR) investigations of infectious diseases that can occur in a specific region/country. MUO requires prolonged immunosuppressive treatment.

Video 6.3

Four-month-old female Malinois affected by spongy degeneration with cerebellar ataxia. The part of the video in slow motion highlights the exaggerated elevation (hypermetria) of all four limbs (particularly obvious in the pelvic limbs), the wide-base stance of the pelvic limbs, and the absence of weakness.

Video 6.4

Sixteen-year-old female mixed-breed dog showing mild signs of vestibular ataxia. Note the marked right head tilt and the tendency to drift towards the right. The dog suffered from idiopathic vestibular disease.

Video 6.5

Eleven-year-old female Hovawart affected by degenerative myelopathy. At this stage of the disease, the dog is showing severe paraparesis (almost nonambulatory) and proprioceptive ataxia of the pelvic limbs. To compensate for the severe weakness in the pelvic limbs, a significant proportion of the body weight is shifted on the thoracic limbs.

Video 6.6

Twelve-year-old male mixed-breed dog with tetraplegia due to a cervical disc extrusion. When supported, the dog shows no voluntary movements of the limbs. Note the normal muscle tone, reflecting an upper motor neuron lesion.

ALGORITHM 6.1

Diagnostic approach to gait abnormalities in dogs.

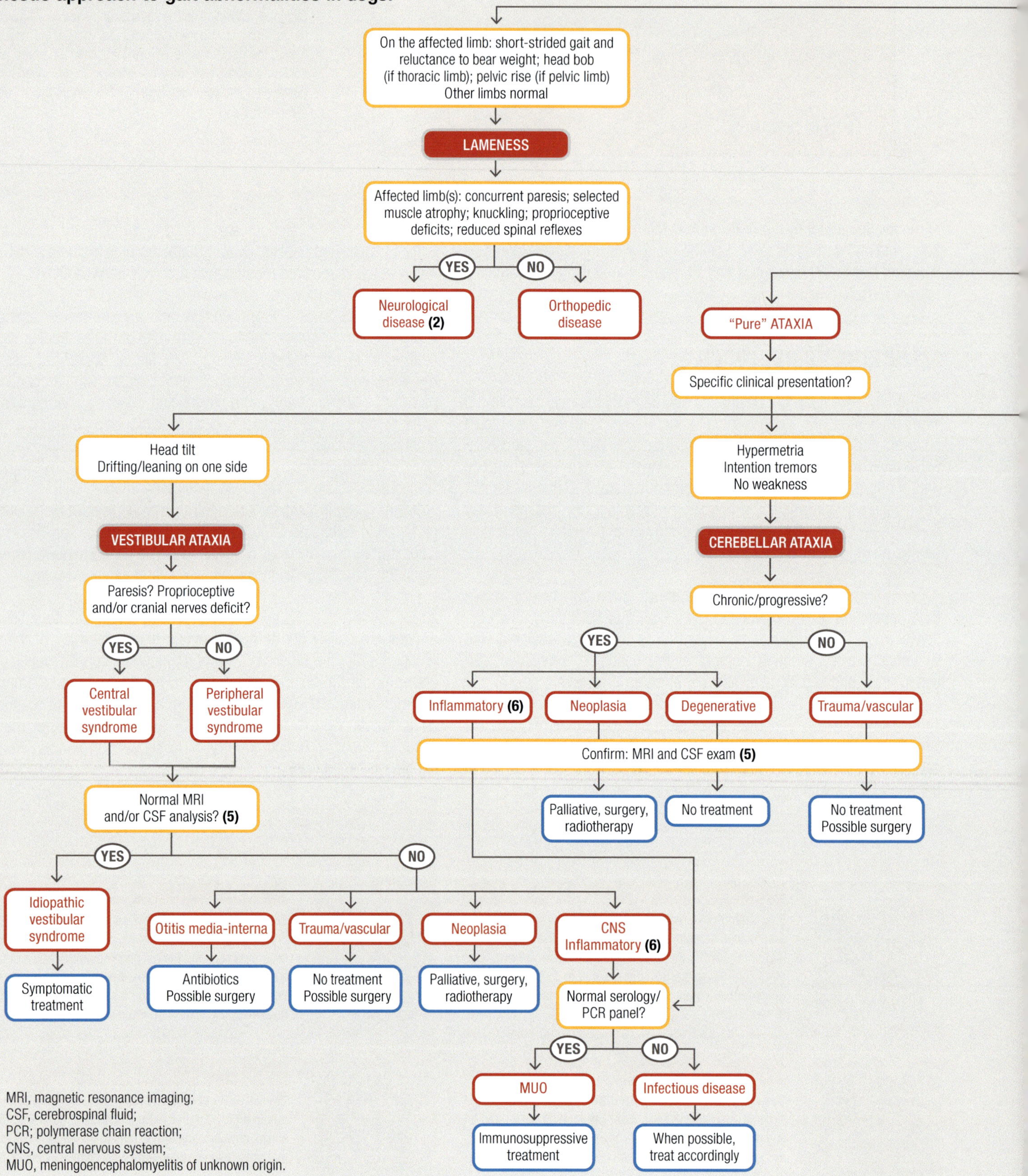

MRI, magnetic resonance imaging;
CSF, cerebrospinal fluid;
PCR; polymerase chain reaction;
CNS, central nervous system;
MUO, meningoencephalomyelitis of unknown origin.

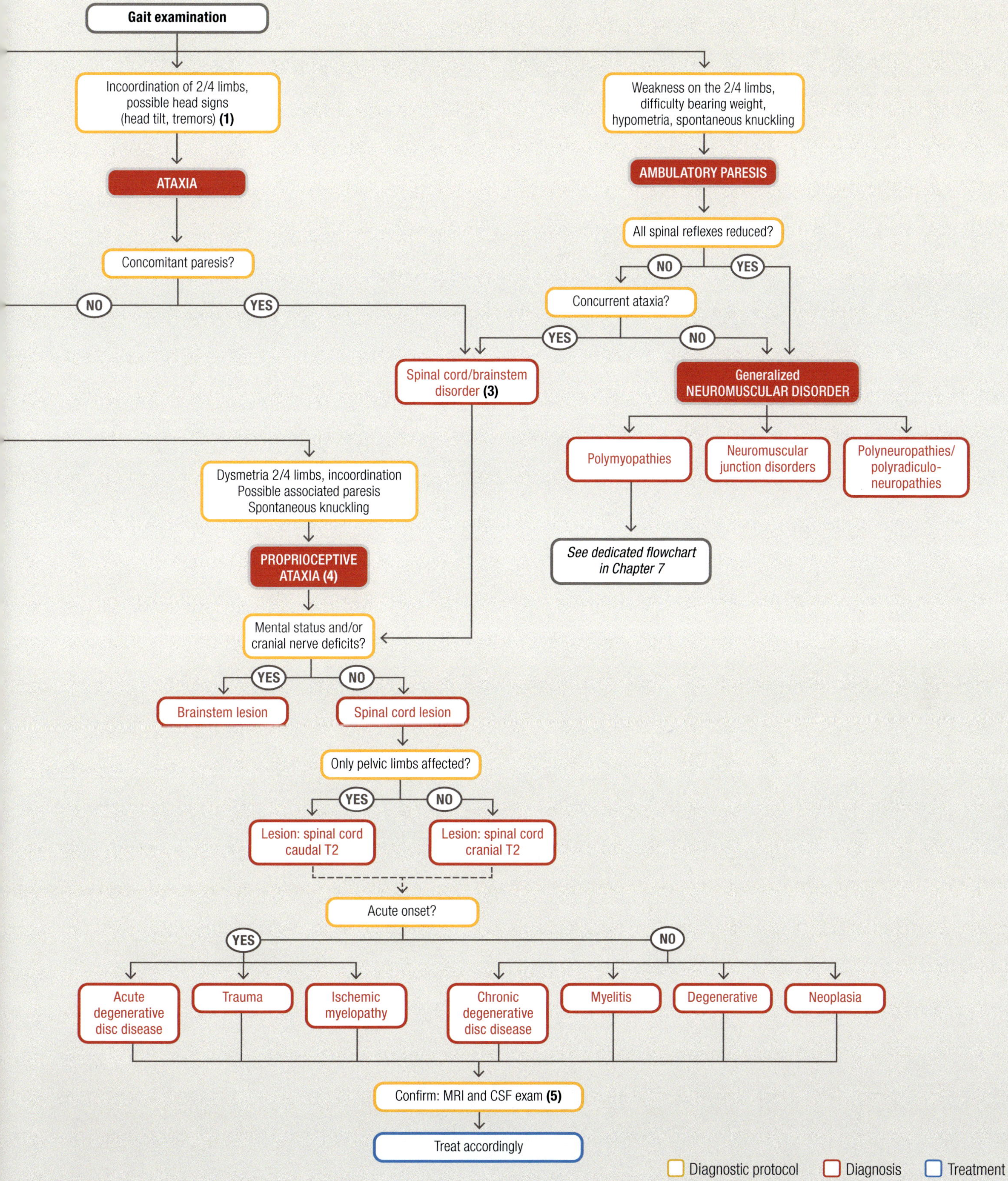
Gait examination
Incoordination of 2/4 limbs, possible head signs (head tilt, tremors) (1)
ATAXIA
Concomitant paresis?
NO
YES
Weakness on the 2/4 limbs, difficulty bearing weight, hypometria, spontaneous knuckling
AMBULATORY PARESIS
All spinal reflexes reduced?
NO
YES
Concurrent ataxia?
YES
NO
Spinal cord/brainstem disorder (3)
Generalized NEUROMUSCULAR DISORDER
Polymyopathies
Neuromuscular junction disorders
Polyneuropathies/ polyradiculo- neuropathies
See dedicated flowchart in Chapter 7
Dysmetria 2/4 limbs, incoordination Possible associated paresis Spontaneous knuckling
PROPRIOCEPTIVE ATAXIA (4)
Mental status and/or cranial nerve deficits?
YES
NO
Brainstem lesion
Spinal cord lesion
Only pelvic limbs affected?
YES
NO
Lesion: spinal cord caudal T2
Lesion: spinal cord cranial T2
Acute onset?
YES
NO
Acute degenerative disc disease
Trauma
Ischemic myelopathy
Chronic degenerative disc disease
Myelitis
Degenerative
Neoplasia
Confirm: MRI and CSF exam (5)
Treat accordingly
Diagnostic protocol
Diagnosis
Treatment

References

1. De Lahunta A, Glass E, Kent M (eds.) *Delahunta's Veterinary Neuroanatomy snd Clinical Neurology*, 5th ed. Philadelphia, USA: Elsevier; 2021.
2. Dewey CW, Da Costa R (eds.). *A Practical Guide to Canine and Feline Neurology*, 3rd ed. Blackwell, Iowa State Press; 2015.
3. Platt SR, Olby NJ (eds.). *BSAVA Manual of Canine and Feline Neurology*, 4th ed. Cheltenham: UK: BSAVA Publications; 2013.

CHAPTER 7

Exercise intolerance

Gualtiero Gandini
DVM, PhD, DECVN

Pathophysiology

Exercise intolerance is defined as the inability or decreased ability of an animal to perform physical activity that is considered normal for the animal's age, breed, and physical condition. In other words, exercise intolerance can also be defined as early and excessive fatigue following a level of exercise that is normal for the individual. In most instances, exercise intolerance is associated with neurological disorders, but it can also be the result of non-neurological conditions such as anemia or cardiovascular and respiratory disorders.

Neurological exercise intolerance is a specific type of paresis and represents the most relevant clinical sign of disorders affecting the *neuromuscular* (NM) *system*, including junctionopathies (e.g., myasthenia gravis), poly(radiculo)neuropathies, and polymyopathies (see Chapters 36 and 37).

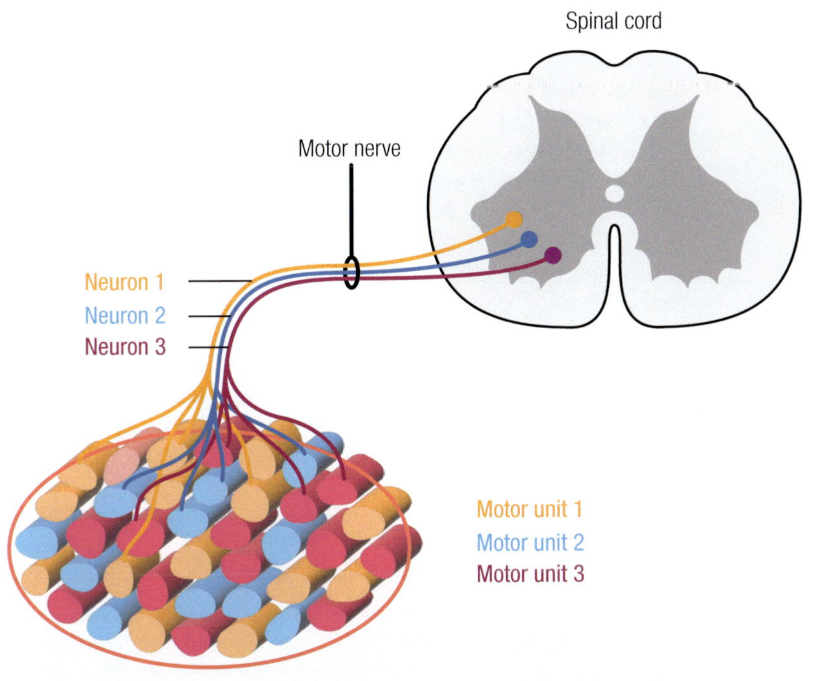

FIG. 7.1 Schematic representation of the organization of three motor units. The motor unit is the morphofunctional unit of the neuromuscular system, consisting of a lower motor neuron and all the muscle fibers innervated by it. Note the multiple muscle fibers innervated by a single motor neuron.

Functional anatomy of the neuromuscular system

The peripheral nervous system (PNS) consists of an efferent part, with motor functions, and an afferent part, with sensory functions. In clinical practice, the efferent part of the PNS is identified with the NM system (or the *lower motor neuron [LMN] system*), which functionally includes the muscle to form a morphofunctional unit of great clinical importance. The functional unit of the NM system is the *motor unit*, which consists of the nerve cell (α-motoneuron), its axon, the neuromuscular junctions, and all the innervated muscle fibers (Fig. 7.1).

The axon of the α-motoneuron emerges from the spinal cord as part of the ventral nerve root, participates in the formation of the spinal nerve, and reaches the neuromuscular junction as part of a specific peripheral nerve (the latter formed by the contribution of several spinal nerves) (Fig. 7.2). Close to the muscle, the axon of the α-motoneuron branches in proportion to the number of innervated muscle fibers. The *neuromuscular junction* (NMJ) is the point of contact between the terminal part of the axon and the skeletal muscle fiber and plays a critically important role in muscle contraction.

Clinical signs

General physical examination

Exercise intolerance may result from non-neurological conditions; therefore, the general physical examination should include special attention to the presence of pale mucous membranes, respiratory distress, cough, abnormal pulse, or peripheral edema, which are all possible signs of an underlying hematological, cardiac, or respiratory disease. It is important to remember that even anemic syndromes and some cardiorespiratory diseases can manifest with weakness. In these patients, exercise rapidly produces signs of fatigue and discomfort, often accompanied by polypnea to the point of respiratory distress. In addition to weakness, exercise may produce more specific signs in dogs with cardiorespiratory disorders, such as coughing fits or abnormal lung sounds

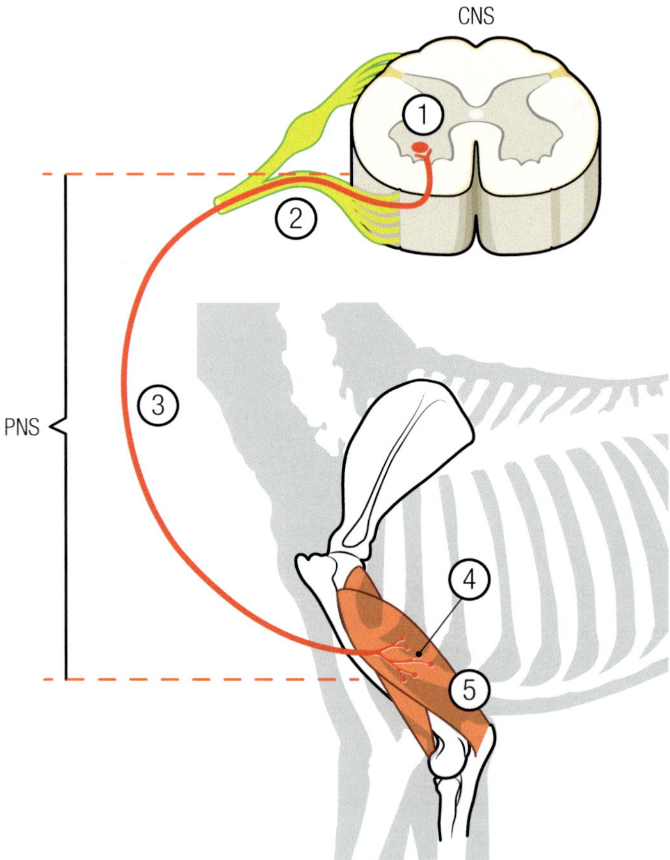

FIG. 7.2 Schematic representation of the neuromuscular system showing its relationship with the central nervous system (CNS) and peripheral nervous system (PNS). The lower motor neuron body (1) is located in the spinal cord (CNS), while the ventral nerve root (2), the peripheral nerve fibers (3), and the neuromuscular junctions (4) are located in the peripheral nervous system (PNS) and represent its efferent part. 5, Striated muscle.

on auscultation. All these signs should be thoroughly considered in an appropriate diagnostic workup. The description of the abovementioned conditions is beyond the scope of this chapter, and the reader is referred to veterinary internal medicine textbooks for further information.

Neurological examination

The NM patient usually has none of the previously described cardiovascular and/or respiratory signs with the exception of polypnea, which is exacerbated by exercise and due to fatigue. In the most severe cases, abnormal breathing can also be observed at rest.

The key word in defining the clinical picture of generalized NM disorders is weakness and specifically LMN weakness. The key points in the neurological examination to define a NM patient are the *gait, spinal reflexes*, and *muscle tone*, all of which are affected by varying degrees of weakness. For educational purposes, the abnormalities observed in NM patients will be presented according to the correct sequence of the different parts of the neurological examination.

Mental status and behavior

Mentation is usually unaltered in NM disorders. Extreme weakness may sometimes give the false impression of drowsiness or lethargy.

Posture

In severe cases, postural changes may be observed and reflect the generalized NM weakness. These include ventroflexion of the neck and head due to the difficulty in supporting the weight of the head. Affected animals may have prolonged recumbency due to their inability to maintain a quadrupedal stance. In extremely severe cases, patients may lie in lateral recumbency (e.g., acute canine polyradiculoneuritis [ACP]).

Although this is more common in cats, dogs can occasionally present with a plantigrade or palmigrade stance, also due to weakness.

Gait and postural reactions

Generalized LMN weakness results in exercise intolerance, which is considered a form of paresis and is not associated with ataxia. In the most severe cases, generalized LMN weakness results in nonambulatory tetraparesis and tetraplegia (Video 7.1).

In case of exercise intolerance, following a period of rest, the gait examination is generally unremarkable on initial assessment, but after exercise (of varying duration and intensity depending on the underlying etiology and its severity), signs of weakness will appear, including hypometria, short strides, joint hyperflexion, limb dragging and nail rubbing on the ground, associated with a lowered tail and progressive neck ventroflexion. In some patients, the weakness does not appear to be evenly distributed, with the pelvic limbs being much more affected than the thoracic limbs (Video 7.2).

Exercise intolerance is characterized by the progressive inability of the animal to support its weight; the animal is forced to lie down to rest and regain the strength needed to walk again. Rest usually improves the condition, which recurs each time the patient is required to exercise. Progressive worsening of generalized tremors, indicating weakness, may also be observed with walking.

Typically, NM patients do not show primary ataxia. This is because selective lesions of the neuromuscular system, which is an efferent motor pathway, do not involve the ascending sensory pathways, which cause ataxia when injured.

In general, the NM dog will show normal postural reactions as long as it has the strength to bear its weight. As the efferent pathways are selectively affected in the NM dog, delayed postural reactions are the result of weakness and not primary proprioceptive dysfunction. To help differentiate a delayed postural reaction due to a problem in the ascending proprioceptive pathways from one caused by a lesion in the descending motor pathways, specific postural reaction tests can be considered. For example, in the NM patient, the wheelbarrowing test with the head in neutral position will reveal greater abnormalities than the same test performed with the head in extension. This is because with the head in extension, the dog receives support and is therefore more able to counteract the weakness. The opposite occurs in dogs with lesions of the proprioceptive pathways: extending their head removes the contribution of vision, which normally causes greater difficulty in performing the test.

Video 7.1

Fourteen-year-old female spayed Galgo mix in lateral recumbency due to extreme weakness. When supported, note the generalized hypotonia, the almost complete absence of voluntary movement in the four limbs, and the hypotrophy of the appendicular muscles. The clinical diagnosis was acute canine polyradiculoneuritis.

Video 7.2

Gait examination of a 6-year-old female Golden Retriever. The gait, almost normal at the beginning of the examination, deteriorates progressively, with more pronounced weakness in the pelvic limbs. Note the progressive short-strided gait, hyperflexion of the joints, dragging of the toes, inability to bear weight on the pelvic limbs, and the need to sit and rest. Postural reactions were normal, and spinal reflexes were uniformly decreased. A nerve biopsy showed that the dog was affected by chronic inflammatory demyelinating polyneuropathy.

Spinal reflexes

Examination of the spinal reflexes may show different results depending on whether the disease is a poly(radiculo)neuropathy, a generalized NM junction disorder, or a generalized muscle disease. Spinal reflexes are uniformly decreased mainly in poly(radiculo)neuropathies (Video 7.3). In the other two forms of the condition, spinal reflexes are usually preserved, although there are some important exceptions to this.

Cranial nerves

Cranial nerve dysfunction may occur in the NM patient.

Poly(radiculo)neuropathies may involve cranial nerve dysfunction in addition to spinal nerve dysfunction.

Some patients, due to involvement of the vagus nerve (cranial nerve [CN] X) may present with voice changes, dysphonia, inspiratory stridor, and dyspnea associated with laryngeal paralysis. Acquired myasthenia gravis is often associated with a reduced palpebral reflex and lip tone (due to the involvement of the facial nerve –CN VII) (Video 7.4), and there may be regurgitation due to the presence of a megaesophagus.

Muscular tone and trophism

In general, NM patients present with varying degrees of muscle hypotonia and hypotrophy. Neuropathic disorders that primarily affect axonal integrity are characterized by a reduction in both muscle tone and muscle trophism. However, if the polyneuropathy is the result of the demyelination process alone, muscle trophism may be almost normal. Generalized myasthenia gravis, with the exception of its fulminant form, is characterized by normal muscle tone and trophism.

Diagnostic approach

Algorithm 7.1 reflects the diagnostic approach to exercise intolerance in dogs. Please refer to chapters 36 and 37 for further information.

Algorithm 7.1 Note 1 Some NM patients may have normal reflexes. In this case, the clinical suspicion of a NM disorder is based on the presence of exercise intolerance (more generally, the presence of paresis) in the absence of ataxia. See Chapter 6 for specific information.

Algorithm 7.1 Note 2 Very few NM diseases have an acute onset, the most important being ACP. ACP predominantly affects the ventral roots of the nerves. The pathophysiology is immune-mediated, and the diagnostic process is often frustrating as blood results are normal and electrodiagnostic tests and muscle and nerve biopsies only show generic signs of abnormality. The disease has a spontaneous benign course and requires symptomatic treatment, including physiotherapy and general care. Less common acute-onset NM disorders include acute fulminant myasthenia gravis, botulism, and tick paralysis (see Chapters 36 and 37).

Algorithm 7.1 Note 3 Electrodiagnostic tests (electromyography, nerve conduction velocity, repetitive nerve stimulation) are useful for confirming the localization, determining the most affected areas, and differentiating between primary myopathy and neuropathy. Unfortunately, electrodiagnostic tests are rarely able to provide an etiological diagnosis.

Muscle and nerve biopsies are useful to confirm the diagnosis, although, as with electrodiagnostic studies, they rarely help to clarify the etiology. This is especially true for neuropathies because the manifestations of nerve pathology are basically limited to axonopathy and demyelination, even in very different neuropathic diseases. Muscle biopsy may be more accurate in differentiating primary myopathies. Because of its specificity, it is important to emphasize the need to send samples to qualified laboratories (see Chapters 36 and 37).

Algorithm 7.1 Note 4 The neostigmine test is rapid and safe and can be used to support the suspicion of acquired myasthenia gravis. A positive test shows a dramatic reversal of the clinical signs a few minutes after administration of the drug (Video 7.5). Unfortunately, the test is neither sensitive nor specific. Confirmation of acquired myasthenia gravis is obtained by a positive result when measuring the concentration of anti-acetylcholine receptor antibodies (see Chapter 36).

Algorithm 7.1 Note 5 Endocrine/metabolic polyneuropathies represent an important group of NM diseases, including diabetic, hypothyroid, and hyperadrenocorticoid neuropathy. The diagnosis is made based on the

Video 7.3

Same dog as in Video 7.1. Spinal reflexes are uniformly decreased/absent. The mental status is normal, even though it could be confused with drowsiness due to the severe weakness.

Video 7.4

Eight-year-old mixed-breed female spayed dog showing multiple cranial nerve deficits. Note the bilaterally decreased palpebral reflex, loss of muscle tone at the lip commissures, and paretic jaw. The video focuses on the cranial nerve examination and does not show the severe exercise intolerance. The dog was affected by generalized acquired myasthenia gravis.

Video 7.5

Same dog as in Video 7.4. The video shows how the exercise intolerance and cranial nerve deficits disappear after the administration of neostigmine (40 μg/kg intramuscularly).

ALGORITHM 7.1

Diagnostic approach to exercise intolerance in dog.

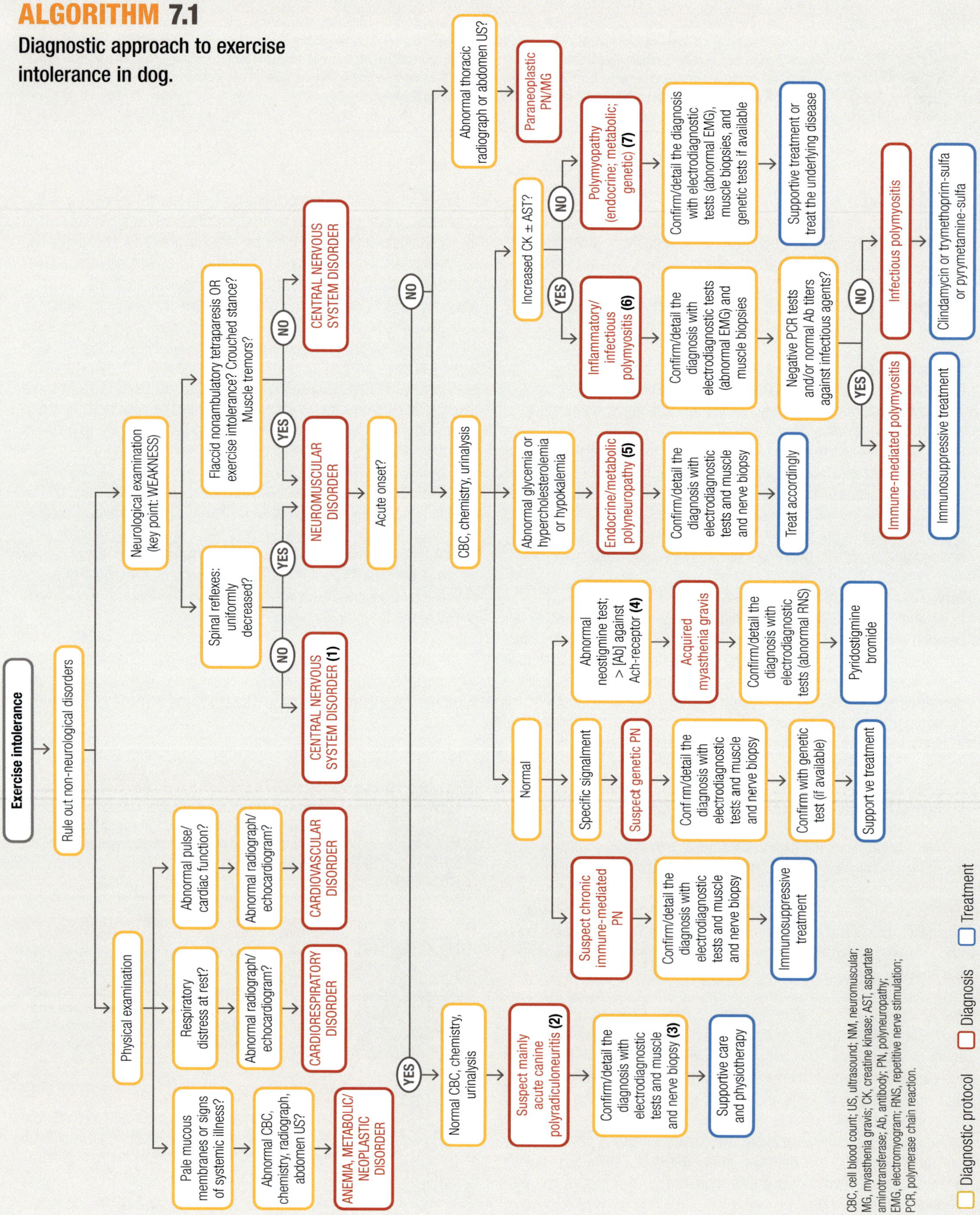

CBC, cell blood count; US, ultrasound; NM, neuromuscular; MG, myasthenia gravis; CK, creatine kinase; AST, aspartate aminotransferase; Ab, antibody; PN, polyneuropathy; EMG, electromyogram; RNS, repetitive nerve stimulation; PCR, polymerase chain reaction.

results of the biochemical profile and specific blood tests. Electrodiagnostic and muscle/nerve biopsies are of little value in establishing the diagnosis as they only show generic signs of nerve/muscle dysfunction (see Chapter 37).

Algorithm 7.1 Note 6 Generalized inflammatory/infectious myopathies are relatively rare in dogs. Polymyositis is an immune-mediated disorder that requires immunosuppressive treatment. Masticatory muscle myositis and extraocular muscle myositis are well-known specific forms of canine immune-mediated myositis. Neosporosis is the most important transmissible disease, causing polymyositis in the dog (see Chapter 36).

Algorithm 7.1 Note 7 Many noninflammatory polymyopathies are degenerative inherited disorders. The most important include, among others: centronuclear myopathy, muscular dystrophy, and myotonia congenita. Metabolic myopathy, characterized by type II fiber atrophy, is a well-documented result of spontaneous or iatrogenic Cushing's syndrome, the latter due to chronic glucocorticoid treatment (see Chapter 36).

References

1. Dewey C, da Costa R (eds.). *Practical Guide to Canine and Feline Neurology*, 3rd ed. Ames, USA: Wiley Blackwell; 2015.
2. Glass EN, Kent M. The clinical examination for neuromuscular disease. *Vet Clin North Am Small Anim Pract.* 2002 Jan;32(1):1–29, v.
3. de Lahunta A, Glass E, Kent M. Lower motor neuron: spinal nerve, general somatic efferent system. In: *de Lahunta's Veterinary Neuroanatomy and Clinical Neurology*, 5th ed. de Lahunta A, Glass E, Kent M (eds). St Louis, USA: Elsevier; 2021, pp. 106–165.

Approach to the neurological patient

Alberta de Stefani
DVM, MRCVS,
PhD, DECVN,
PGDipVetEd, FHEA

Several elements of stress usually surround neurological cases: owners are concerned about their pets' affliction; dogs find themselves in an unfamiliar environment, might be in discomfort, and often mirror their owners' anxiety; and the attending vet might feel uneasy about managing neurological cases. It is, therefore, no surprise the combination of these factors could lead to an unnecessarily unpleasant experience for all parties involved. So, how can we reduce stress and improve the owners' and the dogs' experience as well as our own as veterinarians? Three strategies can be considered: improving communication to make owners better partners in their pets' care, assessing the environment and putting in place small changes that could have a great impact on reducing the stress levels of both owners and dogs, and improving our confidence in the management of neurological cases by familiarizing with a clinical reasoning framework. Note that for the purpose of this chapter, "owners" means the main caregivers and carers of the dog.

Communication

Clear, effective, and compassionate communication is fundamental in developing a strong relationship based on trust and respect between vets and clients. Communication represents a key part of the daily life of vets working in practice, and ample evidence exists to support that effective communication can improve clinical outcomes.[1–3] The owners of neurological patients might feel vulnerable, worried, sad, upset, or frustrated, and our role is to reassure them by acknowledging their concerns and making them feel confident that the problem is in hand. Different communication styles and roles have been identified in human medicine that can be translated into the veterinary consulting room: paternalistic or guardian, consultant or teacher, and shared or collaborator.[1,4] Because the latter communication style is client-centered, it is considered the best way of turning owners into partners in the decision-making process, with a shared goal of maximizing the patient's outcome.[4] The client-centered approach, also known as relationship-centered communication style, aims at building a strong connection between the client and the veterinarian to achieve a wide range of benefits, such as the improvement of the patient's outcomes, the client's satisfaction levels, and the vet's career satisfaction. Building a strong owner–vet relationship can be critical when managing neurological patients. Think of the enormous financial, emotional, and physical commitment we ask owners to adhere to when we offer spinal surgery as a treatment option or when we discuss referral to a different veterinary center. Think of the life-long commitment owners are asked to make when managing a dog with idiopathic epilepsy, the cost of the medications, the emotional burden of caring for an epileptic dog, or the lifestyle changes that this implies. This is without mentioning the challenges of breaking bad news and making end-of-life decisions. To best manage neurological patients, we need to optimize communication and create a strong connection with our clients.

The **relationship-centered communication style** is based on the following principles: engagement, empathy, education, and enlistment (also known as the 4-E model), first introduced by Keller and Carroll in human medicine in 1994.[1,5]

- In the **engagement** phase, the vet creates a connection with the client. Useful communication tools include greeting the client and introducing oneself and anyone else present in the room. A general open question such as "How are you doing today?" might be useful; however, it may not always be appropriate depending on the circumstances of the visit. Once the initial connection has been made, relationship building must continue while the clinical history is collected. Open-ended questions are usually preferable (what, when, where, how, etc.), as the client is given the opportunity to present their views and perceptions (they are after all the experts on their pet), and they feel their concerns are acknowledged. In this phase, **reflective listening** works very well. Reflective listening is the skill of summarizing or paraphrasing what the owners have just told us; this reassures them that they are actively being listened to and their concerns are acknowledged and allows us to check the information is correct while providing an opportunity for the owners to expand, clarify, or rectify any misunderstanding. Understanding their expectations is a critical step in any consultation. This is the time when the vet and owners need to come to an agreement regarding what is achievable so they can develop a shared agenda.

- **Empathy** is the skill that allows us to understand and share the feelings another person is experiencing. During a consultation, acknowledging the owners' feelings allows a rapport to be built and the consultation to move in the right direction. Carson states that "clinical experience shows that until people are allowed to express their emotions, they are usually not ready to take steps toward solving their (or their animals') problems."[6] Demonstrating empathy can take different forms; this could include verbally acknowledging the emotions the owners are feeling with sentences such as "it is totally understandable to be worried about this" or more impersonal statements such as "most people in your situation would be worried about this." However, empathy can also be expressed by respecting the owners' silence while they are composing themselves if they feel overwhelmed by emotions. The vet will have to make the call according to the situation.
- **Education**. There is a point in the consultation when the vet provides relevant medical information, lays out options and opinions, and makes recommendations. The language used is titrated to the degree of medical knowledge of the interlocutor, and jargon is to be avoided if the owners have no medical background. It is critical at this point that the owners reach full understanding of the condition and of the plan of action. The use of open-ended questions (e.g., "How does this sound?"), again, can be invaluable to understand the level of the owners' engagement. Expressing empathy at this stage is essential. Different communication models have been reported to support medical staff in embracing difficult conversations, and it might be a good idea to familiarize with some of them. A useful model is the SPIKES (Setting, Perception, Invitation, Knowledge, Empathy, Summary/Strategy) protocol. This is a six-step communication model that provides a structured approach to delivering difficult news.[7,8]
- **Enlistment** is the principle by which owners become partners in the decision-making process. Shared decision making is the process through which clinicians and owners jointly participate in making a treatment decision after discussing the options, benefits, and harms and considering the pet owner's values, preferences, and circumstances.[9] Shared decision making promotes compliance and adherence (i.e., where the owner demonstrates long-term responsibility for the treatment).[10] For the partnership to work, there has to be mutual trust and respect, and it is critical at this stage to ensure the owners have a clear understanding of the problem and believe in us and our "diagnosis".

TABLE 8.1 SPIKES protocol as a communication model to break "bad news".

SPIKES	
Setting up	This stage involves getting the setting right, preparing what to say and how to say it, becoming mindful of the body language (ours and the owners'), and creating rapport, physical spaces to induce collaboration, and a private space to deliver the news.
Perception	It is crucial to assess the owners' perception of what is happening, while demonstrating empathy throughout, and to determine their level of understanding regarding the problem and their desire to receive more information regarding the condition.
Invitation	After establishing the owners' understanding of the condition, permission can be asked to disclose further details and clarifications regarding the problem in hand.
Knowledge	It is best to deliver "bad news" in stages using verbal and nonverbal cues to help us communicating effectively. It is also important to deliver the news in small chunks and check all along that the owners are following the explanation and coping emotionally (a method called "chunk and check"). Using visual aids (e.g., plastic models, diagnostic images, etc.) can be helpful but only after checking the owners are OK with it. Jargon should be avoided to prevent confusion.
Emotions	Receiving "bad news" can cause a wide range of emotions. It is important to allow the owners to express their emotions by acknowledging and validating their feelings. Empathy is at the core of communication.
Strategy	In this stage, it is important to provide a summary of what has been discussed and make a plan that acknowledges the owners' desires, the pet's needs and welfare, and our professional opinion as veterinarians.

During our communication with the owners, it is also important to pay attention to body language, always ensuring verbal and nonverbal communications are aligned. About 80% of all communication between individuals is nonverbal and generally involuntary.[6] Paying attention to nonverbal cues can help veterinarians to identify the clients' emotional state, for example, if they are comfortable, frightened, or confused. This, however, can work both ways, and clients can read our body language to develop their impressions regarding our confidence, trustworthiness, and reliability. Learning to read, and to some extent, to control nonverbal cues is important to improve communication.

Four sets of nonverbal cues have been identified: kinesics, proxemics, paralanguage, and autonomic shift. Kinesics refers to the ways our body moves, its position, the level of tension in our muscles, and our specific movements or gestures. Proxemics refers to how the space that the vet, client, and dog share during the consultation is organized. Factors such as vertical height differences, the angle of facing while talking, physical barriers (e.g., a table or the animal itself), and interpersonal distance can all affect and reflect the emotional state of the parties involved. Paralanguage includes volume, tone, pitch, intonation of the voice as well as pauses and emphasis while we are communicating our message. Lastly, autonomic shifts are those changes that are under the control of the autonomic nervous system; these may include changes in face color, palms sweating, or changes in breathing pattern. These are usually associated with strong emotions.

Basic behavioral patterns such as the feeling of safety or fight or flight mode will cause changes in our body language.[6] A client or a veterinarian who feels relaxed will have little body tension, perform gestures of openness, and talk in a warm tone of voice, while a client in a fight mode will show tension in their facial and body muscles and might lean forward in an attack posture or create a vertical height difference by standing. The pitch and volume of their voice may be altered, and autonomic shifts such as flushes or sweating may become apparent. A client in flight mode might appear disengaged and show signs of closeness by folding arms or leaning away from the interlocutor; their body might be tense; and they might create a physical barrier between them and the vet by using their pet or folding their arms or legs. Learning to read and becoming aware of these body language cues can help us understand if the consultation is going the way we intended and, if not, implement changes before it is too late. It is important to remember that if we become aware of nonverbal cues, we can use them to our advantage to create a relaxed and safe environment that will establish a productive, collaborative atmosphere. Few small changes can make a huge difference: become mindful of how you greet and welcome owners into the consult room (smile, relaxed facial expression), create a safe interpersonal distance, assess angles of facing to create a collaborative environment (best to avoid direct/confrontational angles), and consider vertical height differences and how they might influence the owners' basic behavior. Creating a safe environment and demonstrating empathy with verbal and nonverbal cues is essential to establishing rapport with the owners. This is a fundamental step in building a strong and productive relationship with our clients.[1,6,11]

Managing the environment

Reducing the stress associated with vet visits in dogs and their owners might be a challenge. However, measures can be put in place to try to minimize anxiety and improve both the dogs' and the owners' experience. While the benefits of effective communication are immense, attention should also be paid to the environment at the veterinary practice in relation to three key parts of the client's visit: the arrival at the practice, the wait in the waiting room, and the consultation.

Arrival at the practice

Because some neurological patients might have mobility or balance issues and cannot walk very far (or at all), easy access to a nearby parking space as well to the clinic (no steps, a ramp, and wide automatic doors) can be very helpful to make the arrival at the practice as stress free as possible.

In the waiting room

A welcoming atmosphere in the reception area and an easy check-in process are also important elements. While delays are inevitable, creating a safe environment for both the dogs and their owners in the waiting room can make waiting less daunting. Nonslippery floors can be useful, particularly for patients with mobility or balance issues. The presence of soft beds at the reception for dogs to use while waiting for an appointment might be well received by the clients and their pets. Reducing the level of noise in the reception area, arranging the waiting area to minimize dog-to-dog interactions, and ideally avoiding interspecies interactions (for example, with cats or exotics) can reduce the dogs' anxiety or excitement. Easy access to water for clients and their dogs, and access to educational leaflets to read or videos to watch on large screens while waiting could make the experience more pleasant. A small area for young children to be entertained could also be a useful addition. On arrival, having a triage system in place for neuro-emergency appointments can also be of great benefit. This not only allows the vets to make a quick assessment of the severity of the condition but also reassures the owners that their dog is given prompt attention. An early assessment also allows us to determine the dog's and the owners' stress levels and to take appropriate action. An example could be a brachycephalic dog showing signs of a brachycephalic obstructive airway syndrome crisis or an overwhelmed owner needing a private space to recompose.

In the consult room

Welcoming the owners and their dogs into a clean and tidy consult room sets the right scene. Nonslippery floors are preferable, and the dog should be given the opportunity to explore and familiarize with

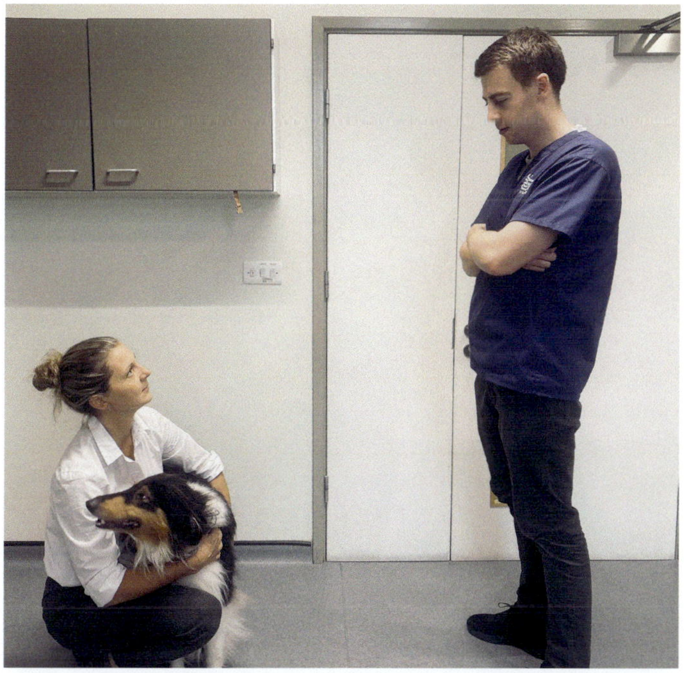

FIG. 8.1 The vertical height difference creates a hierarchical imbalance with the vet imposing physically and emotionally on the client and the pet. The body language is tense and so are the facial features. The client feels intimidated, and the dog is used to create a physical barrier between client and vet. The dog also looks uneasy, with its head turned away from the vet.

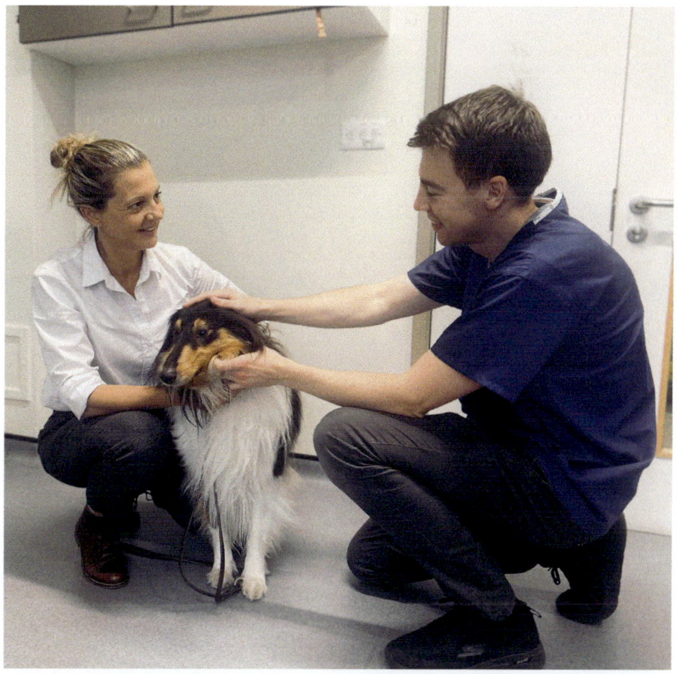

FIG. 8.2 The interaction shown in this picture indicates a collaborative atmosphere. The body language is relaxed, and the client appears engaged in the conversation. Both the client and the vet are touching the dog, which in this case becomes a point of physical and emotional connection. There is symmetry of body expression, with both parties smiling. Even the dog seems to be more relaxed.

the environment before any vet interaction begins. The Dog Friendly Clinic Scheme is a collaborative project between Dogs Trust and the British Veterinary Behaviour Association that aims to provide extensive and detailed advice and guidance on how to improve the experience during vet visits for all parties involved. More information can be found on their website (https://www.dogstrust.org.uk/how-we-help/professionals/vet-clinics).

Clinical reasoning framework

From the veterinarian's perspective, approaching a neurological case can feel overwhelming. We might believe our knowledge and understanding of neurology and neurosciences is not good enough to achieve a neurolocalization, and even if we manage to neurolocalize the lesion, then the list of differentials is way too long to be remembered in full. These, among other factors, can contribute to a sense of discomfort when approaching neurological cases, a phenomenon known as "neurophobia", the fear of clinical neurology and neurosciences.[12]

Thus, which tactics can we put in place in order to not only safely manage neurological patients but also enjoy the process and improve the patients' outcome, our job satisfaction, and ultimately our well-being? A few strategies can be considered, the first being "work smarter, not harder". Being organized and prepared can save lots of stress. For example, condition-specific history taking sheets can allow us to focus on the answers without worrying about remembering what we want to ask. Owners can also be asked to fill in specific questionnaires while waiting for the appointment; this will provide the vet with a wealth of information. Another transformative strategy is to develop a structured and logical approach to neurological cases, in other words, to familiarize with a clinical reasoning framework. Clinical reasoning is a problem-based, systematic approach to clinical cases that provides the clinician with a set path and a framework through which clinical information can be acquired, stored, and analyzed. At the end of the process, a ranked list of differential diagnoses can be reached without the need to overload our memory.[13]

Clinical reasoning also allows the integration of clinical information with our existing knowledge and experience, helping us to create a mental algorithm that, in turn, enables us to produce a sound diagnostic plan or elect an empirical treatment.

Clinical reasoning can take different forms. One well-established structure involves the following four steps: define and refine the problem; define and refine the system; define the location within the system (where appropriate); and define the lesion. However, in recent years, a combination of clinical variables has been studied to assess neurological patients and has resulted in the development of the "five-finger rule" clinical reasoning framework.[14–16] The starting point in this framework is the patient's signalment (represented by the palm of the hand) followed by:

1. Onset of the clinical signs
2. Progression of the clinical signs
3. Presence or absence of pain
4. Presence or absence of lateralization in the clinical signs
5. Neurolocalization

The combination of these clinical variables can help us to develop algorithms, which in turn will enable us to create a sensible and prioritized list of differential diagnoses. One key element is that any form of clinical reasoning must be seen as a cyclical process. Clinical reasoning must be applied and reapplied in light of new clinical information for it to support the development of an accurate list of differentials.

General questions to guide history taking in neurological patients

- What is your main concern with *(name of the pet)*?
- When is the first time you noticed something was not right?
- When is the last time *(name of the pet)* was his/her normal self?
- Have you notice any changes in personality/behavior? If so when is *(name of the pet)* displaying this unusual behavior? All the time, episodically, or after specific tasks (e.g., walks, sleep, eating)?
- How do you think *(name of the pet)* is doing now? Better, worse, the same?
- Has this ever happened before?
- Do you think *(name of the pet)* is in pain?
- Does *(name of the pet)* have any ongoing medical problems?
- Is *(name of the pet)* taking any medications?
- Any previous surgeries?
- Has *(name of the pet)* ever been involved in an accident (hit by a car, fall from a height)?
- Has *(name of the pet)* ever travelled abroad?
- Is *(name of the pet)* up to date with vaccination and parasite prevention?
- Has *(name of the pet)* been with you since he/she was a puppy? If rescued, ask about previous history.

Questions to guide history taking for patients presenting with suspected spinal problems/gait abnormalities

- What is your main concern with *(name of the pet)*?
- When is the first time you noticed something was not right?
- What did you notice first?
- When is the last time *(name of the pet)* was able to walk independently?
- How do you think *(name of the pet)* is doing now? Better, worse, the same?
- Do you think *(name of the pet)* is in pain?
- Has this ever happened before?
- Any previous trauma (falls, road traffic accident)?
- Has *(name of the pet)* been with you since he/she was a puppy? If rescued, ask about previous history.
- Is *(name of the pet)* showing any signs of incontinence/problems urinating/defecating? When is the last time you observed *(name of the pet)* urinating a large volume?
- Has *(name of the pet)* had any previous surgeries?
- Does *(name of the pet)* have any ongoing medical problems?
- Is *(name of the pet)* taking any medications?

KEY POINTS

- Clear, effective, and compassionate communication can improve the clinical outcome and is a key step in developing a strong relationship, based on trust and respect, between vets and clients.

References

1. Cornell KK, Kopcha M. Client-veterinarian communication: skills for client centered dialogue and shared decision making. *Vet Clin North Am Small Anim Pract.* 2007 Jan;37(1):37–47.
2. Frankel RM. Pets, vets, and frets: what relationship-centered care research has to offer veterinary medicine. *J Vet Med Educ.* 2006 Spring;33(1):20–27.
3. Adams CL, Frankel RM. It may be a dog's life but the relationship with her owners is also key to her health and well being: communication in veterinary medicine. *Vet Clin North Am Small Anim Pract.* 2007 Jan;37(1):1–17.
4. Charles C, Gafni A, Whelan T. Decision-making in the physician-patient encounter: revisiting the shared treatment decision-making model. *Soc Sci Med.* 1999 Sep;49(5):651–661.
5. Keller VF, Carroll JG. A new model for physician-patient communication. *Patient Educ Couns.* 1994 Jun;23(2):131–140.
6. Carson CA. Nonverbal communication in veterinary practice. *Vet Clin North Am Small Anim Pract.* 2007 Jan;37(1):49–63.
7. Shaw JR, Lagoni L. End-of-life communication in veterinary medicine: delivering bad news and euthanasia decision making. *Vet Clin North Am Small Anim Pract.* 2007 Jan;37(1):95–108.
8. Rosenzweig MQ. Breaking bad news: a guide for effective and empathetic communication. *Nurse Pract.* 2012 Feb 12;37(2):1–4.
9. Ito Y, Ishikawa H, Suzuki A, Kato M. The relationship between evaluation of shared decision-making by pet owners and veterinarians and satisfaction with veterinary consultations. *BMC Vet Res.* 2022 Aug 2;18(1):296.
10. Abood SK. Increasing adherence in practice: making your clients partners in care. *Vet Clin North Am Small Anim Pract.* 2007 Jan;37(1):151–164.
11. Levinson W, Roter DL, Mullooly JP, et al. Physician-patient communication. The relationship with malpractice claims among primary care physicians and surgeons. *JAMA.* 1997 Feb 19;277(7):553–559.
12. Moreno-Zambrano D, Sandrone S, Meza-Venegas J, et al. Exploring the key factors behind neurophobia: A systematic review of the English, Spanish and Portuguese literature. *Brain Disord.* 2021 Jun;2:100011.
13. Maddison Jill E, Volk Holger A, Church David B. *Clinical Reasoning in Small Animal Practice.* Chichester, UK: Wiley Blackwell; 2015.
14. Cardy TJ, De Decker S, Kenny PJ, Volk HA. Clinical reasoning in canine spinal disease: what combination of clinical information is useful? *Vet Rec.* 2015 Aug 15;177(7):171.
15. Harrison E, Grapes NJ, Volk HA, De Decker S. Clinical reasoning in canine vestibular syndrome: Which presenting factors are important? *Vet Rec.* 2021 Mar;188(6):e61.
16. Armaşu M, Packer RM, Cook S, et al. An exploratory study using a statistical approach as a platform for clinical reasoning in canine epilepsy. *Vet J.* 2014 Nov;202(2):292–296.

CHAPTER 9

Fundamentals of the neurologic examination

Ronaldo Casimiro da Costa
DVM, MSc, PhD,
DACVIM (Neurology)

The neurologic examination is the basis of clinical neurology. Only with a thorough examination can the clinician define the exact clinical problem(s), determine the lesion localization, establish a differential diagnosis list, and design a logical diagnostic plan. Technological advances have made high-field magnetic resonance imaging (MRI) widely available. While this is an extraordinary advance, MRI of the incorrect region is not only poor practice, but also dangerous to the patient and its family, because treatment plans could be designed based on the imaging findings of a wrongly identified problem.

The goals of the neurologic examination are to:

- Confirm that the patient does have a neurologic problem. Orthopedic problems are very common. Unfortunately, many believe that one problem excludes the possibility of others, which could not be farther from the truth. Most middle-aged and older large breed dogs will have concurrent orthopedic and spinal disorders.
- Determine the neurologic findings to localize the lesion(s).
- Establish the severity of the neurologic dysfunction. This is a key point because another common misconception is to assume that neuroimaging findings correlate with neurologic dysfunction, and they typically do not. The extent of neurologic dysfunction should be determined by the neurologic examination.

There are six main components of the neurologic examination: mental status and behavior, gait and posture, cranial nerves, postural reactions, spinal reflexes, and sensory examination (palpation of the spine and, if necessary, assessment of pain perception).[1] The order of each component needs to be respected.

Mentation, behavior, gait, and posture can and should be initially assessed during history taking, ideally with the patient on the floor. Either postural reactions or cranial nerve function can then be assessed (depending on the dog's behavior); this should be followed by evaluation of spinal reflexes, spinal palpation and, only if the patient is plegic (tetra-, para- or monoplegic), pain perception (nociception). Procedures that are more likely to upset the patient should always be performed at the end of the examination. If the clinician upsets the patient early on, it may be difficult to complete the examination. In addition, once pain is elicited, the patient often anticipates further painful stimuli, making it difficult to determine if other procedures are truly painful.

It is essential to pay close attention to all findings and repeat each test as many times as needed to be able to be certain of a neurologic deficit.

Very few tools are required to perform a complete neurologic examination. A nonslippery floor is very important because weak and/or ataxic dogs might refuse to walk on a slippery surface. Acutely "down" dogs often still have motor function in the pelvic limbs, but they may need to be assessed in an open area with a nonslippery floor to observe voluntary movement. A rubber mat is invaluable in evaluating postural reactions. A rubber hammer is used to test myotatic reflexes in most dogs; in small dogs, a hemostat may be helpful. A hemostat is also important when testing the cutaneous trunci (formerly panniculus) reflex as well as pain perception in the limbs. A strong light source is necessary to elicit pupillary light reflexes in excited dogs. A cotton-tipped applicator or a piece of cotton to cover a hemostat is useful to evaluate the nasal sensation.

Definitions of motor deficits

There are significant misunderstandings regarding the definitions of motor deficits. Since proper communication of medical terms is very important for patient care, here are some important definitions:

- Ataxia: loss of coordination. Defined as the inability of the patient to coordinate the position of its head, trunk, and limbs in space.
- Paresis: partial loss of motor function. Paresis should be always defined as ambulatory or nonambulatory.
- Plegia: complete loss of motor function (the same as paralysis). Terms such as "nonambulatory paraplegia" must be avoided, as any paralyzed patient will not be able to walk. "Complete paralysis" is also redundant.
- Tetra-: means involving all four limbs (not legs, quadrupeds do not have legs).
- Para-: involving the pelvic limbs.
- Hemi-: involving the limbs on one side of the body.
- Mono-: involving one limb only.

The most common mistake made by clinicians is to call a dog paraplegic (or paralyzed in the pelvic limbs) when in fact the dog has nonambulatory paraparesis. Although the dog is unable to walk in both cases, nonambulatory paraparesis is dramatically different from paraplegia from a diagnostic and prognostic standpoint. For instance, there is no need to test for pain perception in the limbs of a nonambulatory paraparetic dog due to intervertebral disc extrusion, as the chances of a fast and complete recovery in these patients are high. A true paraplegic dog will have a more severe spinal cord injury, which requires testing for pain perception in the limbs; the absence of pain perception will be associated with a guarded prognosis for recovery of voluntary ambulation.

Performing the neurologic examination

Mental status

Ideally, the dog should be placed on the floor and be allowed to freely explore the examination room. Mental status can be divided into level of consciousness and behavior.

The level of consciousness is primarily a function of the brainstem, and a patient can be classified as follows:

- Alert: The patient responds appropriately to environmental stimuli.
- Obtunded/drowsy: The animal is less reactive to auditory and visual stimuli but arousable.
- Stuporous: The patient is in a profound sleep state, unresponsive to environmental stimuli but responsive to a nociceptive stimulus.
- Comatose: The patient is unconscious and cannot be aroused even with painful stimuli.

Behavior is primarily a function of the forebrain (also known as thalamocortex or prosencephalon). Abnormal behavior is identified by comparing the patient's behavior with the expected behavior for animals of a similar breed and age. The client is usually able to bring subtle behavioral changes to the veterinarian's attention. However, if the owners had never owned a dog before, they may not be able to know what "normal" behavior is, or they may just be used to an abnormal behavior. Therefore, critically assessing the patient's behavior during examination is very important. The most common behavioral changes seen clinically include compulsive behavior, disorientation (inability to contextualize oneself within the environment), and abnormal responses to external stimuli (e.g., exaggerated fear, aggression, and anxiety), the latter due to an inability to adequately process the information from the environment and respond accordingly.

Posture

The ability to maintain a normal posture depends largely on the integrity of the proprioceptive system (general and specific proprioception) and the motor system. Postural changes are mainly due to three categories of problems:

- Antalgic posture
- Mechanical impairments
- True neurological disorders

It is very important to observe the posture of the head, limbs, and trunk during examination. Abnormal head posture is often manifested as a head tilt or a head turn (Fig. 9.1). To ensure that a head tilt is detected, it is important for the clinician to look at the position of the eyes and not the ears, as "ear tilt" can be misleading. Unilateral vestibular dysfunction will often cause head tilt. When an animal develops a head turn, the head is held level, but the nose is turned right or left. Animals with lateralized forebrain lesions may tend to turn their heads and circle in one direction. A head turn is suggestive, but not exclusive of forebrain diseases.[2]

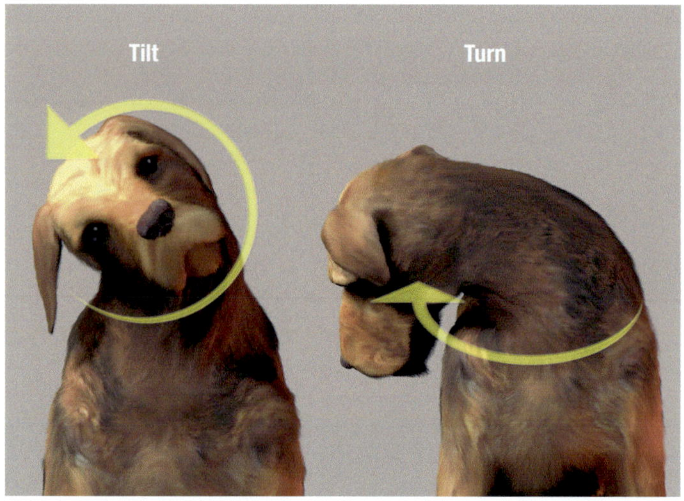

FIG. 9.1 A head tilt posture should be differentiated from head turn. Head tilt (image on the left) typically indicates vestibular disease, whereas head turn (image on the right) suggests a forebrain (thalamocortical) lesion. Exceptions do exist to both situations.

Kyphosis, lordosis, and scoliosis are frequently observed abnormal spinal postures. A kyphotic posture is commonly seen with painful conditions of the thoracolumbar vertebral column (Fig. 9.2). Scoliosis may be seen with congenital malformation and in cases of caudal occipital malformation (Chiari-like syndrome and syringomyelia). Lordosis is infrequently seen and reflects weakness of the epaxial musculature.

A low head carriage (with or without cervical spasms) is also a common posture observed in dogs with painful diseases of the cervical vertebral column (Fig. 9.3). This posture is quite different from that of patients with

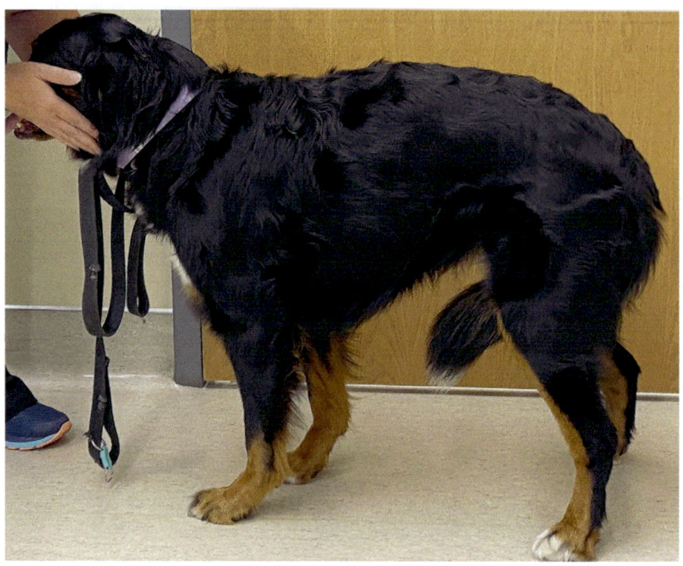

FIG. 9.2 Kyphotic posture in a Bernese Mountain dog with thoracolumbar vertebral column pain.

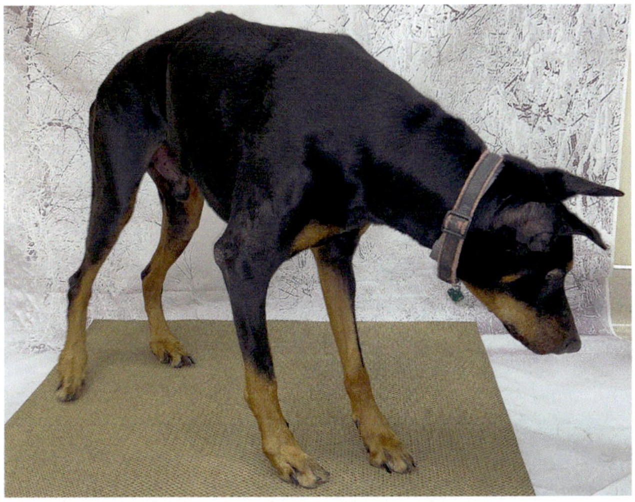

FIG. 9.3 Doberman pinscher dog demonstrating a guarded neck posture indicative of cervical pain.

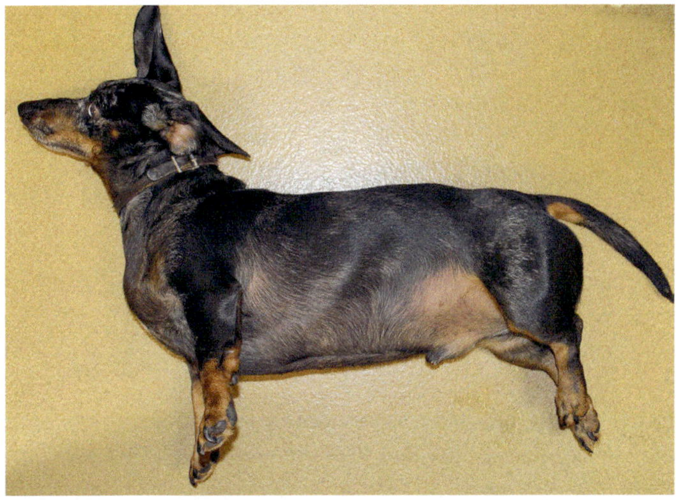

FIG. 9.4 Schiff-Sherrington posture in a Dachshund with thoracolumbar intervertebral extrusion. Note the opisthotonic posture with hyperextension of the cervical spine and thoracic limbs. The dog was paraplegic, with decreased extensor tone and normal patellar and flexor reflexes.

cervical ventroflexion (a posture seen much more commonly in cats). It is typically associated with neuromuscular conditions, but it can also be observed with intramedullary cervical myelopathies (e.g., myelitis, ischemic myelopathies) leading to lower motor neuron signs in the cervical region. Schiff–Sherrington posture is commonly observed with severe spinal cord injuries between the T2 and L5 spinal cord regions. It is characterized by extension of the cervical region and thoracic limbs (best appreciated in lateral recumbency) with paralysis of the pelvic limbs (Fig. 9.4). Importantly, this posture does not have prognostic significance. Patients in lateral recumbency may also adopt two pathological postures:

- Decerebrate rigidity: This posture is due to a brainstem lesion and is characterized by extension of all limbs and sometimes opisthotonus (dorsiflexion of the head and neck). A decreased level of consciousness (often stupor or coma) usually accompanies this posture (Fig. 9.5).
- Decerebellate rigidity: This posture is due to an acute cerebellar lesion and is characterized by opisthotonus, thoracic limb extension, and flexion of the hips. Consciousness is not impaired due to the lack of brainstem involvement.

Plantigrade and palmigrade postures are abnormal postures of the pelvic and thoracic limbs, respectively. They are frequently seen in cases of neuromuscular diseases, primarily polyneuropathies, but can also be seen in patients with musculoskeletal diseases.

Gait

Gait examination along with assessment of mental status are the most important components of the neurologic examination.

The best way to evaluate the gait is by allowing the patient to walk freely in the examination room. This not only enables gait assessment, but also the observation abnormal behaviors, such as circling or even head pressing. While this is ideal, it may not be practical depending on the type and size of the exam room. Thus, leading the patient to walk at a normal pace in hallways is the norm. Contrary to what is typically done for an orthopedic examination, walking the dog at a faster pace does not help to reveal gait abnormalities; it actually tends to mask mild changes. Thus, the dog should be walked at a normal pace or slower, not faster. The gait can be assessed from different angles (front, back, sideways), paying increasing attention to the thoracic limbs, pelvic limbs, or those in one side of the body. Posture can and should be assessed during gait examination. In animals that are very reluctant to walk on the hospital's or clinic's floors, bringing them outside and enticing them to walk on a concrete floor or grass might make them show much more voluntary movement than when observed indoors. The author has seen many cases of dogs referred as paraplegic that showed robust voluntary movement of their pelvic limbs when gait evaluation was repeated outside the hospital. Food can also occasionally be used to entice dogs to get up and walk.

The gait examination should take several minutes, i.e., enough time to see progressive weakness in dogs with lower motor neuron disease, such as myasthenia.

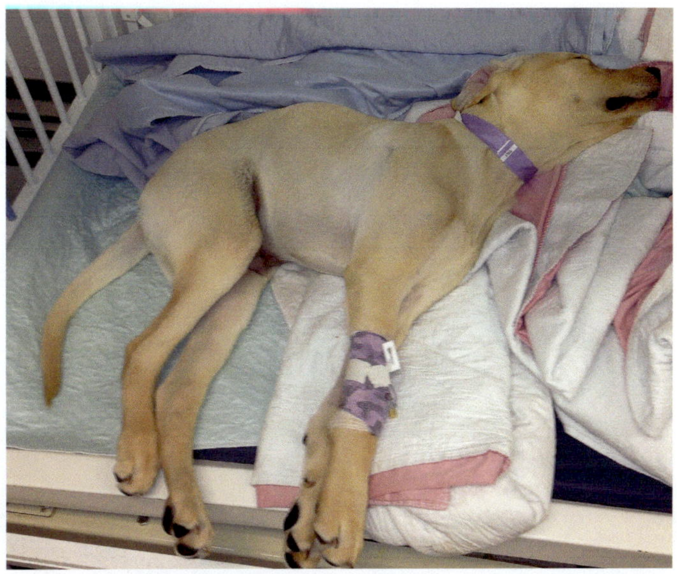

FIG. 9.5 Labrador retriever puppy showing a decerebrate posture with hyperextension of all the four limbs and cervical spine.

Considering the importance of the gait examination, a methodic approach helps to interpret all gait changes appropriately.[3] A useful approach is to start by answering these questions:

- Is the animal able to walk?
- Is the gait normal or abnormal?
- If abnormal, which limb(s) are affected?
- What is the gait problem? Incoordination (ataxia), weakness (paresis or paralysis), or lameness?

All these gait changes are covered in detail in Chapter 6; the reader is invited to refer to that chapter for further information.

Postural reactions

Testing postural reactions is very useful to detect subtle neurologic deficits. They are very sensitive, but not specific to localize lesions, as they test the entire central and peripheral nervous systems. They are also useful in discriminating between orthopedic and neurologic disorders. Often, only two postural reaction tests are needed: proprioceptive positioning (also known as paw placement) and hopping (Video 9.1).

Video 9.1

Examination of postural reactions.

Proprioceptive positioning test

Overall, the proprioceptive positioning test would be the most sensitive and reliable postural reaction test; however, proper patient support is key for reliable results. This can be very challenging in giant breed dogs. Testing over a nonslippery floor also helps. Weight should ideally be evenly distributed in the other limbs. The test is performed by gently turning one paw over so that the dorsal surface is in contact with the ground (it should not be pressed against the ground). The patient should immediately return the foot to a normal position (Fig. 9.6). When properly supported, most patients with orthopedic disease will have normal proprioceptive positioning.

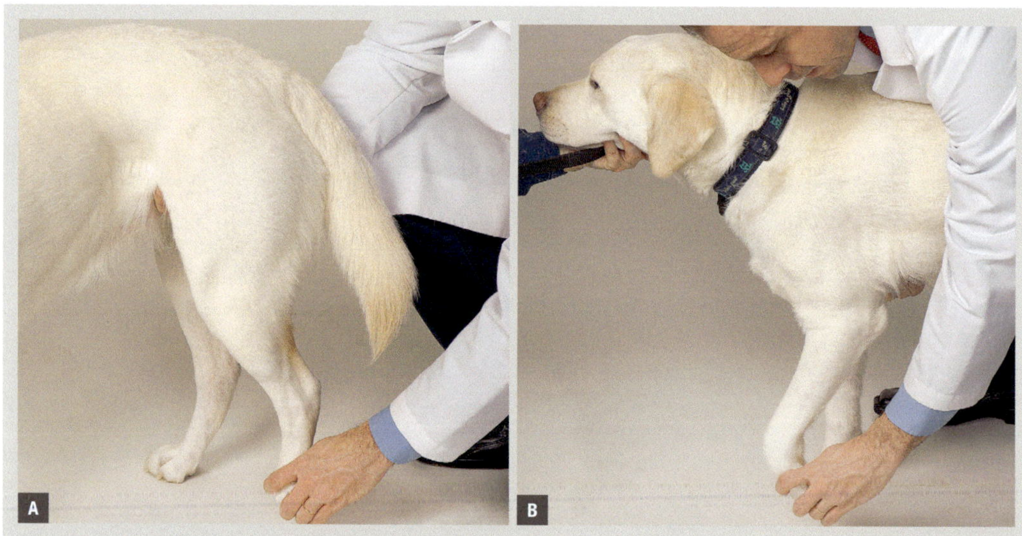

FIG. 9.6 Proprioceptive positioning is evaluated with the patient supported in a standing position in the pelvic (**A**) and thoracic limbs (**B**). Proper support of the patient is essential. The dorsal surface of the paw is placed on the floor without pushing it down. The patient should immediately replace the paw to a normal position.

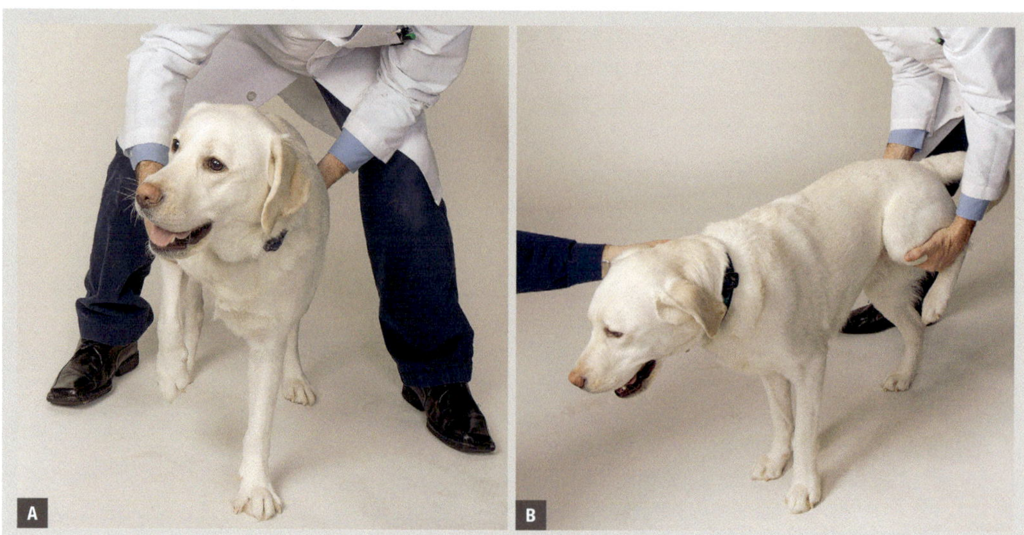

FIG. 9.7 The hopping response in large dogs can be tested by just lifting the contralateral limb and moving the patient laterally to test the thoracic limb (**A**) and pelvic limb (**B**). In small dogs it is preferred to lift 3 limbs off ground to test just the selected limb. It is unnecessary to try to hop medially or cranially.

Hopping test
Performing the hopping test on a nonslippery surface is also helpful. The patient should be held so that its weight is supported by one limb and moved laterally (Fig. 9.7). Normal animals will hop on the limb while keeping the foot under their body for support. Each limb is tested individually, and responses on the left and right are compared. This is a sensitive test for subtle weakness or asymmetry.

Placing response
The placing response test is mostly useful in cats but can also be used in small dogs, although it is not as reliable as proprioceptive positioning. It is performed by making sure the patient's eyes are covered, picking the animal up, and moving it gently towards the edge of a table. When the paw touches the table, the animal should immediately place the limb forward to rest the paw on the table surface. Do not let the patient see the table because then it becomes a visual placing test, which does not assess the proprioceptive pathways.

Wheelbarrowing, extensor postural thrust test, and hemiwalking
Wheelbarrowing, extensor postural thrust, and hemiwalking can be performed if other postural reactions are equivocal.

Wheelbarrowing in the thoracic limbs is done by supporting the patient under its abdomen so that the pelvic limbs do not touch the ground and moving the patient forward. Normal animals will walk with symmetrical, alternate movements of the thoracic limbs.

Extensor postural thrust is tested by lifting the patient by the thorax and lowering the pelvic limbs to reach the floor. When the patient reaches the ground, it is normal to observe a reflex of hyperextension of the pelvic limbs. The animal is then gently moved backwards. Normal patients will feel that their center of gravity is moving caudally, and they will move their pelvic limbs in the same direction to maintain their balance.

Hemiwalking involves lifting the limbs on one side of the body and moving the patient laterally (similar to the technique shown in Figure 9.7. The normal reaction is as described for the hopping response.

Cranial nerves

Mammals have 12 cranial nerves. Not all are routinely tested. Hand-on examination involves testing cranial nerves II through VIII (optic to vestibulocochlear nerves). The preferred order can vary; the author follows the order described below (with the corresponding cranial nerves tested):

- Menace response – optic nerve (sensory), facial nerve (motor), forebrain and cerebellum also involved (Fig. 9.8).
- Eye position – vestibulocochlear nerve (sensory); oculomotor, trochlear, and abducens nerves (motor).
- Size and symmetry of pupils – optic nerve (sensory), oculomotor nerve (parasympathetic).

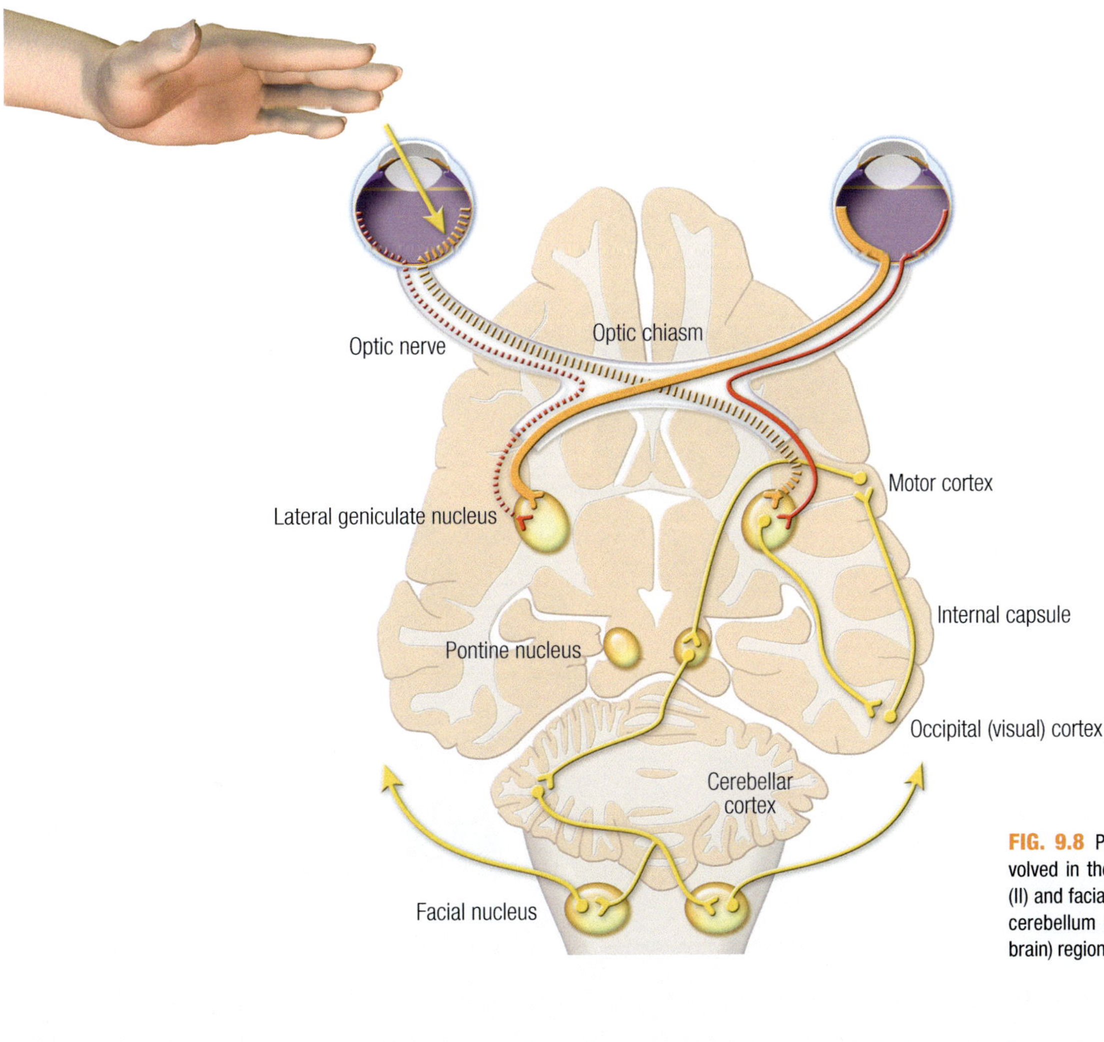

FIG. 9.8 Pathways and structures involved in the menace response – optic (II) and facial (VII) nerves, as well as the cerebellum and thalamocortical (forebrain) regions.

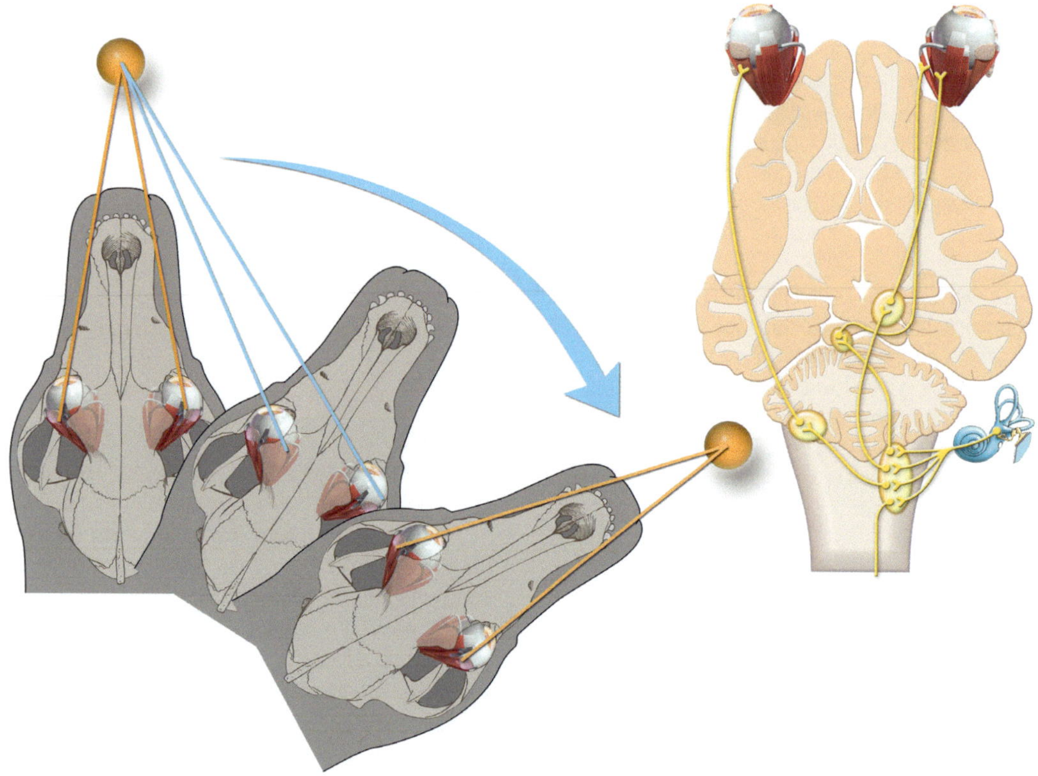

FIG. 9.9 Pathways and structures involved in the oculocephalic reflex or vestibulo-ocular reflex. This test evaluates cranial nerves VIII (sensory) and III, IV, and VI (motor).

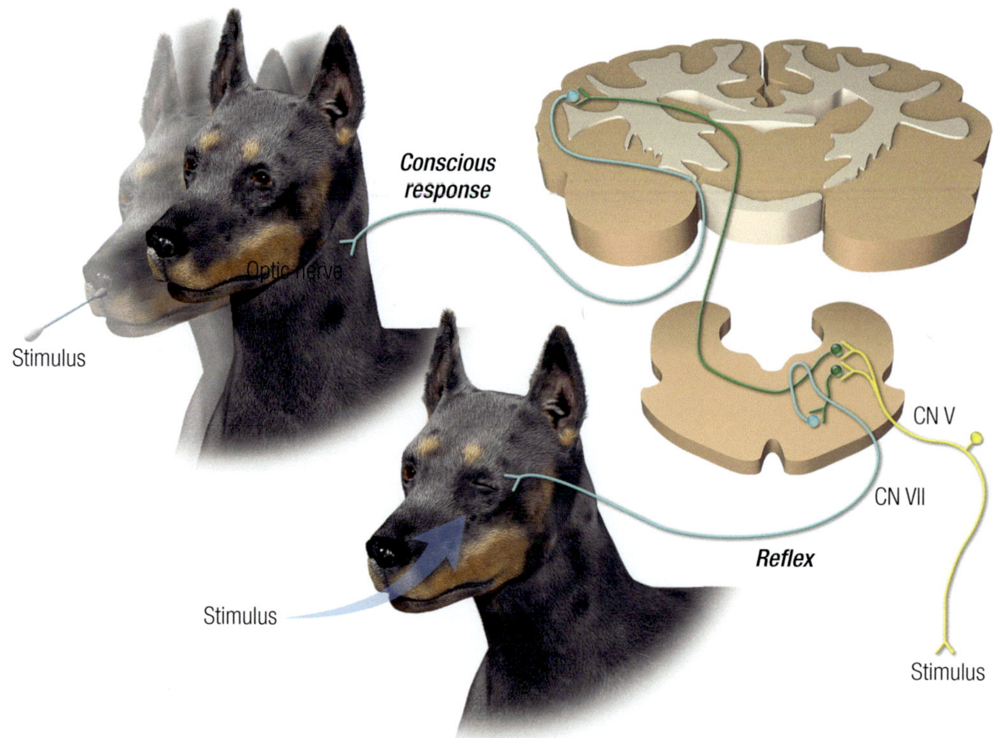

FIG. 9.10 Pathways and structures involved in the nasal sensation testing showing how the cortical response is triggered.

- Pupillary light reflex – optic nerve (sensory), oculomotor nerve (parasympathetic).
- Vestibulo-ocular (oculocephalic) reflex – vestibulocochlear nerve (sensory), oculomotor, trochlear, and abducens nerves (motor) (Fig. 9.9).
- Palpebral reflex – trigeminal nerve (sensory), facial nerve (motor).
- Nasal sensation – trigeminal nerve (sensory), brainstem and forebrain (Fig. 9.10).
- Size and symmetry of muscles of mastication – trigeminal nerve (motor – mandibular branch).
- Facial symmetry – facial nerve.
- Head position – vestibulocochlear nerve.

Proper technique is essential to achieve reliable results; to aid readers in this regard, critical components to perform and interpret the tests are outlined below (Video 9.2).

It is important to remember that the menace response test elicits a conscious response and not a reflex. To evaluate the menace response, move your hand toward the patient's eyes in a threatening manner and observe for a blink response; it does not need to be a complete blink (Fig. 9.11). Make sure you test the ability to blink before menacing the patient. The menacing hand should stop about 30 cm away from the patient's face. This would avoid generating air currents that would stimulate the ophthalmic branch of the trigeminal nerve and cause false positive results. By covering the contralateral eye, you can test the nasal (medial) and temporal (lateral) visual fields of each eye. The menace response may be deficient in puppies and kittens (less than 12 weeks old) due to cerebellar immaturity and the possibility that they have not yet learned the threatening meaning of this stimulus. Consider that normal animals may also display a lack of menace response. This test is one of the most important parts of the neurological examination to evaluate the forebrain.

Video 9.2

Cranial nerve examination.

Observe the eye position, note if strabismus is present and the direction (lateral, ventral, dorsal, medial). Elevating the head to see if it elicits positional strabismus (typically ventral strabismus); its presence is a consistent sign of vestibular dysfunction (Fig. 9.12). Nystagmus can also be observed and should be classified as spontaneous or induced (by elevating the head, for example). The direction (horizontal, rotary, vertical) of nystagmus should also be recorded.

Note the size of the pupils and any difference in pupil size between one eye and other (anisocoria) before actually testing the pupillary light reflex (Fig. 9.13). Bring the light source as close as possible to achieve better miosis before quickly switching the light to the opposite side to see if a consensual reflex is present (Fig. 9.14). Repeat the procedure in the opposite eye.

The oculocephalic or vestibulo-ocular reflex (also known as physiologic nystagmus) is elicited by moving the patient's head side to side and up and down. Normal physiologic nystagmus has a fast phase in the direction of head movement (Fig. 9.15).

The palpebral reflex can be assessed by testing all three branches of the trigeminal nerve. Touching the medial and lateral canthus of the eye tests the ophthalmic and maxillary branches, respectively (Fig. 9.16). The mandibular branch can be tested by touching the base of the ear; this is the least reliable of the three branches. The sensory part of the palpebral reflex is mediated by the trigeminal nerve, and the motor response (blinking) is mediated by the facial nerve.

The temporalis and masseter muscles should be examined and palpated to detect any swelling, atrophy, or asymmetry (Fig. 9.17). If there is severe bilateral weakness, the patient may not be able to close the mouth.

Evaluation of nasal sensation can assess the ophthalmic branch of the trigeminal nerve if the stimulus is directed towards the nasal septum, or the maxillary branch if the stimulus is directed towards the external parts of the nostril. To be able to detect subtle deficits, it may be better to use a cotton-tipped instrument to evaluate the response (Fig. 9.18). This test is performed to assess the conscious cortical response (in the contralateral side of the nostril being stimulated) with withdrawal of the head. The degree of response is variable among animals, so it is important to alternate testing sides to compare the response of the right and left sides.

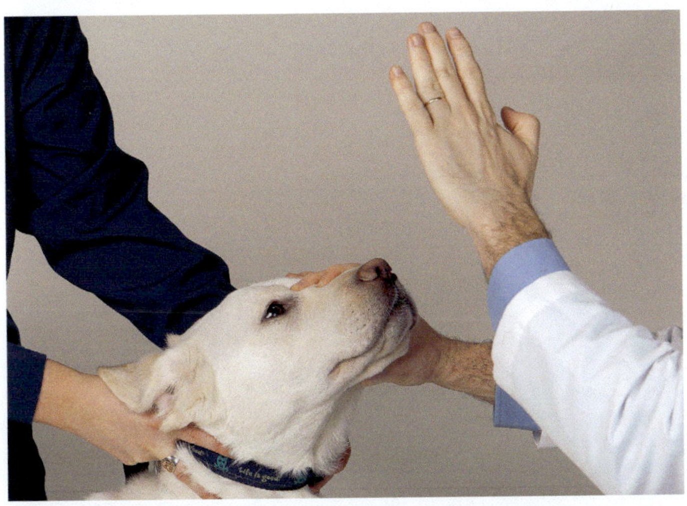

FIG. 9.11 The menace response is elicited by making a threatening gesture at the eye, which should induce a blink. Be careful not to get too close to the eye.

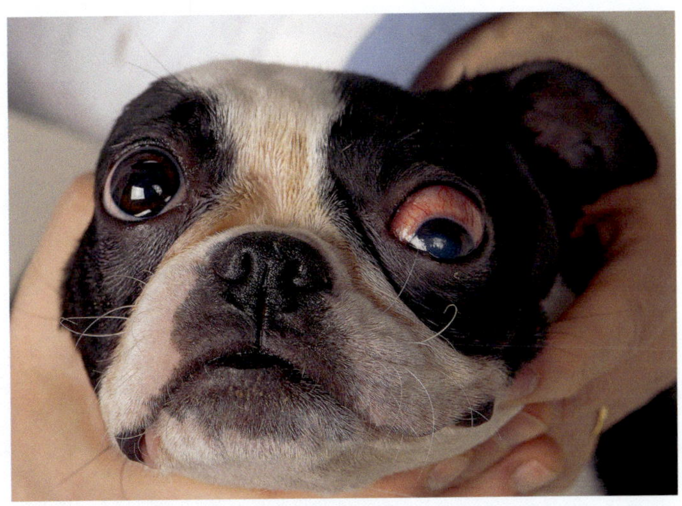

FIG. 9.12 Positional strabismus of the left eye in a dog with vestibular dysfunction. The ventral strabismus is ipsilateral to the side of the head tilt.

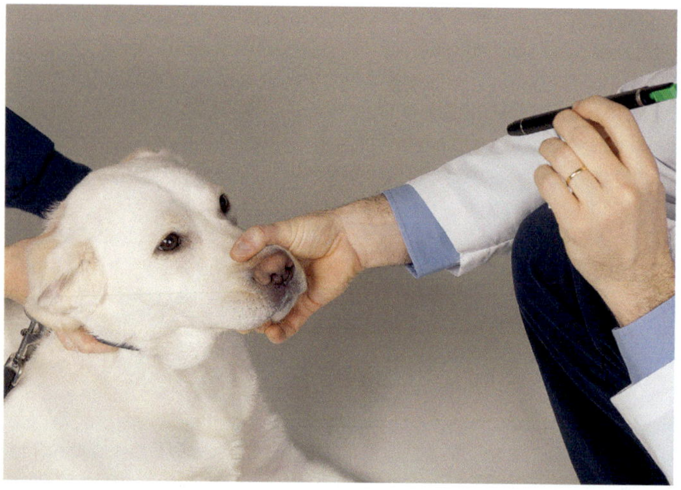

FIG. 9.13 The size and pupillary symmetry are tested by holding a good light source approximately half meter away from the patient's face so that the light shines equally on both eyes.

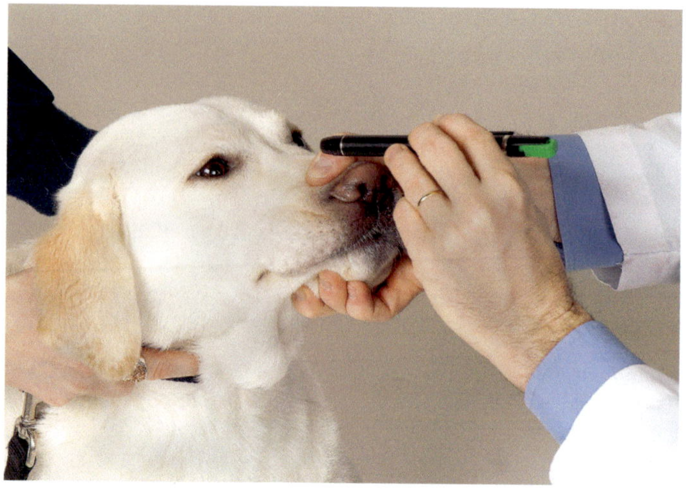

FIG. 9.14 The pupillary light reflex is elicited by shining a bright light in each eye. Normally, there is brisk constriction of the ipsilateral (direct pupillary light reflex) and contralateral pupil (indirect, or consensual pupillary light reflex). There is no need to cover the contralateral eye when testing the direct pupillary light reflex. Ideally, this test should be performed in a dimly lit room.

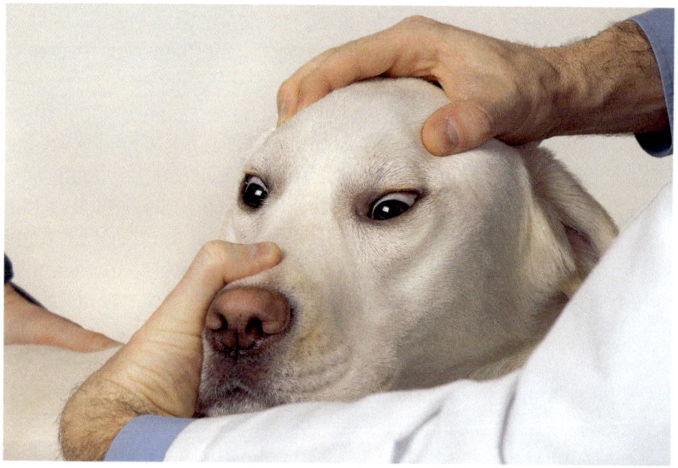

FIG. 9.15 The oculocephalic or vestibulo-ocular reflex is elicited by moving the patient's head side to side or up and down and observing the eye movements. Normal response is to see a nystagmus with the fast phase toward the direction of movement.

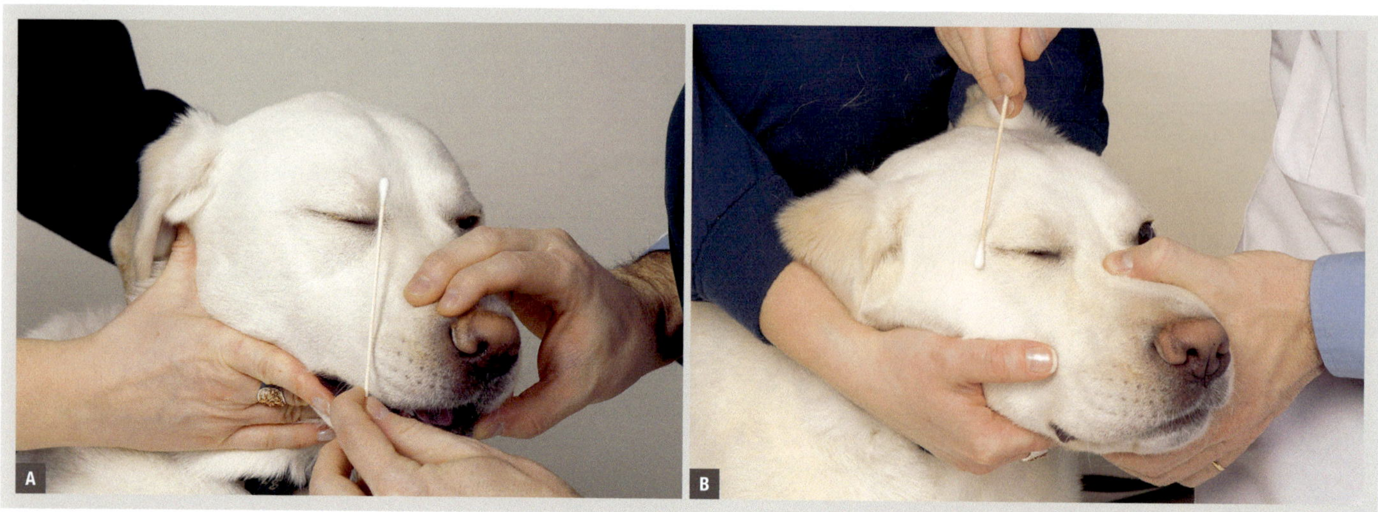

FIG. 9.16 The palpebral reflex is elicited by touching the skin medial to the eye (ophthalmic branch, of the trigeminal nerve) (A) and lateral to the eye (maxillary branch of the trigeminal nerve) (B). Normally, this will induce a blink mediated by the facial nerve. It is recommended to always test both the lateral and medial canthi of the eye to evaluate both branches of the trigeminal nerve.

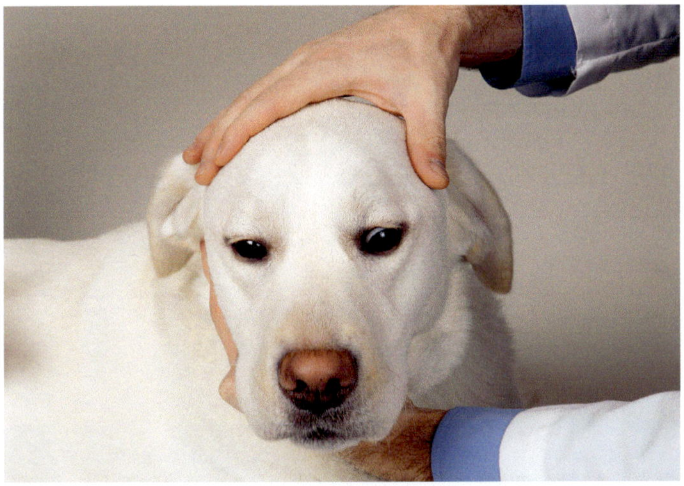

FIG. 9.17 The motor function of the trigeminal nerve is evaluated by palpating the masticatory muscles (temporalis and masseter). Compare the muscles on both sides of the face in relation to the zygomatic arch.

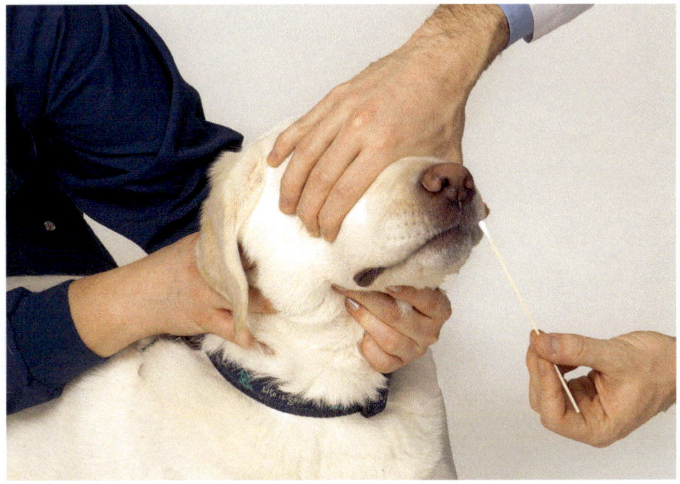

FIG. 9.18 The sensory portion of the trigeminal nerve (CN V) is tested by stimulating the nasal mucosa with an instrument such a forceps or a cotton-tipped applicator. Start with the lightest possible stimulus and progressively increase it, alternating sides, until getting a response. The eyes should be covered to avoid the patient see and anticipate the touch. The normal response is to pull their head away. Decreased sensation or exaggerated responses are abnormal.

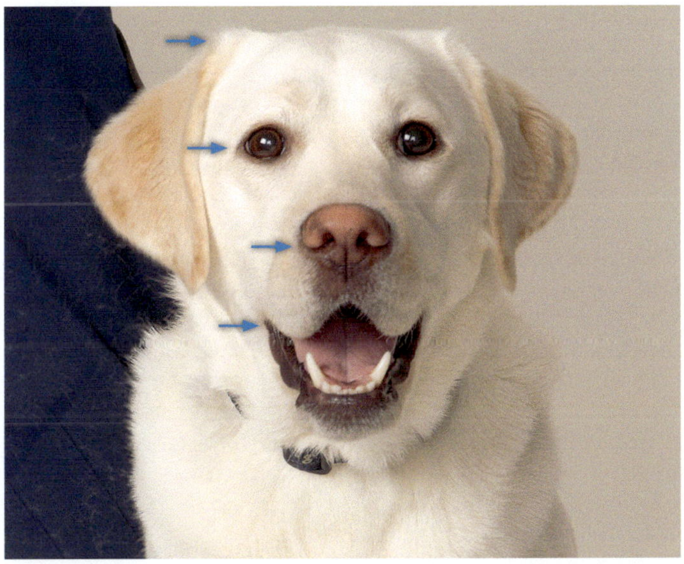

FIG. 9.19 Evaluation of the motor function of the facial nerve involves assessment of muscles of facial expression. Pay attention to the position of the upper lip, eyes, ears, and nostrils (arrows) comparing both left and right sides.

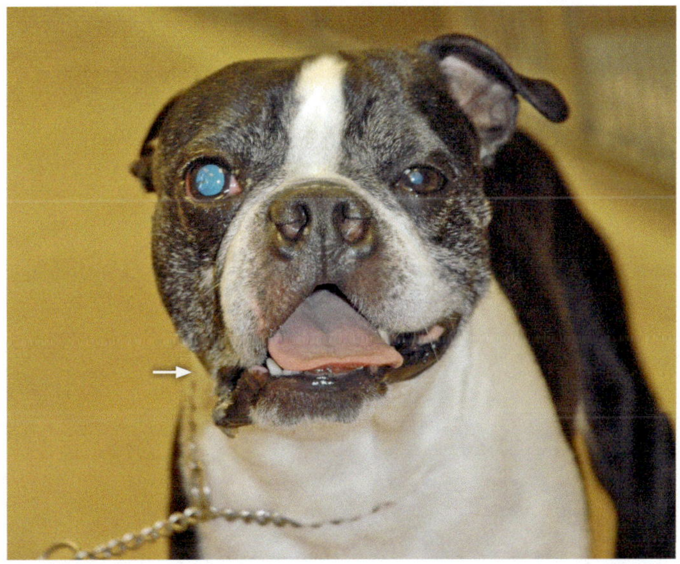

FIG. 9.20 Facial nerve paralysis in the right side demonstrated by the facial asymmetry with a droopy upper lip (arrow) and a widened palpebral fissure. Observe saliva accumulation in the right lip commissure.

Observe the patient's face carefully (preferably stepping back to see it from a distance) and compare the position of the upper and lower lips, eyes, ears, and nostrils (Fig. 9.19). Watch for asymmetrical deficits such as a droopy upper lip, a widened palpebral fissure, spontaneous blinking, or a drooping ear (Fig. 9.20). Because the facial nerve controls the muscles of facial expression, facial asymmetry indicates a facial nerve deficit. As the face is watched, note the alignment of the position of the eyes, and if needed draw a horizontal line centered at both pupils to determine if a head tilt is present. This is not needed in obvious head tilts (Fig. 9.21). Mild degrees of head tilt are frequently missed, but assessing the head position carefully is important to not miss mild head tilts. Do not use the position of the ears as a sign of head tilt, as "ear tilts" can occur without head tilt (Fig. 9.22), and ear tilt does not qualify as a vestibular sign.

Cranial nerves IX (glossopharyngeal nerve) and CN X (vagus nerve) can be indirectly assessed asking the owner about any dysphagia, regurgitation, voice change or inspiratory stridor. Many textbooks describe the swallowing reflex, which can be elicited by touching gently the surface of the base of the tongue or by manually stimulating the external projection of the pharyngeal area. Nevertheless, the author finds this test

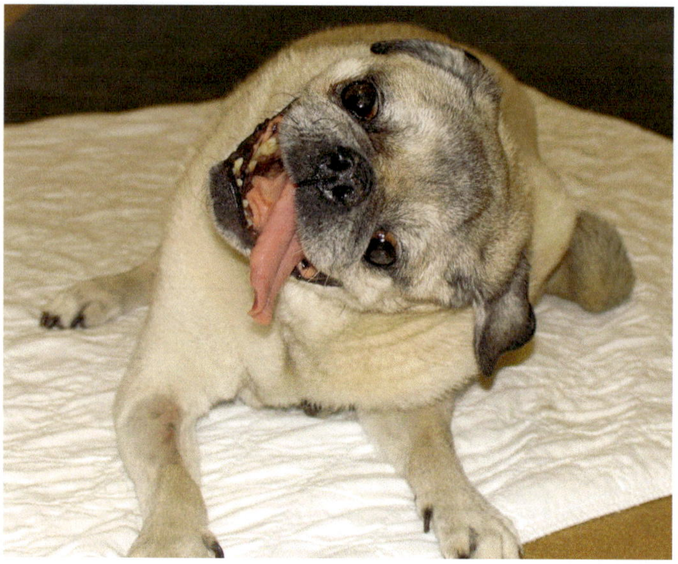

FIG. 9.21 Pug dog with central vestibular disease showing a left-sided head tilt.

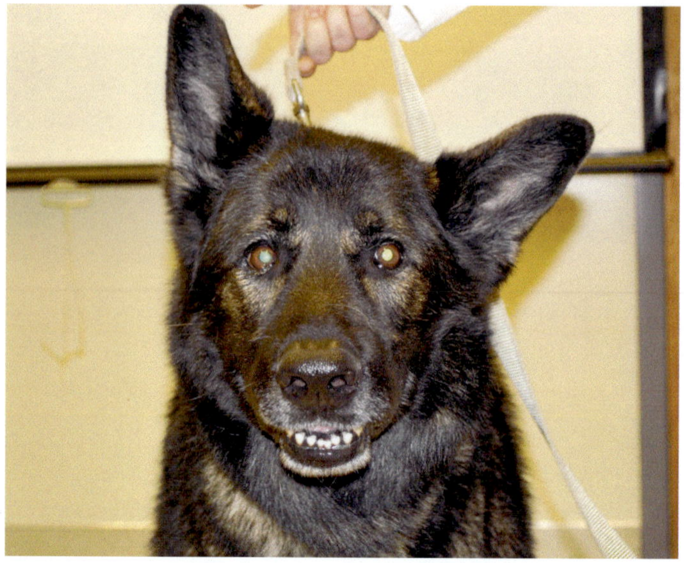

FIG. 9.22 German shepherd dog illustrating a case of "ear tilt", which can be confused with head tilt. Looking at the eye level, one will see that the head does not show evidence of head tilt.

not particularly useful and prefer to refer to the observation of signs of dysphagia and regurgitation.

Deficits involving the olfactory nerve (anosmia, hyposmia) are very uncommon. Testing should be performed with food.

Equally uncommon are deficits involving the hypoglossal nerve (CN XII). Observe the tongue for atrophy, asymmetry, or deviation.

Spinal reflexes

Spinal reflexes assess the integrity of the sensory and motor components of the reflex arc and the influence of descending upper motor neuron pathways.

Many reflexes can be tested, but only a few provide consistent and reliable valid clinical information, namely extensor tone, patellar reflex, flexor (withdrawal reflex), perineal and cutaneous trunci reflexes (Video 9.3). Lesion localization can be effectively achieved performing only these reflexes. Other reflexes can be performed if one chooses to do so. The order of reflex testing can facilitate testing all of them and have better patient cooperation. It is recommended to start with assessment of muscle tone, proceed with myotatic reflexes next, and leave the flexor (withdrawal) reflexes last. It is recommended to begin testing the pelvic limbs before testing the thoracic limbs. The perineal reflex and cutaneous trunci reflex are the last reflexes tested.

Muscle tone (extensor tone)

Extensor tone is one of the most reliable spinal reflexes. It can be performed with the patient standing or in lateral recumbency. Testing should be performed by gently applying pressure in the plantar or palmar surface of the pelvic or thoracic limbs, respectively (Fig. 9.23).

In normal dogs it should be easy to flex the limb when pressure is applied. When pressure is applied, and the extensor tone becomes increased (hypertonic or spastic) this is an indication of an upper motor neuron lesion. Extensor tone is a more reliable indicator of upper motor neuron lesion, as it is not as dependent of the sensory component to be elicited, as the patellar reflex is.

Patellar reflex

Before testing the patellar reflex always palpate the stifle to make sure that the patient does not have severe medial patellar luxation. In cases of patellar luxation, the patellar tendon is not under enough tension and the patellar reflex may be decreased or absent.

With the patient in lateral recumbency, place one hand under the thigh to support the limb with the stifle in a partially flexed position. With the other hand, briskly strike the patellar ligament (located between the patella and tibial tuberosity) with a reflex hammer. The normal response is a single, quick extension of the stifle. An alternative to see and "feel" the patellar reflex is to hold the limb and extend the digits. This may be useful to adjust the degree of limb flexion and extension in cases where the patellar reflex appears decreased (Fig. 9.24). The patellar reflex can also be tested with the patient standing, but this requires more skill and experience, and it is not recommended for the novice examiner. The patellar reflex assesses the integrity of the femoral nerve and L4—L6 spinal cord segments.

Flexor (withdrawal) reflex

With the limb loosely extended, pinch the interdigital skin lightly with your finger (Fig. 9.25). The normal response is flexion of the hip, stifle, and hock (pelvic limb) and the shoulder, elbow, and carpus (thoracic limb). Observe the contralateral limb for extension (crossed-extensor reflex). A crossed-extensor reflex is abnormal in a recumbent animal and usually denotes upper motor neuron disease.

The withdrawal reflex assesses the integrity of spinal cord segments C6—T2 for the thoracic limb, and L6—S2 (primarily L7, S1) for the pelvic limb. The efferent arc of the thoracic limb withdrawal reflex is

Video 9.3

Evaluation of spinal reflexes.

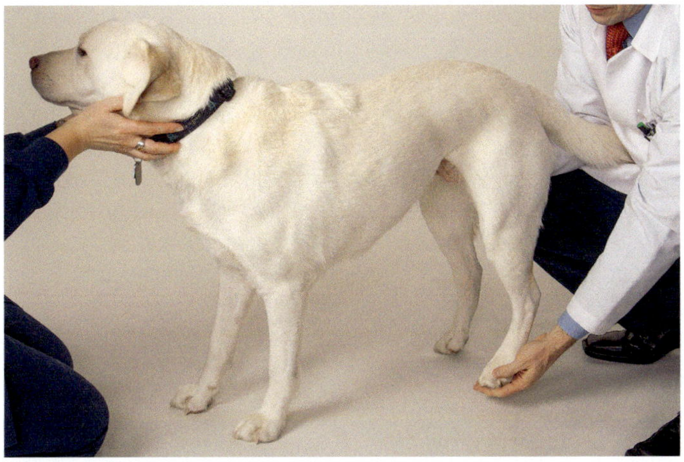

FIG. 9.23 Evaluation of extensor tone is performed by applying pressure in the plantar or palmar surfaces with the patient standing on in lateral recumbency.

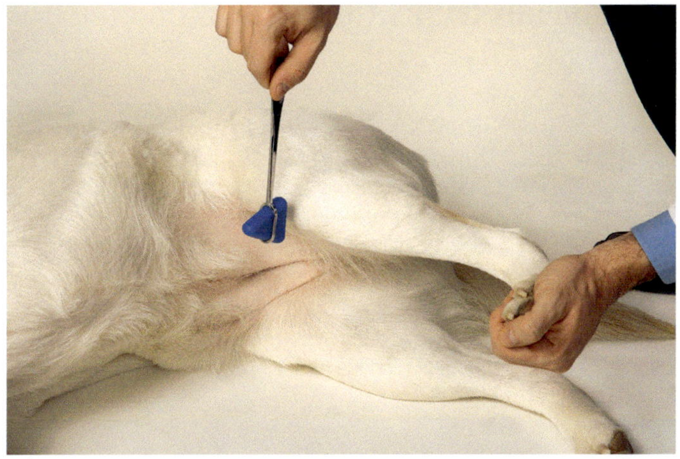

FIG. 9.24 The patellar reflex is elicited by percussing the patellar ligament between the patella and tibial tuberosity.

mediated by the musculocutaneous (the most important nerve for biceps flexion), as well as the axillary, median, ulnar, and radial nerves. In the pelvic limb, the efferent arc is mediated mainly by the sciatic nerve; the femoral nerve contributes to the flexion of the hip.

Other spinal reflexes

The gastrocnemius, cranial tibial, triceps, biceps and extensor carpi radialis reflexes are not reliably identified as the other reflexes listed above,[4] and there are questions whether theses reflexes are true reflexes as they have been shown to be present in animals 30 minutes after euthanasia, after nerve transection or anesthetic block of the plexus.[5,6] The reader can find information about these reflexes elsewhere).[1]

Perineal reflex

To elicit the perineal reflex, lightly touch or stroke the perineum (Fig. 9.26). The left and right sides should be tested. The normal response is contraction of the anal sphincter and tail flexion. The perineal reflex assesses the integrity of sacral (S1—S3) and caudal (tail flexion) spinal cord segments, as well as perineal and caudal rectal nerve branches (both are branches of the pudendal nerve).

Spinal reflexes are graded as follows:

- Absent
- Weak (present but reduced)
- Normal
- Exaggerated
- Clonus (repetitive flexion and extension of the joint in response to a single stimulus)

These grades are translated into numbers used to fill the neurologic examination form. A normal reflex is graded as "2", whereas a decreased reflex is assigned "1", an absent reflex "0", an increased "3", and a clonic reflex "4".[7] See end of chapter for an example of neurologic examination form.

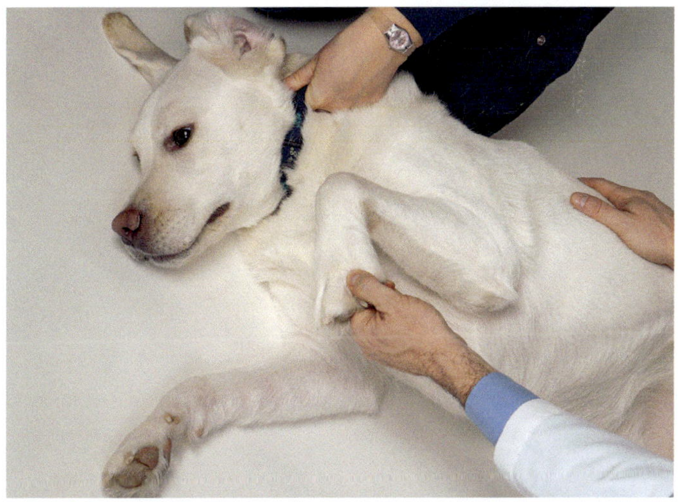

FIG. 9.25 The flexor reflex is tested by pinching the skin between the digits. Normal response is flexion of the hip, stifle, and hock in the pelvic limbs, and carpus, elbow and shoulder in the thoracic limbs. This is a reflex mediated at the level of the spinal cord and does not indicate conscious perception of pain (which happens at a cortical level).

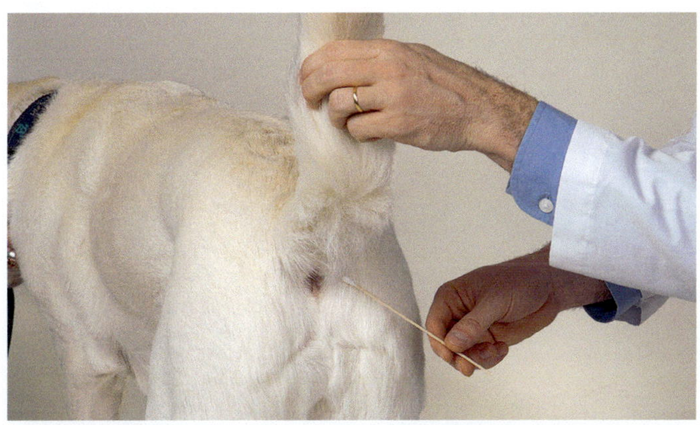

FIG. 9.26 Gently stroking or pinching the perineum tests the perineal reflex. The normal response is flexion of the tail and contraction of the external anal sphincter.

Cutaneous trunci (formerly panniculus) reflex (CTR)

The CTR assesses the sensory integrity of all dermatomes over the thoracolumbar vertebral column (with their corresponding spinal cord segments and nerves). The efferent component is mediated by the lateral thoracic nerve and C8–T1 spinal cord segments (Fig. 9.27).

With the patient standing or in straight sternal recumbency, gently pinch the skin just lateral to the vertebral column (Fig. 9.28). Start just cranial to the lumbosacral region and proceed cranially, one vertebral level at a time. The opposite side is tested similarly. The normal response is a bilateral contraction of the cutaneous trunci muscle, resulting in a twitch of the skin over the thorax and abdomen. If a response is obtained at L6, there is no need to continue pinching more cranially. This reflex is present in the thoracolumbar region and is absent in the neck and sacral regions. An obvious cutoff point suggests a spinal cord lesion typically two vertebral segments cranial to level of cutoff. A lesion affecting the brachial plexus may cause a loss of the ipsilateral CTR with a normal response on the other side, regardless of the level at which the skin is stimulated. Thoracotomies typically transect the lateral thoracic nerve, also causing ipsilateral loss of the CTR. It is very important to document the cut-off point of the CTR in paraplegic dogs with absent nociception, as cranial migration of the CTR has been associated with 145 times higher odds of the patient developing progressive myelomalacia (Fig. 9.29).[8]

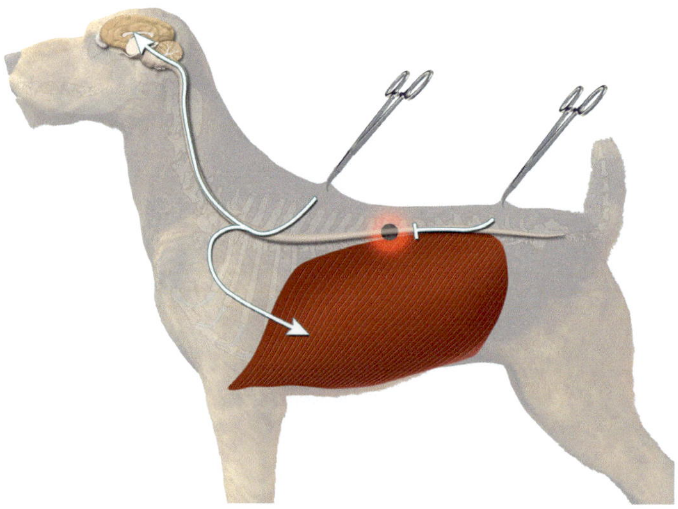

FIG. 9.27 With spinal cord lesions along the thoracolumbar region, the ascending pathway of the cutaneous trunci reflex is interrupted, and the reflex is absent approximately 2 vertebral bodies caudal to the lesion. Testing the reflex cranial to the lesion point will elicit a response.

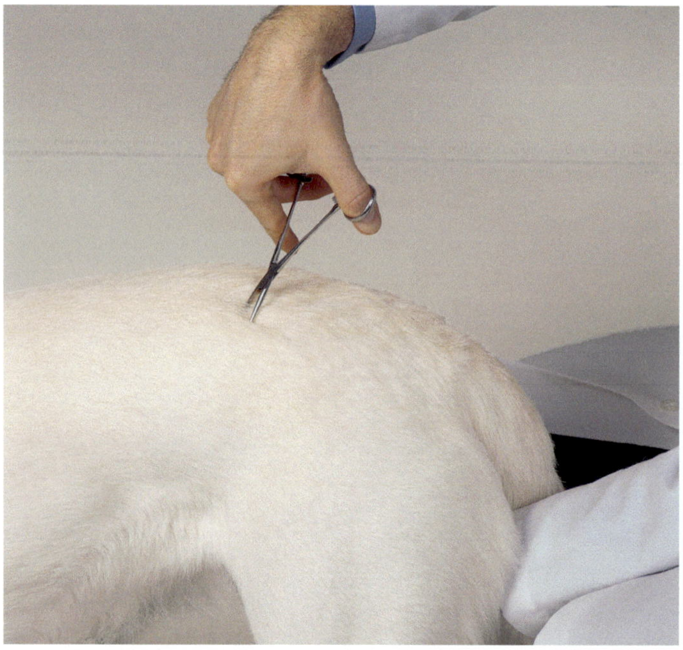

FIG. 9.28 The cutaneous trunci reflex is evaluated by lightly pinching the skin just lateral to the vertebral column, starting over the lumbosacral region and proceeding cranially, one vertebral level at a time. The normal response is a bilateral contraction of the cutaneous trunci muscle resulting in a twitch of the skin over the thorax and abdomen.

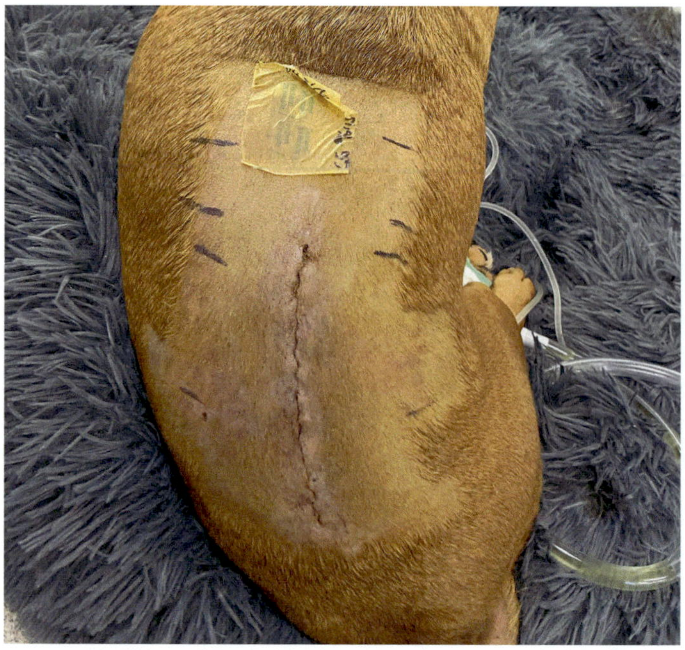

FIG. 9.29 Markings indicating multiple cut-offs of the cutaneous trunci reflex along the thoracolumbar spine of a Dachshund after decompressive surgery for thoracolumbar intervertebral disc extrusion. Monitoring the cutaneous trunci reflex is useful for early identification of progressive myelomalacia.

Vertebral column palpation

Palpation of the vertebral column is very important to determine if the patient has a painful spinal condition (Video 9.4). Deeply palpate the paraspinal muscle for pain. To be effective the palpation should be performed with the correct technique. For palpation of the thoracolumbar region it is recommended to start in the cranial thoracic area, as spinal problems are less common there, and proceed caudally until the lumbosacral region (a region much more commonly affected with spinal problems). Pressure should be directed ventrally and the patient should ideally be supported under the sternum and pelvic regions (Figs. 9.30 and 9.31).
Cervical palpation is more technically challenging. It should be performed by pressing against the ventral aspect of the vertebral column, while supporting the dorsal neck with the opposite hand (Fig. 9.32).

Video 9.4

Palpation of the vertebral column/assement of spinal pain.

The advantages of this technique are that subtle pain can be detected, presumably by applying pressure more directly to the problem area, and anatomic landmarks (e.g., caudal ventral midline protuberances, lateral processes of C6) can be readily palpated. If palpation does not induce pain, gently extend and flex the head with one hand while placing the other hand on the cervical muscles to detect muscle tensing.

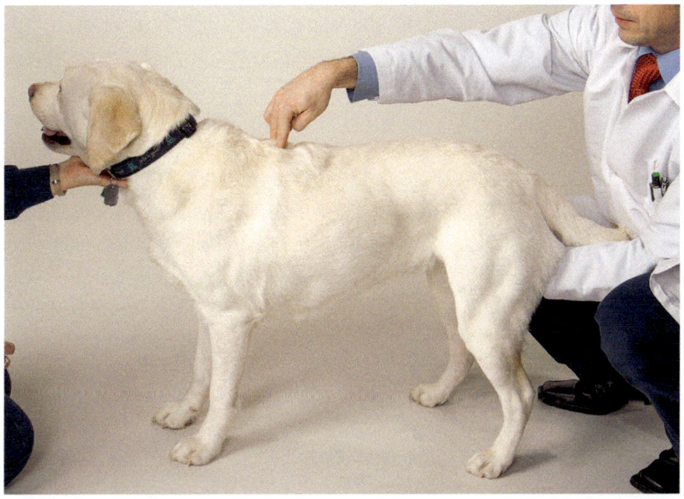

FIG. 9.30 Palpation of the thoracolumbar vertebral column is performed applying direct pressure ventrally, starting in the cranial thoracic region and moving caudally until reaching the lumbosacral region.

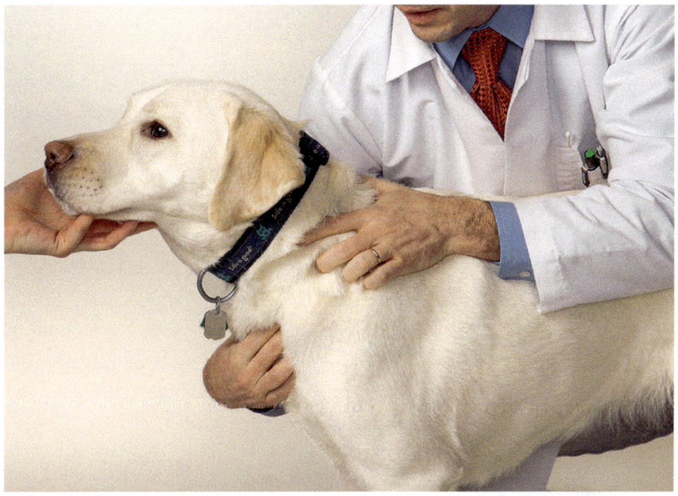

FIG. 9.31 Direct application of pressure to the ventral aspect aiming at the spaces in between the transverse processes as close as possible to the foraminal level is a sensitive method of detecting and localizing cervical hyperesthesia in dogs.

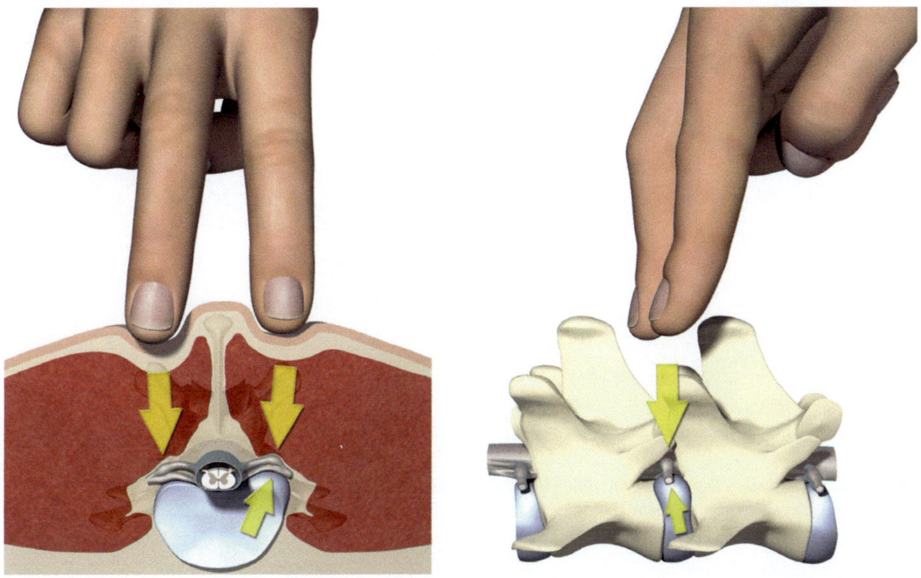

FIG. 9.32 Diagram illustrating the position of the fingers in relation to the spinous processes for palpation. The fingers should be kept relatively close to each other, and pressure should be performed between the spinous processes because most disease processes involve the intervertebral discs.

This has to be done carefully and avoiding forcing it excessively as severe neurologic deterioration can ensue if the patient has potentially unstable vertebral conditions (such as atlantoaxial subluxation). A safer method is to use a food treat and make the dog follow it in all directions. This would more closely assess the natural cervical range of motion and the patient will stop if the movement becomes painful. The main advantage of this technique is that it does not carry the risk of neurologic deterioration.

Palpation of the head can be performed for masses, defects, or persistent fontanelles. Lightly squeezing the head by grasping above the zygomatic arch often elicits a painful response in dogs with structural brain disease.

Limbs are initially palpated with the patient standing. Contralateral limbs are compared for symmetry. The limbs are more closely examined with the animal in lateral recumbency, when the spinal reflexes are tested.

Pain perception (nociception)

Pain perception, or nociception, should be performed in any limb(s) paralyzed (most commonly tested in paraplegic dogs). Nociception was formerly divided into superficial and deep, but since the nociceptive pathways for these two degrees of noxious stimuli are poorly divided, this differentiation is not typically used anymore. Pain perception at the skin level is best assessed using autonomous zones, these are specific zones where a single nerve provides sensory input for that zone, for example over the skin of the third digit for the radial nerve.[9]

A few key points to keep in mind. Nociception or pain perception with a hemostat should only be tested in plegic patients. If voluntary movement is present, there is no need to test pain perception. Equally important, if one already observed response to pain during the withdrawal reflex, there is no need to repeat it (Fig. 9.33A). Hemostatic forceps can be used to test pain perception and both the medial and lateral digits of the pelvic limbs should be tested (Fig. 9.33B). If no response is seen, evaluate the tail. Absence of conscious response indicates a guarded to poor prognosis for intervertebral disc extrusion and other transverse myelopathies.[10] Withdrawal of the limb indicates only an intact reflex arc (peripheral nerve and spinal segments). A behavioral response such as turning the head or vocalization indicates conscious perception. When testing specifically for pain perception, forget "limb responses" and focus on the head!

Conclusion

Many people feel that performing a complete neurologic examination in general practice is an unachievable goal. The goal of keeping the neurologic examination to the most essential and reliable tests is to just to hopefully have more clinicians being willing to perform an examination. With that in mind, it is still better to perform a limited examination than no examination altogether. For example, in a patient with a history of seizures, paying special attention or performing only the menace response, nasal sensation, proprioceptive positioning, and carefully assessing the behaviour, would assess the clinicians in identifying those dogs likely to have idiopathic epilepsy, versus, those with structural epilepsy. Similarly, in a "down dog", identifying whether the dog does or does not have spinal pain as well as nociception (pain perception in the limbs), has key diagnostic and prognostic purposes. Finally, the basis of clinical neurology is lesion localization. The list of differential diagnoses and the diagnostic approach are completely dependent on the lesion localization. And lesion localization can only be achieved with a good neurologic examination.

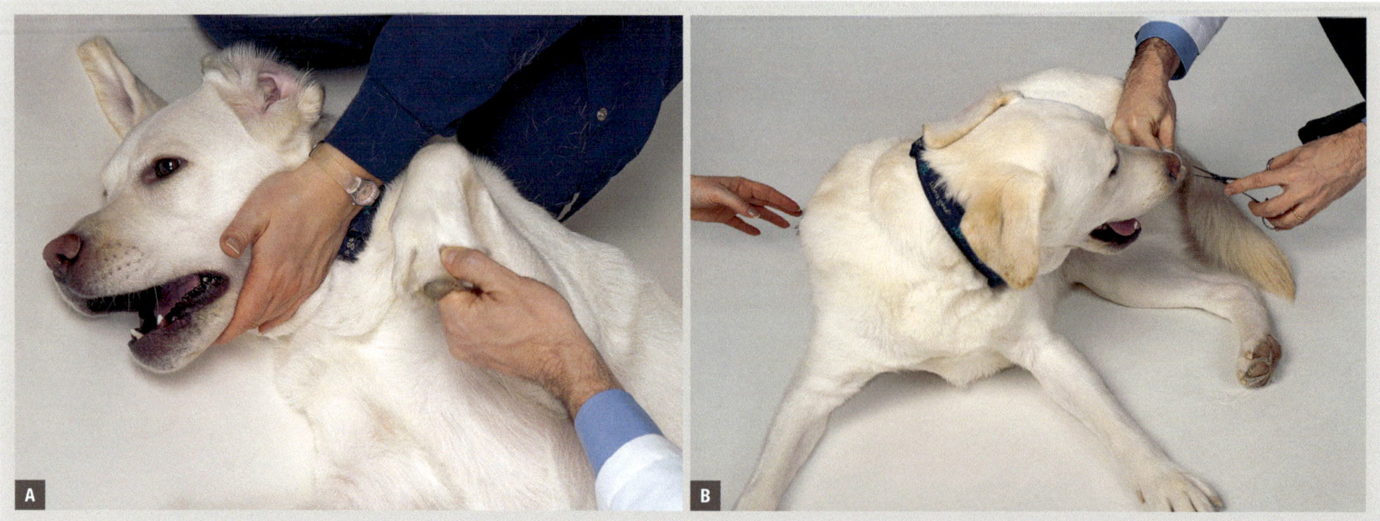

FIG. 9.33 Assessment of pain perception can be performed manually during testing the withdrawal reflex (A) or with a hemostat (B). If the patient does not respond to manual pressure, a hemostat must be used before calling the nociception absent. In the pelvic limbs it is recommended to test the lateral and medial digits as their sensory innervation is mediated by the sciatic and femoral nerves, respectively. A conscious response, such as crying or turning the head, indicates that nociception is present. Simple flexion of the limb without a conscious response means that the flexor reflex is present but nociception is absent.

KEY POINTS

- Learn to first to just observe the patient. The hands-off observation of gait, posture, behavior and mentation can be done in all patients, and are the most informative components of the neurologic examination
- Always remember to put the patient on the floor. Many "down/non-ambulatory" animals will ambulate when placed on the floor, primarily if the floor is non-slippery.
- Postural reactions, primarily proprioceptive positioning, are excellent to confirm the presence of a neurologic abnormality, even though they are of limited value to localize lesions. Remember to support them very well. This is primarily important (and challenging) in large and giant breed dogs.
- Spinal reflexes are of crucial importance to localize spinal cord lesions, but they do not provide information about its severity.
- Any dog with a history of seizures (which indicates a functional or structural dysfunction of the forebrain), should have these 4 items assessed very carefully – behavior, menace response, nasal sensation and proprioceptive positioning. Most cranial nerve tests will be unaffected, only menace and nasal sensation are sensitive to forebrain dysfunction (technique is key, however, to achieve reliable results for both)!
- Spinal palpation is very important to allow us to narrow down our list of differential diagnosis.
- Deep pain perception, or nociception, should always be done in paraplegic patients (but not in ambulatory animals). Make sure you do not incorrectly interpret a normal flexor reflex as the presence of deep pain perception (a normal response of deep pain involves conscious/behavioural response) and not only flexing the limb.

References

1. Dewey CW, da Costa RC, Thomas WB. Performing the Neurologic examination. In: Dewey, CW, da Costa RC (eds.). *Practical Guide to Canine and Feline Neurology*, 3rd ed. Wiley; 2015, pp. 9–29.
2. Nagendran A, José López R, Suñol A, et al. The value of a head turn in neurolocalization. *J Vet Intern Med.* 2024 Jan-Feb;38(1):268–276.
3. Parent J. Clinical approach and lesion localization in patients with spinal diseases. *Vet Clin North Am Small Anim Pract.* 2010 Sep;40(5):733–753.
4. Giebels F, Pieper L, Kohn B, Volk HA, Shihab N, Loderstedt S. Comparison of interobserver agreement between the evaluation of bicipital and the patellar tendon reflex in healthy dogs. PLoS One. 2019 Jul 10;14(7)
5. Tudury EA, Araújo B, Fernandes T, et al. Carpi radialis and cranial tibial reflexes:myotatic or muscular response? *Proceedings of the 16th ESVOT Congress,* Bologna, Italy, 2012.
6. Tudury EA, de Figueiredo ML, Fernandes TH, et al. Evaluation of cranial tibial and extensor carpi radialis reflexes before and after anesthetic block in cats. *J Feline Med Surg.* 2017 Feb;19(2):105–109.
7. de Lahunta A, Glass EN, Kent M. The Neurologic examination. In: de Lahunta A, Glass EN, Kent M. Veterinary Neuroanatomy and Clinical Neurology. 4th ed, 2015. Elsevier, Philadelphia, PA. p. 525–539.
8. Muguet-Chanoit AC, Olby NJ, Lim JH, et al. The cutaneous trunci muscle reflex: a predictor of recovery in dogs with acute thoracolumbar myelopathies caused by intervertebral disc extrusions. *Vet Surg.* 2012 Feb;41(2):200–206.
9. Bailey, C. S. and R. L. Kitchell. Cutaneous sensory testing in the dog. *J Vet Intern Med.* 1987 Jul-Sep;1(3):128-35.
10. Olby NJ, da Costa RC, Levine JM, Stein VM; Canine Spinal Cord Injury Consortium (CANSORT SCI). Prognostic Factors in Canine Acute Intervertebral Disc Disease. *Front Vet Sci.* 2020 Nov 26;7:596-059.

CHAPTER 10

Neurolocalization and differential diagnoses

Alberta De Stefani
DVM, MRCVS, PhD, DECVN, PGDipVetEd, FHEA

Reaching a neurolocalization might feel intimidating and overwhelming, and the general perception is that neuroanatomy (and functional neuroanatomy) is too complex and beyond reach. However, an in-depth knowledge of neuroanatomy is not necessary for daily clinical work. This chapter will elucidate the functional and dysfunctional anatomy of different parts of the nervous system and highlight how specific locations within the nervous system consistently produce clinical signs that, once identified, will support a neurolocalization. Investing a small amount of time and effort in reaching a basic understanding of neuroanatomy will significantly increase your confidence and enjoyment when managing neurological cases. Neurolocalization is also a fundamental step in the clinical reasoning framework. Together with the anamnestic information and clinical findings, neurolocalization enables us to develop a prioritized list of differential diagnoses, which in turn helps us choose the most appropriate diagnostic plan or empirical treatment and make sense of the diagnostic test results. The neurological examination enables us to determine if a patient is neurological or not and, together with their history, to record the presence or absence of specific neurological deficits. It should be highlighted that, for reaching a neurolocalization, recording the "normal" is as important as recording the "abnormal".[1,2] Think, for example, of the relevance of finding a normal pupillary light reflex in the context of a blind patient, or how identifying normal spinal reflexes can help us further refine a spinal cord neurolocalization. As a general rule, an attempt should always be made to justify all the clinical/neurological findings with one location. However, this might not always be possible and in such cases more than one localization (i.e., multifocal or diffuse neurolocalization) should be considered.

To support our interpretation of the clinical/neurological findings, it is essential to have a grasp of the organization of the nervous system and the function of each of the main components.

Neurolocalization

The nervous system can be broadly divided into central nervous system (CNS), peripheral nervous system (PNS) and autonomic nervous system.[3,4] The CNS can be further divided into intracranial (forebrain, brainstem, and cerebellum) and extracranial (spinal cord) structures. The PNS can be divided into peripheral nerves, neuromuscular junctions, and muscles. The two major divisions of the autonomic nervous system are the sympathetic and parasympathetic systems; these will only be briefly mentioned in this chapter.

Reaching a neurolocalization is a step-by-step process; it usually feels less intimidating to localize to broad regions first. Following the physical and neurological examination and after determining that the problem is definitively neurological, it may be helpful to proceed towards a definitive neurolocalization by excluding those neuroanatomical regions that are less likely to be involved and moving to progressively smaller regions until a single area is identified. For example, an initial step could include determining whether the lesion affects the PNS or CNS. The vast majority of PNS disorders affect its efferent (motor) part. This is why, when localizing a lesion at the PNS, neurologists refer to the neuromuscular (or lower motor neuron [LMN]) system. In the case of generalized peripheral LMN dysfunction, it is possible to observe generalized weakness, various degrees of paresis in the absence of primary ataxia, decreased spinal reflexes (not always), and muscle tone.

If the clinical presentation does not match with a neuromuscular localization, the lesion is localized to the CNS. It is then useful to determine whether it affects the intracranial or extracranial nervous system by assessing for mental status and behavioral and/or cranial nerve/menace response abnormalities. If such abnormalities are observed, a spinal cord neurolocalization can be ruled out. Further fine tuning to specific areas within the intracranial structures might then be possible based on the neurological examination findings.

Intracranial CNS localization

The three major intracranial functional areas of interest for the neurologist are the prosencephalon (forebrain), the brainstem, and the cerebellum (Fig. 10.1)

Forebrain (prosencephalon)

The forebrain is anatomically located in the rostrotentorial portion of the neurocranium and includes the cerebrum

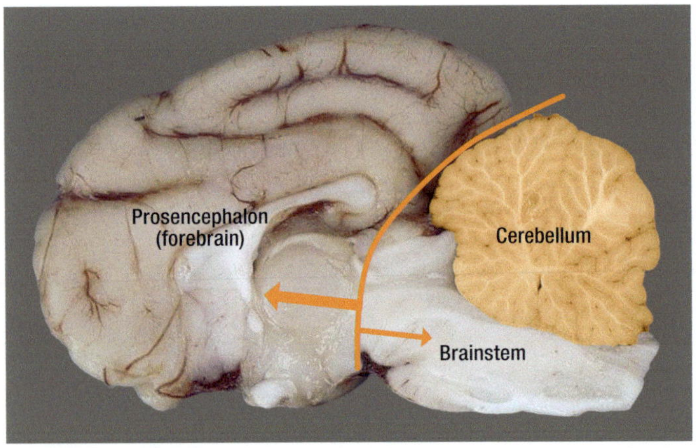

FIG. 10.1 Three anatomofunctional regions (prosencephalon, brainstem, and cerebellum) into which the brain is divided for the purpose of the neuroanatomical localization of the lesion. Picture courtesy of Dr. Carlo Cantile.

(or telencephalon) and the diencephalon. From a functional perspective, the cerebrum can be divided into five paired regions or lobes: the frontal, parietal, temporal, and occipital lobes and the rhinencephalon (olfactory bulbs, piriform lobe, and hippocampus).[1,3,5]

The cerebrum is important for the control of behavior, consciousness, learning, and memory. The forebrain receives proprioceptive and nociceptive sensory inputs and oversees conscious proprioception and pain perception. Additionally, the occipital lobes are in charge of vision, and the rhinencephalon (phylogenetically the oldest part of the telencephalon) is important for the perception of smell and is in close association with the limbic system.

The diencephalon is considered a major relay center with visual, auditory, proprioceptive, and nociceptive sensory information transiting through this structure before being projected to the relevant parts of the cerebral cortex. The diencephalon is also involved in the control of sleep and the level of consciousness and wakefulness (it is part of the ascending reticular activating system [ARAS] projecting to the cerebral cortex) and in behavioral patterns due to its connection with the limbic system. Autonomic and endocrine functions, such as thirst, appetite, temperature, and electrolyte balance, are controlled in the diencephalon. Olfactory, visual, and pupillary light reflex (PLR) functions are also controlled in the diencephalon: olfaction, via a projection of cranial nerve I (CN I) on the hypothalamus and limbic system; and vision and PLR via CN II (optic nerve) and the optic chiasm, which are located ventral to the hypothalamus.[5]

Considering the significant overlap of clinical signs referable to the cerebrum and diencephalon, these two regions will be considered together and will be referred to as a forebrain neurolocalization. It is important to remember that forebrain diseases may produce very mild and insidious neurological signs even in the presence of extensive lesions. Based on the author's clinical experience and the published literature, up to 1 in 5 dogs with an intracranial lesion may have a normal neurological examination.[6,7] Therefore, if a forebrain lesion is suspected, great importance should be given to any of the signs described below, even if they are very mild.

Neurological examination findings that might help in reaching a forebrain neurolocalization are related to:

- **Mental status**. Forebrain lesions are more likely to cause mild mentation changes such as drowsiness. More dramatic changes in mental status, however, are not impossible, particularly if there is significant involvement of the diencephalon or if the cerebrum is diffusely affected (e.g., in case of increased intracranial pressure).
- **Behavioral changes.** Aggressive, apathetic, disoriented, anxious, or overexcited behavior may be observed. Aimless pacing, compulsive gait, circling in wide or tight circles, becoming trapped in furniture, and head pressing can also be seen with diseases affecting the forebrain.
- **Posture**. The presence of head and/or body turn (usually toward the lesion) can be documented.
- **Gait**. The forebrain is of minor importance when it comes to gait generation, regulation of posture, and maintenance of muscle tone. In dogs, these functions are delegated to subcortical structures (mostly brainstem nuclei). Gait abnormalities are therefore uncommon or very subtle with forebrain lesions in this species. Compulsive walking may be observed, and lateralizing forebrain lesions can lead to ipsilateral compulsive circling. Compulsive walking should be considered a behavioral change rather than a true gait abnormality.
- **Postural reactions** deficits can be recorded in dogs with forebrain lesions. If present, these occur contralateral to the side of the lesion. The combination of postural reaction deficits and a normal (or nearly normal) gait is an important indicator of forebrain dysfunction.
- **Spinal reflexes** as well as muscle tone are usually unaffected in dogs with forebrain lesions.
- **Cranial nerve assessment**. When evaluating the cranial nerves, the most typical presentation of a forebrain lesion is an abnormal menace response and cotton ball test in the absence of other cranial nerve deficits. An abnormal menace response test does not necessarily imply that the dog is blind. In most cases, a lack of response indicates a cognitive deficit and an inability to "recognize" the threat and act accordingly. The menace response and cotton ball test enable us to check a long pathway involving the cerebrum. Most cranial nerve tests evaluate the brainstem.

In the case of a forebrain lesion, the cranial nerve examination may also detect visual, olfactory (rare), and facial sensory deficits. Visual deficits can manifest as a reduced or absent menace response contralateral to the lesion. Blindness can be confirmed by walking the dog in a room with obstacles, by performing the cotton ball test or, in small patients, by performing visual placements.

Palpation of the head and spine may lead to the detection of head or cervical pain. This may be secondary to meningeal stretching and referred pain. Pain as a clinical sign has also been associated with diencephalic lesions (thalamic pain syndrome).

Episodic events such as epileptic seizures or movement disorders (dyskinesias) may not be directly observed by the attending veterinarian during the consultation, but a history or video recording of such events supports a forebrain neurolocalization.

Brainstem

Anatomically, the brainstem is made of the diencephalon, mesencephalon, pons, and medulla oblongata (or medulla). The brainstem represents the connection between the cerebral hemispheres and the spinal cord. Despite the brainstem having a multitude of complex functions, anatomically and functionally it resembles the spinal cord, with dorsally located sensory areas, ventrally located motor areas, and autonomic areas situated in between the sensory and motor areas.[1–3,5] The brainstem oversees and regulates the level of consciousness (via the ARAS), contains cardiovascular and respiratory control centers (medullary reticular formation), sees the transit of ascending sensory and descending motor tracks, and comprises the (paired) nuclei of ten cranial nerves, CN III through CN XII.

It is important to note that, although the diencephalon is anatomically part of the brainstem, from a functional point of view it forms a unit with the cerebrum (forebrain). For this reason, when we localize the lesion to the brainstem, the word "brainstem" refers to the mesencephalon (midbrain), the pons, and the medulla oblongata.[1,8]

Lesions of the brainstem may produce abnormalities in mental status, from mild drowsiness to stupor and coma; this is due to the involvement of the ARAS, which extends along the entire length of the brainstem. Sensory and upper motor neuron (UMN) tracts also course through the entire brainstem; a lesion in this area can therefore lead to unilateral or bilateral postural reaction deficits and tetraparesis (or plegia). In addition, lesions in different areas of the brainstem may produce specific signs:

- **Midbrain**. The nuclei of the oculomotor nerve (CN III; both motor and parasympathetic) and trochlear nerve (CN IV) reside in this area of the brainstem. Lesions in the midbrain can thus lead to deficits in the innervation of the extraocular muscles and consequent strabismus. Lateral strabismus in the ipsilateral eye can be observed in case of CN III dysfunction, and dorsolateral strabismus of the contralateral eye in case of CN IV involvement (it is the only cranial nerve that decussates). If the parasympathetic nucleus of CN III is involved, PLR deficits will be present. The midbrain also houses the (paired) red nuclei, a very important structure for gait generation and control in the UMN system.
- **Pons**. The motor nuclei of the trigeminal nerve (CN V) reside in the pons (the sensory nuclei of CN V extend along the entire length of the brainstem). Lesions in this region can therefore lead to motor deficits of CN V.
- **Medulla oblongata**. The remainder of the cranial nerve nuclei are located in the medulla. From cranial to caudal, these include the abducent nerve (CN VI), facial nerve (CN VII), and four paired vestibular nuclei (CN VIII) in the cranial medulla, and the glossopharyngeal nerve (CN IX), vagus nerve (CN X), accessory nerve (CN XI), and hypoglossal nerve (CN XII) in the caudal medulla. CNs VII, IX and X also have a parasympathetic component. The medulla oblongata also contains respiratory and autonomic centers for heart and blood pressure control. Lesions in the cranial medulla are likely to cause vestibular signs plus or minus facial paralysis, while lesions of the caudal medulla are more likely to cause dysphagia, dysphonia, and tongue paresis/paralysis. Respiratory dysfunction and alteration of heart rate and blood pressure can also be observed with lesions of the medulla oblongata.

Neurological findings that might help reach a brainstem neurolocalization include:

- **Mental status**. When the ARAS is involved, brainstem lesions can cause significant and severe mentation changes, such as stupor and coma. Normal mentation can however be documented.
- **Behavior**. Behavioral changes are not expected with brainstem lesions. However, if the mental status is severely affected, dogs may appear quiet and apathetic and show inadequate interaction with the environment.
- **Posture**. Depending on the location of the lesion within the brainstem, the posture may be normal. However, a head tilt and wide base stance may be observed with involvement of the vestibular nuclei. Very severe midbrain lesions can also cause decerebrate rigidity, usually associated with very severe mentation changes (stupor/coma).
- **Gait**. Brainstem lesions can cause from very subtle to marked alterations of the gait. Tetra- or hemiparesis/-plegia can be seen if the UMN system is involved. Ataxia associated with a variable degree of paresis may be observed due to the involvement of the vestibular nuclei and proprioceptive pathways.
- **Postural reactions**. Mild to severe deficits may be documented, especially in cases with proprioceptive ataxia.
- **Spinal reflexes** are usually not affected, though mild hyperreflexia may be seen.
- **Cranial nerve** deficits can be expected from CN III to XII.
- **Palpation** of the cervical region might identify hyperesthesia.
- **Abnormal movements**. Pathological nystagmus can be observed. Convergence-retraction nystagmus has been documented with midbrain lesions,[9] and horizontal, rotatory, and vertical nystagmus is usually part of vestibular dysfunction.

Cerebellum

The cerebellum is located in the caudal fossa and is separated from the cerebrum by the osseus tentorium and tentorium cerebelli. Three pairs of peduncles (rostral, middle, and caudal) attach the cerebellum to the brainstem. The main function of the cerebellum is to regulate movement (rate, range, and force). The cerebellum also has a direct connection with the vestibular nuclei and therefore contributes to the regulation of equilibrium and body posture at rest and during movement. The cerebellum does not initiate movement; rather, it coordinates and regulates movement, exerting an inhibitory action mainly. Lesions in the cerebellum may cause a specific type of ataxia (cerebellar ataxia), characterized by hypermetria and truncal ataxia (body sway), intention tremors, and difficulty in initiating movements. Vestibular dysfunction can also be documented.[1–3,5]

Neurological findings that may help to reach a cerebellar neurolocalization include:

- **Mental status and behavior** are unaffected. The cerebellum has no influence on the mental status and behavior.
- **Posture**. A wide base stance is often recorded with cerebellar lesions. A head tilt may be present and may be paradoxical. When in lateral recumbency, the dog may display decerebellate rigidity. This posture is characterized by opisthotonos and extensor rigidity of the thoracic limbs with flexed hips.
- **Gait**. Cerebellar ataxia, characterized by hypermetria (ipsilateral in case of a focal lesion), and truncal ataxia without paresis are observed.
- **Postural reactions** are usually unaffected. A delay in the initiation of movement, for example while testing hopping, can be present, usually followed by an exaggerated (dysmetric) response.
- **Spinal reflexes** are unaffected with cerebellar lesions.
- **Cranial nerve** assessment might identify ipsilateral decreased/absent menace response with normal vision.
- **Palpation** is usually normal.
- **Abnormal movement**. Intention tremors can be present as well as pathological nystagmus depending on the location of the lesion within the cerebellum.

Extracranial CNS (spinal cord) localization

If a dog does not display mental status, behavioral, and/or cranial nerve/menace response abnormalities and does not have generally decreased spinal reflexes and/or pure paresis, the lesion is localized to the extracranial CNS, and specifically the spinal cord.

The spinal cord is fully contained in the vertebral canal; it begins at the foramen magnum and terminates at the 6th or 7th lumbar vertebra in most dogs. However, variations exist between dog sizes and breeds.[3,10]

The spinal cord can be seen as a tubular structure, with white matter tracts forming the outer portion and grey matter forming the center. The white matter can be divided into dorsal, lateral, and ventral funiculi; broadly speaking, the dorsal funiculus carries ascending (sensory) information regarding proprioception, the lateral funiculus carries ascending (sensory) information regarding proprioception, touch, pressure, temperature and pain as well as descending motor input, and the ventral funiculus mainly carries descending motor information.

The spinal cord grey matter is made of the cell bodies of the efferent neurons, interneurons, and sensory neurons. The efferent motor neuron (LMN) cell bodies lie in the ventral horn, the preganglionic neuronal cell bodies for the autonomic system (sympathetic in the thoracolumbar region and parasympathetic in the sacral segments) lie in the intermediate horn, and the sensory cell bodies lie in the dorsal root ganglia.[5]

Four spinal cord functions are clinically relevant to the neurologist: transmission of proprioception, motor function, bladder function, and transmission of deep pain perception. Most spinal cord injuries result from compressive lesions, as in the case of disc extrusion; in such cases, some or all of the spinal cord functions may be lost, typically in the order listed above (proprioception is lost first, followed by motor function, bladder control, and deep pain perception).[1,3,4]

The spinal cord is divided into segments. With few exceptions, a specific spinal cord segment lies cranial to the vertebral body carrying the same name. This is an important concept to keep in mind when interpreting neurological findings to ensure a correct neurolocalization. Each spinal cord segment receives sensory information from a specific surface area of the body (dermatometer) and conveys motor input to a specific group of muscle fibers. It is important to remember that for spinal cord lesion localization, we refer to the spinal cord segment, not the vertebral body.

Functionally, the spinal cord is divided into five regions:

- C1–C5: cervical region
- C6–T2: cervicothoracic region
- T3–L3: thoracolumbar region
- L4–S3: lumbosacral region
- Cd1–5: caudal or coccygeal region

This division is based on the observation that lesions within the same region tend to cause consistent clinical signs. Also, it should be noted that when assessing spinal cord lesions, the neurological deficits develop caudal to the lesion.

When evaluating a spinal cord lesion, it is important to first determine whether the lesion affects all four limbs or only the pelvic limbs. In the former case, the lesion localization should be cranial to T3; in the latter case, the lesion is localized in any spinal cord segment caudal to T2. Evaluation of the spinal reflexes will help the clinician to further localize the lesion to one of the aforementioned regions.

Cervical region, C1–C5 spinal cord segments

Lesions at this level may cause gait abnormalities in all four limbs including, depending on the severity, proprioceptive ataxia, and tetraparesis/-paralysis. In lateralizing lesions, gait dysfunction can be confined to the limbs on the ipsilateral side of the body and produce, in severe cases, hemi-paresis/paralysis. Lesions in the C1–C5 spinal cord segments will interfere with the UMN pathway reaching both the thoracic and pelvic limbs, leading to normal or increased muscle tone and normal or increased spinal reflexes in all four limbs (thoracic and pelvic) (Fig. 10.2A). Spinal reflexes are not reduced/absent because the lesion does not involve the spinal cord intumescences. However, it should be noted that a reduced thoracic limb flexor reflex may be observed in approximately 30% of cervical (C1–C5) lesions.[11] Muscle atrophy in cervical lesions usually develops in chronic stages and is due to disuse, not to denervation. It is also important to note that the phrenic nerve originates in this region, more specifically from cell bodies in the C5–C7 spinal cord segments. Severe lesions in these segments can therefore lead to respiratory (diaphragmatic) dysfunction.

Urinary retention, although uncommon, may be observed.

Cervicothoracic region C6–T2 spinal cord segments

Lesions at this level also have the potential to cause gait abnormalities in all four limbs including, depending on the severity, proprioceptive ataxia, and tetraparesis/-paralysis. In case of lateralizing lesions, gait dysfunction may only affect the limbs on the ipsilateral side of the body and produce, in severe cases, hemi-paresis/paralysis. It should be noted that lesions in the C6–T2 spinal cord segments will interfere with the LMN system in the thoracic limbs and simultaneously affect the UMN system reaching the pelvic limbs. This may result in decreased to absent

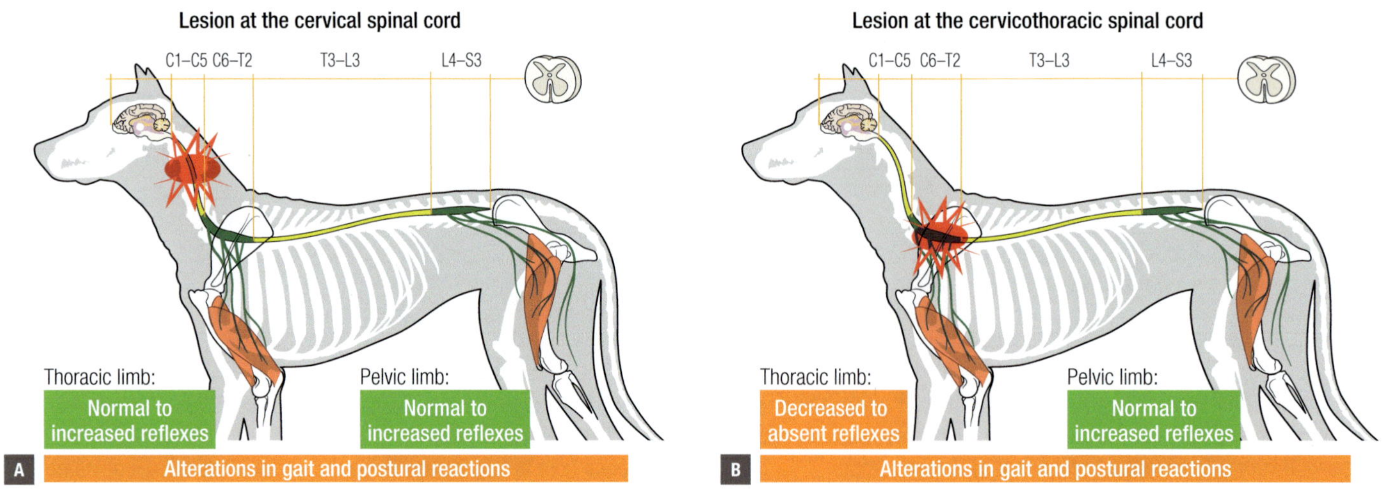

FIG. 10.2 Illustration showing the clinical presentation in the case of a lesion affecting the cervical (A) or cervicothoracic (B) spinal cord.

muscle tone and decreased to absent spinal reflexes in the thoracic limbs, and normal to increased muscle tone and normal to increased spinal reflexes in the pelvic limbs (Fig. 10.2B). The C6–T2 segments are also known as the cervical intumescence, since the cell bodies of the neurons that form the brachial plexus nerves reside in the grey matter of this region. This is why a lesion at this level can affect the LMNs reaching the thoracic limbs. The cutaneous trunci reflex may be absent with lesions affecting the caudal segments of the C6–T2 region, given that the lateral thoracic nerve (efferent arm of this reflex) originates from neurons in the C8–T1 segments.

The LMNs are somatotopically arranged, so that the most cranial segments of the intumescence supply the cranial and proximal muscles of the limbs and the caudal segments supply the caudal and distal muscles. In severe lesions, neurogenic muscle atrophy in C6–T2 lesions may develop rapidly in the thoracic limbs where the LMNs are compromised. Urinary retention, although not common, may be observed.

Thoracolumbar region, T3–L3 spinal cord segments

Lesions in this region will cause neurological deficits only in the pelvic limbs; the thoracic limbs will be normal. In the dog, the most common spinal cord lesions occur at the thoracolumbar level.

Lesions at this level may cause different degrees of gait abnormalities in the pelvic limbs including, depending on the severity, pelvic limb proprioceptive ataxia and paraparesis to paraplegia. The UMN axons directed to the pelvic limbs course through the T3–L3 region, and lesions at this level therefore have the potential to disrupt this system and cause normal to increased muscle tone and normal to increased spinal reflexes in the pelvic limbs (Fig. 10.3A). The presence of a cutaneous trunci reflex cutoff may further assist in narrowing down the lesion localization to the T3–L3 spinal cord segments. Another important clinical sign to be aware of is urinary retention. This is often associated with the severity of the spinal cord lesion and may represent an additional challenge in the management of paraplegic dogs.

In acute T3–L3 spinal cord injuries, a Schiff–Sherrington posture may be documented. This is due to disruption of the cell bodies of border cells (L2 to L4) or of their ascending tract, leading to thoracic limb disinhibition. Clinically, dogs display increased extensor tone in the thoracic limbs, which is more notable when the patient is in lateral recumbency. In such cases, it is important to note that the thoracic limbs are neurologically normal. The presence of a Schiff–Sherrington posture should not mislead the clinician in reaching the wrong neurolocalization.

Spinal shock is a phenomenon that can develop in peracute and acute severe myelopathies affecting the T3–L3 spinal cord segments. This phenomenon is characterized by a transient reduction in segmental spinal reflexes (lasting a few hours) and muscle tone (lasting up to several days) of the pelvic limbs, giving a false impression of a LMN (L4–S3) lesion.[11,12]

Lumbosacral region, L4–S3 spinal cord segments

The L4–S3 segments are also known as the lumbosacral intumescence. The cell bodies of the neurons that form the nerves supplying the pelvic limbs reside in the grey matter of this region. Lesions in this region will cause LMN dysfunction in the pelvic limbs, tail, perianal area, and bladder, which can manifest as reduced/absent muscle tone and reduced/absent spinal reflexes (Fig. 10.3B). Muscle atrophy may develop quickly. As in the cervical intumescence, the LMNs in the lumbosacral intumescence are somatotopically arranged, so that the most cranial segments of the intumescence supply the cranial and proximal muscles of the limbs and the caudal segments supply the caudal and distal muscles. The lumbosacral region can be further divided into the L4–L6 spinal cord segments, which give rise to the femoral nerve, and the L6–S3 spinal cord segments, which give rise to the sciatic (L6–S1), pudendal (S1–S3), and pelvic (S1–S3) nerves. Neurological deficits referrable to the femoral nerve (e.g., a reduced/absent patellar reflex and a reduced [proximal] withdrawal reflex) may be observed with lesions affecting the L4–L6 spinal cord segments. Neurological deficits referrable to the sciatic, pudendal, and pelvic nerves (e.g., a reduced/absent withdrawal reflex, a reduced/absent perianal reflex, and bladder dysfunction, respectively) can be seen with lesions affecting the L6–S3 spinal cord segments. Bladder dysfunction (urinary incontinence) and fecal incontinence may be present.[3,12]

Caudal or coccygeal region, Cd1–5 spinal cord segments

The cell bodies of the neurons that form the nerves supplying the tail reside in the grey matter of this region. Damage to these spinal cord segments may lead to the development of LMN dysfunction of the tail, flaccid paresis, or paralysis.

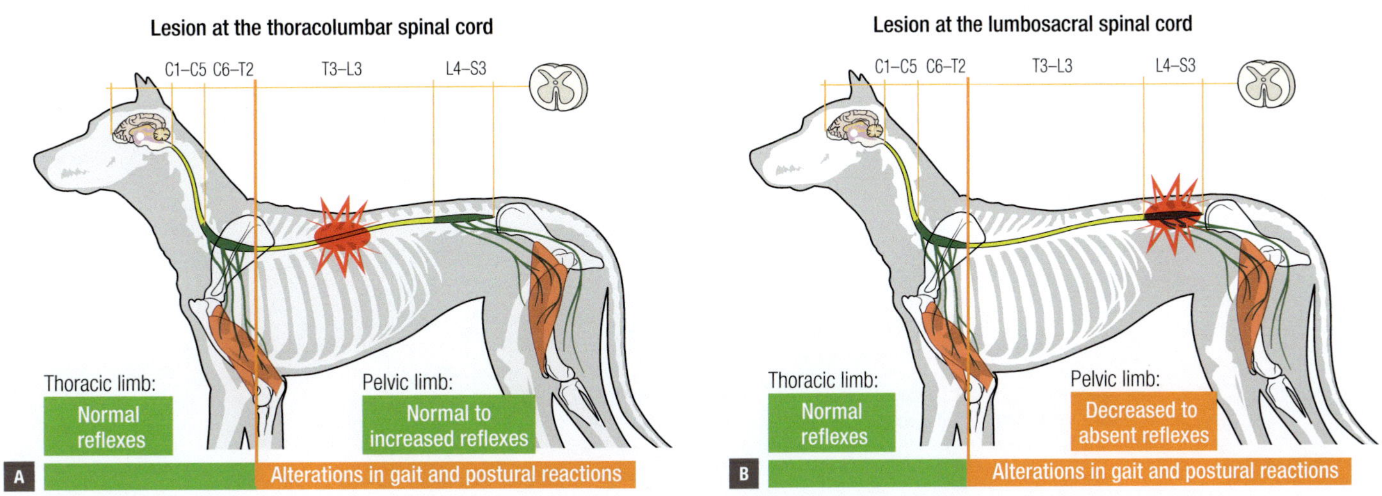

FIG. 10.3 Illustration showing the clinical presentation in the case of a lesion affecting the thoracolumbar (A) or lumbosacral (B) spinal cord.

Localization in the neuromuscular system (efferent part of the PNS)

The functional unit of the neuromuscular system is the motor unit, made of the LMN, its axon, the neuromuscular junction, and its innervated muscle fibers.

Since almost no spinal cord disorders selectively affect the LMN in the dog, in neurology, localization in the neuromuscular system refers to the efferent part of the PNS, which includes the peripheral nerves (including the cranial nerves), the neuromuscular junctions, and the muscles.[1–3]

The hallmark feature of a neuromuscular lesion localization is weakness, which can be focal or generalized and mild or severe depending on the distribution and severity of the lesion. Weakness produces gait dysfunction consistent with paresis in absence of primary ataxia. Dogs with neuromuscular disorders have normal mentation unless they are systemically unwell.

It is important to stress that, in many instances, it is not possible to differentiate, from a clinical point of view, between neuromuscular disorders affecting the nerve, the neuromuscular junction, or the muscle.

Peripheral nerves

The hallmark of peripheral neuropathies is LMN weakness, which is clinically manifest as reduced to absent muscle tone and reduced to absent reflexes, resulting in flaccid paresis/paralysis of the muscles supplied by the affected nerve or nerves and rapidly developing muscle atrophy (1–2 weeks).[3] One single nerve (mononeuropathy) or multiple nerves (polyneuropathy) can be affected depending on the underlying disease process.[13,14]

With very few exceptions (e.g., rare sensory neuropathies), primary ataxia is not a feature of polyneuropathies because only the efferent part of the nerve is affected. Postural reactions can be variably affected; however, they are normally preserved if the dog is adequately supported when tested.[5] The presence of motor deficits in the absence of abnormal postural reactions can help support a neuromuscular neurolocalization. Postural reactions will be, of course, absent in flaccid nonambulatory tetraparetic to tetraplegic dogs, as they are too weak to perform the correcting movement. Ambulatory patients may display a short-strided gait, difficulty to bear weight, and palmigrade and/or plantigrade stance. Polyneuropathies cause muscle tone and spinal reflexes to be significantly

TABLE 10.1 Clinical signs observed depending on the affected spinal cord segments.

Neurological examination	Spinal cord segments				
	C1–C5	C6–T2	T3–L3	L4–S3	Cd1–Cd5
Mental status	■ Normal	■ Normal	■ Normal	■ Normal	■ Normal
Posture	■ Normal, low head carriage possible	■ Normal, low head carriage possible	■ Normal, kyphosis possible ■ Schiff–Sherrington possible with peracute and acute myelopathies	■ Normal, kyphosis possible in lumbosacral region	■ Normal, kyphosis possible in lumbosacral region
Gait Sensory and motor functions	■ Proprioceptive ataxia all four limbs ■ Tetraparesis/-plegia ■ Hemiparesis/-plegia	■ Proprioceptive ataxia all four limbs ■ Tetraparesis/-plegia ■ Hemiparesis/-plegia ■ TLs may appear weaker than PLs	■ TLs normal ■ Proprioceptive ataxia in PLs ■ Paraparesis/-plegia	■ TLs normal ■ L4–L6 lesions: proprioceptive ataxia in PLs, mild paraparesis/-plegia possible ■ L7–S3 lesions: no ataxia, paraparesis only	■ TLs normal ■ No ataxia ■ Paresis/plegia of the tail
Postural reactions	■ May be reduced or absent in all four limbs or one side of the body with lateralizing lesions	■ May be reduced or absent in all four limbs or one side of the body with lateralizing lesions	■ Normal TLs ■ May be reduced or absent in PLs	■ Normal TLs ■ May be reduced or absent in PLs	■ Normal in TLs and PLs
Cranial nerves	■ Normal, possible Horner's syndrome	■ Normal, possible Horner's syndrome	■ Normal	■ Normal	■ Normal
Spinal reflexes and muscle tone	■ Normal to increased spinal reflexes and muscle tone in all four limbs	■ Reduced spinal reflexes and muscle tone in TLs particularly with C8–T2 lesions. ■ Normal to increased spinal reflexes and muscle tone in PLs	■ Normal TLs ■ Normal to increased spinal reflexes and muscle tone in PLs	■ Normal TLs ■ Reduced spinal reflexes and muscle tone in PLs	■ Normal TLs and PLs reflexes and muscle tone Hypotonic/flaccid tail
Bladder control	■ Usually preserved, possible urinary retention	■ Usually preserved, possible urinary retention	■ Urinary retention possible, usually associated with severe neurological dysfunction (paraplegia)	■ Loss of bladder control, sphincter hypo-/areflexia (urine leaking)	■ Normal

TLs, thoracic limbs; PLs, pelvic limbs.

decreased to absent in all four limbs. Significant weakness affecting the cervical muscles may also be observed, and dogs may be struggling to keep the head up. Generalized LMN weakness, together with adequate postural reactions leads to a LMN neurolocalization.[3]

Neuromuscular junction

Weakness is also the most important feature of a neuromuscular junction lesion localization (junctionopathy). Weakness in this group of conditions is due to a disruption in transmission between the nerve terminal and the muscle. Depending on the type of junctionopathy (presynaptic vs. postsynaptic) and severity of the clinical presentation, muscle tone and spinal reflexes may be variably affected. Presynaptic junctionopathies, such as botulism, cause an inadequate release of acetylcholine in the synaptic cleft and usually lead to rapid development of severe muscle hypotonia and reduced to absent reflexes, a clinical presentation that is very similar to polyneuropathies. The cranial nerves can also be involved. In postsynaptic junctionopathies, such as myasthenia gravis, acetylcholine is normally released in the synaptic cleft; however, this neurotransmitter cannot bind to its receptors. Myasthenia gravis can have different clinical presentations and is classified as focal, generalized, and fulminant. In dogs still able to walk, exercise-induced weakness/collapse (exercise intolerance) may be observed; this weakness usually improves following a short period of rest. In these dogs, reflexes may be initially normal but weaken or fatigue with repeated testing. In this case, they will return to normal following a period of rest. Regurgitation may be reported by the owners or observed during the examination due to the presence of megaesophagus.[3,15,16]

Muscles

Generalized myopathies can cause exercise intolerance, weakness, and muscle atrophy. Muscle pain, dysphagia, and regurgitation can also be observed depending on the underlying condition, its distribution, and the severity of the clinical presentation. Muscle tone can be normal, increased, or decreased depending on the condition and stage of the disease process (acute vs. chronic). Spinal reflexes are usually unaltered but may become reduced with severe muscle atrophy and fibrosis. Postural reactions are usually unaffected unless there is very severe weakness.[17,18]

Differential diagnoses

Once the history has been collected, the physical and neurological examinations have been performed, and a neurolocalization has been reached, the next critical step in the management of a neurological patient is to develop a list of differential diagnoses.

Not only will this help us choose the most appropriate diagnostic plan, it will also help us make sense of the results of our investigations. The risks of embarking on a diagnostic plan without a clear idea of what we are searching for are many; one of them is the risk of misinterpreting incidental findings as clinically relevant: an example is mistaking ventriculomegaly for clinical hydrocephalus. Diagnostic tests also represent a financial and emotional investment for the owners, who may feel frustrated and distressed if these tests are not necessary or meaningful. This may ultimately compromise trust in the vet–owner relationship.

In cases in which diagnostic tests cannot be performed (due to financial, logistic, or medical reasons), a prioritized list of differential diagnoses is also what allows us to draw a sensible empirical treatment plan.[19]

Reaching a prioritized list of differential diagnoses does not have to be daunting. All we need is to combine the information previously collected in the diagnostic process (signalment, history, neurolocalization) with our knowledge of how different disease processes affecting the nervous system naturally progress over time. Having a structured approach at this stage is essential, as the final goal of applying clinical reasoning is to systematically organize clinical information so that a prioritized list of differentials (by disease process) can be created.[19–22]

This task can be made easier using an acronym that includes all the disease processes affecting the nervous system. VITAMIN D or DAMNIT V are the most popular acronyms to establish a list of differentials in neurology.

For the purpose of this book, we will use the VITAMIN D mnemonic: vascular (ischemic or hemorrhagic), inflammatory or infectious, traumatic, anomalous, metabolic (nutritional and toxic), idiopathic, neoplastic, degenerative.

Each disease process may be associated with a specific signalment and have a specific onset, progression, distribution, and neurolocalization (Fig. 10.4). A peracute onset of nonprogressive (or spontaneously improving) cerebellar signs, for example, would point towards a vascular event as the most likely underlying disease process, while an insidious (chronic) onset of progressive cerebellar signs could indicate a neoplastic or degenerative process.

It is therefore important to always pay attention and enquire about the onset and progression of the clinical signs, as this is a fundamental step in the development of a prioritized list of differential diagnoses.

Vascular

Disruption of the vascular supply can lead to significant tissue damage in the affected CNS area. Vascular disorders can be secondary to ischemic events or, less commonly, due to the development of hemorrhage within the CNS. Vascular ischemic events usually present as peracute or acute; the clinical signs are typically static (nonprogressive) and spontaneous improvement usually occurs in the following 24–72 hours. The resulting neurological deficits are usually lateralized (focal and asymmetrical), and pain is not a typical feature.[23–25]

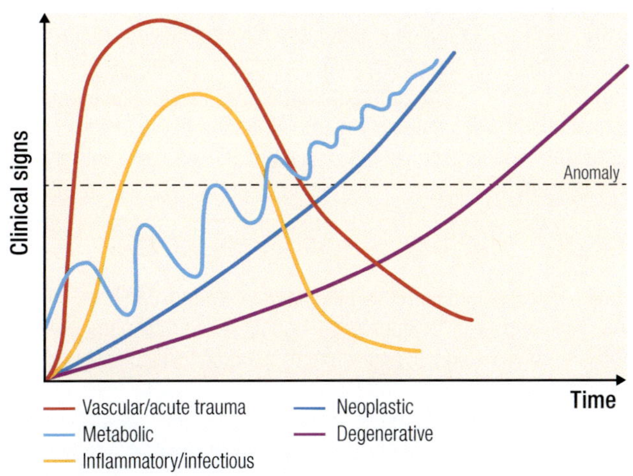

FIG. 10.4 Progression of clinical signs depending on the disease etiology. This graph illustrates what is commonly observed in most cases, but exceptions are seen in all categories.

Inflammatory and infectious

Inflammatory diseases can be secondary to a sterile inflammatory process (meningoencephalomyelitis of unknown origin),[26,27] or they may be due to an infection.[2] The onset of the clinical signs can range from acute to subacute and chronic. In a minority of cases, the clinical signs may also be reported to wax and wane in the early stages or have a very insidious onset. One common feature, however, is the progressive nature of the clinical signs if the patient is left untreated. The distribution of the lesions can vary from focal to multifocal, and pain may be present on palpation of the head or spine.

Traumatic

Trauma can be subdivided into exogenous and endogenous trauma.
Exogenous traumatic events, such as road traffic accidents or falls from heights, will cause a peracute/acute onset of clinical signs. Depending on the severity of the traumatic injury, the clinical signs may remain static or improve; however, deterioration is also possible in cases of edema or unstable fracture/luxation in spinal trauma. The distribution of the lesions will determine if the clinical signs are focal, multifocal, or diffuse. Pain can be a prominent and important feature in traumatic injuries.[2,3]
Endogenous trauma includes conditions such as acute intervertebral disc hernation and is characterized by an acute onset of often bilateral, although not necessarily symmetrical, possibly progressive neurological deficits. Endogenous trauma also includes degenerative structural disorders (e.g., degenerative lumbosacral stenosis, chronic disc protrusion, cervical stenotic myelopathy), which are characterized by an insidious onset and progressive signs.
It should be noted that some authors include structural degenerative disorders such as disc extrusion due to degenerative disc disease in the "degenerative" category.

Anomalous

Congenital malformations can affect the neuroparenchyma, as occurs in hydrocephalus or spinal cord dysraphism, or the surrounding bony structures such as the skull and vertebral column. Congenital malformations are not always clinically significant and need to be cautiously assessed in the context of the patient's clinical presentation.
When congenital malformations are clinically relevant, the clinical signs are often seen early in life and can have a static or, more rarely, a slowly progressive nature. Exceptions exist, however; an example is the sudden onset of peracute/acute signs due to the exacerbation of congenital atlantoaxial instability. The distribution of the lesions can be focal or diffuse depending on the specific diagnosis, and pain may be variably present.[2,5]

Metabolic (including nutritional and toxic)

Metabolic derangements affecting the nervous system can have multiple causes, including organ failure (e.g., hepatic encephalopathy), energy metabolism issues (e.g., hypoglycemia), electrolyte disturbances, and hormonal imbalances. Even though many of these metabolic derangements can be chronic, the onset of neurological signs is often acute, with a waxing and waning pattern, particularly in the early stages. Pain is not a feature. Intracranial structures (more commonly the forebrain) and the PNS can be affected.[2]

Nutritional disorders usually cause bilateral, symmetrical neurological signs that are acute (occasionally insidious) in onset and progressive in nature if not addressed. Some nutritional disorders, such as thiamine deficiency, can affect targeted areas in the CNS. Although pain is not a common feature, nutritional disorders such as nutritional hyperparathyroidism can lead to pathological bone (vertebral) fractures and severe pain.[28]
The "metabolic disorder" category also includes toxic disorders. They are typically characterized by an acute onset of diffuse and symmetrical neurological signs. A multitude of toxins exist that can lead to various degrees of intracranial structure dysfunction.

Idiopathic

Several idiopathic conditions affecting the nervous system have been identified, including idiopathic facial nerve paralysis, idiopathic vestibular syndrome, and idiopathic epilepsy. The clinical signs in this category tend to have an acute onset and generally a benign, self-limiting nature.[2]
Great variability however exists between these syndromes, and for the "idiopathic" category, it is not possible to define common characteristics in terms of onset and progression of clinical signs.

Neoplastic

Both primary and metastatic tumors can affect the nervous system. Middle-aged to older dogs are mainly affected, and the clinical signs typically have a chronic onset and progressive nature. An acute onset of clinical signs is sometimes observed, particularly with the forebrain neurolocalization. Factors contributing to acute deterioration of a chronic condition include a mass lesion reaching a critical size and a consequent lack of residual intracranial compensatory mechanisms (Monro–Kellie law), the sudden development of a spontaneous intratumor hemorrhage (e.g., pituitary apoplexy), or vascular compromise secondary to mass effect. The clinical signs can reflect a focal lesion; however, multifocal or diffuse localizations are possible. The CNS and PNS can be affected, and pain can be variably detected.[2,5]

Degenerative

Those degenerative conditions that primarily affect the nervous tissue fall under the degenerative disease category. Most of them have an underlying genetic base (e.g., lysosomal storage diseases, mitochondrial encephalopathies, organic acidurias, degenerative myelopathy). They are characterized by a chronic, progressive, bilateral (symmetrical or asymmetrical) nonpainful presentation. Given the hereditary/familial nature of many of these conditions, the patient's signalment is a crucial piece of information. These diseases can have both a juvenile and late onset (e.g., degenerative myelopathy).[3,12] An important senile degenerative disorder is senile cognitive dysfunction, which has an insidious onset and slowly progressive course.[29,30]
It is undoubtedly difficult to clearly classify these diseases as "traumatic" or "degenerative". Acute endogenous trauma, such as intervertebral disc extrusion, does not produce strictly degenerative lesions of the nervous tissue; in disc extrusion, the true degenerative process is that affecting the disc, not the nervous tissue. Chronic endogenous trauma producing chronic micropressures on adjacent neural tissues (as in cervical stenotic myelopathy) can cause degeneration of the more superficial white matter of the spinal cord.

KEY POINTS

- The neuroanatomical localization of a lesion is a fundamental step-by-step process to be taken at the end of the neurological examination.
- A neurological lesion can be localized to the CNS (intra- or extracranial) or PNS (nerve, neuromuscular junction, or muscle); some lesions may have a multifocal localization.
- Intracranial CNS lesions can be furtherly localized to the forebrain, brainstem, or cerebellum.
- Extracranial CNS lesions can be localized to the cervical (C1–C5), cervicothoracic (C6–T2), thoracolumbar (T3–L3), lumbosacral (L4–S3), or caudal (Cd 1–5) segments of the spinal cord.
- Spinal reflexes are important to determine whether a lesion is localized to the neuromuscular system or to the segments of the spinal cord. However, they are not important in assessing the severity of a lesion.
- VITAMIN D and DAMNIT V are two acronyms that can be used to establish a list of the possible differential diagnoses.
- The onset and progression of the clinical signs are of crucial importance to create a prioritized list of differential diagnoses.

References

1. Thomson C, Hahn C. *Veterinary Neuroanatomy: A Clinical Approach. Veterinary Neuroanatomy.* Edinburgh: Saunders Elsevier; 2012.
2. Platt SR, Olby NJ. *BSAVA Manual of Canine and Feline Neurology.* 4th ed. Gloucester, UK: British Small Animal Veterinary Association; 2013.
3. Dewey Curtis W, Da Costa Ronaldo C. *Practical Guide to Canine and Feline Neurology.* 3rd ed. Ames, Iowa, USA: Wiley Blackwell; 2016.
4. Uemura E. *Fundamentals of Canine Neuroanatomy and Neurophysiology.* Ames, Iowa, USA: Wiley Blackwell; 2015.
5. de Lahunta A, Glass E, Kent M. *Veterinary Neuroanatomy and Clinical Neurology.* 4th ed. St. Louis, MO: Elsevier Saunders; 2015.
6. Loncarica T, Balducci F, Bernardini M. Prevalence of idiopathic epilepsy and structural epilepsy in 74 Boxer dogs in a referral hospital. *Front Vet Sci.* 2022 Aug 19;9:956648.
7. Bush W, Barr C, Darrin E, et al. Results of cerebrospinal fluid analysis, neurologic examination findings, and age at the onset of seizures as predictors for results of magnetic resonance imaging of the brain in dogs examined because of seizures: 115 cases (1992–2000). *J Am Vet Med Assoc.* 2002 Mar 15;220(6):781–784.
8. Evans HE, de Lahunta A. *Miller's Anatomy of the Dog.* 4th ed. St. Louis, Missouri: Elsevier Saunders; 2013.
9. Crawford AH, Beltran E, Lam R, Kenny PJ. Convergence-Retraction Nystagmus Associated with Dorsal Midbrain Lesions in Three Dogs. *J Vet Intern Med.* 2016 Jul 1;30(4):1229–1234.
10. Khan Z, Munro E, Shaw D, Faller KM. Variation in the position of the conus medullaris and dural sac in adult dogs. *Vet Rec.* 2019 Jul 6;185(1):20.
11. Forterre F, Konar M, Tomek A, et al. Accuracy of the withdrawal reflex for localization of the site of cervical disk herniation in dogs: 35 cases (2004-2007). *J Am Vet Med Assoc.* 2008 Feb 15;232(4):559–563.
12. Lorenz MD, Coates JR, Kent M. *Handbook of Veterinary Neurology.* Saint Louis, Mo: Elsevier/Saunders; 2011.
13. Cuddon PA. Electrophysiologic assessment of acute polyradiculoneuropathy in dogs: comparison with Guillain-Barré syndrome in people. *J Vet Intern Med.* 1998 Jul-Aug;12(4):294–303.
14. Añor S. Acute lower motor neuron tetraparesis. *Vet Clin North Am Small Anim Pract.* 2014 Nov;44(6):1201–22.
15. Shelton GD. Myasthenia gravis and disorders of neuromuscular transmission. *Vet Clin North Am Small Anim Pract.* 2002 Jan;32(1):189–206, vii.
16. Shelton GD. Myasthenia gravis and congenital myasthenic syndromes in dogs and cats: A history and mini-review. *Neuromuscul Disord.* 2016 Jun;26(6):331–334.
17. Glass EN, Kent M. The clinical examination for neuromuscular disease. *Vet Clin North Am Small Anim Pract.* 2002 Jan;32(1):1–29, v.
18. Podell M. Inflammatory myopathies. *Vet Clin North Am Small Anim Pract.* 2002 Jan;32(1):147-167.
19. Maddison JE, Volk HA, Church DB. *Clinical Reasoning in Small Animal Practice.* Chichester, West Sussex: Wiley-Blackwell; 2015.
20. Cardy TJ, De Decker S, Kenny PJ, Volk HA. Clinical reasoning in canine spinal disease: what combination of clinical information is useful? *Vet Rec.* 2015 Aug 15;177(7):171.
21. Harrison E, Grapes NJ, Volk HA, De Decker S. Clinical reasoning in canine vestibular syndrome: Which presenting factors are important? *Vet Rec.* 2021 Mar;188(6):e61.
22. Gruppen LD. Clinical Reasoning: Defining It, Teaching It, Assessing It, Studying It. *West J Emerg Med.* 2017 Jan;18(1):4–7.
23. Garosi LS. Cerebrovascular disease in dogs and cats. *Vet Clin North Am Small Anim Pract.* 2010 Jan;40(1):65–79.
24. Garosi L, McConnell JE, Platt SR, et al. Results of diagnostic investigations and long-term outcome of 33 dogs with brain infarction (2000-2004). *J Vet Intern Med.* 2005 Sep-Oct;19(5):725–731.
25. Wessmann A, Chandler K, Garosi L. Ischaemic and haemorrhagic stroke in the dog. *Vet J.* 2009 Jun;180(3):290–303.
26. Granger N, Smith PM, Jeffery ND. Clinical findings and treatment of non-infectious meningoencephalomyelitis in dogs: a systematic review of 457 published cases from 1962 to 2008. *Vet J.* 2010 Jun;184(3):290–297.
27. Talarico LR, Schatzberg SJ. Idiopathic granulomatous and necrotising inflammatory disorders of the canine central nervous system: a review and future perspectives. *J Small Anim Pract.* 2010 Mar;51(3):138–149.
28. Tal M, Parr JM, MacKenzie S, Verbrugghe A. Dietary imbalances in a large breed puppy, leading to compression fractures, vitamin D deficiency, and suspected nutritional secondary hyperparathyroidism. *Can Vet J.* 2018 Jan;59(1):36–42.
29. MacQuiddy B, Moreno JA, Kusick B, McGrath S. Assessment of risk factors in dogs with presumptive advanced canine cognitive dysfunction. *Front Vet Sci.* 2022 Oct 18;9:958488.
30. Osella MC, Re G, Odore R, et al. Canine cognitive dysfunction syndrome: Prevalence, clinical signs and treatment with a neuroprotective nutraceutical. *Appl Anim Behav* Sci. 2007 Jul;105(4):297–310.

Laboratory investigations

Giulia Cagnotti
DVM, MRCVS, PhD, DECVN

The laboratory evaluation of dogs affected by neurological diseases is often complicated. Primary diseases of the nervous system rarely exhibit specific minimum database findings. However, the minimum database can prove extremely useful when systemic illnesses that may cause central nervous system (CNS) involvement are suspected, such as metabolic or infectious diseases.

A routine standard minimum database is also essential in the diagnostic workup of patients with neuromuscular signs. In these patients, a complete blood count (CBC), biochemistry panel, and urinalysis can help identify systemic abnormalities that may result in neuromuscular weakness and/or exercise intolerance, such as severe anemia and electrolyte imbalances, endocrinopathies, or myopathies.

The wide range of available assays and the common finding of nonsignificant abnormalities for the problem at hand are two other challenges of clinical pathology applied to neurology. The veterinarian should always assess the relevance and significance of laboratory data in conjunction with other clinical findings and diagnostic tests results.

Standard minimum database

A minimum database should always be included in the diagnostic workup of neurological patients to assess their general health status, before moving to more invasive diagnostic procedures such as magnetic resonance imaging (MRI), cerebrospinal fluid (CSF) sampling, and electrodiagnostic investigations. A minimum database may also serve as an initial point in the monitoring of patients undergoing treatment or suggest metabolic or infectious diseases that may also involve the nervous system. The standard minimum database generally includes a CBC and examination of blood smears, serum biochemistry, and a urinalysis.[1–3]

Complete blood cell count (CBC)

CBC abnormalities include changes in red blood cells (RBCs), white blood cells (WBCs), and platelets (PLTs). Both increased and decreased concentrations of RBCs, namely polycythemia and anemia, may be directly or indirectly associated with neurological signs.

While polycythemia is usually associated with a hyperviscosity syndrome due to a myeloproliferative disorder (either primary or secondary to cardiovascular, renal, or neoplastic disease), anemia can occur in a variety of pathological conditions and can be classified as regenerative or nonregenerative. An algorithm for interpreting anemia in relation to the most frequently associated neurological disorders in dogs is shown in Figure 11.1.

An increase in WBCs, or leukocytosis, is a common finding in infectious diseases as well as in some metabolic disorders. The most common changes include neutrophilia with lymphopenia, monocytosis, and eosinopenia. An algorithm for their interpretation in canine neurology is shown in Figure 11.2. An exception to this general rule is the occurrence of malignant leukocytosis (leukemia), for which further diagnostic tests such as cytofluorometry or polymerase chain reaction for antigen receptor rearrangements (PARR) are needed.

A reduced number of WBCs in the bloodstream is defined as leukopenia. Neutropenia is usually encountered in cases of severe sepsis or endotoxemia, while an absolute lymphopenia (associated with neutropenia or neutrophilia with a left shift and toxic changes) and mild anemia are typical of the viremic phase of viral infections and are commonly observed in acute canine distemper. In this case, eosinophilic RBC and WBC inclusions may be found on cytological evaluation.

The term thrombocytopenia defines a decrease in circulating PLTs. If severe enough (<30,000 PLTs/µL), it may be the cause of spontaneous bleeding that could involve the CNS. However, thrombocytopenia in a patient with neurological signs is most commonly associated with increased PLT consumption during an infectious process (see Figs. 11.1 and 11.2).

Serum biochemistry

To facilitate the interpretation of the biochemistry panel, the tested parameters can be grouped together based on the body system or physiological process to allow for pattern recognition. Grouping tests can also aid in the selection of additional tests to identify disease processes. One possible way of grouping basic chemistry tests in relation to the most common neurological disorders may be as follows:

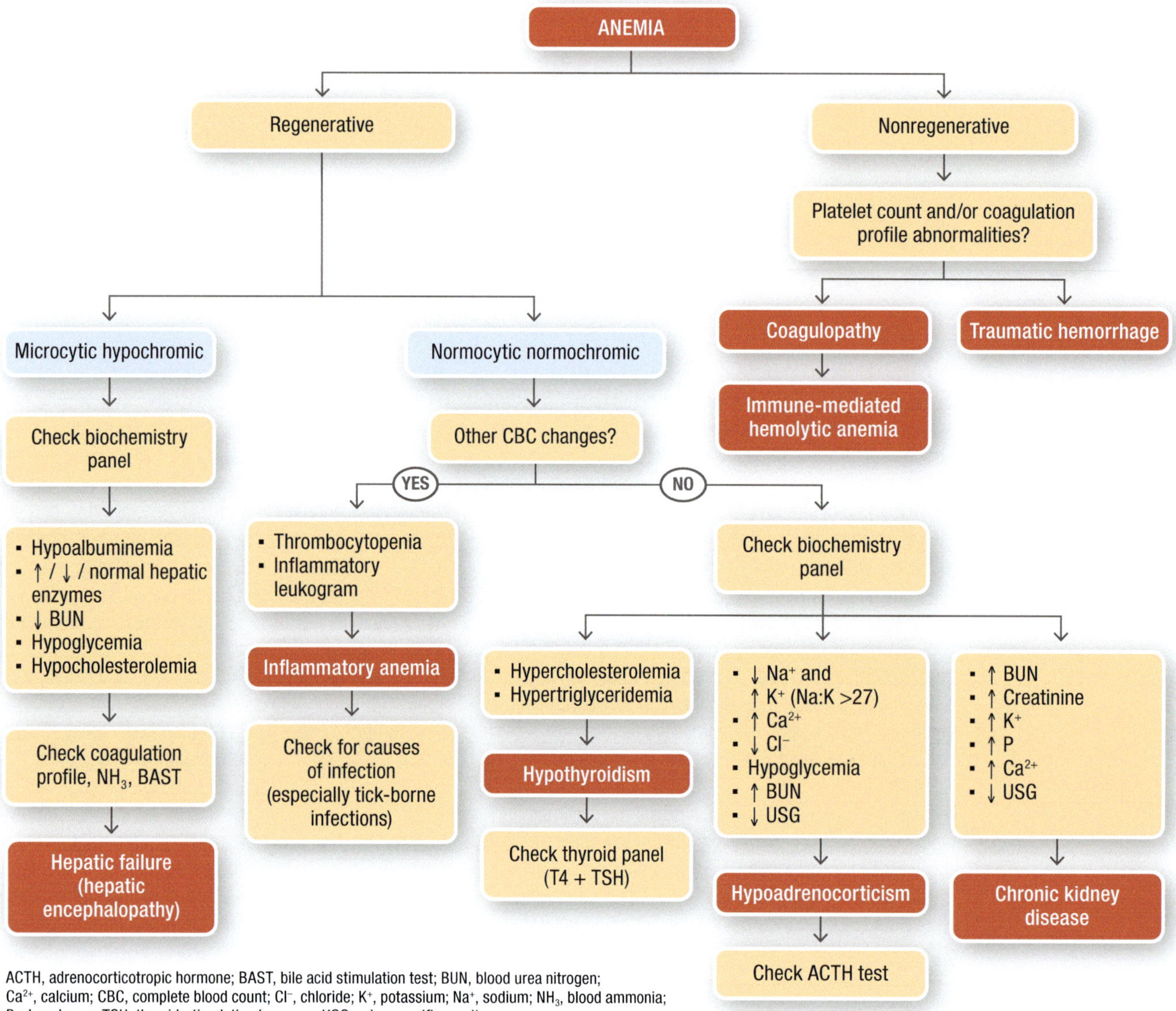

ACTH, adrenocorticotropic hormone; BAST, bile acid stimulation test; BUN, blood urea nitrogen; Ca^{2+}, calcium; CBC, complete blood count; Cl^-, chloride; K^+, potassium; Na^+, sodium; NH_3, blood ammonia; P, phosphorus; TSH, thyroid-stimulating hormone; USG, urine specific gravity.

FIG. 11.1 Algorithm for the interpretation of anemia in relation to the most frequently associated neurological diseases in dogs.

- Electrolytes and glucose: sodium (Na^+), potassium (K^+), chloride (Cl^-), magnesium (Mg^{2+}), calcium (Ca^{2+}), phosphorus (P), and glycemia.
- Protein metabolism: albumin, globulin, and serum protein electrophoresis (SPE).
- Kidney function: blood urea nitrogen (BUN) and creatinine (to be assessed in conjunction with protein metabolism, electrolytes, and urinalysis).
- Liver function: hepatic enzymes, bilirubin, blood ammonia concentration (NH3), and bile acid stimulation test (BAST) (to be assessed in conjunction with protein metabolism and coagulation profile).
- Muscle injury: creatine kinase (CK) and aspartate aminotransferase (AST).

Electrolyte and glucose

Electrolyte and glucose abnormalities that can cause neurological signs in dogs are reported in Table 11.1.

Protein metabolism

Serum total protein consists of albumin and globulins. Disturbances in albumin concentrations are generally not associated with neurological signs. However, hyperglobulinemia, while not primarily associated with neurological signs, can be suggestive of systemic diseases that may affect the nervous system. More particularly, two abnormal patterns can be recognized in this context:

- Polyclonal gammopathy: It indicates an acquired immune response to an antigenic stimulus, inflammation, or infection and is the result of immunoglobulin production by lymphocytes B, which occurs up to 7–10 days after the antigenic stimulus. This results in an increase in both β and γ globulins. Many pathological conditions can result in a polyclonal gammopathy, including systemic chronic infectious or immune-mediated diseases and systemic neoplasia.
- Monoclonal gammopathy: In this case, a single clone of immunoglobulins is produced by lymphocytes B or plasma cells and results in a

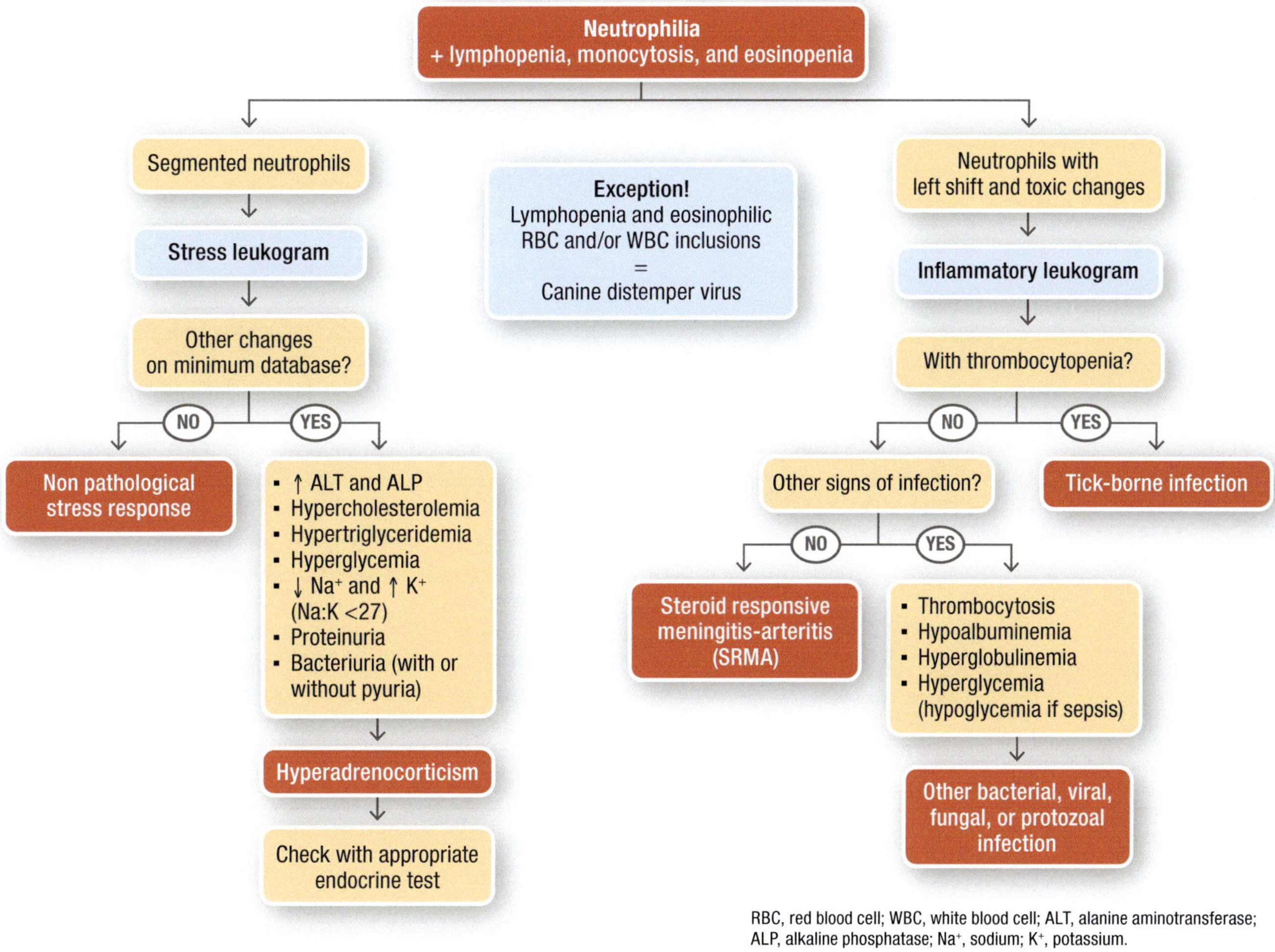

FIG. 11.2 Algorithm for the interpretation of leukocytosis in relation to the most frequently associated neurological diseases in dogs.

specific peak of the β or γ region of the electrophoretogram. In canine neurology, the most common causes include neoplastic disorders of lymphocytes or plasma cells that can involve the CNS (i.e., leukemias, lymphoma, plasmacytoma, multiple myeloma).

Acute-phase proteins (APPs) are a class of blood proteins that can increase (positive APPs) or decrease (negative APPs) in response to inflammation. C-reactive protein (CRP) is a marker of acute inflammation and may aid in differentiating inflammatory from immune-mediated neurological diseases. CRP is usually increased in steroid responsive meningitis-arteritis (SRMA), but there is debate as to the diagnostic value of its concentration in meningoencephalitis of unknown origin (MUO).[4]

Kidney function

Renal function is primarily assessed by combining the results of serum biochemistry (BUN and creatinine), which are indicators of glomerular function, with those of urinalysis to evaluate tubular function. Increased concentrations of serum creatinine and BUN, indicative of renal failure, may lead to neurological sequelae. Indeed, uremic encephalopathy is one of the most severe complications of renal failure in humans and has been reported anecdotally in dogs.[5]

Liver function

The assessment of liver function requires interpreting biochemistry findings in conjunction with the CBC and urinalysis results. The hepatic enzymes found in a biochemistry panel can be categorized as follows:

- Alanine aminotransferase (ALT) and aspartate aminotransferase (AST): found in high concentrations in the hepatocytes, released in case of injury. ALT is considered largely liver-specific, whereas AST is present in both the liver and the skeletal muscles.
- Alkaline phosphatase (ALP) and gamma-glutamyl transferase (GGT): biliary epithelial cell membrane-associated enzymes, induced (ALP) or released from the membrane (GGT) in cholestasis.

Neurological signs of liver failure, referred to as hepatic encephalopathy, develop when liver function is compromised due to organ failure, hepatic microvascular dysplasia, or portosystemic shunt. Abnormalities in liver enzyme concentrations alone are not sufficient to detect liver dysfunction, and they must be supported by abnormal liver function tests, namely serum bile acid (SBA) and NH_3 testing.[6,7]

Serum bile acids (SBAs)

In companion animals, a BAST, which involves the evaluation of both fasting and postprandial samples, is suggested in case of suspected hepatic failure as its sensitivity is superior to that of the single measurement

TABLE 11.1 List of the main electrolyte and glucose abnormalities responsible for neurological signs in dogs.

Substrate	CNS (seizures and intracranial abnormalities)	PNS (weakness)
Glucose	**Hypoglycemia** <2.5 mmol/L (<45 mg/dL) **Hyperglycemia** >55.5 mmol/L (>1,000 mg/dL)	**Hypoglycemia** <2.5 mmol/L (<45 mg/dL)
Na^+	**Hyponatremia** <125 mmol/L **Hypernatremia** >170 mmol/L	
K^+		**Hypokalemia** <3 mmol/L **Hyperkalemia** >8 mmol/L
Ca^{2+}	**Hypocalcemia** tCa <1.6 mmol/L (<6.5 mg/dL) iCa <0.8 mmol/L (<3.2 mg/dL) **Hypercalcemia** tCa >3.5–4 mmol/L (>14–16 mg/dL) iCa >1.6 mmol/L (> 6.4 mg/dL)	**Hypocalcemia** (*clinical sign: muscle cramps*) tCa <1.6 mmol/L (<6.5 mg/dL) iCa <0.8 mmol/L (<3.2 mg/dL) **Hypercalcemia** tCa >3.5–4 mmol/L (>14–16 mg/dL) iCa >1.6 mmol/L (>6.4 mg/dL)
P		**Hypophosphatemia** <0.32 mmol/L (<1 mg/dL)
Mg^{2+}		**Hypomagnesemia** <0.4 mmol/L (<1 mg/dL)

CNS, central nervous system; PNS, peripheral nervous system; Na^+, sodium; K^+, potassium; Mg^{2+}, magnesium; Ca^{2+}, calcium; P, phosphorus; tCa, total calcium; iCa, ionized calcium.

of a fasting sample. The fasting sample must be collected usually after an overnight fast, while the postprandial sample should be taken 2 hours after the patient has eaten a small fatty meal. Both samples should be collected into tubes with no anticoagulants, and prompt separation of the serum should be performed.

In case of lipemia and hemolysis, SBA concentrations should be interpreted with caution because these disorders can cause falsely increased or decreased results, respectively. These concentrations may also be falsely lower in animals younger than 16 weeks of age.

Both fasting and postprandial SBA concentrations are typically moderately to markedly elevated in cirrhosis, while in portovascular anomalies fasting SBA concentrations can sometimes be normal or mildly elevated, and postprandial concentrations are typically moderately to markedly elevated.[8] One study has reported the sensitivity and specificity of fasting SBA measurements for diagnosing portosystemic shunts (cutoff value of 20 mmol/L) to be 93% and 67% in dogs, respectively.[7]

In up to 20% of dogs, higher fasting than postprandial values may be detected. This finding may be related to a recent meal, gallbladder contraction during fasting, or delayed gastric emptying.[9]

Blood ammonia (NH_3)

This test requires more complex sample handling and specific instrumentation that is not frequently available in general practice. It is also considered less sensitive than a BAST but can be of help in patients in which feeding is not feasible. For the diagnosis of hepatic failure, only increased values are useful. However, physiologically increased values can be observed after a high protein meal or strenuous exercise. The sensitivity of blood NH_3 levels for the detection of congenital portosystemic shunts has been reported to be 81–100% in dogs.[6] In patients with hepatic encephalopathy, however, the NH_3 concentration is not predictive of the severity of the clinical signs.

In summary, the typical abnormalities that can be identified on blood testing in hepatic encephalopathy are:[10]

- Increased bilirubin and SBA concentrations (due to increased uptake and excretion of bilirubin and bile acids).
- Increased blood NH_3 and reduced BUN concentrations (due to increased uptake and conversion of ammonia to urea).
- Hypocholesterolemia (due to altered lipid metabolism).
- Hypoglycemia (due to altered gluconeogenesis).
- Hypoalbuminemia and reduced production of coagulation factors (due to altered protein synthesis).
- Microcytic hypochromic anemia (due to altered iron homeostasis).

Although increased fasting ammonia and SBA concentrations are considered accurate indicators of a portosystemic shunt, it must be emphasized that the diagnosis of hepatic encephalopathy (in particular due to congenital and acquired portosystemic shunts) cannot be made on the basis of elevated SBAs alone but requires further confirmation.

Liver function should also be periodically monitored in epileptic patients receiving antiepileptic medications with hepatic metabolism, especially phenobarbital (PB). Indeed, chronic administration of PB results in increased serum activity of hepatic enzymes (ALP, ALT, and GGT) and hypoalbuminemia. It is however unclear whether these abnormalities reflect PB-mediated induction of hepatic enzymes or a real hepatocellular damage or cholestasis.[11]

Muscle injury

Indicators of muscle injury on the standard minimum database are AST and CK values. While AST elevations can be related to both hepatic and muscular damage, CK activity is considered a specific marker of myofiber damage.

As a rule, normal to mildly increased CK values (0–2,000 UI/L) can be found in focal myopathies (e.g., masticatory muscle myositis), endocrine myopathies, neuropathies, and nondystrophic congenital myopathies. Moderate increases in CK activity (2,000–20,000 UI/L) are usually indicative of generalized inflammatory myopathies, while marked increases (>20,000 UI/L) are typical of necrotizing and dystrophic myopathies.[12]

It is worth remembering that noninflammatory muscle disease such as trauma or epileptic seizures can also lead to increased AST and CK values.

Urinalysis

A routine urinalysis is part of the standard minimum database required in the management of neurological diseases. The results should always be interpreted in conjunction with those of the biochemistry panel, and urine and blood samples should be collected at the same time and before the administration of any kind of treatment, including fluid therapy.

Primary neurological diseases rarely, if ever, cause abnormalities on routine urinalysis. Generally, abnormal findings are seen with systemic diseases (especially endocrine and metabolic diseases) causing secondary neurological disorders (see Figs. 11.1–11.3). Pure proteinuria without any other abnormality can be observed in systemic infectious diseases or multiple myeloma (Bence Jones proteinuria).

Ammonium biurate crystalluria can be present in portosystemic shunts (except in Dalmatians and English Bulldogs), while calcium oxalate crystals can be seen in ethylene glycol intoxication.

CSF collection and analysis

CSF is the product of plasma ultrafiltration, mainly by the choroid plexi within the ventricular system, where it circulates and then flows caudally into the central canal of the spinal cord towards the cauda equina. Most of the CSF flows through the nervous parenchyma into the subarachnoid space, where it is reabsorbed into the venous system by the arachnoid villi.[13]

CSF analysis is a common, simple, and relatively inexpensive procedure, though it is rarely diagnostic by itself in CNS disorders. The presence of abnormalities depends not only on the type of pathological process but also on its location and extent. Usually, lesions involving the meninges and the ependymal layers cause the most dramatic CSF changes, while parenchymal, extradural, or nonexfoliative lesions are associated with only minimal or no alterations.[14] For this reason, quantitative CSF abnormalities are not correlated with the severity of the disease. CSF collection and analysis are therefore indicated in patients with CNS lesions, although the diagnostic value of CSF analysis alone is low. In a retrospective study in 256 dogs in which CSF analysis and MRI were performed, a specific etiological diagnosis was established in only 2% of CSF samples.[15]

As a general rule, congenital malformations, metabolic-toxic, idiopathic, or degenerative diseases are unlikely to cause CSF abnormalities, while relevant alterations may be found in infectious-inflammatory processes and some types of neoplasia (e.g., lymphoma, meningioma).[16]

In small animals, CSF collection can be performed from two sites:[8]

- The atlanto-occipital (AO) cistern (also called cerebellomedullary cistern or cisterna magna). This option is technically less challenging, carries a reduced risk of iatrogenic blood contamination, and ensures collection of an adequate sampling volume. However, it carries a risk of major complications, such as respiratory arrest due to iatrogenic brainstem trauma.
- The caudal lumbar (CL) region. The most common site of collection is between L5–L6; L6–L7 can also be considered in small breed dogs. Collection at L4–L5 is described in some textbooks and refers to large breed dogs. Collection at the CL region is safer than sampling from the AO cistern, but it is more difficult, with a higher risk of iatrogenic blood contamination. In addition, it usually allows the collection of only moderate amounts of fluid.

The choice between the two collection sites should be based on the information on feasibility and safety obtained from the MRI study and the clinical presentation. In focal CNS disorders, CSF sampling is more likely to be representative of the ongoing pathology if collected caudal to the lesion, due to the physiological direction of CSF flow in the CNS. Therefore, in patients with an intracranial pathology, AO collection is more appropriate, whereas the CL site is preferred in diseases involving the spinal cord.

Risks and contraindications

CSF collection is always performed under general anesthesia and therefore carries anesthesia-related risks. In addition, with AO collection, positioning of the head with ventroflexion of the neck may lead to inadvertent loss of airway patency due to kinking of the endotracheal tube. Both collection sites carry the risk of iatrogenic damage due to needle puncture of the underlying nervous parenchyma. While inadvertent penetration into the brainstem parenchyma when collecting CSF from the AO cistern may result in transitory vestibular signs or, in more severe cases, in respiratory arrest and death of the patient, CSF collection at the CL site, despite the high likelihood of puncturing the spinal cord/cauda equina, does not typically cause any relevant complications. In modern practice, CSF collection should always be performed after MRI. CSF sampling must be avoided in patients displaying clinical or MRI signs of increased intracranial pressure. If deemed necessary,

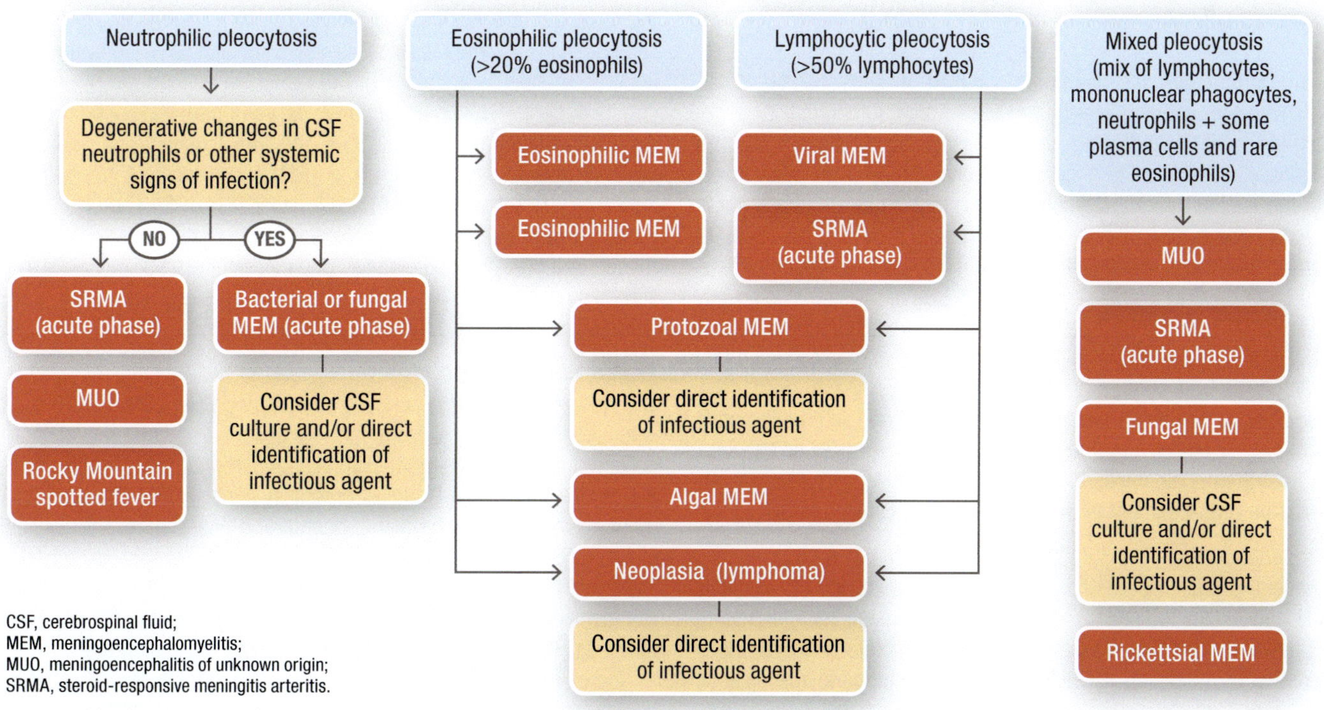

FIG. 11.3 Proposed interpretation for CSF pleocytosis in various CNS disorders.

medical interventions aimed at reducing the intracranial pressure (e.g., administration of mannitol or hypertonic saline solution or hyperventilation to maintain the $PaCO_2$ at approximately 30–35 mmHg) should be performed before CSF collection. CSF collection should be avoided in patients with suspected active intracranial hemorrhage, large lesions occupying the intracranial space, or severe hydrocephalus.

CSF sampling from the AO cistern is not recommended in patients with suspected or confirmed atlantoaxial instability, because the positioning needed for the procedure can severely worsen the clinical signs. Removal of an excessive volume of CSF should be avoided to prevent traumatic hemorrhage of the brain parenchyma or transtentorial or trans–foramen magnum herniation. It is commonly suggested to collect no more than 1 mL/5 kg of bodyweight. To avoid abrupt changes in CSF pressure that can also result in brain hemorrhage and herniation, aspiration of the CSF via a syringe directly from the spinal needle must be avoided.

Procedure

For both collection sites, the patient is placed in lateral recumbency as close as possible to the edge of the table, under general anesthesia. The site of collection is prepared by clipping and surgically scrubbing the area.

AO CSF collection

With the patient in lateral recumbency, the head is ventroflexed with the nose elevated to get the sagittal plane of the muzzle and the table parallel. There are two sets of anatomical landmarks for the identification of the correct site of needle insertion:

- Create an imaginary triangle between the external occipital protuberance and the rostral borders of the wings of the atlas on both sides. The point for needle insertion is at the base of the triangle, at the intersection between the line connecting the two rostral borders of the wings of the atlas and the midline.
- Create an imaginary triangle between the external occipital protuberance and the caudal borders of the wings of the atlas. The location for needle insertion is on the midline, one-third to halfway caudal to the occipital protuberance.

Once the appropriate site has been identified, a spinal needle with a stylet is inserted perpendicular to the skin surface. Although 22-gauge, 38 mm long spinal needles are usually used in small animals, 75 mm long spinal needles may be necessary in giant breed dogs. After insertion of the needle through the skin and the muscle layers, the stylet is removed to check for CSF flow and repositioned if no flow is observed. The needle is advanced slowly 1–2 mm at a time, and the procedure repeated until CSF flow is observed. A sudden loss of resistance is usually noted once the dura mater is penetrated. When the subarachnoid space is entered, CSF will appear in the needle hub. CSF can be collected into a sterile plastic tube by direct dripping.

In case of contact with a bony surface, the spinal needle can be gently retracted a few millimeters and redirected slightly cranially or caudally. If this fails, the needle needs to be removed and a second attempt performed after reassessment of the correct anatomical landmarks.

CL CSF collection

The patient is placed in lateral recumbency, and the lumbar spine is flexed by advancing the pelvic limbs cranially to increase the interarcuate space between the spinous processes. The correct intervertebral space is identified by palpating the iliac crests as a landmark: the spinous process found on the midline immediately cranial to that point is that of L6. The needle is then positioned immediately lateral to the midline at the level of the identified spinous process and inserted in an oblique fashion (30–60° from an imaginary line perpendicular to the long axis of the spine). The needle (22-gauge spinal needle with a length of 38, 75, or 90 mm depending on the patient's size) is then advanced slowly in an oblique cranioventral direction. A mild limb or tail twitch is elicited when passing through the caudal spinal cord or the cauda equina. CSF collection is then performed as described for AO collection.

In case of iatrogenic blood contamination, the first drops may be discarded in order to collect appropriate material for the analysis. In many instances, the blood flow is mild and self-limiting. If the blood contamination does not resolve, the procedure should be repeated from the beginning.

The minimum volume of CSF necessary for a complete analysis is 0.5 mL. It should be collected in a plastic tube and stored refrigerated, avoiding glass containers to prevent adhesion. If samples are hemorrhagic, EDTA tubes may be indicated to avoid clotting. The analysis must be performed within 30 minutes to 1 hour from the collection to preserve cytological details. When this is not feasible, several suboptimal methods have been proposed to preserve the diagnostic quality of canine CSF samples, including refrigeration at 4°C with addition of 10% fresh autologous serum, 20% fresh or frozen fetal calf serum, or 1:1 hetastarch or the use of a TransFix®/EDTA tube.[17] However, if the analysis is going to be delayed, it is recommended to divide the CSF sample into an unaltered aliquot for the assessment of the total nucleated cell count (TNCC) and the protein concentration, and a second aliquot with a preservative for cytological evaluation and differential cell count.[17]

Routine CSF analysis

Gross evaluation

Normal CSF must have the same characteristics as water: clear and colorless. Turbidity is related to an increase in cell number (usually over 200–500 WBCs/µL or 400–700 RBCs/µL) or in protein concentration. In this case, CSF may also become more viscous.

A red discoloration is usually associated with the presence of blood. In this case, it is important to determine whether it is iatrogenic or the result of a pathological hemorrhage. This distinction can be made by both gross and microscopic examination of the sample: a uniform red discoloration can be observed during collection in cases of pathological hemorrhage, while with iatrogenic contamination, the sample is initially colorless and becomes red during collection, and it is likely to clot if put in a plain tube. Xantochromia refers to yellow discoloration of the CSF and indicates the presence of bilirubin. In neurological disorders, xantochromia is mainly related to a previous hemorrhage that can persist for 2–4 weeks in the subarachnoid space. Xanthochromia has also been reported in severe icterus due to systemic hyperbilirubinemia.[8,14,17]

Protein concentration

The normal CSF protein concentration in dogs and cats is <25 mg/dL when CSF is collected from the AO cistern and <40 mg/dL if it is collected at the CL region, with albumin representing approximately 80–90% of the total protein content in normal CSF. However, since different methods for protein concentration assessment are available, results are best interpreted using reference values established by the individual laboratory. The methods described for protein concentration assessment include qualitative (turbidimetric) methods and quantitative methods. The latter are considered by far the most accurate.

An increase in protein concentration can be seen in disorders altering blood–brain barrier (BBB) permeability or in cases of intrathecal production of immunoglobulins. To distinguish between these two conditions, various calculated values have been proposed. Increases in the albumin quotient (AQ) ratio [(CSF albumin/serum albumin) × 100] suggest a disruption of the BBB, while an increase in the IgG index [CSF IgG/serum IgG) × (serum albumin/CSF albumin)] indicates intrathecal globulin production, typical of infectious diseases.[14]

Total RBC and WBC counts

In small animals, the normal CSF contains <5 WBCs/mm^3 and no RBCs.[14] The gold standard for RBC and WBC counts is manual counting using a specific hemocytometer. Recently, the use of automated hematological flow cytometric analyzers has been investigated for automated CSF cell counting in dogs. However, the results of the study do not support the use of these analyzers as an alternative to the manual counting system.[18]

The current literature provides conflicting data on whether blood contamination has a predictable effect on CSF analysis. As a general rule, the TNCC is considered likely reliable with an RBC contamination of up to 5,000 RBC/μL, but when the RBC count is >500/μL, the neutrophil and eosinophil percentages and protein concentration are unreliable.[17]

After determining the RBC and WBC counts, microscopic cytological evaluation of the sample is essential to determine cell morphology and identify potential etiological infectious agents (rarely) or neoplastic cells (especially in lymphoma). Cytological evaluation of CSF is usually performed on slides prepared using cytocentrifugation.

When a cytocentrifuge is not available, a sedimentation chamber can be constructed using a microscope slide, a filter paper, a 1 mL syringe, and a pair of paper clips. A hole of the same diameter as that of the syringe is made in the center of the filter paper. The plunger is removed from the syringe and the barrel of the syringe is cut in half to produce a cylinder open at both ends. The cylinder is then put on the microscope slide and the filter paper in correspondence to the hole. The construction is then secured by clamping the syringe barrel flanges with paper clips on both sides. The sedimentation chamber is then placed on a flat counter, 0.25–0.5 mL of CSF are dropped in the barrel and the chamber is left in place for at least 30 minutes. The fluid will be absorbed by the filter paper, while cells will remain attached to the microscope slide. The slide is then air-dried and routinely stained for cytological evaluation.[19]

Pleocytosis refers to an increased TNCC in CSF. Based on the predominating cell type on microscopic examination, it can be further classified as neutrophilic (>50% neutrophils), eosinophilic (>20% eosinophils), lymphocytic (>50% lymphocytes), and mixed (mixture of lymphocytes, neutrophils, and mononuclear cells with no predominant cell population). Figure 11.3 summarizes the types of CSF pleocytosis in various CNS disorders.

An increased protein concentration with a normal TNCC is defined as albuminocytological dissociation. This abnormal finding has been associated with a wide variety of neurological diseases and different pathophysiological mechanisms have been proposed, including intrathecal production of specific proteins, dysfunction of the BBB, decreased CSF flow, and sequestration of CSF in cases of spinal cord compression.

In addition to the classical analysis, CSF is an optimal substrate for the detection of antigens, antibodies, or, more recently, pathogenic DNA or RNA, which is critical for differentiating between immune-mediated inflammatory and infectious diseases of the CNS.

Infectious disease testing

Inflammatory diseases affecting the CNS in dogs can be due to infectious or immune-mediated causes. According to the available literature, immune-mediated conditions are considerably more common than infectious conditions, comprising over 80% of all inflammatory diseases affecting the CNS in dogs presented to referral centers.[20] The clinical diagnosis of these diseases is based on a combination of signalment, history, neurological examination, and ancillary diagnostic procedures such as blood work, MRI, and CSF analysis. In this context, infectious disease testing (on blood or, preferably, CSF samples) is of utmost importance to exclude infectious causes and allows the establishment of a prompt therapeutic protocol with immunosuppressive medications.

Diagnostic tests for infectious diseases can be broadly divided into:

- Organism detection tests: culture/isolation, antigen detection, pathogenic DNA or RNA detection with polymerase chain reaction (PCR) techniques.
- Antibody detection tests.

Optimizing the diagnosis may require the use of multiple tests simultaneously or sequentially. However, due to factors such as cost and time constraints, not all these diagnostic tests can be routinely performed. Therefore, it is essential for clinicians to carefully select the most appropriate test(s) considering the specific clinical situation.

Historically, serology, which involves the detection of antibodies, has been the primary method to determine exposure to infectious agents in dogs showing specific clinical signs. While serology remains important for diagnosing infectious diseases, it is best used alongside isolation or molecular diagnostic approaches for each organism and individual patient. Serology testing can be performed on serum, CSF, or both. Antibody testing is highly valuable as supportive evidence of infection, but certain factors such as previous exposure, vaccination against the agent, or cross-reactivity with antibodies from other infectious agents can weaken the information, potentially leading to an incorrect diagnosis of the cause of the neurological signs. Antibody titers only indicate exposure to the organism but do not confirm an active infection, as occurs in most cases of positive antibody titers against *Toxoplasma gondii*. Specifically, IgM and IgG antibodies reflect acute and chronic infection, respectively. To support the suspicion of a recent infection, antibody titers can be rechecked after 1–4 weeks to look for seroconversion (a 4-fold increase in the antibody titer, e.g., 1:4 to 1:16, 1:16 to 1:64).

While rarely employed in veterinary medicine, in cases in which there is suspicion of an infectious disease localized to the CNS, calculation of the antibody index (or IgG index) can be performed.

Typically, an elevated IgG index (>1.3) indicates an inflammatory condition. However, normal values may be found in some inflammatory diseases, and increased values can be observed in cases of neoplasia.

Antigen testing is not influenced by confounding factors typical of antibody testing. However, it may lack sensitivity as it requires the presence of the organism itself in the evaluated substrate. The advent of molecular diagnostic tests (e.g., PCR) applied to CSF has significantly enhanced the diagnosis of CNS infections. PCR is based on the precise identification of the pathogen's nucleic acid. Nonetheless, a negative PCR result does not definitively rule out an infection. A false negative result may occur if nucleic acids are present in the nervous parenchyma and not in the CSF, or if they are present in the CSF but at undetectable levels. Additionally, a PCR result could be negative if the disease was caused by a pathogen that is no longer present. Conversely, a positive PCR result does not always indicate active infection, as a pathogen's nucleic acids may be present in latent and subclinical infections or in recovered animals that still retain nonviable pathogens or free nucleic acids. Therefore, PCR results should also always be interpreted in conjunction with the patient's history, clinical signs, and results of other diagnostic tests.

TABLE 12.1 Terminology used in genomics.

Sequence	The string of nucleic acids in a gene or genome. The Sanger sequencing method is the gold standard for accurate DNA sequencing used to confirm other methods.
Reference sequence	The original whole genome sequence that was assembled for a species and provides the baseline from which variants are identified. The reference is updated regularly as new whole genome sequences are compiled. An allele in the reference sequence is often called the "wild-type" allele.
Variant	A portion of the gene sequence that is different from the reference sequence.
Mutation	A change that has occurred in the sequence of a gene that will be perpetuated. This can result in a benign variant, but the term is commonly used to denote a pathogenic variant.
Pathogenic variant	Term preferred by geneticists for a disease-causing variant. The mutation must meet criteria for demonstrating that it is indeed the cause and not a benign variant.
Single nucleotide polymorphisms (SNPs)	Variants where only a single nucleotide is substituted (e.g., A to G); SNPs are the most common type of variant. They are often benign and are used to identify differences between individual chromosomes for association studies. To be classified as pathogenic, they must be clearly associated with the disease and ideally shown to affect protein function and/or cause similar signs in other species or rodent models.
Whole genome sequence (WGS)	A read of the entire sequence of base pairs from an individual animal. It is assembled using the reference sequence and then can be compared to WGSs from other individuals to identify unique variants. Alternatively, only the exons can be sequenced, reducing costs (whole exome sequence).
Exon	A portion of DNA that codes for a section of the messenger RNA that is then translated into a protein (expressed).
Intron	A portion of DNA that is not translated into a protein and is spliced out before the RNA is translated into a protein. It may still contain important regulatory signals, but variants are generally thought to be benign.
Phenotype	The physical manifestation of a trait that can be influenced by genetics, epigenetics, or the environment.
Genotype	The genetic makeup of an individual with respect to a specific gene (allele).
Allele	One of the alternate forms of a gene or locus.
Locus	The location of a gene or genes on a chromosome; often used as a vague proxy for a gene in gene mapping studies before the specific gene is identified.
Recombination	As the pairs of chromosomes line up during meiosis, there can be breakage and exchange of portions between the pair. This results in a change in the sequence of alleles in the chromosomes.
Segregation	The separation of alleles during meiosis that determines which allele is passed to an offspring.
Phenocopy	When an animal shows signs of a hereditary disease but does not have the genotype associated with that disease. Some reserve the term for acquired diseases that mimic a genetic one, while others also apply it to different mutations producing a similar phenotype.

Source: O'Brien and Leeb, 2014.[1]

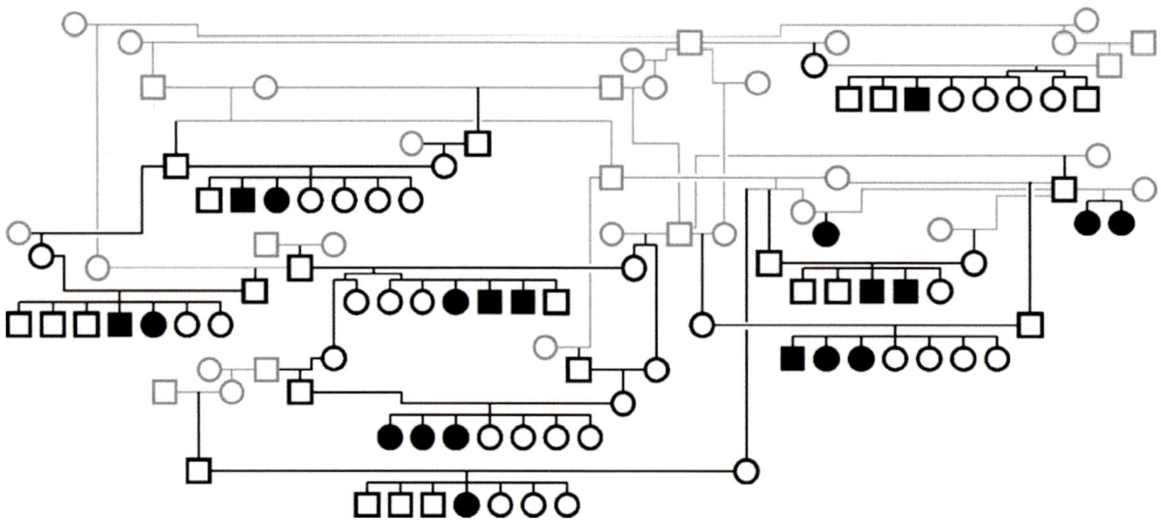

FIG. 12.1 Pedigree showing the spread of a pathogenic variant in family of dogs. Males are shown as squares, females as circles. Filled symbols represent affected dogs. Lines connecting a male and female horizontally indicate a breeding. Brackets extending vertically from that line represent the offspring of that breeding. A popular sire (square, top center) will spread unrecognized pathogenic variants that he carries along with the desirable traits that made him popular. It is not until second (F2) or later generations that the disease becomes apparent as two offspring that are carriers of the pathogenic variant breed producing affected pups. By then, those alleles may be widely disseminated in the population. Source: O'Brien, 2013.[5]

TABLE 12.2 General characteristics of some hereditary neurological diseases. Source: O'Brien, 2011.[6]

Congenital malformations	■ Neonatal or young onset of signs ■ Static or progressive signs ■ Other organs may be involved ■ Diagnosed on advanced imaging or necropsy
Organic acidurias	■ Neonatal or young onset ■ Waxing and waning encephalopathy ■ Dietary influences ■ Ketonuria, acidosis or anion gap, hypoglycemia, or hyperammonemia possible ■ Possible symmetric, gray-matter signal changes on magnetic resonance imaging (MRI) ■ Diagnosed on urine organic acid screens from specialized laboratories
Lysosomal storage diseases	■ Neonatal to middle age onset ■ Varying signs of ataxia, blindness, weakness, dementia, seizures ■ Inexorably progressive course ■ Possible symmetric atrophy on MRI ■ Diagnosed on necropsy or occasionally liver or leukocyte inclusions; rarely urine or cerebrospinal fluid metabolites
Channelopathies	■ Neonatal to adult onset ■ Altered excitability of muscle or nerves ■ Signs of myopathy, collapse, ataxia, or seizures ■ May be episodic ■ Diagnosed on clinical signs and/or electrodiagnostics
Neurodegenerative diseases	■ Young to old age onset and progressive course ■ Selective or diffuse degeneration of neurons, myelin, or muscle ■ Possible selective brain atrophy on MRI in encephalopathies ■ Degenerative changes on biopsy or necropsy

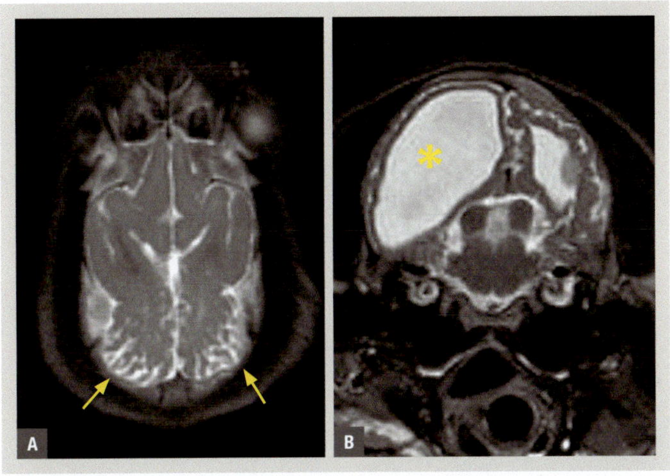

FIG. 12.2 Most hereditary congenital anomalies will be symmetric, such as this polymicrogyria (arrows) of the occipital lobes in Standard Poodles (**A**). Exceptions do occur, however, such as the hydrocephalus (*) also seen in polymicrogyria disease, which is often asymmetric (**B**).[7]

signs may clearly reflect a neurological disease, but the neonatal onset makes it easy to cull the affected pups and ignore the problem. If, on the other hand, the breeders are willing to address the problem, they will be rewarded with increased litter size and improved health. Structural abnormalities of development of the nervous system are best diagnosed through advanced imaging or necropsy. These can be either agenesis (failure of development) or dysgenesis (abnormal development). Most hereditary disorders will be symmetric, although exceptions do occur (Fig. 12.2). Most structural abnormalities are not progressive, but some such as hydrocephalus or vertebral anomalies can progress.

Inborn errors of metabolism occur when a key enzyme in a metabolic pathway is disrupted. This may interfere with the production of energy or synthesis of necessary products (Fig. 12.3). The resulting clinical signs are often encephalopathy and/or weakness and can sometimes be affected by diet. Thus, they could easily be confused with a portosystemic shunt. The intermediary steps in metabolic pathways are often organic acids. When an enzyme deficiency blocks a metabolic pathway and there is no alternative pathway, then the upstream organic acids accumulate. These organic acids are typically excreted in the urine, where they can be detected by specific assays, giving rise to the term organic acidurias. Accumulation of these abnormal byproducts or interference with energy production can result in metabolic acidosis, hypoglycemia, or ketosis, which may suggest an organic aciduria on routine clinical pathology. Some organic acidurias, such as L2-hydroxyglutaric aciduria, will have specific magnetic resonance imaging (MRI) changes typically affecting gray matter.[8]

Alternatively, the enzyme deficiency may affect catabolism of macromolecules in the lysosome. Since these are large, insoluble compounds, they are rarely excreted in the urine but instead accumulate within the lysosome. Because synthesis is not affected, animals with lysosomal storage diseases often have normal development and delayed onset of clinical signs. Signs typically start in young adults, but they can be delayed to much later, as occurs in Tibetan Terriers with neuronal ceroid lipofuscinosis.[9] Signs inexorably progress as more accumulated byproduct interferes with normal central nervous system function; most are fatal. MRI may show generalized brain atrophy. Often, other organs are also affected and sometimes the storage product can be seen in leukocytes, liver, or muscle biopsy. Otherwise, lysosomal storage diseases are typically diagnosed by demonstrating membrane-bound storage material at necropsy. Not all catabolism occurs in lysosomes, and the storage product of some enzyme deficiencies, such as glycogen storage disease, may be free in the cytoplasm.

Mutations affecting ion channel function can alter the excitation/inhibition balance in excitable membranes, producing disease. Since the effects are functional rather than structural, most will not show histological changes and are diagnosed based on clinical signs and/or electrodiagnostic tests. Clinical signs in channelopathies depend on the nature of the change and which part of the nervous system is predominantly affected. In neuromuscular disease, hyperexcitability of the peripheral nerves or muscles can result in myokymia or myotonia, respectively, which would be seen on electrodiagnostic tests. Hyperexcitability of the cerebral cortex could result in epileptic seizures. Ion channel mutations may underly many idiopathic epilepsies, but most probably result from polygenic traits representing a combination of multiple variants that affect excitability. Benign familial juvenile epilepsy in Lagotto Romagnolo dogs is a hereditary epilepsy that also illustrates changes in gene expression during development. A mutation affecting an adhesion molecule in the glutamatergic synapse (LGI2) causes epileptic seizures in young dogs.[10] As the animal matures, however, the gene that codes for this neonatal isoform of the molecule

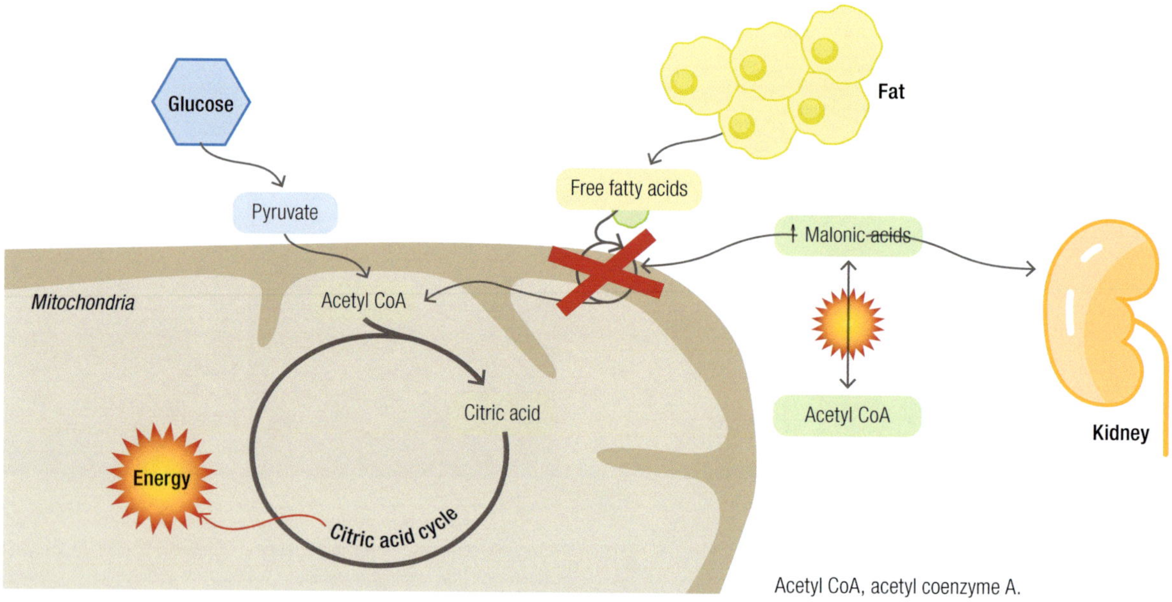

FIG. 12.3 Malonic acid is a byproduct of the citric acid cycle that regulates the transport of free fatty acids into the mitochondria. A deficiency of an enzyme that metabolizes malonic acid leads to a buildup of this organic acid that can be detected in the urine. Increased malonic acid prevents utilization of fatty acids for energy in the fasted state, which results in hypoglycemia, seizures, and encephalopathy if the dog is anorexic. Ensuring a steady source of carbohydrates reverses all the clinical signs.[12]

is inactivated and the gene for the adult form (*LGI1*) is activated, which results in remission of the seizures. Some channelopathies, such as the one affecting the inward-rectifying potassium channel Kir4.1 (*KCNJ10*), affect multiple functions.[11] The mutation disrupts the ability of astrocytes to buffer extracellular potassium, leading to hyperexcitablity of neurons. In the cerebellum, this disrupts the timing of Purkinje cell firing, thereby causing ataxia; in the spinal cord, it affects the lower motor neuron, causing myokymia/neuromyotonia; and in the cerebral cortex, it produces epileptic seizures. Hence, the acronym for the disease is SAMS (spinocerebellar ataxia with myokymia and/or seizures).

While hereditary neurodegenerative diseases can start at a young age, some, such as degenerative myelopathy, have a much older onset.[13] A mutation affects some function necessary for cell maintenance, causing premature cell death and signs of disease. The degeneration can be very specific, as in hereditary cerebellar ataxia in Gordon Setters, in which only Purkinje cells are affected,[14] or more generalized, as in multiple system degeneration in Kerry Blue Terriers and Chinese Crested dogs, in which cell loss occurs in the cerebellum, caudate nucleus, and substantia nigra.[15] In multiple system degeneration, the clinical signs and MRI findings are pathognomonic for the disease, but histopathology is often necessary to identify the distribution and character of the degeneration.

Segregation analysis

Hereditary diseases run in families; thus, family histories can aid in their recognition. Familial, however, does not always mean hereditary.[1] Family members share a common environment. As a result, dietary deficiencies, toxicities, or infections may affect multiple members of a family over generations. Ruling out such acquired diseases may necessitate in-depth testing, including necropsy of one or more affected individuals. If known acquired diseases are ruled out, then a hereditary condition needs to be seriously considered. The next step would be to examine how the disease appears to be passed through the family (segregation analysis). Sometimes, when considered ethically acceptable, trial breedings, including repeating a breeding that produced affected animals, may be helpful. Otherwise, the extended family over multiple generations can be analyzed if that information is available.

Important considerations are the percentage of offspring affected, the sex ratio of affected dogs, and whether parents are affected or not (Table 12.3). The anticipated percentage affected based on the mode of inheritance is compared to the observed percentage affected in the litter(s). The anticipated percentage affected is just a probability, however, and the actual percentage can vary from litter to litter. Since often only affected animals are brought to our attention, an ascertainment bias may affect the perceived percentages.

Several other factors can also complicate the determination of the mode of inheritance. Accurate phenotype determination is probably the most serious source of error of these studies. In some diseases such as epilepsy, acquired diseases can produce clinical signs identical to those of the hereditary disease (phenocopy), or an affected individual may die before clinical signs are manifest, as in degenerative myelopathy, which typically begins at 8–10 years of age. This can lead to misclassification of individuals and to erroneous conclusions. In some diseases, an individual may have the disease genotype but either show no signs (incomplete penetrance) or a mild or variant form (variable expressivity), which can also lead to misclassification.

If the character of the disease or segregation in the family suggests a hereditary condition, then DNA testing should be considered to aid in the diagnosis.

> To interpret DNA test results appropriately, the clinician needs to understand the types of DNA tests available and the chances of false positive or negative results.

TABLE 12.3 Segregation in different modes of inheritance.

	Autosomal recessive	Autosomal dominant	X-linked recessive	Mitochondrial
Parents' genotype	Both carriers	One affected	Mother carrier	Mother carrier or affected
Sex of offspring	Both affected	Both affected	Males affected	Both affected
% Offspring affected	25% of litter	50% of litter	50% of males	Variable*
% Offspring carriers	50% of litter**	No carriers	50% of females	Variable % of females*

*Effect depends on the number of mitochondria with the pathogenic variant passed in the egg.
** If the affected offspring can be identified, then 66% of the normal offspring will be carriers.

DNA test development

Several strategies have been used to identify mutations associated with a hereditary disease and reflect the evolution of the technology to study genomics. To interpret DNA tests appropriately, the clinician needs to understand how tests are developed and the level of confidence they can have in the results. The techniques used to identify the mutation are the candidate gene approach, genome-wide association studies (linkage analysis), or whole genome sequencing.

Candidate gene approach

If mutations in a gene are known to cause the disease in other species or breeds, then that gene could be sequenced in an animal of a different breed or species with a similar phenotype and potentially pathogenic variants identified. For example, if a young dog had signs of muscle wasting, weakness, elevated serum creatine kinase, and dystrophic changes on biopsy, it would be diagnosed with muscular dystrophy. The genes associated with muscular dystrophy could then be sequenced in the affected dog and analyzed for variants likely to affect the function of the related proteins.[16] If that variant were in the gene coding for dystrophin, a gene associated with the phenotype in other species and breeds, then immunohistochemistry for the protein could be performed on a muscle biopsy. If it showed that no dystrophin was present in the muscle, then the variant would be considered pathogenic. However, the protein could be present but not be functional. Then further studies would be needed to prove the variant was indeed pathogenic.

Genome-wide association studies

Not all hereditary diseases have genes already associated with them in other species or may have too many possible candidate genes to sequence all of them. In this case, genome-wide association studies (GWAS or linkage analysis) are used to map the location of the gene associated with disease to a chromosome.[1] In GWAS, thousands of single nucleotide polymorphisms (SNPs) spread throughout the genome of an individual are assayed using an array called a SNP chip. SNPs are benign variants that do not affect function but can be used to detect differences in the chromosomes between individuals. SNPs are compared between a population of affected animals and a population of normal animals of the same breed. The original mutation that led to the disease would have occurred on a chromosome that had a unique collection of SNPs called a haplotype. As that chromosome is passed on through generations, recombinations occur during meiosis that alter the haplotype. When a recombination occurs, SNPs that are close to the pathogenic variant on the chromosome are less likely to be separated from the pathogenic variant than ones further away. Thus, SNPs close to the pathogenic variant in the original haploptype are more likely to be present in affected animals than the normal ones. These are called linked markers. Plotting the probability of SNPs being present in the affected animals versus that in controls results in a graph called a "Manhattan Plot" (Fig. 12.4). The area where this difference is statistically significant defines a locus, an area of that chromosome where the gene responsible is likely to be found. Genes within that area become candidates based on their location and can be sequenced and potentially pathogenic variants identified. One or more of the SNPs within the locus can serve as a proxy for the actual mutation and form the basis for a linked-marker DNA test.

A linked-marker test, however, can lead to misleading results. If another recombination happens to occur between the marker and the pathogenic variant in an individual, then the marker will no longer be linked to the disease in the offspring of that individual, resulting in false negative/positive tests. Even if the marker is relatively rare in the breed, it may still occur in some individuals independent of the pathogenic variant, which will result in false positive tests. This is of particular concern if such a test is applied to another breed. Once the pathogenic variant is identified, a DNA test for that specific mutation will replace the linked marker test.

Whole-genome sequencing

As the cost of whole-genome sequencing (WGS) has decreased, it has become feasible to sequence the entire genome of one or more affected individuals. Each nucleotide in the individual sequence can be compared to those in hundreds of publicly available WGSs from animals without the disease. The pathogenic variant should be homozygous in affected individuals and absent (or very rare) in the controls. Thousands of benign variant SNPs will also meet these criteria. The results are then filtered for variants that are likely to affect the function of a protein. For example, a change from a positively charged to a negatively charged amino acid in the active site of an enzyme would be more likely to affect function than a change from one hydrophobic amino acid to another in a structural component of the enzyme. The biology of the protein is also considered. Altering an ion channel would be more likely to cause a seizure phenotype than altering a component of myelin. The resulting short list of variants that meet these criteria become the candidates that are further evaluated. Even if the computer programs predict that the variant will affect function, it is still possible that it may be a benign variant that is just linked to the actual variant causing the disease. Ideally, further

KEY POINTS

- It has been estimated that any animal carries at least 5–6 potential disease-causing mutations, and the nervous system is frequently affected by hereditary disease.
- Some diseases are well recognized in certain breeds and just the breed and signs will allow selection of the appropriate DNA test. For others, the characteristics of the presentation may suggest that the disease is hereditary.
- DNA testing can aid in the diagnosis of an individual patient, but it is not a substitute for a thorough examination and routine diagnostic tests. As with any diagnostic test, the clinician must understand the strengths and weaknesses of DNA tests to make an accurate diagnosis.
- To interpret DNA test results appropriately, the clinician needs to understand the types of DNA tests available and the chances of false positive or negative results.
- A DNA test is for a specific mutation, not a disease. Other mutations or acquired diseases could cause the same phenotype.
- With genetic counseling, the veterinarian can help breeders maintain the desirable traits that made the stud popular while avoiding further affected animals.

References

1. O'Brien DP, Leeb T. DNA testing in neurologic diseases. *J Vet Intern Med.* 2014 Jul-Aug;28(4):1186–1198.
2. Patterson DF. Companion animal medicine in the age of medical genetics. *J Vet Intern Med.* 2000 Jan-Feb;14(1):1–9.
3. Meyers-Wallen VN. Ethics and genetic selection in purebred dogs. *Reprod Domest Anim.* 2003 Feb;38(1):73–76.
4. Donner J, Anderson H, Davison S, et al. Frequency and distribution of 152 genetic disease variants in over 100,000 mixed breed and purebred dogs. *PLoS Genet.* 2018 Apr 30;14(4):e1007361.
5. O'Brien DP. Translating Next Generation Genomics into a Clinical Diagnosis. In: *Proceedings of the ACVIM Forum*, Indianapolis, IN, 2015.
6. O'Brien DP. Basic Genomics. In: *Proceedings of the 29th American College of Veterinary Internal Medicinc Forum.* Denver, CO, 2011;394–396.
7. Jurney C, Haddad J, Crawford N, et al. Polymicrogyria in standard poodles. *J Vet Intern Med.* 2009 Jul-Aug;23(4):871–874.
8. Abramson CJ, Platt SR, Jakobs C, et al. L-2-Hydroxyglutaric aciduria in Staffordshire Bull Terriers. *J Vet Intern Med.* 2003 Jul-Aug;17(4):551–556.
9. Farias FH, Zeng R, Johnson GS, et al. A truncating mutation in ATP13A2 is responsible for adult-onset neuronal ceroid lipofuscinosis in Tibetan terriers. *Neurobiol Dis.* 2011 Jun;42(3):468–474.
10. Seppälä EH, Jokinen TS, Fukata M, et al. LGI2 truncation causes a remitting focal epilepsy in dogs. *PLoS Genet.* 2011 Jul;7(7):e1002194.
11. Gilliam D, O'Brien DP, Coates JR, et al. A homozygous KCNJ10 mutation in Jack Russell Terriers and related breeds with spinocerebellar ataxia with myokymia, seizures, or both. *J Vet Intern Med.* 2014 May-Jun;28(3):871–877.
12. O'Brien DP, Barshop BA, Faunt KK, et al. Malonic aciduria in Maltese dogs: normal methylmalonic acid concentrations and malonyl-CoA decarboxylase activity in fibroblasts. *J Inherit Metab Dis.* 1999 Dec;22(8):883–890.
13. Awano T, Johnson GS, Wade CM, et al. Genome-wide association analysis reveals a SOD1 mutation in canine degenerative myelopathy that resembles amyotrophic lateral sclerosis. *Proc Natl Acad Sci U S A.* 2009 Feb 24;106(8):2794–2799.
14. Agler C, Nielsen DM, Urkasemsin G, et al. Canine hereditary ataxia in old english sheepdogs and gordon setters is associated with a defect in the autophagy gene encoding RAB24. *PLoS Genet.* 2014 Feb 6;10(2):e1003991.
15. O'Brien DP, Johnson GS, Schnabel RD, et al. Genetic mapping of canine multiple system degeneration and ectodermal dysplasia loci. *J Hered.* 2005;96(7):727–734.
16. Sharp NJ, Kornegay JN, Van Camp SD, et al. An error in dystrophin mRNA processing in golden retriever muscular dystrophy, an animal homologue of Duchenne muscular dystrophy. *Genomics.* 1992 May;13(1):115–121.
17. O'Brien DP. Genomics for Clinicians In: *Fall Conference for Veterinarians.* University of Illinois, Urbana Illinois, 2018.
18. Kolicheski AL, Johnson GS, Mhlanga-Mutangadura T, et al. A homozygous PIGN missense mutation in Soft-Coated Wheaten Terriers with a canine paroxysmal dyskinesia. *Neurogenetics.* 2017 Jan;18(1):39–47.
19. Zeng R, Coates JR, Johnson GC, et al. Breed distribution of SOD1 alleles previously associated with canine degenerative myelopathy. *J Vet Intern Med.* 2014 Mar-Apr;28(2):515–521.
20. Ivansson EL, Megquier K, Kozyrev SV, et al. Variants within the SP110 nuclear body protein modify risk of canine degenerative myelopathy. *Proc Natl Acad Sci U S A.* 2016 May 31;113(22):E3091-100.
21. Buckingham KJ, McMillin MJ, Brassil MM, et al. Multiple mutant T alleles cause haploinsufficiency of Brachyury and short tails in Manx cats. *Mamm Genome.* 2013 Oct;24(9-10):400–408.
22. Mhlanga-Mutangadura T, Johnson GS, Ashwini A, et al. A Homozygous RAB3GAP1:c.743delC Mutation in Rottweilers with Neuronal Vacuolation and Spinocerebellar Degeneration. *J Vet Intern Med.* 2016 May;30(3):813–818.
23. Mhlanga-Mutangadura T, Johnson GS, Schnabel RD, et al. A mutation in the Warburg syndrome gene, RAB3GAP1, causes a similar syndrome with polyneuropathy and neuronal vacuolation in Black Russian Terrier dogs. *Neurobiol Dis.* 2016 Feb;86:75–85.
24. Wiedmer M, Oevermann A, Borer-Germann SE, et al. A RAB3GAP1 SINE Insertion in Alaskan Huskies with Polyneuropathy, Ocular Abnormalities, and Neuronal Vacuolation (POANV) Resembling Human Warburg Micro Syndrome 1 (WARBM1). *G3 (Bethesda).* 2015 Nov 23;6(2):255–262.
25. Mosher DS, Quignon P, Bustamante CD, et al. A mutation in the myostatin gene increases muscle mass and enhances racing performance in heterozygote dogs. *PLoS Genet.* 2007 May 25;3(5):e79.
26. Marsden CD, Ortega-Del Vecchyo D, O'Brien DP, et al. Bottlenecks and selective sweeps during domestication have increased deleterious genetic variation in dogs. *Proc Natl Acad Sci U S A.* 2016 Jan 5;113(1):152–157.
27. Gandolfi B, Daniel RJ, O'Brien DP, et al. A novel mutation in CLCN1 associated with feline myotonia congenita. *PLoS One.* 2014 Oct 30;9(10):e109926.
28. Woelfel C, Meurs K, Friedenberg S, et al. A novel mutation of the CLCN1 gene in a cat with myotonia congenita: Diagnosis and treatment. *J Vet Intern Med.* 2022 Jul;36(4):1454–1459.
29. Schulz A, Ajayi T, Specchio N, et al. Study of Intraventricular Cerliponase Alfa for CLN2 Disease. *N Engl J Med.* 2018 May 17;378(20):1898–1907.
30. Vuillemenot BR, Katz ML, Coates JR, et al. Intrathecal tripeptidyl-peptidase 1 reduces lysosomal storage in a canine model of late infantile neuronal ceroid lipofuscinosis. *Mol Genet Metab.* 2011 Nov;104(3):325–337.

CHAPTER 13

Neuroimaging

Silke Hecht
DVM, DACVR, DECVDI

Clinical signs referable to the nervous system are a common reason for presentation of canine patients to the veterinary practitioner. Diagnostic imaging is a mainstay in the workup of patients with suspected neurological disease. Among the various techniques available, magnetic resonance imaging (MRI) is the gold standard for imaging the nervous system due to its superior soft tissue resolution. In most neurological cases, MRI provides accurate and detailed imaging of the lesion. MRI detects inflammatory or ischemic lesions of the nervous tissue that cannot be detected by other techniques.

Computed tomography (CT) is less frequently used in neurological practice and finds its value especially in the diagnostic evaluation of traumatized patients or those with suspected bone lesions. It is also valuable in the diagnosis of mineralized intervertebral disc extrusions but is inferior to MRI in the ability to identify nonmineralized disc herniations and secondary changes such as spinal cord contusion or myelomalacia.

Radiographs remain a valuable test in the assessment of some spinal diseases.

This chapter will provide an overview of the use of radiography, CT, and MRI in the evaluation of the brain, spine, nerves, and muscles in dogs.

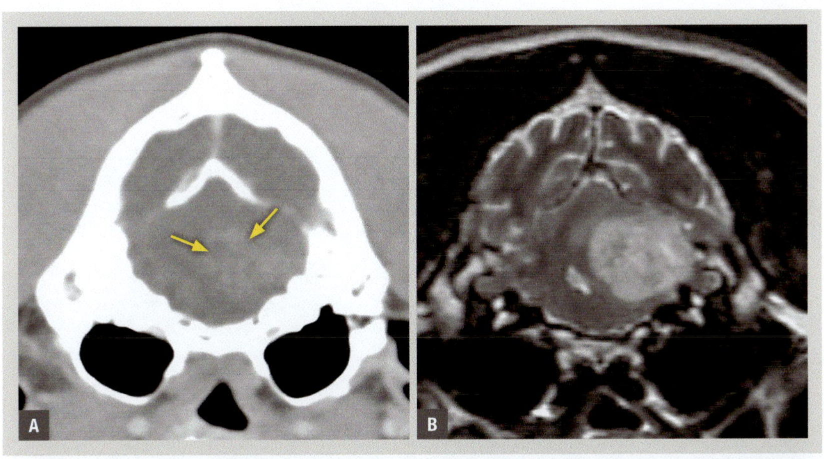

FIG. 13.1 Comparison of transverse postcontrast computed tomography (CT) (**A**) and T2-weighted magnetic resonance imaging (MRI) (**B**) scans of the brain in a 11-year-old Blue Tick Hound with a cerebellar mass (glioma, presumptive). The mass (arrows) is poorly contrast-enhancing on CT and is only faintly visible, while it is easily identified on MRI.

General approach to neuroimaging of the canine patient

Brain

Radiographs of the head may provide some information on osseous abnormalities of the skull but often underestimate the severity of the changes and are inadequate for evaluation of intracranial structures.[1] CT is inferior to MRI in the diagnosis of some brain parenchymal diseases but is typically an adequate diagnostic test for diagnosis of fluid accumulations (e.g., ventriculomegaly/hydrocephalus) and contrast-enhancing intracranial lesions (e.g., many brain tumors). In case of brain trauma, CT may be preferred over MRI due to the speed of image acquisition and excellent imaging capabilities for detection of intracranial hemorrhage, bone lesions, and intracranial foreign bodies.[2] MRI provides excellent soft tissue contrast and is generally considered the gold standard for brain imaging in both humans and dogs.[3] A comparison between MRI and CT images of the brain in the same canine patient are provided in Figure 13.1.

Imaging of the brain can be performed to assess the following elements: size, shape, and symmetry of the forebrain, diencephalon, mesencephalon, cerebellum and brainstem, and gray and white matter; size and appearance of fluid-filled spaces (subarachnoid space and ventricular system); evidence of intracranial mass effect; appearance of associated structures (e.g., cranial nerves, intracranial vessels, choroid plexus, and pituitary gland); and changes to the skull and extracranial structures (e.g., the muscles, nasal cavity, and paranasal sinuses, eyes and orbits, auditory structures, salivary glands, oral cavity, pharynx, larynx, and cranial neck including the spine).[2–5] Mass lesions within the cranial vault are classified, based on their origin, as extra-axial (originating outside the brain parenchyma) and intra-axial (originating from the brain parenchyma). An overview of the possible differential diagnoses for intra- and extra-axial lesions is provided in Table 13.1, and example images of these lesions are provided in Figure 13.2.

Intravenous contrast medium administration is commonly performed for both CT and MRI studies of the brain.[6]

Some intracranial structures are located outside the blood–brain barrier and show physiological contrast-enhancement (intracranial vessels, choroid plexus, pituitary gland, and trigeminal nerves). Contrast enhancement is expected with intracranial lesions that are located outside the blood–brain barrier and vascularized (e.g., meningeal tumors), but is not seen with intracranial lesions protected by the blood–brain barrier (e.g., some glial tumors) or lesions that are completely blood-filled or necrotic. It is important to note that a major advantage of MRI over CT is the ability to detect non-contrast-enhancing lesions on specific precontrast sequences (e.g., T2-FLAIR [fluid-attenuated inversion recovery], see below). Intracranial abnormalities that may be encountered secondary to various disease processes include perilesional vasogenic edema, mass effect, brain herniation, (obstructive) hydrocephalus, hemorrhage, and cerebral necrosis (Fig. 13.3).

Concurrent extraneural abnormalities noted on imaging, such as lymphadenopathy of the head and neck, muscle atrophy, abnormal contents within the tympanic bulla, or soft tissue masses of the head, may or may not be associated with the patient's signs and should be carefully evaluated in light of the patient's presenting neurological complaints. Imaging findings with various intracranial diseases overlap, and the ranking of differential diagnoses for brain lesions seen on imaging is usually influenced by additional information (patient signalment and history) and results of other tests (laboratory and cerebrospinal fluid analyses). It is also important to note that some brain diseases may go undetected on imaging (e.g., degenerative or toxic encephalopathies, vascular events, and some inflammatory conditions), and that a normal imaging study of the brain does not exclude central nervous system disease.[3]

Spine

Radiographs can provide important information especially on abnormalities of the osseous vertebrae and vertebral alignment. They are often the first imaging test performed in patients with spinal trauma or congenital spinal instability (e.g., atlantoaxial subluxation) and in patients with a high

TABLE 13.1 Main differential diagnoses for intracranial lesions.

Extra-axial		Intra-axial			Both extra- and intra-axial
Single	**Multiple**	**Single**	**Multiple symmetric**	**Multiple asymmetric**	
Neoplastic ■ In typical location, e.g., pituitary tumor, choroid plexus tumor, nerve sheath tumor, nasal tumor extending into cranial vault ■ Anywhere, e.g., meningioma, histiocytic sarcoma	**Neoplastic** (e.g., metastatic disease, round cell tumor)	**Neoplastic** (e.g., glial tumor)	**Metabolic, degenerative, nutritional, and toxic encephalopathies**	**Inflammatory** (e.g., meningo-encephalitis of undetermined etiology	**Neoplastic** (e.g., round cell tumor)
Inflammatory (e.g., empyema)	**Inflammatory** (e.g., granulomatous disease)	**Inflammatory** (e.g., granuloma or abscess)	**Inflammatory disease** (rare, e.g., granulomatous meningoencephalitis)	**Neoplastic** (e.g., metastatic disease or round cell neoplasia)	**Inflammatory** (e.g., meningo-encephalitis)
Vascular/traumatic (e.g., epidural hematoma)		**Vascular** (e.g., ischemic event)	**Neoplasia** (rare, e.g., butterfly glioma)	**Vascular** (e.g., multifocal infarcts)	

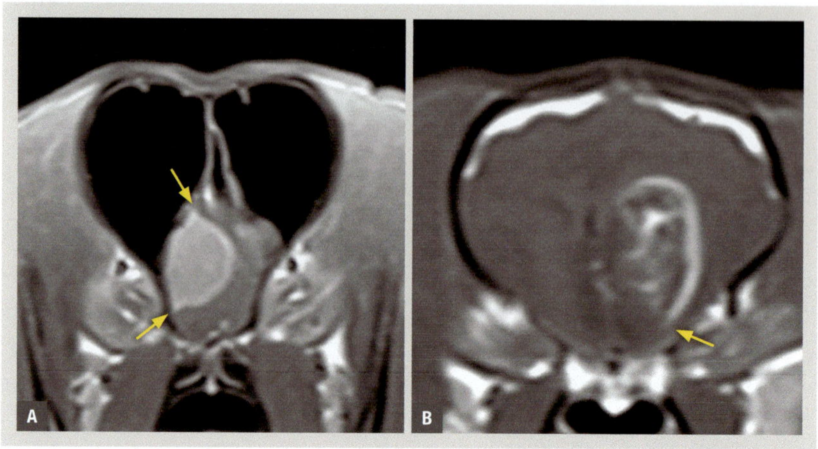

FIG. 13.2 Transverse postcontrast T1-weighted images of the brain in two different dogs illustrating imaging features of extra- versus intra-axial masses. (**A**) In this 7-year-old Weimaraner, there is a large, homogeneously contrast-enhancing peripheral mass associated with the right olfactory bulb. This mass is in broad-based contact with the overlying skull and has linear meningeal enhancement extending from its periphery, consistent with a "dural tail sign" (arrows). (**B**) In this 4-year-old Boston Terrier, there is a large, heterogeneously enhancing mass with partial rim enhancement associated with the left frontal lobe, which is surrounded by brain parenchyma and has an acute angle where it contacts the skull (arrow).

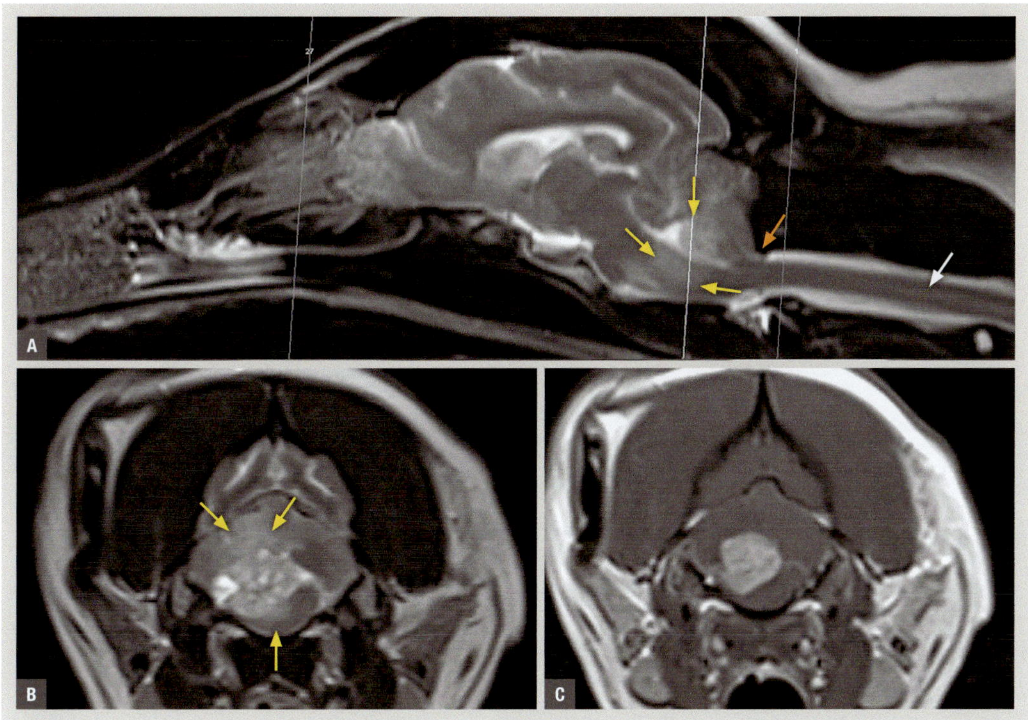

FIG. 13.3 Magnetic resonance images from a 3-year-old Shetland Sheep Dog with a large, strongly contrast-enhancing mass associated with the caudal fossa, likely representing a choroid plexus tumor of the fourth ventricle, and secondary changes. (**A**) Parasagittal T2-weighted image, (**B**) transverse T2-weighted image, (**C**) transverse T1-weighted postcontrast image. The mass itself is strongly contrast-enhancing, well-circumscribed, and contiguous with the choroid plexus of the fourth ventricle (**C**). There is extensive ill-defined perilesional T2 hyperintensity throughout the brain parenchyma bordering the mass, consistent with vasogenic edema (yellow arrows in A and B). There is herniation of the cerebellum through the foramen magnum (orange arrow in A) and mild syringomyelia (white arrow in A).

suspicion of discospondylitis or spinal neoplasia. Myelography is a radiographic contrast procedure that involves the injection of contrast material into the subarachnoid space. It provides information on the contents of the vertebral canal and the spinal cord that cannot be obtained from plain radiographs.[7,8] However, due to its invasive nature and inferiority in the diagnostic yield compared to advanced imaging techniques, this contrast procedure is no longer recommended for the diagnostic workup of small animal neurology patients.

CT is inferior to MRI in the diagnosis of disorders of the spinal cord, abnormal soft tissue lesions within the vertebral canal (e.g., nonmineralized intervertebral disc herniations), and bone marrow abnormalities (e.g., infiltrative neoplasia). However, CT is an excellent diagnostic test for evaluation of the vertebral cortices, vertebral alignment, compromise of the vertebral canal, diagnosis of mineralized intervertebral disc extrusions, and any spinal or paraspinal soft tissue abnormalities associated with contrast-enhancement.[9] CT can be combined with myelography for improved evaluation of the vertebral canal. MRI is generally considered the gold standard for the evaluation of most spinal disorders in dogs, with the possible exception of those with acute spinal trauma, those unable to undergo prolonged anesthesia, or those with primarily bone or mineral abnormalities or metallic material in the area of interest.[3] An example of the information gained by the use of radiographs, MRI, and CT in the evaluation of a canine neurology patient is provided in Figure 13.4.

Imaging studies of the spine are aimed at assessing the number, conformation, alignment, and integrity of the osseous vertebrae; the intervertebral disc spaces; the vertebral canal (epidural fat, subarachnoid space, and spinal cord); and the spinal nerves, regional vasculature, and paraspinal soft tissues. Based on their relationship with the spinal cord and dural sac, spinal lesions are subdivided into extradural lesions (originating outside the dura), intradural-extramedullary lesions (located between the meningeal layers but outside the spinal cord), and intramedullary lesions (originating from the spinal cord). An overview of the possible differential diagnoses for different types of spinal lesions is provided in Table 13.2, and example images of these lesions are provided in Figure 13.5.

Intravenous contrast medium administration with spinal CT or MRI may or may not be necessary. As described for brain lesions, lesions that are located outside the blood–central nervous system–barrier and vascularized will show contrast enhancement. Vertebral anomalies, mineralized intervertebral disc extrusion with or without associated extradural hemorrhage, and acute spinal trauma are usually adequately evaluated on noncontrast images. However, contrast medium administration is helpful in the evaluation of soft tissues and inflammatory or neoplastic lesions. Some spinal lesions tend to occur in a typical location (e.g., articular process hypertrophy in the caudal cervical spine with the osseous form of caudal cervical spondylomyelopathy, or signal intensity changes in the spinal cord gray matter with fibrocartilaginous embolism). Additional findings in the field of view, such as a paraspinal abscess, lymphadenopathy, or an abdominal mass, may aid in prioritization of differential diagnoses for spinal lesions. As occurs with brain imaging studies, the findings in various diseases overlap, and additional information or tests may be needed to establish an appropriate list of differential diagnoses. It is also important to note that some spinal diseases may not cause abnormalities on imaging studies (e.g., degenerative myelopathy, meningomyelitis, ischemic events), and that a normal imaging study does not rule out spinal disease. As previously mentioned for the brain, it is important to stress that MRI is far superior to CT in the identification of spinal and paraspinal soft tissue lesions and of bone lesions centered on the medullary cavities of the vertebrae. This is especially true for non-contrast-enhancing lesions (e.g., ischemic myelopathies, certain degenerative diseases, myelomalacia, and some types of meningomyelitis and intramedullary neoplasia), which can be detected on certain precontrast MRI sequences but not on CT.

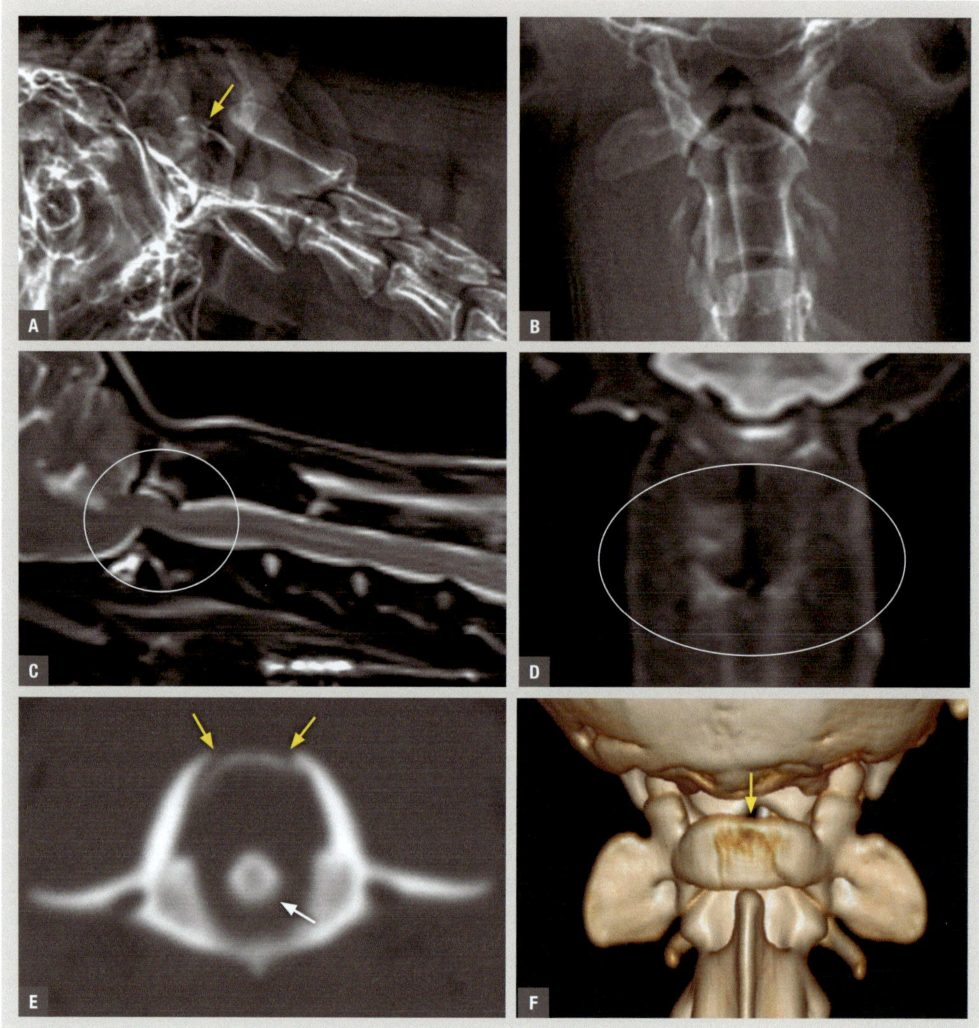

FIG. 13.4 Radiographs (**A, B**), magnetic resonance (MR) images (**C, D**), and computed tomography (CT) images (**E, F**) of the cervical spine of a 10-year-old Yorkshire Terrier presented after trauma (dog attack). (**A, B**) Oblique lateral and ventrodorsal radiographs obtained at the referring veterinarian; there was concern for possible spinal fractures. A focal step in the dorsal lamina of C1 (yellow arrow) is seen on the lateral view (**A**). The appearance of C2 and C3 on the ventrodorsal view (**B**) was attributed to superimposition of the airways and surrounding soft tissues. The dens axis appears normal. (**C**) Sagittal T2-weighted MR image showing evidence of mild traumatic atlantoaxial subluxation, with focal compression of the cranial cervical spinal cord from ventral (circle). There is also evidence of impingement on the cervical spinal cord by the caudal margin of the dorsal arch of the atlas. There is mild intramedullary hyperintensity associated with the spinal cord at this level, and the central canal is visible throughout the length of the field of view. (**D**) Dorsal STIR (short tau inversion recovery) MR image showing marked paraspinal muscle hyperintensities associated with the cervical spine, consistent with soft tissue trauma (circle). (**E, F**) Transverse and 3D reconstructed CT images showing a focal compression fracture of the dorsal arch of the atlas, causing mild compromise of the vertebral canal from dorsally (yellow arrows). The mild dorsal subluxation of the dens of C2 identified on MRI is again noted (white arrow in E).

TABLE 13.2 Main differential diagnoses for spinal lesions.

Extradural	Intradural-extramedullary	Intramedullary
■ Disc herniation ■ Vertebral and epidural neoplasia (e.g., primary bone tumor, multiple myeloma, lymphoma, metastatic disease) ■ Inflammatory lesions (e.g., empyema) ■ Hemorrhage/hematoma ■ Vertebral fracture/luxation ■ Vertebral anomaly ■ Hypertrophied spinal ligaments ■ Articular facet degenerative joint disease	■ Neoplasia (nerve sheath tumor, meningioma, nephroblastoma, other) ■ Hemorrhage/hematoma (rare) ■ Intradural disc extrusion (rare)	■ Spinal cord neoplasia (e.g., ependymoma, glioma, lymphoma, metastases) ■ Edema ■ Inflammatory lesions (myelitis) ■ Hemorrhage ■ Ischemic vascular event (e.g., fibrocartilaginous embolism) ■ Specific types of intervertebral disc disease (acute noncompressive nucleus pulposus extrusion or intramedullary disc extrusion)

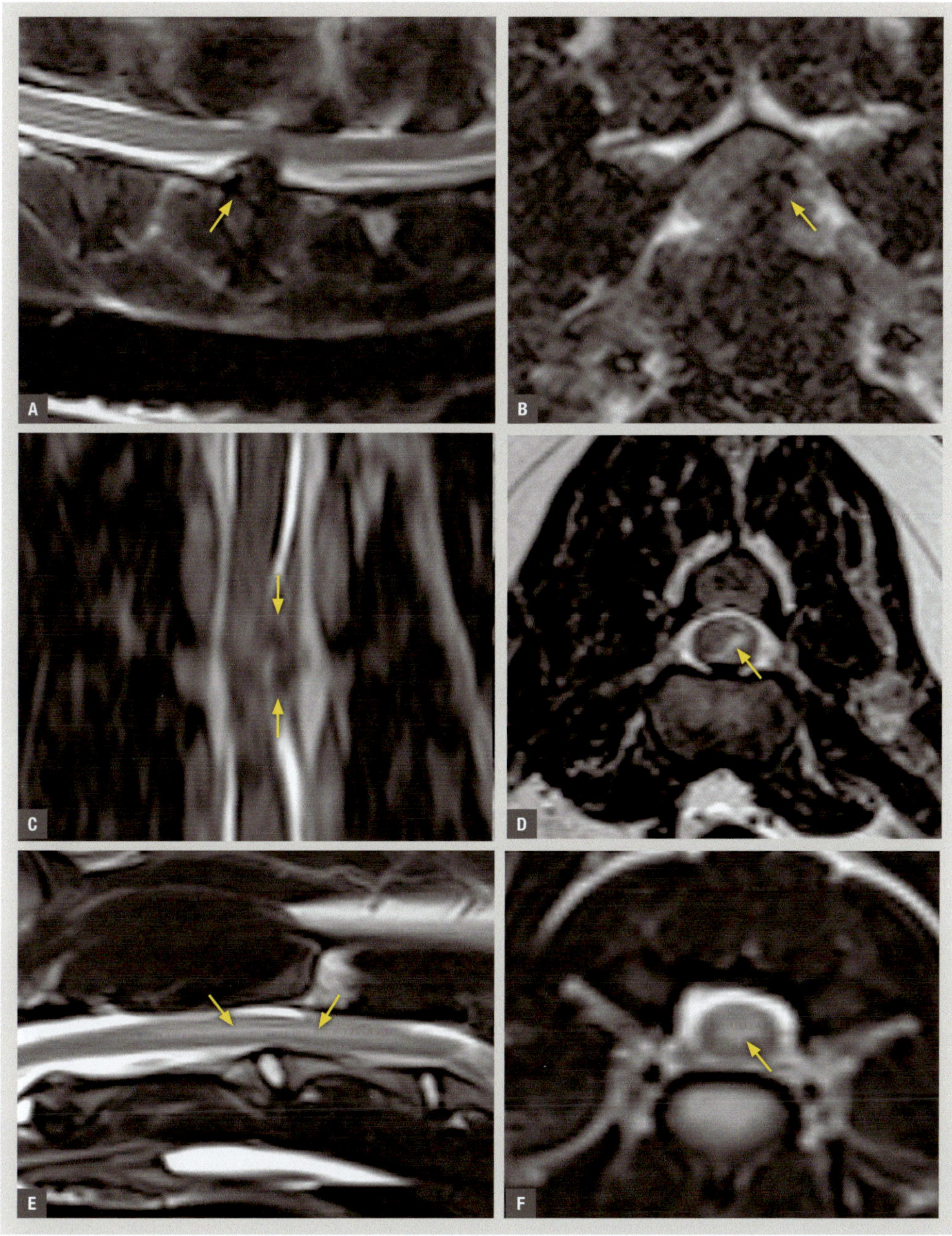

FIG. 13.5 Magnetic resonance imaging studies in three different dogs (sagittal/dorsal and transverse T2-weighted images) showing examples of extradural (**A, B**), intradural-extramedullary (**C, D**), and intramedullary (**E, F**) lesion location. Note the location of the abnormality (arrows) with respect to the subarachnoid space. (**A, B**) Intervertebral disc extrusion causing extradural spinal cord compression in a 7-year-old Golden Retriever. (**C, D**) Intradural-extramedullary mass (meningothelial meningioma, confirmed) with left-sided paraspinal muscle atrophy in a 9-year-old Labrador Retriever. (**E, F**) Intramedullary lesion (presumptive ischemic myelopathy) in a 5-year-old mixed breed dog.

Nerves

Evaluation of the cranial nerves and their associated skull foramina is part of a routine CT or MRI examination of the brain.[10] As for other soft tissue structures, MRI is the preferred imaging modality in the assessment of cranial neuropathies and allows evaluation of the actual nerves along with their associated intracranial nuclei. The role of CT is limited to the identification of mass lesions arising from the nerves and secondary changes (bone abnormalities and muscle atrophy). The optic nerves, optic chiasm, and trigeminal nerves are typically visible in normal dogs. The facial and vestibulocochlear nerves are small but can usually be well evaluated due to their characteristic location within the facial canal and close to the inner ear, respectively. While the other cranial nerves are not typically individually visible in normal dogs unless special thin-section techniques are used, they can be identified as extra-axial nodules or masses in a characteristic location when enlarged. Enlargement of the cranial nerves, often associated with increased contrast-enhancement, can be seen with inflammatory conditions (neuritis) or neoplasia (e.g., nerve sheath tumor).[11] Unilateral enlargement points towards a neoplastic lesion rather than inflammation. Widening of the associated skull foramen due to pressure atrophy is also more common with neoplasia. Muscle atrophy can be seen secondary to inflammatory or neoplastic conditions but is generally more severe and asymmetric with neoplasia. Bilateral nerve enlargement or involvement of multiple nerves (polyneuropathy) are more common with inflammatory conditions.

Similarly, evaluation of the spinal nerves is part of a routine CT or MRI examination of the spine. However, it is important to note that the brachial plexus and lumbosacral plexus are physically distant from the actual spine, necessitating an adjustment of the field of view and scan planes to make sure these anatomical structures are included in the examination if their assessment is indicated based on the physical and neurological examinations.[12] The spinal nerves are seen originating from the spinal cord within the vertebral canal and exiting the vertebral canal at their intervertebral foramina (at the level of their respective spinal cord segment) or, in the case of the cauda equina, further caudally after travelling some distance in the vertebral canal. Normal nerve roots and spinal nerves are thin and inconspicuous, and are better identified on MRI than on CT. As described for the cranial nerves, inflammatory conditions and neoplasia will result in enlargement, increased conspicuity, and contrast medium uptake of the nerves.[13] When they affect the nerve at the level of the vertebral canal, mass lesions (e.g., peripheral nerve sheath tumors) can be extradural and/or intradural-extramedullary in location and can even infiltrate into the spinal cord. Over time, nerve root enlargement can result in pressure atrophy of the bone and widening of the intervertebral foramen. Dependent on the duration of the disease process, secondary muscle abnormalities (neurogenic atrophy) may also be present. Examples of MRI findings in inflammatory and neoplastic neuropathies are shown in Figure 13.6.

Muscles

The musculature of the head and spine is evaluated along with the other structures. While major lesions such as masses or mineralization may be evident on radiographs, cross-sectional imaging (especially MRI) provides improved information. CT may provide information on muscle mass and symmetry, presence of masses (e.g., neoplasia or paraspinal abscess), mineralization, presence of foreign material or gas, and overall density. MRI provides the best soft tissue contrast. Muscle abnormalities on MRI can be grouped into three categories.[14] Muscle edema can be seen with acute myositis or trauma and is characterized by signal intensity changes on MRI but an otherwise normal appearance of the affected muscle. Similar abnormalities have been reported with muscle degeneration and inflammation in dogs affected by intervertebral disc disease.[15] Fatty infiltration may be observed with increasing age, chronic myopathies such as denervation (as seen with nerve sheath tumors or degenerative lumbosacral stenosis), or severe prior trauma. This is

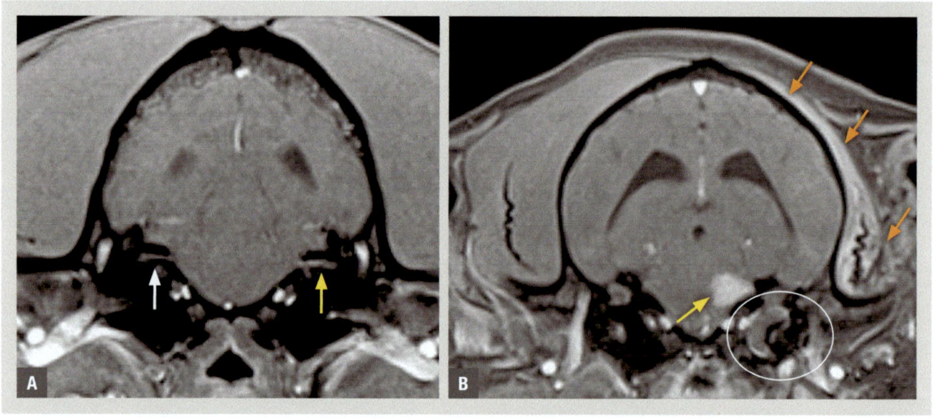

FIG. 13.6 Examples of magnetic resonance imaging findings in inflammatory and neoplastic neuropathies. Transverse T1-weighted postcontrast images with fat saturation. (A) Left-sided facial neuritis in an 11-year-old mixed breed dog. The left facial nerve (yellow arrow) is mildly thickened and contrast enhancing compared to the normal nerve on the right (white arrow). (B) Left-sided trigeminal nerve sheath tumor in a 10-year-old Pembroke Welsh Corgi. The left trigeminal nerve is markedly enlarged and contrast-enhancing (yellow arrow). Note the severe atrophy of the left masseteric and temporalis muscles (orange arrows) and the presence of fluid within the left tympanic bulla, secondary to denervation of the tensor veli palatini muscle (circle).

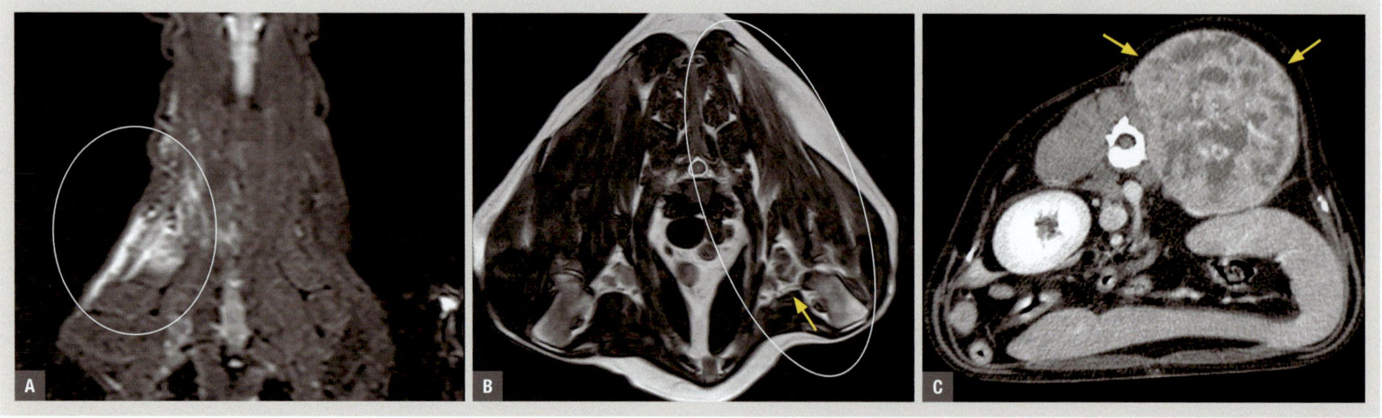

FIG. 13.7 Examples of different types of myopathies on magnetic resonance (A, B) and computed tomography (C) images. (A) Edema pattern in a dog with spinal trauma (dog attack). On the dorsal plane STIR (short tau inversion recovery) image, there is diffuse hyperintensity of the musculature on the right side of the neck and right forelimb (circle), with maintained normal muscle volume, representing a combination of edema and contusion/hemorrhage. (B) Muscle atrophy and fatty infiltration in an 8-year-old mixed breed dog with a brachial plexus tumor. This transverse T2-weighted image shows a decreased volume of the left shoulder girdle and forelimb musculature in comparison with the right side, with a diffuse increase in T2 signal intensity (circle). The brachial plexus tumor is indicated by the arrow. (C) Mass lesion pattern. This transverse postcontrast image of the lumbar spine in a 6-year-old Pitbull shows a large mass associated with the left epaxial musculature (soft tissue sarcoma; arrows).

characterized by a change in signal intensity on MRI or a density change on CT with an increase in intramuscular fat, a decrease in lean muscle mass, and an overall decreased muscle volume (atrophy). The third type of muscle lesion is a mass lesion pattern that can be seen with trauma, abscessation, and neoplasia. This type of lesion is characterized by muscle enlargement combined with loss of normal muscle pattern and a change in signal intensity (MRI) or tissue density (CT), respectively. Many mass lesions will show increased contrast medium uptake compared to normal musculature.

Examples of MRI and CT findings in different types of myopathies are shown in Figure 13.7 (see also Figs. 13.4–13.6).

Imaging modalities

Survey radiographs

Radiographs are generally of little value in the evaluation of patients with intracranial disease, with the possible exception of those with head trauma (e.g., fractures), bony mass lesions (e.g., multilobular tumor of bone), lesions resulting in extensive bone lysis of the skull (e.g., frontonasal tumors), or opaque foreign bodies (e.g., migration of an ingested metallic needle). Even if an obvious lesion is identified on survey radiographs of the head, the extent of the disease process and secondary intracranial changes are usually underestimated, and cross-sectional imaging is required for further evaluation. Head radiography will not be discussed further in this chapter, and the reader is referred to alternate resources for further information.[1]

Radiographs also have limitations in the evaluation of the spinal and paraspinal soft tissues but can provide important information on various diseases of the osseous vertebrae. An adequate radiographic examination of the spine typically requires acquisition of at least two well-positioned and collimated orthogonal radiographs, sometimes with the addition of oblique projections. To achieve adequate patient positioning, spinal radiographs are usually obtained under anesthesia or at least sedation. Acquisition of radiographs in only one plane (typically, lateral views) may occasionally suffice for diagnosis, for example, in cases of obvious spinal instability, spinal trauma, or aggressive bone lesion (Fig. 13.8). The radiographic evaluation of the spine should include an assessment of the paraspinal soft tissues, vertebral formula and any anatomical variants, vertebral alignment, overall bone opacity and opacity of individual vertebrae, cortical integrity, intervertebral disc space width, and size and opacity of the intervertebral foramina.[7]

Disorders that can be diagnosed on survey radiographs include congenital anomalies (e.g., atlantoaxial instability, articular process dysplasia, and transitional vertebrae), inflammatory conditions (e.g., discospondylitis), extradural spinal neoplasia (e.g., osteosarcoma and multiple myeloma), traumatic lesions (e.g., vertebral fractures, trauma from projectiles, and spinal instability), and degenerative changes (e.g., intervertebral disc mineralization and spondylosis deformans). Identification of a site of disc herniation may be possible on radiographs; however, advanced imaging is needed for full evaluation and surgical planning.

Myelography

Myelography involves the injection of positive contrast medium into the subarachnoid space followed by acquisition of radiographs to allow evaluation of the vertebral canal and spinal cord. A myelogram can also be combined with a CT examination (see below). A myelographic examination requires general anesthesia and should only be performed in practices/hospitals where appropriate further steps (e.g., surgery) can be taken following completion of the imaging procedure. It is generally considered a safe procedure. However, important contraindications include inflammatory conditions within the vertebral canal (meningitis), increased intracranial pressure, and known allergy to iodinated contrast media (rare in dogs). The most common adverse effect of myelography is postprocedural seizure activity (reported in up to 20% of patients).[7,16,17]

Before the advent of CT and MRI, myelography was considered an excellent test to evaluate the contents of the vertebral canal and categorize a lesion as intramedullary, intradural-extramedullary, or extradural (Fig. 13.9).[18] As mentioned above, this technique has largely been replaced by cross-sectional imaging modalities today, but the myelographic terminology to describe lesion location in relation to the dura and spinal cord has been retained.

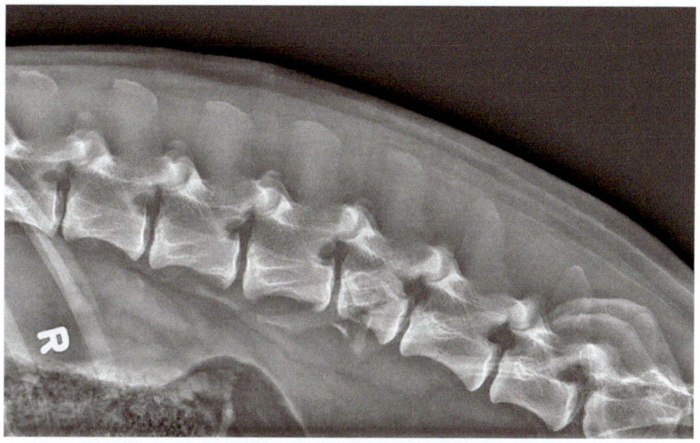

FIG. 13.8 Lateral radiograph centered on the caudal lumbar spine in a 2-year-old old English Sheepdog that had been hit by a car. An orthogonal view was not obtained at the time of presentation. The L5 vertebra is foreshortened, with discontinuity of the ventral cortex and numerous small bone fragments superimposed with the vertebra and adjacent sublumbar soft tissues. Note also the presence of material of bone opacity obscuring part of the vertebral canal at this level. The imaging findings are consistent with a compression fracture of L5 with comminution, likely resulting in extradural spinal cord compression.

Computed tomography (CT)

As mentioned above, even though CT is inferior to MRI in the evaluation of soft tissues, it is able to provide important information on many diseases and is frequently performed in the assessment of small animal neurology patients.[2,5,8,9,17] It is fast and may be preferred in patients unable to undergo prolonged anesthesia for MRI. Metallic material in the area of interest (e.g., metallic implants or ballistic projectiles) may cause significant artifacts on MRI, with CT being preferred in this case. CT may also be preferred over MRI in cases of acute head and/or spinal trauma, for the evaluation of known or suspected cortical bone lesions, and in chondrodystrophic dogs with a clinical suspicion of mineralized intervertebral disc extrusion. It is important to reiterate that CT is inferior to MRI in the ability to identify nonmineralized disc herniations and secondary changes such as spinal cord contusion or myelomalacia.

The CT scan of the brain is typically repeated after intravenous administration of iodinated contrast medium at a dose of 600–880 mg I/kg. Contrast medium administration may or may not be performed for a spinal CT study. Intravenous contrast medium administration should be

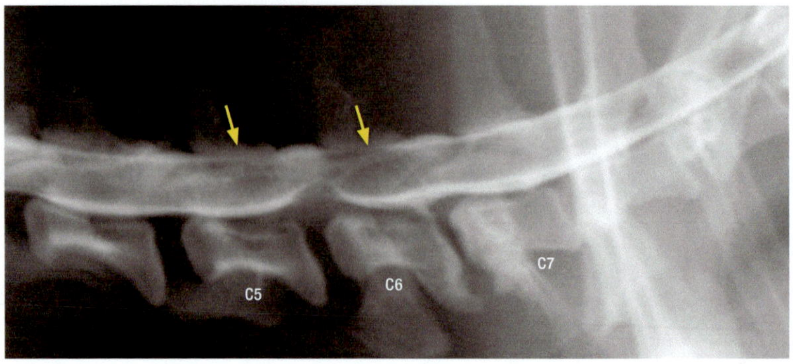

FIG. 13.9 Lateral myelographic view of the cervical spine in a 9-year-old Shi Tzu with an intervertebral disc extrusion at C5–C6. There is dorsal deviation and attenuation of the ventral contrast column dorsal to the C5–C6 intervertebral disc space. There is also attenuation of the dorsal contrast column, from cranial C5 to caudal C6 (arrows), indicative of an acute disc herniation. The C5–C6 intervertebral disc space is mildly narrowed compared to C4–C5. Also, note the marked intervertebral disc space narrowing at C6–C7, with endplate sclerosis and ventral spondylosis deformans. This is indicative of chronic degenerative intervertebral disc disease. There is no evidence of a compressive myelopathy at this level.

avoided in dehydrated animals and judiciously performed in dogs with multiorgan dysfunction. If CT of the spine is performed, the study can be combined with a myelogram for improved evaluation of the vertebral canal contents. In addition to being a diagnostic imaging test, CT can be used to facilitate tissue sampling of the head or (para)spinal tissues and allows for surgical and radiation therapy planning.

Like radiography, CT utilizes X-rays for image generation. Unlike in conventional radiography, the X-ray tube is not stationary with respect to the patient but rotates around the animal.[19] Detectors located opposite the X-ray tube receive the X-rays after they have gone through the patient, allowing reconstruction into transverse images. While older generation scanners were only able to generate individual slices, often with a large slice thickness, newer (multislice) scanners are able to acquire submillimeter slices that can be reconstructed into multiplanar (sagittal, oblique, and dorsal planes) and even three-dimensional (3D) images. The CT examination can typically be performed under sedation; however, general anesthesia is recommended for longer studies, if a CT angiogram is planned (uncommon for neurological conditions in small animals), or if CT-guided sampling (e.g., of a spinal or paraspinal mass) is planned following the imaging study.

Following acquisition of a surview image (topogram), transverse images of the area of interest are acquired. It is important to set up the scan so that images are reconstructed with both edge enhancing (sharp/bone) and soft tissue algorithms for adequate evaluation of the osseous and soft tissue structures. It is important to do this during or immediately after the scan, as adjustment of an algorithm can no longer be performed after raw data have been deleted from the actual CT scanner. The algorithm should not be confused with the "window setting", which is aimed at maximizing the contrast between different tissues and can be adjusted in any viewing software without a time limit as long as images are available in DICOM (Digital Imaging and Communications in Medicine) format. Windowing is based on the concept that tissues have a specific density/attenuation value on CT images that correlates with the degree of X-ray attenuation. This value is expressed in Hounsfield units (HU). The basis of Hounsfield unit calculation is the average attenuation of water, which was assigned the value of 0 HU. The degree of X-ray attenuation of other tissues is compared to that of water. As with radiography, cortical bone strongly attenuates X-rays, resulting in a "white" (hyperattenuating) appearance on CT images. Cortical bone density is high (variable but approximately 1000 HU). Soft tissues cause less X-ray attenuation, resulting in a gray appearance on CT images (average density 30 to 60 HU). It should be noted that while fluid and soft tissues have the same opacity on radiographs and cannot normally be distinguished, the difference in their density on CT is enough to allow them to be differentiated. Fat and gas attenuate X-rays to a lesser degree than fluid, resulting in a dark (fat) or completely black (gas) appearance on CT images, with HU values in the negative range (fat, -70 to -100 HU; air/gas, approximately -1000 HU).[19] As both standard computer monitors and the human eye are limited in their ability to differentiate shades of gray, CT images are "windowed" to maximize the visual difference between the tissues of interest. This is accomplished by adjusting the window center (WC) and window width (WW). A bone window (e.g., WC 500 HU, WW 2500) provides excellent contrast of osseous structures, while a soft tissue window (e.g., WC 50 HU, WW 350 HU) maximizes density differences between soft tissues. Visualization of subtle brain lesions can be further improved using a modified soft tissue window with an even lower WC (e.g., 30 HU) and narrower window width (e.g., 200 HU). Example images demonstrating the effects of the choice of algorithm and window levels on CT images are shown in Figure 13.10.

For a CT study of the head, the patient is usually positioned in sternal recumbency as this is helpful to ensure straight positioning. The scan should be planned to include the cranial vault from at least the level of the cribriform plate to the foramen magnum. Extension of the scan field rostrally (to include the nasal cavity) and/or caudally (to include the cranial cervical spine and regional lymph nodes) may be warranted based on scan indication and clinical suspicion. The skull, cranial vault, and brain are fairly symmetric in most animals. The skull is of bone density (average, 1000 HU). Cerebrospinal fluid within the ventricular system is fluid attenuating (0 to 5 HU). The white matter tracts may be visible if a brain window is used and are hypoattenuating compared to the adjacent gray matter (25–35 HU vs. 35–50 HU). Most intracranial lesions appear hypoattenuating to normal brain parenchyma on precontrast images. Mineralized brain lesions (e.g., chronic granulomas) appear hyperattenuating. Acute and subacute intracranial hemorrhage will also appear hyperattenuating (40 to 100 HU), which supports the choice of CT as the first-line imaging test for dogs presented with acute head trauma.[20] Following intravenous contrast medium administration, there is physiological enhancement of some intracranial structures located outside the blood–brain barrier (pituitary gland, choroid plexus, trigeminal nerves, and to some degree meninges). Most brain tumors in dogs are also located outside the blood–brain barrier (i.e., extra-axial tumors, which include, among others, meningiomas, pituitary tumors, choroid plexus tumors, and tumors extending into the cranial vault such as sinonasal carcinomas) and will show contrast medium uptake (Fig. 13.11). In fact, the sensitivity of contrast-enhanced CT for the identification of canine brain tumors is as high as 92%.[21] However, intra-axial lesions may or may not be contrast-enhancing, and CT has limited ability in the identification of nonenhancing brain lesions (e.g., infarcts, metabolic

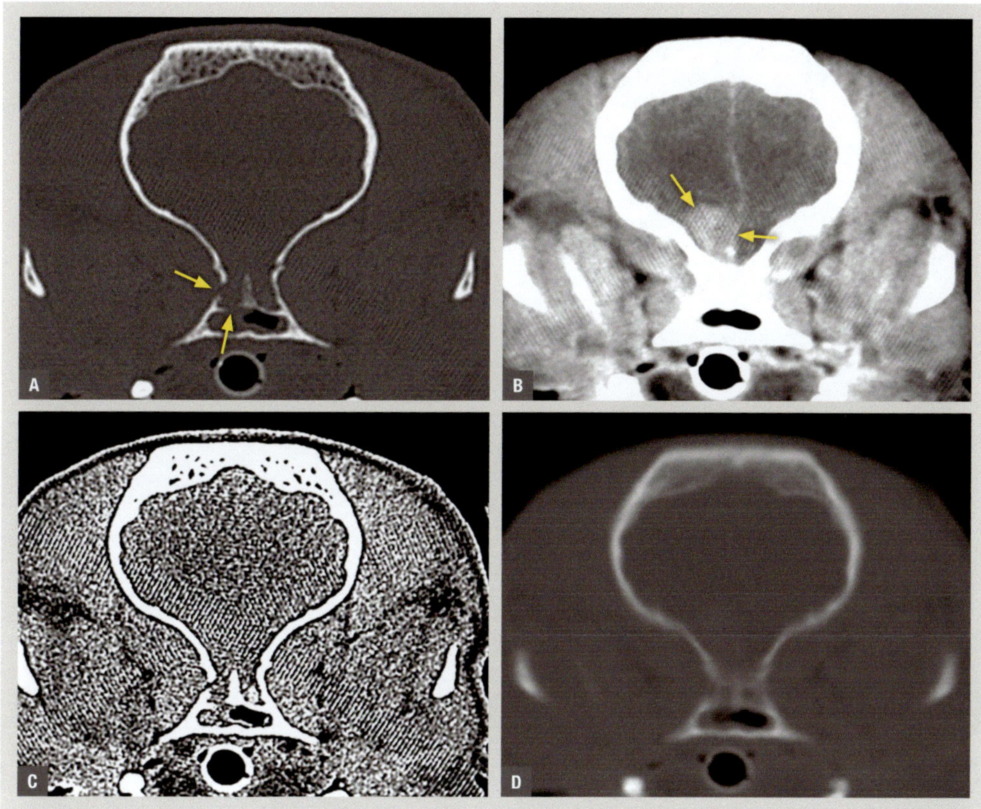

FIG. 13.10 Appropriate (A, B) and inappropriate (C, D) combinations of CT algorithms and windows for examination of the brain of a dog (14-year-old Shi Tzu) with a nasal tumor crossing the cribriform plate and extending into the cranial vault. (A) This image was reconstructed with a bone algorithm and is displayed in a bone window (WC 600 HU, WW 2600 HU). There is excellent bone detail, and several regions of bone lysis are identified (arrows). (B) This postcontrast image was reconstructed with a soft tissue algorithm and is displayed in a soft tissue window (WC 35 HU, WW 150 HU). Soft tissue contrast is excellent. There is a contrast-enhancing mass associated with the right ventral aspect of the cranial vault (arrows). Note the diffuse hypoattenuation of the white matter tracts of the right cerebral hemisphere, consistent with vasogenic edema, and midline shift towards the left. (C) This image was reconstructed with a bone algorithm (same algorithm as A) but was combined with a soft tissue window (same window as B). Neither the bone nor the soft tissue structures can be adequately evaluated on this image. (D) This postcontrast image was reconstructed with a soft tissue algorithm (same algorithm as B) and is displayed in a bone window (same window as A). Neither the bone nor the soft tissue structures can be adequately evaluated on this image.

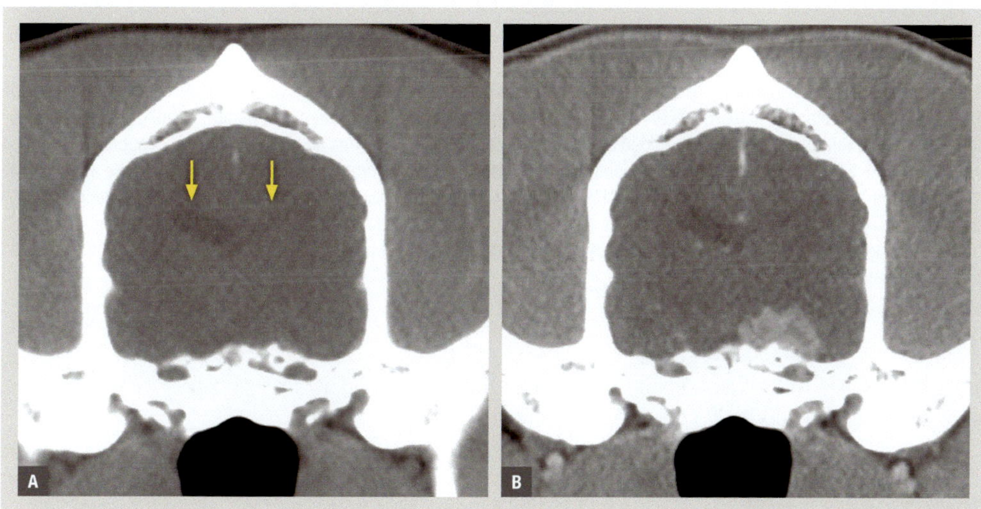

FIG. 13.11 Transverse pre- (A) and postcontrast (B) computed tomography (CT) images of the brain in an 8-year-old mixed breed dog. There is a moderately contrast-enhancing mass lesion associated with the left ventral aspect of the cranial vault, which is in broad-based contact with the underlying skull, consistent with a meningioma. The asymmetry of the lateral ventricles (arrows) was attributed to a congenital anomaly rather than mass effect from the brain tumor, as there was no evidence of perilesional edema or a midline shift on this CT study or the magnetic resonance examination performed by the primary veterinarian prior to referral.

encephalopathies, some brain tumors such as gliomas, and some inflammatory lesions of the central nervous system; see Fig. 13.1).[22,23] In addition to image evaluation in the transverse plane, evaluation of multiplanar reconstructed images (e.g., sagittal plane) is helpful to better evaluate the overall extent of the lesion and gain a 3D understanding of the anatomical relationships within the cranial vault. 3D reconstruction of a head CT data set may potentially improve visualization of bone abnormalities such as skull fractures, but it is unlikely to provide additional information about the brain.

For a CT study of the spine, the dog is typically placed in dorsal recumbency to minimize respiratory motion artifacts. Exceptions may include some cases of spinal trauma, instances of known or strongly suspected vertebral or paraspinal mass lesions when CT-guided sampling is considered, or when distortion of soft tissues due to positioning would interfere with surgical planning. As described for the brain, an initial topogram is acquired, followed by acquisition of transverse images of the area of neurolocalization.[5,8,9] The spine, vertebral canal, and paraspinal soft tissues appear fairly symmetric on transverse images. As cortical bone

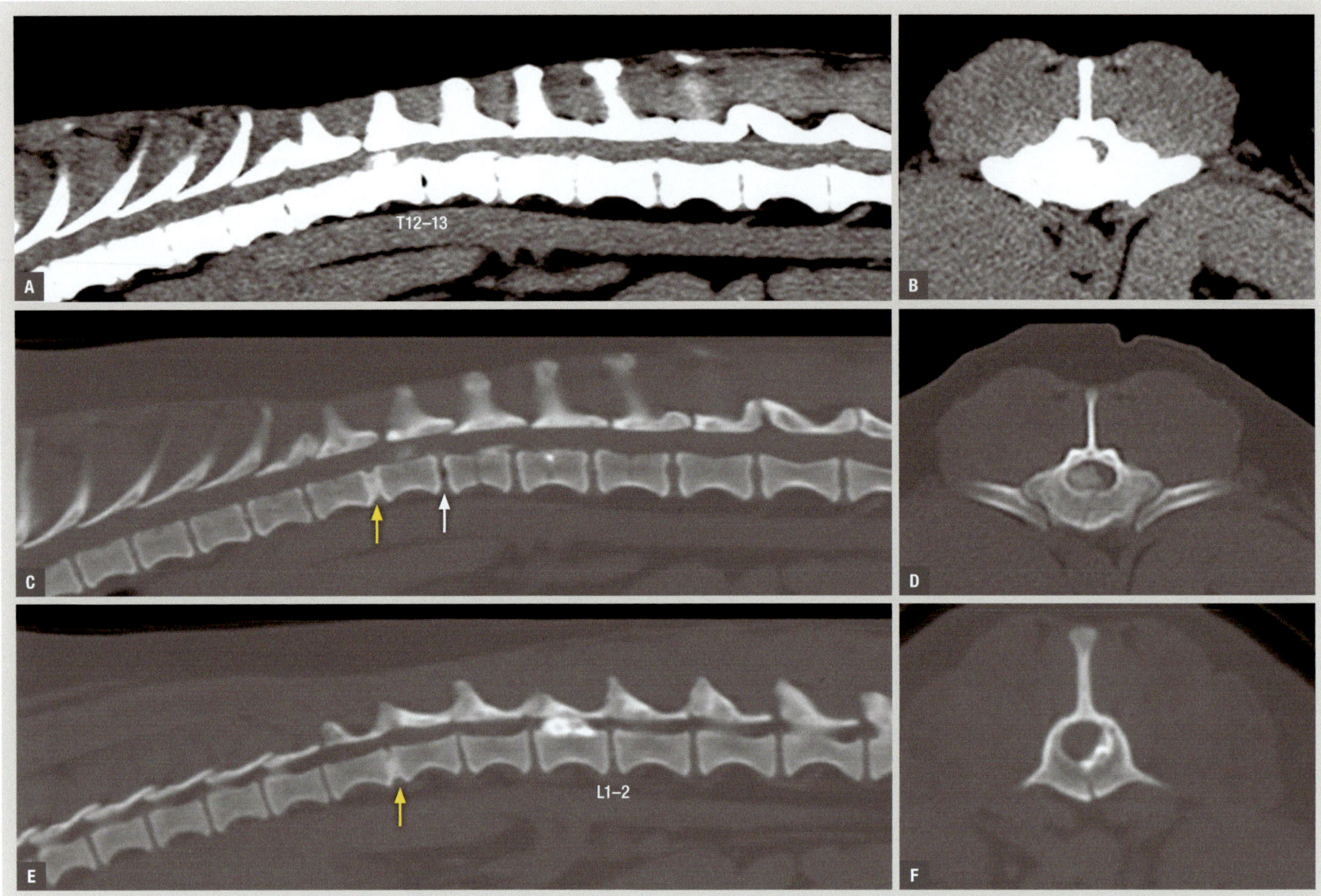

FIG. 13.12 Acute and chronic intervertebral disc extrusions in a 5-year-old Dachshund. Sagittal/parasagittal reconstructed (**A, C, E**) and transverse (**B, D, F**) images in soft tissue (**A, B**) and bone (**C–F**) algorithm and window. There is an acute intervertebral disc extrusion at T12–T13, with cranial migration of extruded disc material. Note the large volume of mineralized disc material over the midbody of T12. This material is ventral and mostly right-sided on the transverse images (**B, D**), has an irregular margin, occupies more than 50% of the transverse vertebral canal diameter, and results in severe left dorsal displacement and compression of the spinal cord from right ventral. There is complete effacement of the epidural fat at this level. Note also the focal gas attenuating focus within the T12–T13 intervertebral disc space (white arrow), consistent with a "vacuum phenomenon". (**E, F**) There is also a chronic intervertebral disc extrusion of L1–L2 with cranial migration of extruded disc material. The extruded disc material is strongly hyperattenuating and smoothly marginated and can be seen within the ventral and left side of the vertebral canal, resulting in mild to moderate spinal cord compression. The epidural fat at this level is maintained. Note the presence of in situ intervertebral disc mineralization at T11–T12 (yellow arrow).

elsewhere, the vertebral cortex has a density of approximately 1000 HU. The intervertebral discs in young dogs are soft tissue attenuating but may show increasing mineralization with age, especially in chondrodystrophic breeds. The vertebral canal contains the soft tissue–attenuating spinal cord (approximately 40 to 60 HU), which is bordered by a variable amount of epidural fat (approximately -100 HU). Differentiation of the spinal cord gray and white matter is typically not possible. Normal spinal nerves are inconspicuous but may be visible, especially in the caudal lumbar spine, where the nerve roots of the cauda equina appear as thin, soft tissue attenuating bands bordered by epidural fat. The central canal is not identified unless dilated. The subarachnoid space may be identified on non-contrast-enhanced images as a fluid attenuating region at the level of the cranial cervical spine (cisterna magna) but is otherwise best evaluated on a CT myelogram when it is filled with positive contrast medium. The paraspinal musculature is normally soft tissue attenuating but can show a variable degree of fatty infiltration, especially in older dogs. Following intravenous contrast medium administration, contrast enhancement of the vasculature and, to a lesser degree, of the paraspinal soft tissues will be observed.

CT is a useful diagnostic test in the evaluation of dogs with (acute) thoracolumbar myelopathies. According to one study, less than 8% of dogs required additional imaging tests (myelography or MRI) following a thoracolumbar CT examination.[24] The most common spinal disease in dogs is intervertebral disc disease, which is accurately diagnosed in many cases using CT (81.8–100%).[17,25–27] It is however inferior to MRI in the detection of nonmineralized disc herniations and secondary changes with prognostic implications, such as spinal cord contusion or myelomalacia. It is also important to note that the identification of the most significant lesion in a dog with multifocal disc herniations may be challenging. In case of mineralized intervertebral disc herniation (with or without associated hemorrhage), any abnormal extradural material causing a variable degree of spinal cord compression will be hyperattenuating and easily visualized within the vertebral canal. In acute cases, effacement of the epidural fat may also be observed. A CT diagnosis of herniation of nonmineralized intervertebral disc material is more challenging and may be aided by either intravenous or intrathecal contrast medium administration (CT myelogram). CT is also useful in the evaluation of congenital spinal anomalies/malformations; inflammatory conditions of the osseous vertebrae; paraspinal soft tissues and/or vertebral canal (discospondylitis, paraspinal abscess, or epidural empyema); vertebral, paraspinal, or epidural neoplasms, including muscle masses and nerve sheath tumors; spinal trauma; and degenerative conditions. It is important to note the following considerations:[5,8,28]

- Determination of the exact anatomical location of a lesion with respect to the spinal cord (extradural, intradural-extramedullary, or intramedullary) may be challenging on CT.
- Nonenhancing lesions, such as herniated nonmineralized disc material, myelitis, or some intramedullary tumors (e.g., gliomas), may not be detectable on CT.
- Degenerative and metabolic myelopathies do not typically result in CT abnormalities.

In addition to image evaluation in the transverse plane, assessment of multiplanar reconstructed images is greatly helpful in evaluating conformation and alignment of the osseous vertebrae and intervertebral disc spaces and the vertebral canal. 3D reconstruction of a spinal CT data set can contribute to a better understanding of the conformation of the osseous vertebrae and vertebral alignment and is commonly performed for surgical planning of congenital or traumatic spinal abnormalities (see Fig. 13.4). An example of a spinal CT study in a dog with intervertebral disc extrusion is provided in Figure 13.12.

Magnetic resonance imaging (MRI)

MRI has superior soft tissue imaging capabilities compared to radiographs or CT and is considered the gold standard for the evaluation of most disorders of the central nervous system in dogs. Possible exceptions include animals unable to undergo prolonged anesthesia, acute head or spinal trauma patients, and patients with metallic material in the area of interest or primarily osseous or mineral abnormalities. A detailed discussion of the physics and basic principles of MRI is beyond the scope of this chapter; however, a brief overview of the principles of image formation, MRI sequences and techniques, and interpretation principles is provided. The reader is referred to other texts for more detailed information.[3,29]

MRI is a modality that aims at the visualization of mobile hydrogen protons. Hydrogen is the most common element in the body. MRI can distinguish hydrogen protons within different tissues and structures (e.g., soft tissue, fat, and fluid). When placing a patient in the gantry of an MRI scanner, most of the patient's hydrogen protons align with the main magnetic field. These hydrogen protons can now be manipulated by the application of targeted radiofrequency pulses. After the radiofrequency pulses are switched off, hydrogen protons return to their original alignment while releasing energy that is received and used for image generation. Different tissues and materials will behave differently depending on the distribution and number of hydrogen protons and other factors such as magnetic field variations, leading to different levels of brightness ("intensities") on the resulting images. Modifying scan parameters (most importantly, the time of repetition [TR] between successive radiofrequency pulses and the time of echo [TE] between the radiofrequency pulse and signal generation, although there are many others) generates image data sets in which different tissues appear with different intensities, thereby allowing identification of the type of tissue and any intrinsic tissue abnormalities. These different types of image data sets are termed "sequences", and the parameters used for their acquisition determine their "weighting". Most soft tissue materials contain a large amount of mobile hydrogen protons, giving a strong signal on most MRI sequences. On the contrary, regions that do not contain hydrogen protons at all (e.g., air-filled spaces) and structures containing nonmobile/tightly bound hydrogen protons (e.g., cortical bone, mineralization, tendons, and ligaments) will show no signal on MRI and appear black.

The indications for intravenous contrast medium administration in MRI and the requirements for a lesion to show contrast enhancement are the same as in CT studies. MRI contrast agents are gadolinium based, paramagnetic, and produce signal intensity changes in enhancing tissues due to their effect on the local magnetic field. The standard dose is 0.2 mmol/kg, which can be increased when performing vascular studies. With the exception of a few isolated reports of adverse effects, MRI contrast agents are considered safe for use in dogs.[30]

Important MRI sequences include the following:

- ***T1-weighting:*** On T1-weighted images, fluid is dark, fat is bright, and soft tissues are intermediate. Most lesions will appear T1 hypointense prior to contrast medium administration. Exceptions include, among others, fat-containing lesions, certain stages of hemorrhage, some types of mineral deposits (e.g., manganese), some melanocytic lesions, and occasionally vascular events. Contrast-enhancing lesions will appear hyperintense on postcontrast T1-weighted images.
- ***T2-weighting:*** On T2-weighted images, fluid is bright. Even though fat should in theory appear dark, recent modifications to T2 techniques and the introduction of fast and turbo spin echo techniques have changed the appearance of fat, which now typically appears hyperintense on these sequences. Soft tissues are intermediate in intensity. Most central nervous system lesions will result in an increase in mobile hydrogen protons, resulting in increased T2 signal intensity of the affected tissue. For this reason, T2-weighted imaging has also been termed a "pathology scan". Exceptions include lesions containing mineral substances, certain stages of hemorrhage, some granulomatous and neoplastic lesions, and others.
- ***Intermediate or proton-density (PD) weighting:*** This technique is characterized by excellent anatomic detail and has improved bone imaging abilities compared to many other MRI sequences.
- ***Fluid-attenuated inversion recovery (FLAIR):*** On FLAIR images, pure fluid is suppressed and will appear hypointense (dark or "black"). While FLAIR images can in theory be generated with either T1- or T2-weighting, T2-weighted FLAIR is more commonly used. On T2-FLAIR, structures and lesions containing pure/cystic fluid (e.g., normal ventricles and cysts) are suppressed, while T2 hyperintense noncystic structures and abnormalities (most brain lesions, such as inflammatory, vascular, edematous, and neoplastic abnormalities) will remain hyperintense. This not only allows classification of a lesion as cystic or solid, it also increases the conspicuity of lesions adjacent to fluid-filled structures. Fluids containing cells and/or protein will not suppress on FLAIR, constituting a potential pitfall.
- ***Short tau inversion recovery (STIR):*** On STIR images, fat is suppressed and will appear hypointense (dark). Fluid and T2 hyperintense structures and lesions will appear hyperintense. This sequence aids in the classification of a lesion as fatty and increases conspicuity of soft tissue infiltrates in fatty tissues by suppressing the background signal. STIR sequences are excellent for the evaluation of bone

marrow, paraspinal muscle/soft tissue, and brachial or lumbosacral plexus lesions.

- ***Single shot techniques:*** Heavily T2-weighted images provide excellent delineation of fluid-filled spaces and structures and, when used for imaging of the spine, provide similar information as a conventional myelogram. Names used for these sequences in the literature are often specific to a particular vendor (e.g., HASTE, SS-FSE, SSH-TSE, FASE), and the neutral term "magnetic resonance (MR) myelogram" should be given preference. These techniques are excellent not only to classify spinal lesions as intramedullary, intradural-extramedullary, or extradural, but also to differentiate acute from chronic compressive myelopathies and identify dilatation of the subarachnoid space (e.g., with subarachnoid diverticula). They may also provide prognostic information in dogs suspected of myelomalacia.
- ***T2*-weighting:*** T2*-weighted images are very sensitive to magnetic field inhomogeneities. This is an advantage in the diagnosis of hemorrhagic lesions, which will focally distort the magnetic field and result in a markedly hypointense region on these images ("susceptibility artifact"). Similar hypointensities can be caused by proximity of air-filled spaces or the presence of mineralization.
- ***Susceptibility weighted imaging*** is a newer, similar technique believed to provide improved differentiation between truly hemorrhagic and mineralized lesions compared to T2*-weighted images.

TABLE 13.3 Suggested protocols for magnetic resonance examination of the canine brain and spine.

Brain	Spine
■ Sagittal T2 ■ Transverse T2 ■ Transverse T1 ■ Transverse T2-FLAIR ■ Transverse T2* ■ Diffusion weighted imaging ■ Postcontrast T1 (transverse, sagittal and/or dorsal plane; +/- fat saturation) ■ +/- Dorsal T2 ■ +/- PD-W ■ +/- 3D T2-W sequence ■ +/- 3D T1-W sequence ■ +/- STIR ■ +/- Others	■ Dorsal STIR ■ Sagittal T2 ■ Sagittal T1 ■ Sagittal STIR ■ Sagittal MR myelogram ■ Transverse T1 ■ Transverse T2 ■ +/- Postcontrast T1 (transverse, sagittal and/or dorsal plane; +/- fat saturation) ■ +/- T2* ■ +/- 3D T2-W sequence ■ +/- 3D T1-W sequence ■ +/- PD-W ■ +/- Others

STIR, short tau inversion recovery; FLAIR, fluid-attenuated inversion recovery; MR, magnetic resonance; PD-W, proton density–weighting; T2-W, T2-weighted; T1-W, T1-weighted.

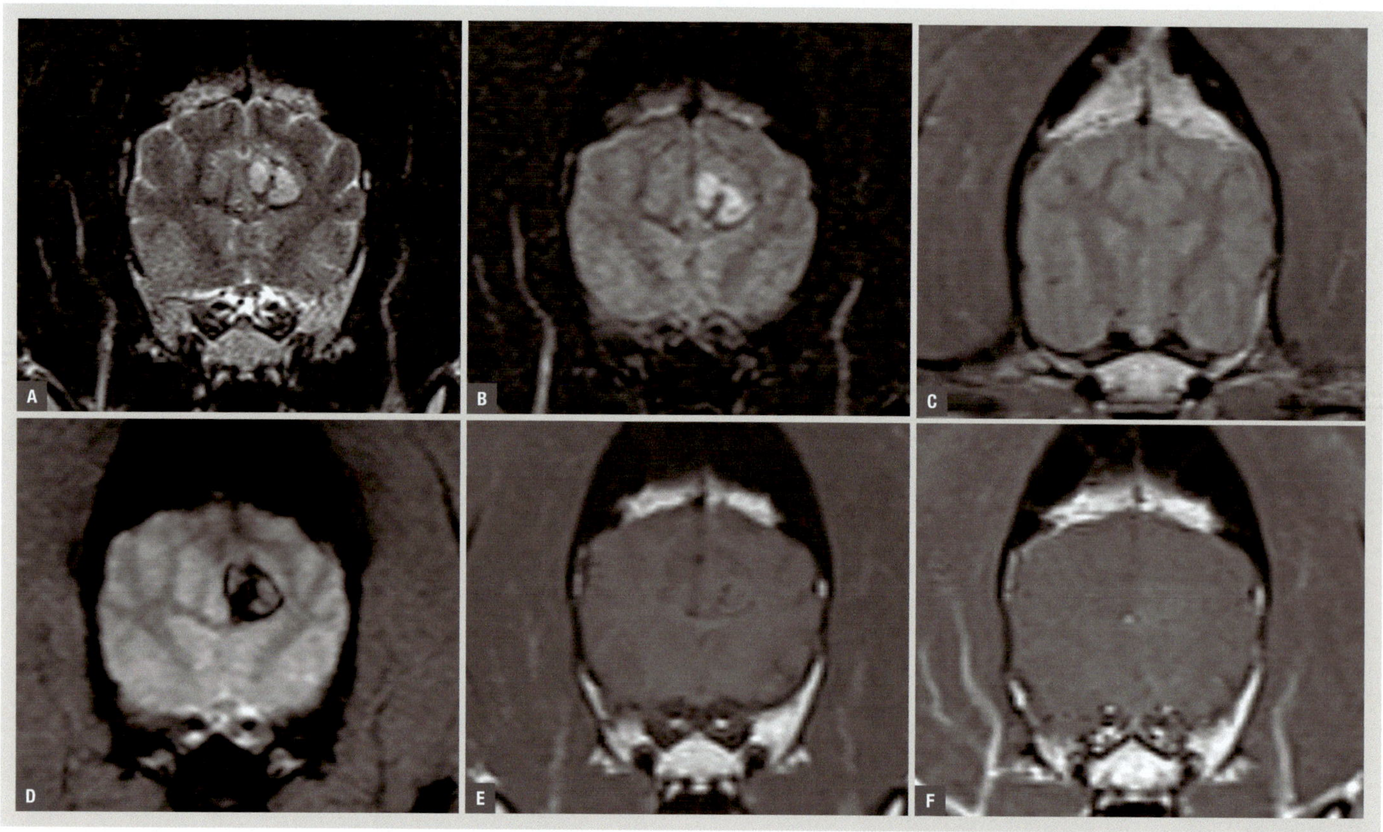

FIG. 13.13 Magnetic resonance imaging study of the brain in a 3-year-old Rottweiler presented with acute onset seizures. Transverse T2-weighted (**A**), T2-FLAIR (fluid-attenuated inversion recovery) (**B**), proton-density-weighted (**C**), T2*-weighted (**D**), and pre- (**E**) and postcontrast (**F**) T1-weighted images at the level of the forebrain. There is a focal mass associated with the left frontal lobe. The lesion is bilobed, with a hyperintense center and hypointense rim on T2 and FLAIR images (**A, B**). On T2*-weighted images (**D**), the lesion is markedly hypointense, consistent with a susceptibility artifact. The lesion is inconspicuous and isointense to brain parenchyma on proton-density and T1-weighted images (**C, E**) and does not show evidence of contrast-enhancement (**F**). Based on imaging findings and follow-up, a diagnosis of hemorrhagic stroke was made.

- *Diffusion-weighted imaging (DWI) and apparent diffusion coefficient (ADC) map:* This technique allows the identification of tissues affected by cytotoxic edema. It is most commonly used to identify ischemic events (infarcts), which will appear hyperintense on DWI and hypointense on ADC map. It is important to note that this technique is most useful in the acute stage of ischemic lesions, and that subacute or chronic infarcts will present with pseudonormalization or even reversal of signal intensities. DWI has other possible applications, including the identification of intracranial abscesses and evaluation of certain intracranial neoplastic diseases.
- *Fat suppression:* Unlike STIR, which is a standalone sequence with a specific weighting, fat suppression can be added onto any sequence. If added to a T2-weighted or proton density–weighted sequence, it will result in suppression of fat, increasing the conspicuity of any bone marrow or adjacent soft tissue lesions. If added onto postcontrast T1-weighted images, it will suppress signal from fat, and any residual hyperintense region will most likely represent contrast-enhancement. This increases the conspicuity of contrast-enhancing lesions. Fat suppression techniques are limited to high-field magnets.

Numerous MRI sequences exist, and more are being constantly developed. Additional sequences that are gaining popularity and are increasingly being used in small animal neuroimaging include 3D volume acquisitions with various weightings (which allow acquisition of very thin slices and reconstruction of images into different planes), subtraction techniques (most commonly subtraction of pre- and postcontrast T1-weighted images to increase conspicuity of contrast-enhancing lesions), and vascular imaging techniques.

An MRI study of the brain can be performed with the patient in dorsal or sternal recumbency. An MRI study of the spine (including the brachial and lumbosacral plexus) is typically performed in dorsal recumbency, with possible exceptions including spinal trauma cases, in which distortion of paraspinal muscular/soft tissues would interfere with image interpretation and surgical planning, and others. Various recommendations for optimal brain and spine imaging can be found in the literature.[31,32] Some suggested protocols can be found in Table 13.3. Examples of MRI studies of the brain and spine in canine patients are provided in Figures 13.13 and 13.14 and Videos 13.1 and 13.2.

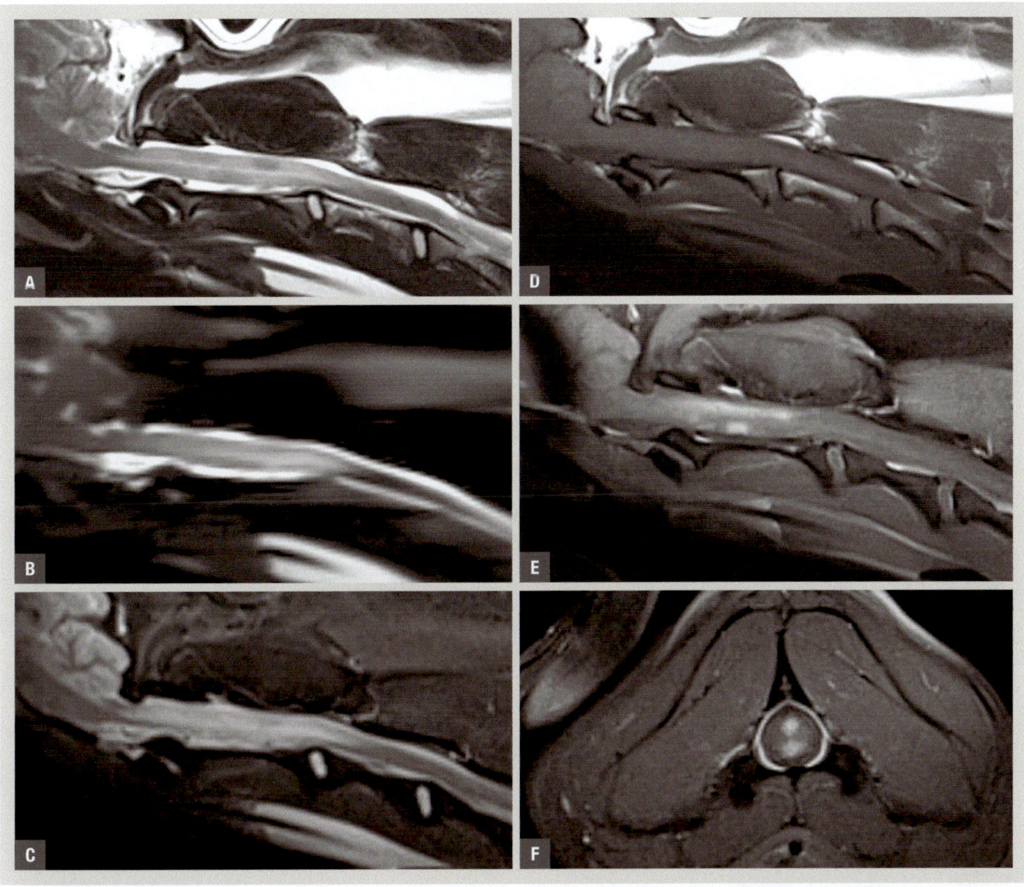

FIG. 13.14 Magnetic resonance imaging study of the cervical spine in a 9-year-old mixed breed dog with progressive C1–C5 myelopathy. Sagittal T2-weighted (**A**), magnetic resonance myelogram (**B**), STIR (short tau inversion recovery) (**C**), precontrast T1-weighted (**D**), and postcontrast sagittal (**E**) and transverse (**F**) T1-weighted images with fat saturation. There is an intramedullary lesion associated with the cranial cervical spinal cord, extending from the foramen magnum to the midbody of C3. The lesion is T2 hyperintense, with multifocal foci that are isointense to the normal spinal cord (A through C). There is mild circumferential attenuation of the subarachnoid space (**B**). The lesion is T1 isointense to the spinal cord (**D**). On postcontrast images, there are multifocal rounded to linear regions of strong contrast-enhancement within the cord, corresponding to the T2 isointense regions. A large portion of the adjacent intramedullary T2 hyperintensity is nonenhancing, consistent with perilesional edema. A diagnosis of meningomyelitis of unknown origin was made based on imaging findings, inflammatory cerebrospinal fluid tap, negative infectious disease testing, and response to treatment.

Video 13.1

Approach to magnetic resonance imaging of the brain.

Video 13.2

Approach to magnetic resonance imaging of the spine.

KEY POINTS

Diagnostic imaging is an integral part of the workup of dogs with neurological diseases.

Survey radiographs

- May allow identification of major skull lesions but are inadequate for evaluation of intracranial structures.
- Useful for spinal imaging, specifically for:
  – Providing a general overview of the anatomical conformation and vertebral alignment.
  – Evaluating obvious bone lesions (e.g., fractures, discospondylitis, or bone neoplasms).
  – Assessing the patient for suspected spinal instability.

Computed tomography

- Fast.
- Can be performed under sedation.
- Excellent test to identify cortical bone lesions, mineralized lesions such as intervertebral disc extrusions, and spinal or intracranial hemorrhage.
- Modality of choice in the evaluation of trauma patients and patients with congenital or acquired bone lesions.
- Generally adequate in the evaluation of contrast-enhancing soft tissue lesions.
- Lacks accuracy in the evaluation of subtle and non-contrast-enhancing soft tissue abnormalities as well as bone marrow lesions.

Magnetic resonance imaging

- Generally considered the gold standard for the evaluation of the brain and spine in dogs.
- Possible exceptions include cases of acute trauma, patients unable to undergo prolonged anesthesia, and patients with primarily bone or mineral abnormalities or metallic material in the area of interest.
- More sensitive compared to other techniques in detecting ischemic vascular and inflammatory lesions, and intraparenchymal non-enhancing, space-occupying lesions.
- Slower than CT.

References

1. Drees R. Head. In: Hecht S (ed.). *Diagnostic Radiology in Small Animal Practice*, 2nd ed. Sheffield: 5m Publishing Ltd; 2020. pp. 53–71.
2. Hecht S. Brain. In: Schwarz T, Saunders J (eds.). *Veterinary Computed Tomography.* West Sussex: Wiley-Blackwell; 2011. pp. 185–196.
3. Mai W. *Diagnostic MRI in Dogs and Cats.* Boca Raton: CRC Press (Taylor and Francis); 2018.
4. Joslyn S, Hague D. Magnetic resonance imaging of the small animal brain. *In Practice.* 2016;38.
5. Wisner E, Zwingenberger A. *Small Animal CT and MRI.* Ames: Wiley Blackwell; 2015.
6. Owen M. Radiographic, Computed Tomography, and Magnetic Resonance Contrast Media. In: Thrall DE (ed.). *Veterinary Diagnostic Radiology*, 7th ed. St. Louis: WB Saunders; 2018. pp. 96–109.
7. Hecht S, Morandi F. Spine (Neuroradiology including Contrast procedures). In: Hecht S (ed.). *Diagnostic Radiology in Small Animal Practice*, 2nd ed. Sheffield: 5m Publishing Ltd; 2020. pp. 72–105.
8. Widmer WR, Thrall DE. Canine and Feline Vertebrae. In: Thrall DE (ed.). *Veterinary Diagnostic Radiology*, 7th ed. St. Louis: WB Saunders; 2018. pp. 249–270.
9. Seiler G, Kinns J, Dennison S, et al. Vertebral column and spinal cord. In: Schwarz T, Saunders J (eds.). *Veterinary Computed Tomography.* West Sussex: Wiley-Blackwell; 2011. pp. 209–228.
10. Couturier L, Degueurce C, Ruel Y, et al. Anatomical study of cranial nerve emergence and skull foramina in the dog using magnetic resonance imaging and computed tomography. *Vet Radiol Ultrasound.* 2005;46:375–383.
11. Parry AT, Volk HA. Imaging the cranial nerves. *Vet Radiol Ultrasound.* 2011;52:S32-41.
12. Mai W. MRI of the Brachial and Lumbosacral Plexuses. In: Mai W (ed.). *Diagnostic MRI in Dogs and Cats.* Boca Raton: CRC Press; 2018. pp. 603–617.
13. Kraft S, Ehrhart EJ, Gall D, et al. Magnetic resonance imaging characteristics of peripheral nerve sheath tumors of the canine brachial plexus in 18 dogs. *Vet Radiol Ultrasoun.* 2007;48:1–7.
14. May DA, Disler DG, Jones EA, et al. Abnormal signal intensity in skeletal muscle at MR imaging: Patterns, pearls, and pitfalls. *Radiographics.* 2000;20:S295-S315.
15. Morrison EJ, Baron-Chapman ML, Chalkley M. MRI T2/STIR epaxial muscle hyperintensity in some dogs with intervertebral disc extrusion corresponds to histologic patterns of muscle degeneration and inflammation. *Vet Radiol Ultrasoun.* 2021;62:150–160.
16. Barone G, Ziemer LS, Shofer FS, Steinberg SA. Risk factors associated with development of seizures after use of iohexol for myelography in dogs: 182 cases (1998). *J Am Vet Med Assoc.* 2002 May 15;220(10):1499–1502.
17. Robertson I, Thrall DE. Imaging dogs with suspected disc herniation: pros and cons of myelography, computed tomography, and magnetic resonance. *Vet Radiol Ultrasound.* 2011;52:S81-84.
18. Roberts RE, Selcer BA. Myelography and epidurography. *Vet Clin North Am Small Anim Pract.* 1993;23:307–329.
19. Schwarz T, Saunders J. *Veterinary Computed Tomography.* West Sussex: Wiley-Blackwell; 2011.
20. Chai O, Peery D, Bdolah-Abram T, et al. Computed tomographic findings in dogs with head trauma and development of a novel prognostic computed tomography-based scoring system. *Am J Vet Res.* 2017;78:1085–1090.
21. Turrel JM, Fike JR, LeCouteur RA, Higgins RJ. Computed tomographic characteristics of primary brain tumors in 50 dogs. *J Am Vet Med Assoc.* 1986;188:851–856.
22. Gielen I, Kromhout K, Gavin P, et al. Agreement between low-field MRI and CT for the detection of suspected intracranial lesions in dogs and cats. *J Am Vet Med Assoc.* 2013;243:367–375.
23. Vitale S, Foss K. Immune-Mediated Central Nervous System Disease-Current Knowledge and Recommendations. *Top Companion Anim Med.* 2019 Mar;34:22–29.
24. Emery L, Hecht S, Sun X. Investigation of parameters predicting the need for diagnostic imaging beyond computed tomography in the evaluation of dogs with thoracolumbar myelopathy: Retrospective evaluation of 555 dogs. *Vet Radiol Ultrasound.* 2018;59:147–154.
25. Hecht S, Thomas WB, Marioni-Henry K, et al. Myelography Vs. Computed Tomography in the Evaluation of Acute Thoracolumbar Intervertebral Disk Extrusion in Chondrodystrophic Dogs. *Vet Radiol Ultrasoun.* 2009;50:353–359.
26. Israel SK, Levine JM, Kerwin SC, et al. The Relative Sensitivity of Computed Tomography and Myelography for Identification of Thoracolumbar Intervertebral Disk Herniations in Dogs. *Vet Radiol Ultrasoun.* 2009;50:247–252.
27. Olby NJ, Munana KR, Sharp NJH, Thrall DE. The computed tomographic appearance of acute thoracolumbar intervertebral disc herniations in dogs. *Vet Radiol Ultrasoun.* 2000;41:396–402.
28. Kinns J, Mai W, Seiler G, et al. Radiographic sensitivity and negative predictive value for acute canine spinal trauma. *Vet Radiol Ultrasoun.* 2006;47:563–570.
29. Hecht S. Update on Magnetic Resonance Imaging of the Brain and Spine. *Advances in Small Animal Care.* 2022:73–94.
30. Scarabelli S, Cripps P, Rioja E, Alderson B. Adverse reactions following administration of contrast media for diagnostic imaging in anaesthetized dogs and cats: a retrospective study. *Vet Anaesth Analg.* 2016 Sep;43(5):502–510.
31. Dennis R. Optimized technique: Spine. In: Mai W (ed.). *Diagnostic MRI in Dogs and Cats.* Boca Raton: CRC Press; 2018. pp. 106–129.
32. Hecht S. Optimized technique: Brain. In: Mai W (ed.). *Diagnostic MRI in Dogs and Cats.* Boca Raton: CRC Press; 2018. pp. 88–105.

CHAPTER 14

Electrodiagnostic investigations

Ezio Bianchi
DVM, DECVN

Video 14.1

Primary orthostatic tremor in a Siberian Husky. Note the intense muscle tremor of the hindlimbs when standing and the difficulty in transitioning to a sitting position. The electromyogram recorded with monopolar electrodes in the awake dog while standing shows typical discharges with a frequency of 19 Hz. Muscle silence is observed during electromyography in lateral recumbency.

Electrodiagnostic (EDX) investigations, when applied to the nervous system, provide information about the function of neural structures. These tests are also known as clinical electrophysiological studies because they basically consist in recording the electrical activity produced spontaneously (electroencephalography [EEG] or electromyography [EMG]) or as a result of the application of specific stimuli (motor nerve conduction studies [MNCS], sensory nerve conduction studies [SNCS], F waves, and others) by neurons or muscle fibers. Depending on the type of EDX test, electrical, magnetic, acoustic, or visual stimuli may be required.[1,2]

EDX investigations are a very sensitive and objective extension of the neurological examination, which can be used to study the function of specific structures.[2] Some tests, such as EMG, MNCS, F-wave testing, repetitive nerve stimulation (RNS), and motor evoked potentials (MEPs), examine in detail specific parts of the somatic efferent (motor) structures (central and/or peripheral nervous system, neuromuscular junction, muscles). Other tests such as SNCS and recording of cord dorsum potentials (CDPs) and somatosensory evoked potentials (SSEPs) are used to investigate specific segments of the peripheral or central part of the somatic afferent (sensory) pathways. There are also tests that assess both the afferent and the efferent arms of a particular reflex arc, such as the H reflex and the blink reflex.

Finally, some tests are specifically designed to assess special senses, such as electroretinography (ERG) or the assessment of brainstem auditory evoked potentials (BAEPs) and visual evoked potentials (VEPs).[1]

Because of its characteristics, EDX testing can help to localize and assess the severity of the dysfunction of the affected nervous structures. An important limitation of EDX testing is that it rarely provides etiological information. Other diagnostic tests, such as imaging, laboratory investigations, or examination of tissue biopsies are often needed to determine the nature of the lesions.[2,3]

EDX studies are performed using specific equipment. Needle electrodes of various types and lengths are commonly used for electrical stimulation and as recording and grounding electrodes. These tests are painful, and voluntary muscle contractions and tremors can make interpretation of the tracings difficult. Therefore, they are usually performed under general anesthesia. Body temperature should be monitored during an EDX study, as hypothermia and hyperthermia affect the results. Other important sources of interference are artifacts from other electrical devices located close to the patient.[3] Electrical noise should be reduced at least to an acceptable level, especially when recording smaller sensitive potentials such as SSEPs or BAEPs, or during SNCS.[3,4]

The first part of this chapter introduces the tests used to investigate neuromuscular disorders: EMG, MNCS, RNS, F wave and H reflex testing, SNCS, and assessment of cord dorsum potentials. The second part of the chapter addresses BAEP, transcranial MEP and SSEP testing. These techniques provide information about the function of the central nervous system, among other things.

Electrodiagnostic tests performed in the diagnostic evaluation of neuromuscular disorders

Electromyography (EMG)

EMG records the electrical activity produced by striated muscles. EMG potentials can result from voluntary muscle contractions or from spontaneous depolarization of muscle cells. Obtaining EMG recordings of voluntary contractions requires the patient's cooperation. In small animals, EMG is therefore usually performed under general anesthesia and only spontaneous electrical activity is evaluated.[1,3] An exception is the study of involuntary pathological tremor. In these cases, recording the muscle potentials responsible for the tremor syndrome in the conscious dog can help to define the type of tremor (e.g., orthostatic tremor; Video 14.1).[5]

Muscle potentials are usually recorded using standard concentric needles inserted at different points and to different depths to map most of the volume of the muscle under study. These special needles record the potentials generated by the muscle fibers near the tip of the needle. The interpretation of the recorded electrical activity is done by the operator looking at the screen and listening to the sounds produced by the loudspeaker of the device.[3,6]

When the dog is under anesthesia, normal muscles are relaxed and therefore electrically silent, resulting in a flat tracing. Insertional activity, miniature endplate potentials (MEPPs), and endplate spikes (EPS) are the only (physiological) potentials that can be recorded in normal muscles. Insertional activity is recorded during needle insertion as a result of the irritation of muscle fibers. MEPPs and EPS can be recorded in normal muscles when the needle tip is close to the endplate.[7]

Abnormal findings on EMG tracings are the result of spontaneous depolarization of single muscle fibers or of the spontaneous activation of a motor unit (motor unit action potential [MUAP]).[8]

Fibrillation potentials and *positive sharp waves* are the most common pathological potentials that can be recorded as a consequence of spontaneous depolarization of single muscle fibers. These potentials have characteristic morphologies and a regular firing rate. *Complex repetitive discharges* (CRDs) are the result of the spontaneous activation of multiple muscle fibers firing in synchrony, producing a uniform repetitive polyphasic pattern (Fig. 14.1). They typically start, stop, or change their waveform abruptly. *Myotonic potentials* are discharges from a single muscle fiber (Video 14.2). They can be distinguished from CRDs, fibrillations, and positive sharp waves by the waxing and waning of the amplitude and frequency of the individual potentials (Table 14.1).[3,8,9]

Fibrillation potentials, positive sharp waves, and CRDs are classified as spontaneous pathological activity (SPA) and indicate the presence of a pathological condition affecting the motor nerve fibers innervating the muscle (neuropathy) or directly affecting the muscle (myopathy). With denervation, at least 5 days are required for SPA to occur.[3] Myotonic discharges are recorded in myotonia congenita and myotonic dystrophy, but also in myotonia secondary to pituitary-dependent hypercortisolism.[8,10]

MUAPs result from the synchronous activation of a single motor unit's muscle fibers. A single MUAP is usually defined as a fasciculation. When a single motor unit fires two, three, or more times in a very short interval, the terms doublets, triplets, and multiplets are used (see Fig. 14.1). These potentials reflect the spontaneous activation of a lower motor neuron or its axon and are occasionally recorded in motor neuron diseases, radiculopathies, entrapment neuropathies, and polyneuropathies (see Table 14.1).[8,11]

Myokymic and neuromyotonic discharges are spontaneous discharges from a single motor unit with distinct characteristic patterns that have been reported in several disorders such as channelopathies (Video 14.3; see Table 14.1).[8,11]

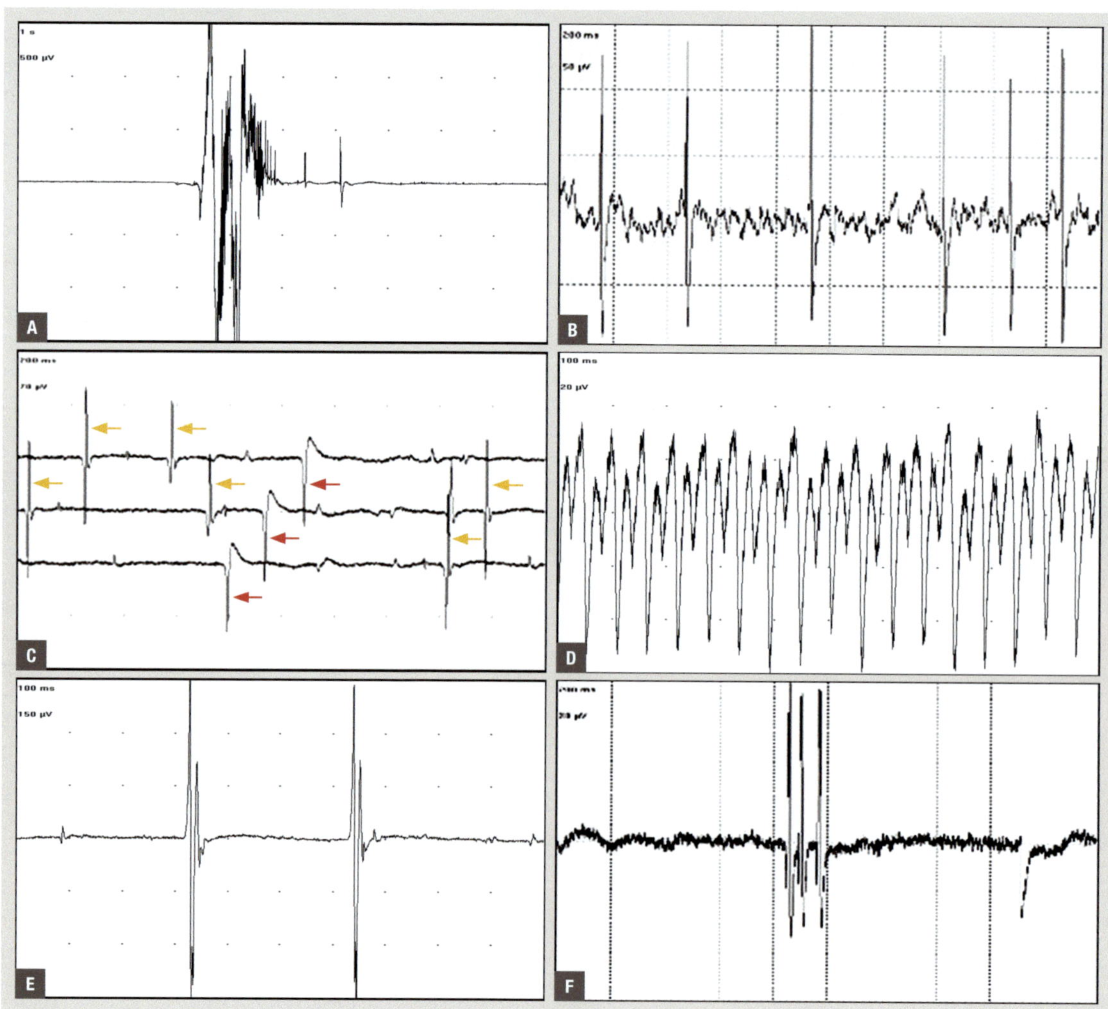

FIG. 14.1 Examples of spontaneous potentials on electromyography (EMG). **(A)** Insertional activity in a normal muscle. 100 ms/Div; 500 µV/Div. **(B)** Six endplate spikes on a background of miniature endplate potentials. 20 ms/Div; 50 µV/Div. **(C)** Spontaneous pathological activity consisting of fibrillations (orange arrows) and positive sharp waves (red arrows). 20 ms/Div; 70 µV/Div. **(D)** Complex repetitive discharge. 10 ms/Div; 20 µV/Div. **(E)** Triphasic motor unit action potential (MUAP). 10 ms/Div; 150 µV/Div. **(F)** Single MUAP firing three times in about 15 ms (triplet). 20 ms/Div; 20 µV/Div.

Motor nerve conduction studies (MNCS)

As reported in the previous paragraph, pathological findings on EMG are often similar in myopathic and neuropathic disorders. MNCS and other tests that evaluate nerve fibers (F wave testing, SNCS, recording of CDPs) provide useful information to detect neuropathies and characterize the lesion.

Specifically, MNCS assess the function of motor fibers in the peripheral nerves. The most commonly assessed nerves are the radial and ulnar nerves for the forelimb and the sciatic–tibial and sciatic–peroneal nerves for the hindlimb.[3] The stimulation and recording points for these nerves are the same as for the other tests that evaluate motor and/or sensory fibers (Fig. 14.2). The nerve is electrically stimulated using two monopolar needle electrodes (cathode and anode) placed approximately 2–3 cm apart.[3,13] Depolarization of the nerve fibers under the cathode produces a nerve impulse that travels along the nerve fibers. The result of motor fiber activation is a compound muscle action potential (CMAP), which is recorded in a target muscle innervated by the nerve under study. A CMAP is the sum of the action potentials of the muscle fibers activated by the nerve impulse. A CMAP therefore reflects muscle fiber function and, indirectly, motor nerve fiber function and transmission at the neuromuscular junction. Supramaximal stimuli are used to ensure all axons are activated. A stimulus is considered supramaximal if the increase in intensity does not result in an increase in CMAP amplitude. To obtain a conduction velocity value of the motor nerve fibers only (avoiding a conduction delay at the nerve terminals, neuromuscular junction, and muscle fibers), the nerve must be stimulated in at least two sites (Fig. 14.2). Motor nerve conduction velocity is the difference in latency between the two CMAP responses divided by the surface distance between the two stimulation points. This value reflects the speed of the fastest motor nerve fibers.[1,3]

In addition to motor nerve conduction velocity, the other parameters necessary for interpretation of a MNCS are derived from accurate examination and measurement of distal and proximal CMAPs. In particular, the amplitude, area, duration, and morphology of CMAPs are evaluated and compared to normal values reported in the literature or, ideally, to values obtained from a group of normal dogs tested using the same methodology.[14]

When interpreting MNCS findings, it is also very important to consider the effect of physiological factors such as limb temperature, limb length, volume of the target muscle and age of the dog.[1,3] To aid in the interpretation of MNCS findings, the nerves of the contralateral limb should be tested for comparison if the disorder is limited to one limb.

TABLE 14.1 Main features of the spontaneous physiological and pathological potentials that can be recorded by electromyography.[8,9]

	Origin	Morphology, firing rate, and pattern	Sound	Interpretation
Insertional activity	Muscle fibers	High-frequency discharge associated with needle insertion	Crisp static	Normally present in muscles
Miniature endplate potential (MEPP)	Endplate	Small-amplitude monophasic negative potentials/20–40 Hz	Seashell	Normally present in muscles
Endplate spikes (EPS)	Muscle fibers near endplate	Biphasic, 1–5 ms, initial negative (upward) deflection, irregular	Sputtering	Normally present in muscles
Fibrillations	Muscle fibers	Biphasic/triphasic, duration 1–5 ms, initial positive (downward) deflection, regular 0.5–10 Hz	Rain on roof, frying eggs	Neuropathy, myopathy
Positive sharp waves	Muscle fibers	Biphasic, long duration, initial positive (downward) deflection, regular 0.5–10 Hz	Dull pops	Neuropathy, myopathy
Complex repetitive discharges	Multiple muscle fibers, time-linked	Repetitive high frequency polyphasic/complex discharges; uniform frequency, amplitude, and shape	Machine gun	Neuropathy, myopathy (chronic)
Myotonic potentials	Single muscle fiber	Repetitive discharges of a single myofiber, waxing and waning of amplitude and frequency	Dive bomber	Myopathies (e.g., myotonia, "Cushing's myotonia")
Fasciculations, doublets, triplets, multiplets	Muscle fibers of a motor unit	High-amplitude long duration (>5 ms) biphasic, triphasic or polyphasic potentials. The MUAP can be single or the motor unit may fire two, three or more times in a very short interval	Corn popping, horse trotting	Tetanus, motor neuron disease, radiculopathies, polyneuropathies
Myokymic discharges	Muscle fibers of a motor unit	Rhythmic, grouped discharges of the same motor unit (MUAP); rate interburst 1–5 Hz	Marching soldiers	Myokymia, radiculopathy, neuropathy, channellopathies
Neuromyotonic discharges	Muscle fibers of a motor unit	High-frequency decrementing, repetitive discharges of a single motor unit (MUAP)	Pinging sound	Neuromyotonia, channellopathies

Video 14.2

Example of myotonic potentials. Note the waxing and waning of the discharges of the individual muscle fibers.

Video 14.3

Example of myokymic discharges. Note the rhythmic, clustered discharges of the motor unit muscle fibers.

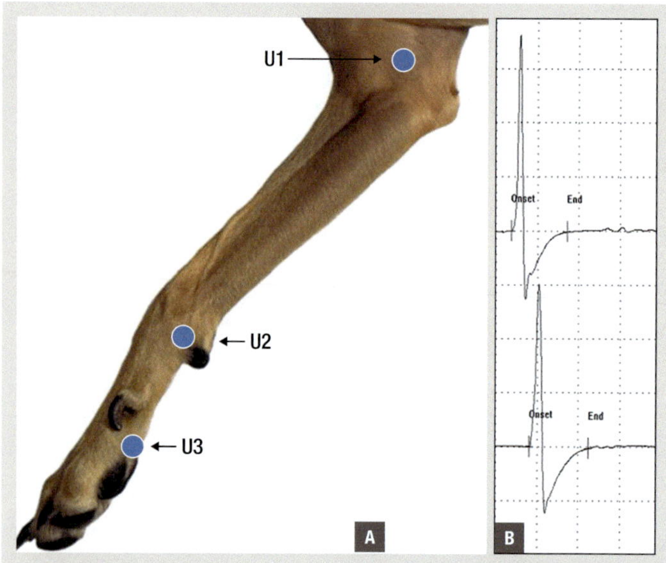

FIG. 14.2 (**A**) Schematic representation of the most common points of stimulation and recording in electrodiagnostic studies of the ulnar nerve. U1, proximal stimulation point of motor nerve conduction studies (MNCS), recording point of sensory nerve conduction studies (SNCS); U2, distal stimulation point of MNCS, stimulation point of F waves and repetitive nerve stimulation (RNS), point of stimulation or of recording of SNCS; U3, MNCS recording point (palmar interossei muscle), SNCS stimulation point. (**B**) MNCS of a normal ulnar nerve. Upper tracing: compound muscle action potential (CMAP) with distal stimulation (U2). Lower tracing: CMAP with proximal stimulation (U1). Conduction velocity, 63 m/s; 5 ms/Div; 5 mV/Div.

To avoid recording falsely reduced CMAP amplitudes, the use of monopolar needle electrodes during MNCS, RNS and F wave testing is recommended. In particular, it is ideal to place the recording electrode in the belly of the target muscle, close to the motor point, and the reference electrode on the tendon (belly-tendon placement) or distally in the subcutaneous tissue in small muscles such as the interossei muscles.[1,3] Identifying the prevalence of signs of axonal or demyelinating lesions of nerve fibers is important in the diagnosis of neuropathies. Signs suggestive of a demyelinating lesion are:

1. Severely reduced conduction velocity with no significant reduction in CMAP amplitude/area.
2. Increased duration of CMAPs (temporal dispersion), often with abnormal morphology (polyphasia).
3. CMAP amplitude/area to proximal stimulation is less than 50% of CMAP amplitude/area to distal stimulation. This condition is suggestive of a "conduction block" and occurs particularly when there is focal demyelination between the two stimulation points (Fig. 14.3).[1,3,13]

The main feature of axonopathy in MNCS is a reduction in the amplitudes/areas of the distal and proximal CMAPs without significant temporal dispersion and with only a mild or moderate reduction in conduction velocity (Fig. 14.3). Similar findings may be seen in disorders affecting neuromuscular transmission such as botulism or very severe myopathies.[1,3,13]

Interpretation of MNCS findings is often complicated by the simultaneous presence of axonopathy and demyelination. The appearance of SPA on EMG at least 5–7 days after the onset of the neuropathy and the grading of the signs of denervation may help to determine which of demyelination or axonopathy is the predominant lesion.

In case of traumatic nerve injury, the aim of MNCS is to classify the functional lesion into one of three categories: neurapraxia (i.e., focal segmental demyelination without disruption of axon continuity and of surrounding connective tissues), axonotmesis (i.e., damaged axons +/- disruption of surrounding connective tissues) and neurotmesis (i.e., complete nerve transection). This distinction is of great therapeutic and prognostic importance. MNCS should be performed at least 5–7 days after the injury, as Wallerian degeneration secondary to nerve fiber transection may occur in the first week. In neurapraxia, MNCS are usually normal, or a conduction block may be present at the level of the lesion. In axonotmetic lesions, the amplitude and area of the distal and proximal CMAPs are reduced. In the presence of neurotmesis, no CMAP can be recorded in the target muscle. The prognosis for recovery of function of the injured nerve is usually poor in cases of neurotmesis or axonotmesis with severely reduced amplitudes/areas.[15,16]

F waves and H reflex

Like MNCS, F wave testing assesses motor nerve fiber function. Specifically, F waves are the result of antidromic activation of the motor fibers of peripheral nerves.[1,3] Supramaximal electrical stimuli produce impulses that travel orthodromically (towards the periphery) along the fibers and trigger the generation of a CMAP (M wave), and other impulses that travel antidromically (towards the spinal cord) and reach the cell bodies of the lower motor neurons. At this level, a new signal is generated that travels orthodromically along the nerve and stimulates activation of the target

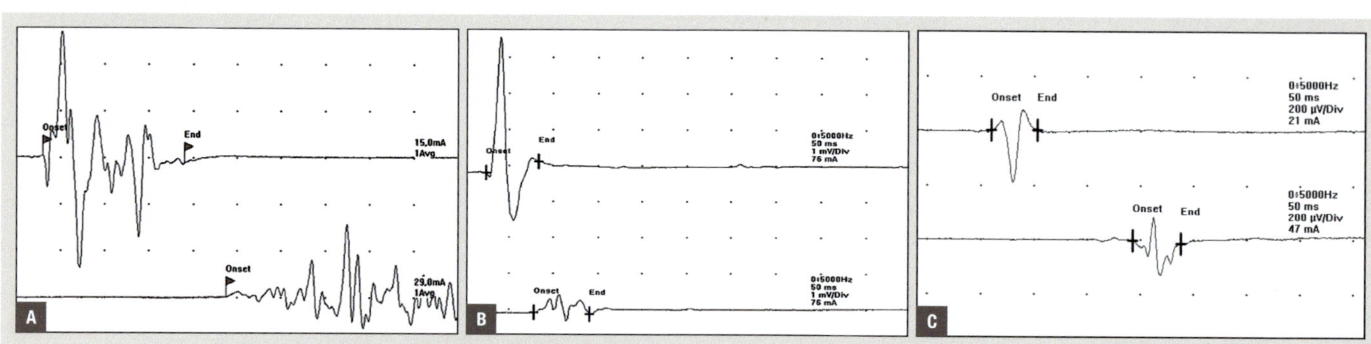

FIG. 14.3 Examples of abnormal motor nerve conduction studies (MNCS) of the ulnar nerve. (**A**) Compound muscle action potentials (CMAPs) with polyphasia and temporal dispersion. Conduction velocity, 10 m/s (demyelination); 5 ms/Div; 2 mV/Div. (**B**) CMAP amplitude to proximal stimulation is less than 50% of CMAP amplitude to distal stimulation (conduction block). Conduction velocity, 45 m/s (focal demyelination); 5 ms/Div; 1 mV/Div. (**C**) Reduced CMAP amplitude to proximal and distal stimulation. Conduction velocity, 50 m/s (axonopathy); 5 ms/Div; 200 µV/Div.

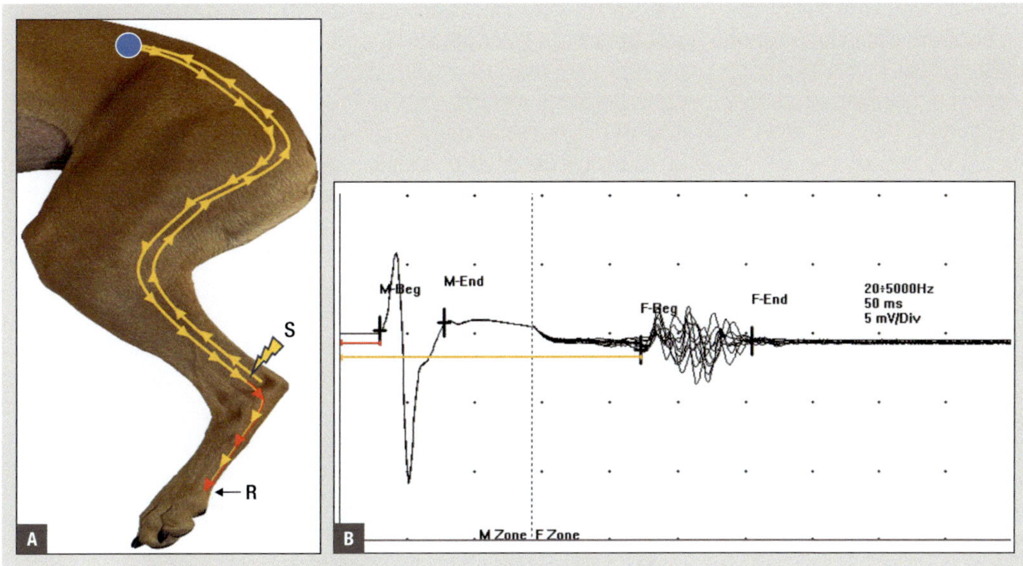

FIG. 14.4 (**A**) Schematic representation of the F wave circuit of the sciatic tibial nerve. S, stimulation at the hock; R, recording at the plantar interossei muscles. (**B**) Example of normal F waves. Red line, M wave latency; yellow line, F wave minimum latency. 5 ms/Div; 5 mV/Div.

muscle, producing specific muscle potentials called F waves (Fig. 14.4). Compared to CMAPs, F waves have a longer latency because of the circuit the action potential has to travel through. The reduced amplitude of F waves compared to that of CMAPs is due to the fact that only 1–5% of the lower motor neurons that are antidromically activated "backfire" to produce orthodromic impulses.[17] As each waveform varies slightly in amplitude, latency, and F wave configuration, a minimum of 10–20 tracings are recorded. Parameters such as minimum latency, F-ratio, and persistence (expressed as a percentage) are then measured. The circuit responsible for the generation of F waves involves only the motor fibers of motor and mixed peripheral nerves, but unlike MNCS, F wave testing also evaluates the proximal portions of these fibers. Therefore, F waves are very useful to study plexopathies and radiculopathies involving the ventral roots.[1,3,17]

An increase in the minimum latency compared to the expected latency based on limb length and a decrease in F wave persistence are usually reported in disorders affecting motor fibers.[18] In these cases, if the (demyelinating) lesions of the motor fibers are not evenly distributed along the nerve, the F-ratio will be abnormal. In particular, the F-ratio will be increased compared to normal values if the proximal segment of the nerve is more affected, and decreased if the distal portion of the nerve is more affected.[19]

The H reflex involves the same circuit as the stretch reflex. The electrical stimulus activates 1A sensory fibers, which synapse with (alpha) lower motor neurons. From the lower motor neurons, the impulse travels along motor axons and induces the generation of muscle potentials (H reflex), which appear in the waveform after the M wave and before the F waves.[1,3,17,20] Similar to F wave testing, the H reflex test evaluates the proximal part of the peripheral nerves. In this case, both the sensory and motor roots are involved in the generation of the recorded potentials. Some technical implications make the identification and interpretation of the H reflex more complex than for F waves. For this reason, the H reflex has little clinical relevance and is rarely recorded in clinical practice.

Repetitive nerve stimulation (RNS)

RNS is an electrodiagnostic test commonly used to assess neuromuscular junction function. Like MNCS, it consists in supramaximal electrical stimulation of a mixed or motor nerve and the recording of CMAPs in a target muscle. However, unlike MNCS, RNS records a series of 9 or 10 stimuli. The variations in CMAP amplitude and area are automatically measured by the EDX equipment.[3,21] In particular, the differences in the amplitude and area between the last and first CMAPs and between the fifth and first CMAPs are reported on the screen as a percent decrement or increment. Stimulation rates of 2 and 3 Hz are commonly used. In a normal dog, at these low stimulation frequencies, no decrements in the amplitude or area (or decrements of less than 10%) are recorded between the first and subsequent CMAPs (Fig. 14.5).[3,22,20] In a dog affected by generalized myasthenia gravis, the amplitude and area of CMAPs usually decrease by significantly more than 10%, especially within the

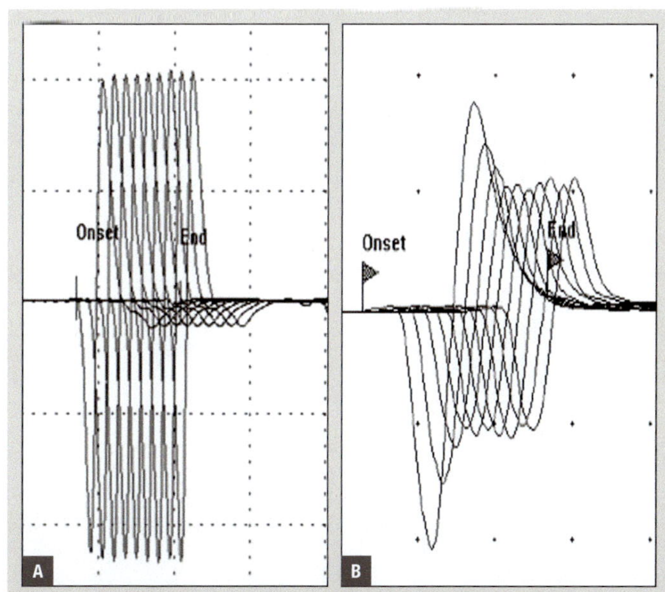

FIG. 14.5 Repetitive nerve stimulation (RNS) in a normal dog stimulated at a low frequency (3 Hz). 2 ms/Div; 2 mV/Div. (**B**) RNS in a dog with myasthenia gravis at a stimulation rate of 3 Hz. Note the decremental response (44% amplitude decrease between waves 5 and 1). 2 ms/Div; 2 mV/Div.

first 5 stimuli (Fig. 14.5).[3,22] Similar decreases can be seen in presynaptic neuromuscular junction disorders such as botulism, and occasionally in individuals with severe myopathies.[23] High stimulation frequencies of up to 30 Hz can be used to confirm the suspicion of botulism, which may cause increases in CMAP amplitude and area.[21,23]

Sensory nerve conduction studies (SNCS)

SNCS are used to investigate the function of sensory fibers in peripheral nerves.[13] Sensory nerve action potentials (SNAPs) are recorded with monopolar needle electrodes directly from sensory nerves (e.g., saphenous nerve or lateral superficial radial nerve) or mixed nerves (e.g., tibial nerve, peroneal nerve, ulnar nerve). The stimulation is delivered either directly to the nerve or through the distal skin.[3,24] In general, SNAP amplitudes are about 1000 times smaller than CMAP amplitudes (Fig. 14.6A). Therefore, SNAPs can easily be abolished by background noise, electrical interferences, or stimulus artefacts. A technique that is always used to extract SNAPs (and other small amplitude potentials) from the electrical and physiological background noise is signal averaging.[24] Signal averaging involves mathematically averaging a variable number of recordings. The purpose is to remove random background noise and to "highlight" the potential of interest (SNAP), which is time-locked to the stimulus. The sensory conduction velocity is calculated by dividing the distance between stimulus and recording by the latency of the SNAP.[24] The value obtained reflects the speed of the fastest sensory fibers. As with MNCS, a reduction in sensory conduction velocity indicates a demyelinating disorder or loss of the fastest sensory nerve fibers.[13] Unfortunately, identification of sensory axonopathies is often difficult due to the high variability of normal SNAP amplitudes.[24] In focal lesions, the SNCS is abnormal only if the damage is distal to the spinal ganglion (postganglionic lesions).

Assessment of cord dorsum potentials (CDPs)

CDPs are generated by interneurons of the lumbosacral and cervicothoracic intumescences when the sensory fibers of the peripheral nerves are electrically stimulated. Their assessment is useful for examining the function of the proximal/dorsal radicular portion of sensory fibers.[25] The active recording electrode is placed as close as possible to the interarcuate ligament between L4 and L5 or L5 and L6 for the tibial and peroneal nerves and to the C7-T1 interarcuate ligament or to the dorsal lamina of T1 for the ulnar and radial nerves. The reference recording electrode is placed in the subcutis on the contralateral side at 1–2 cm from the active electrode.[25] As with SNCS, signal averaging is necessary to extract the CDP from the background noise. Another trace should be obtained using the same method to check the reproducibility of the potential of interest (Fig. 14.6B). Expected normal values of CDP onset latency can be calculated based on limb length.[25] An increase in latency compared to the expected value indicates the presence of a demyelinating lesion. As occurs with SNAPs, CDP amplitudes are highly variable even in normal individuals.[3,25] For this reason, the identification of axonopathies involving sensory fibers is often difficult or impossible. In focal lesions, CDPs are affected in both preganglionic and postganglionic lesions.

General guidelines for interpreting the results of thorough electrodiagnostic studies in generalized neuromuscular patients are given in Algorithm 14.1.

Electrodiagnostic tests performed in the diagnostic evaluation of auditory pathways and central nervous system disorders

Brainstem auditory evoked potential (BAEP) testing

BAEP testing, also known as BAER (brainstem auditory evoked response) and ABR (auditory brainstem response) testing, assesses auditory function by recording potentials evoked by acoustic stimuli along the auditory pathway. BAEPs are generated within 10 ms of the stimulus and can be air conducted (produced by headphones or inserted earphones) or bone conducted (produced by special transducers).[26,27] To avoid unwanted cross-stimulation, the nonstimulated contralateral ear is masked with white noise. Stimulation intensity is measured in dB NHL (decibels normal hearing level). Zero dB NHL represents the hearing threshold of a group of people with normal hearing.[28] The intensity of the stimulus directly affects the BAEP trace. As the intensity is increased, the latencies of the waves of the waveform decrease while their amplitudes increase.[26]

Recordings are made with monopolar needle electrodes. Typically, the active electrode is placed at the vertex of the skull (midway between the eyes and the nuchal crest) and the reference electrode is placed just

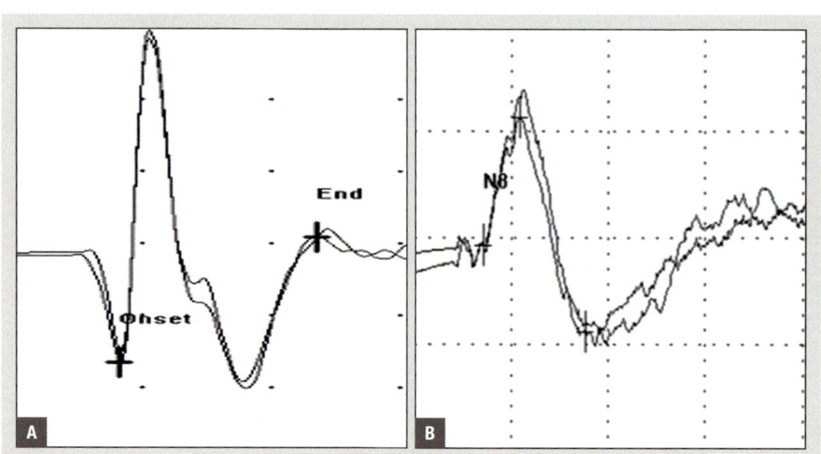

FIG. 14.6 (A) Normal tibial nerve sensory nerve conduction studies (SNCS). Conduction velocity, 65 m/s; 2 ms/Div; 2 μV/Div. (B) Normal cord dorsum potential (CDP) of the tibial nerve. 2 ms/Div; 2 mV/Div.

ALGORITHM 14.1

Guidelines for interpretation of electrodiagnostic (EDX) investigation in generalized neuromuscular patients.

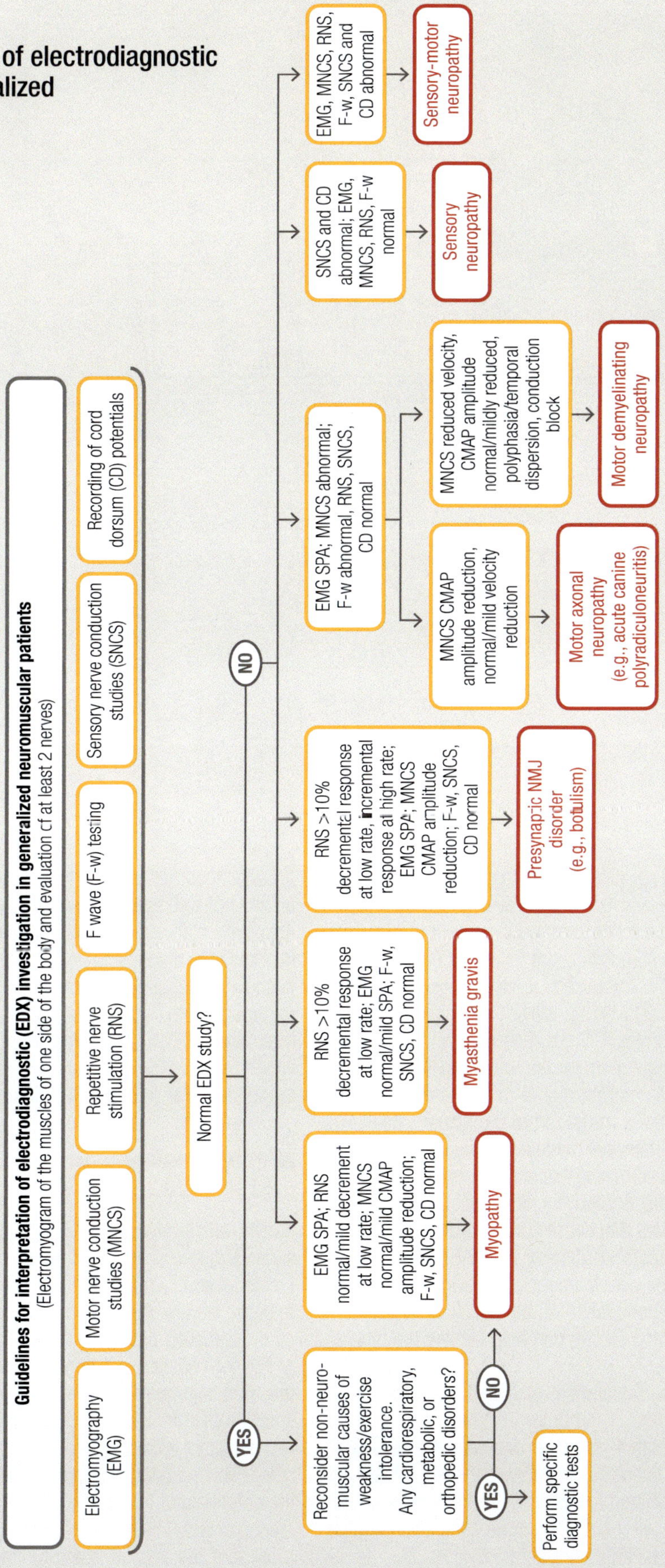

SPA, spontaneous pathological activity;
CMAP, compound muscle action potential;
NMJ, neuromuscular junction.

Diagnostic protocol | Diagnosis | Treatment

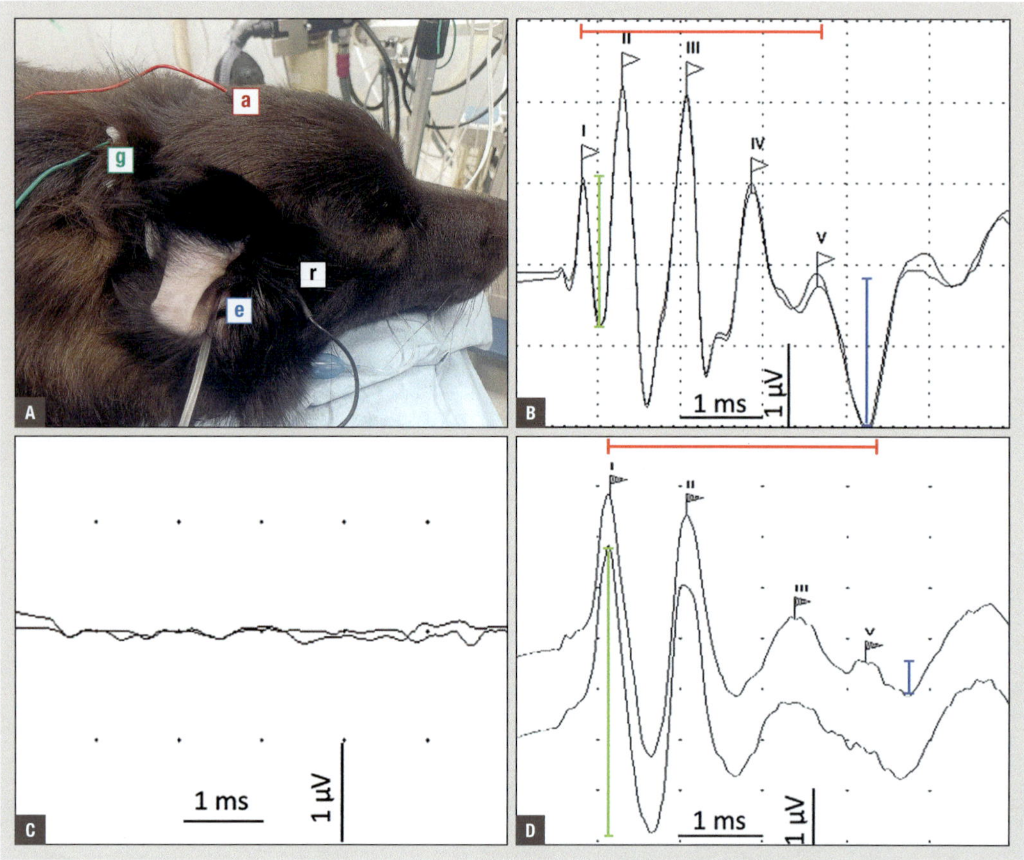

FIG. 14.7 (**A**) Assessment of auditory function using the brainstem auditory evoked potential (BAEP) test in an adult dog; a, active electrode; r, reference electrode; g, ground; e, insert earphones. (**B**) Example of a normal BAEP trace. (**C**) Flat trace from the ear of a dog with profound sensorineural (cochlear) deafness. (**D**) BAEP tracing of a Jack Russel with hereditary ataxia. Note the increased interpeak latencies (IPLs) I-V, the reduced wave III and wave V amplitudes and, consequently, the reduced wave V/wave I amplitude ratio. 90 dB NHL. Red line, IPL I-V; green line, wave I amplitude; blue line, wave V amplitude.

rostral to the base of the tested ear (Fig. 14.7).[26] To obtain a clear waveform, the signal is recorded several times and "averaged". Ideally, the repeatability of the waveform should be checked by superimposing two traces obtained using the same stimulation and recording parameters.[28]

The BAEP waveform is usually composed of vertex-positive waves, labelled with Roman numerals (Fig. 14.7). Wave I originates from the ipsilateral cochlear nerve, and waves II–V are generated with the contribution of various auditory brainstem structures, including the cochlear nuclei and caudal colliculi.[26] The morphology of the waveform and the amplitude and latency of the waves measured at the positive peak are important in the clinical interpretation of the test.

BAEP testing is a very important screening test used in puppies of breeds potentially affected by pigment-associated (cochlear-saccular) deafness. In this and other hearing disorders that cause complete degeneration of the cochlea (profound sensorineural deafness), the BAEP waveform in the affected ear is flat. In fact, no waves are recorded, regardless of the intensity and type (air- or bone-conducted) of the stimulus.[26]

In the presence of hypoacusia, the BAEPs can help identify the type of hearing loss.

In conductive hearing loss (i.e., impairment of sound transmission to the inner ear caused by disorders of the outer or middle ear), BAEPs recorded with air-conducted stimuli show an increase in the BAEP threshold and in absolute peak latencies, and a wave V latency-intensity curve with a normal slope but shifted to the right.[26,29] In these patients, the thresholds and waveforms recorded using bone stimulation, which bypasses the outer and middle ear, are normal.[26,27]

In sensorineural (cochlear) hearing loss, the threshold is elevated for both air and bone stimuli, and the latency-intensity curve of wave V is steeper, especially at lower stimulus intensities.[26,29]

In addition to diagnosing hearing loss, BAEPs can be used as a diagnostic tool for neurological disorders. In particular, they can help differentiate peripheral from central vestibular disorders. In the presence of a central/brain stem lesion, abnormalities such as the absence of one or more waves, a decrease in the wave V/wave I amplitude ratio and an increase in the interpeak latencies (IPLs) may occur.[1]

Motor evoked potentials (MEPs) and somatosensory evoked potentials (SSEPs)

SSEPs and transcranial MEPs can be used to study the function of ascending and descending spinal pathways, respectively.[30,31]

Electrical stimuli applied to sensory or mixed peripheral nerves are used to evoke SSEPs. Ascending impulses can be recorded at different levels of the sensory pathway. While cord dorsum potentials are recorded at the intumescences, sensory evoked potentials can be recorded at the thoracolumbar and cervical spine and at the scalp. As with other small amplitude sensory potentials, the SSEPs requires the "averaging" technique to extract the evoked potentials from random background noise, and recordings are made twice to assess the reproducibility of the potentials of interest.[30]

Transcranial MEPs are muscular potentials evoked by a magnetic or electrical stimulus applied to the motor cortex. From the brain, the impulse travels along the entire descending motor pathway to the target muscle. The resulting CMAP is recorded with monopolar needles, as in MNCS, or with a standard concentric needle. Due to the greater amplitude of the CMAPs, averaging is not required in MEPs, but the potentials produced by 10–20 stimuli are usually recorded.[31]

Both transcranial MEPs and SSEPs, especially cortical recordings, are affected by anesthetics. Therefore, these tests are usually performed with different sedation protocols. As usual, the latency and amplitude of evoked potentials are measured and compared with published normative values.[30,31] Severe spinal cord lesions often result in the absence of motor and/or sensory evoked potentials.[33]

Transcranial MEPs and SSEPs are often used as part of research protocols in studies of specific neurological disorders to provide objective information on spinal cord function. In particular, they have been used in degenerative and traumatic disorders.[32,33]

KEY POINTS

- Electrodiagnostic (EDX) investigations are a very sensitive and objective extension of the neurological examination.
- EDX studies rarely provide etiological information, but they are used primarily for their ability to assess the function of specific nervous structures.
- EDX studies for neuromuscular disorders should ideally be performed at least 5–7 days after the onset of the disorder. They can help to differentiate myopathies from neuromuscular junction disorders and neuropathies.
- EDX investigations can help classify neuropathies based on the functional lesion present.
- Brainstem auditory evoked potential testing is the test most commonly used for the diagnosis of hearing loss in dogs.

References

1. Poncelet L, Poma R. Electrophysiology. In: Platt S, Olby N. (eds.) *BSAVA manual of canine and feline neurology.* 4th edition. Gloucester: BSAVA; 2013. p. 59–76.
2. Preston DC, Shapiro BE. Approach to nerve conduction studies and electromyography. In: Preston DC, Shapiro BE (eds.) *Electromyography and muscular disorders.* 3rd edition. Philadelphia: Elsevier; 2013. p. 1–7.
3. Cuddon PA. Electrophysiology in neuromuscular disease. *Vet Clin North Am Small Anim Pract.* 2002; 32(1):31–62.
4. Chiappa KA. Principles of evoked potentials. In: Chiappa KA (ed.) Evoked potentials in clinical medicine. 3rd edition. Philadelphia: Lippincott-Raven; 1997. p. 1–30.
5. Liatis T, Gutierrez-Quintana R, Mari L, et al. Primary orthostatic tremor and orthostatic tremor-plus in dogs: 60 cases (2003-2020). *J Vet Intern Med.* 2022 36(1):179–189.
6. Preston DC, Shapiro BE. Basic overview of electromyography. In: Preston DC, Shapiro BE (eds.) *Electromyography and muscular disorders.* 3rd edition. Philadelphia: Elsevier; 2013. p. 125–128.
7. Kimura J. Techniques to assess muscle function. In: Kimura J, (ed.) *Electrodiagnosis in Diseases of Nerve and Muscle Principles and Practice.* 3rd edition. Oxford: Oxford University Press; 2001. p. 307–338.
8. Preston DC, Shapiro BE. Basic electromyography: analysis of spontaneous activity. In: Preston DC, Shapiro BE (eds.). *Electromyography and muscular disorders.* 3rd edition. Philadelphia: Elsevier; 2013. p. 220–234.
9. Kimura J. Types of electromyographic abnormalities. In: Kimura J (ed.). *Electrodiagnosis in Diseases of Nerve and Muscle Principles and Practice.* 3rd ed. Oxford: Oxford University Press; 2001. p. 339–369.
10. Golinelli, S, Fracassi, F, Bianchi, E, et al. Clinical features of muscle stiffness in 37 dogs with concurrent naturally occurring hypercortisolism. *J Vet Intern Med.* 2023; 37(2):578–585.
11. Vanhaesebrouck AE, Bhatti SF, Franklin RJ, Van Ham L. Myokymia and neuromyotonia in veterinary medicine: a comparison with peripheral nerve hyperexcitability syndrome in humans. *Vet J.* 2013 Aug;197(2):153–162.
12. De Risio L, Zavattiero S, Venzi C, et al. Focal canine tetanus: diagnostic value of electromyography. *J Small Anim Pract.* 2006 May;47(5):278–280.
13. Kimura J. Principles and variations of nerve conduction studies. In: J Kimura (ed). *Electrodiagnosis in Diseases of Nerve and Muscle: Principles and Practice.* 3rd edition Oxford: Oxford University Press; 2001. p. 91–129.
14. Walker TL, Redding RW, Braund KG. Motor nerve conduction velocity and latency in the dog. *Am J Vet Res.* 1979;40(10):1433–1439.
15. Menchetti M, Gandini G, Bravaccini B, et al. Clinical, Electrodiagnostic Findings and Quality of Life of Dogs and Cats with Brachial Plexus Injury. *Vet Sci.* 2020 Jul 31;7(3):101.
16. Troupel T, Van Caenegem N, Jeandel A, et al. Epidemiological, clinical, and electrophysiological findings in dogs and cats with traumatic brachial plexus injury: A retrospective study of 226 cases. *J Vet Intern Med.* 2021;35(6):2837–2845.
17. Kimura J. The F wave and the A wave. In: Kimura J, (ed.) *Electrodiagnosis in Diseases of Nerve and Muscle Principles and Practice.* 3rd edition. Oxford: Oxford University Press; 2001. p. 439–465.
18. Okuno S, Kobayashi T, Orito K. F-wave latency and F-wave conduction velocity for the tibial nerve in clinically normal dogs. *Am J Vet Res.* 2002; 63(9):1262–1264.
19. Poncelet L, Balligand M. Nature of the late potentials and F-ratio values in dogs. *Res Vet Sci.* 1991 Jul;51(1):1–5.
20. Knecht CD, Redding RW. Monosynaptic reflex (H wave) in clinically normal and abnormal dogs. *Am J Vet Res.* 1981;42(9):1586–1589.
21. Kimura J. Techniques or repetitive stimulation. In: Kimura J, (ed.) *Electrodiagnosis in Diseases of Nerve and Muscle Principles and Practice.* 3rd edition. Oxford: Oxford University Press; 2001. p. 257–278.
22. Gödde T, Jaggy A, Vandevelde M, Gaillard C. Evaluation of repetitive nerve stimulation in young dogs. *J Small Anim Pract.* 34(8):393–397.
23. van Nes JJ, van der Most van Spijk D. Electrophysiological evidence of peripheral nerve dysfunction

TABLE 15.1 Summary of the Finnish neurological functional testing battery (FINFUN).

Functional task	0	1	2	3	4
Lying sternal	Unable to lie in sternal position	Able to lie in sternal position strongly supported	Able to lie in sternal position lightly supported	Able to lie in sternal position independently for 5 seconds	Able to lie in sternal position for 5 seconds and follow the surrounding environment
Standing up from lying	Not able to stand up from lying	Stands up from lying strongly supported	Stands up from lying lightly supported	Stands up from lying into standing position independently	Stands up from lying into a balanced standing position
Sitting	Not able to sit or maintain sitting position	Able to sit strongly supported	Able to sit lightly supported	Able to maintain sitting position independently for at least 5 seconds	Able to sit in a balanced position for at least 5 seconds
Standing up from sitting	Not able to stand up from sitting	Stands up from sitting strongly supported	Stands up from sitting and able to maintain the standing position lightly supported	Stands up from sitting independently and is able to independently maintain the standing position for at least 3 seconds	Stands from sitting position into a balanced standing position, symmetrical thrust in both pelvic limbs
Standing	Not able to stand	Able to stand strongly supported	Able to stand lightly supported for at least 5 seconds	Able to maintain standing position for at least 5 seconds independently	Stands balanced for 5 seconds or more and is able to follow the environment
Proprioceptive positioning	Proprioceptive positioning is absent in all affected limbs	Proprioceptive positioning is decreased in all affected limbs	Proprioceptive positioning is mildly decreased in all affected limbs	Proprioceptive positioning is normal in one of the affected limbs	Proprioceptive positioning is normal in all four limbs
Start to walk from standing	Needs heavy support in standing, is not able to start walking without strong support	Stands with light support, needs strong support when walking	Stands independently, needs light support when walking	Stands and starts to walk independently, walks 3 meters	Starts to walk from a normal/near-normal standing position, and walks 3 meters or more
Walking	Not able to walk 30 meters	Walks 30 meters or less, strongly supported	Walks more than 30 meters, lightly supported	Walks 30 meters or more independently	Walks 30 meters back and forth (60 meters total)
Running	Not able to run	Able to run with light support 30 meters or less	Runs 30 meters or more, but struggles to do it independently	Runs 30 meters or more, but struggles to do it independently	Runs 30 meters back and forth effortlessly (60 meters total)
Walking turns	Able to walk with light support on a straight line	Able to walk the turns with light support, may fall in both directions	Walks the turns independently, may fall in one direction	Walks the turns in both directions independently without falling	Walks the turns independently in both directions and effortlessly
Walking stairs	Not able to climb stairs	Climbs the stairs strongly supported	Climbs up and down stairs, needing support climbing up or down	Climbs up and down stairs independently	Climbs up and down the stairs effortlessly

Principles

Principles of neurological rehabilitation in humans have focused on finely adjusted movements and skill acquisition characteristic of the pyramidal system and corticospinal tract. The pyramidal system is less developed in dogs than it is in humans, and therefore treatment is focused predominantly on gait reeducation and gross movement patterns for function.

The rationale for neurological rehabilitation

Acute spinal cord injury is the most common neurological disease in small animals. The spinal cord may experience compression (through inflammation, hemorrhage, or debris [e.g., extruded disc material]), contusion, shearing, or distraction. Early intensive rehabilitation, often performed from day one post surgery and for short periods a few times a day, has shown to accelerate the recovery of motor function and restore independent mobility.[4]

Cell death may occur at the injury site due to the disrupted cell body function and loss of axonal transport. Connectivity to adjacent neurons is poor, and neuron degeneration may occur distal to the injury site. There are also several endogenous mechanisms that can influence the survival or death of a neuron (including inflammatory mediators, free radicals, nitric oxide, trophic factors, chemokines, and cytokines); neurological rehabilitation is thus key in delaying, limiting, and modifying these changes.

Neural inflammation, modulated by microglia and astrocytes, occurs secondary to the original injury and can impact function.

Neuroplasticity defines the ability of the nervous system to change its activity in response to intrinsic or extrinsic stimuli by reorganizing its structure, functions, or connections after injuries such as a spinal cord injury. In the case of neurological disease or trauma, it is possible to influence the remaining neurons and thus strengthen their survival and generate new neural networks. Exercise strengthens skeletal muscle following neurogenic muscle atrophy, reinforces the pyramidal and therefore corticospinal pathways, and promotes neuroplasticity for functional improvements.[5] Consequently, rehabilitation and its ability to enhance neuroplasticity and reduce neural inflammation, thus optimizing functional recovery, has been the strong focus in research.[4]

Enhancing neurotrophin production in the spinal cord and skeletal muscle, particularly brain-derived neurotrophic factor (BDNF) and neurotrophic factor-3 (NT-3), stimulates neuronal cell survival and can be achieved through physical activity and exercise.[6–7] Implementing exercise early following injury will enhance improvements in function through neuroplasticity. The type and duration of exercise are key components in raising BDNF and NT-3 production, with gait reeducation that is task specific and repetitive having the greatest effect.[8]

Gait reeducation for spinal cord injuries may be performed with the use of a treadmill or over land, neither of which has a greater benefit in functional improvement over another.[9] When comparing body weight supported treadmill (BWST) training to traditional treadmill training, 60% of dogs in the former group and only 10% of dogs in the latter group recovered motor function after 4 weeks.[10] Gait reeducation is easier to execute on a treadmill, allowing for repeated simulated stepping in a rhythmical fashion. Underwater treadmills are becoming increasingly popular, particularly for the weaker, paretic patient. The buoyancy and hydrostatic pressure effects can enhance the stability of the patient, while the limbs may be manually facilitated to promote normal movement patterns. Gait reeducation in any form will activate neural networks, which results in the recovery of walking.[9]

Exercise should not be the only treatment technique considered in neurological rehabilitation, since it has demonstrated to produce only a minimal increase in BDNF that may not be enough to optimize neuroplasticity. Studies have looked at the effect of neural inflammation on functional recovery and highlighted the importance of addressing this in addition to the downregulation of neurotrophins as seen in spinal cord injuries.[11] While gait reeducation and exercise can modulate neural inflammation and stimulate neurotrophin production, the effects of these treatment methods can be enhanced by combining them with the use of photobiomodulation therapy (PBMT), neuromuscular electrical stimulation (NMES), and acupuncture.

Neurological physical rehabilitation treatment

Supportive care

Supportive care, particularly in the recumbent large breed or obese patient, is required to prevent secondary complications such as pressure sores, urine scald, urine infection, or respiratory complications. Pressure relief bedding needs to be provided, a turning regime implemented in order to minimize the risk of pressure sores, and regular checks for soiling of the bedding performed, with the bedding immediately changed if indicated. Positional changes should occur every 4–6 hours, and the patient should be supported with additional bolsters or a rolled-up towel or blanket for example, when required. For large dogs, positional changes should be more frequent. Left and right half sternal lying are common positions, but sternal recumbency may also be tolerated for shorter periods. Sternal recumbency allows the patient to see what is going around them more easily and the patient to eat in a safer position and increases lung volumes, thereby minimizing the risk of respiratory complications such as hypoventilation, lung atelectasis, and mucus retention.

Assistive devices such as hoists, quad carts, harnesses, slings, or slide sheets may be used to reduce the risk of injury to the patient or handler when transferring, mobilizing, and rehabilitating the neurological patient. They should be correctly fitted and used, causing the patient no unnecessary discomfort. For the weak and ataxic patient, harnesses that provide thoracic and pelvic support are used to support them until they regain independent mobility. They should not be used to lift them clear of the ground.

Patients with reduced or absent proprioceptive input are at a high risk of skin abrasions to the digits and bony prominences of the limbs. These may be caused by long periods of recumbency in one position, knuckling or scuffing of the digits while mobilizing (assisted or unassisted), or self-mutilation. Protection is often required in the form of dressings or boots (Fig. 15.1), though these can limit sensory input to the distal limbs, inhibiting the recovery of proprioceptive input and motor output. For patients with good proximal limb function, devices that facilitate correct placement of the distal limb may be worn for short periods of supervised exercise.

Manual therapies

Sensory stimulation activities are designed to stimulate and enhance sensory input. Largely following the Rood neurological approach to rehabilitation from human medicine,[12] they are used to facilitate specific responses. The application may be through a cutaneous application of stroking, brushing, tapping, or vibration; thermal application with ice (to enhance neuromuscular tone) and warmth (to reduce neuromuscular tone); proprioception with stretch, resistance, and joint compression; in addition to labyrinthine, visual, auditory, olfactory, and taste stimuli. Any motor response is then used in developmental sequences from sternal recumbency to sit, stand, and walking. Feedback and repetition are crucial for motor learning to occur.

Passive range of motion (PROM) exercises are employed to flex and extend peripheral joints in the tetra- or paraplegic or very weak patient. For some patients, stretching of the periarticular structures is also required. Combined, these techniques enhance synovial fluid production and local circulation, preventing joint stiffness and soft tissue fibrosis, and

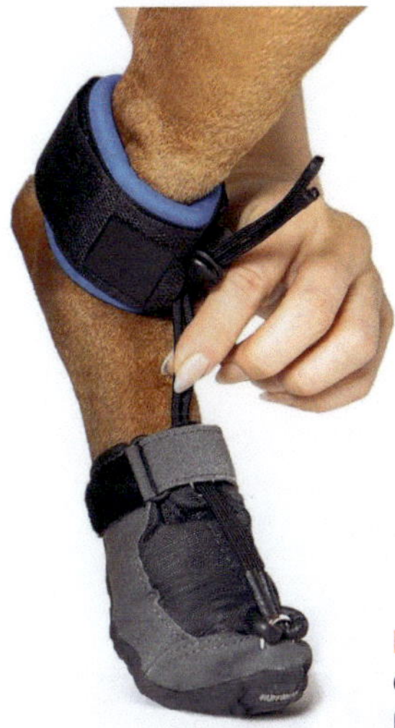

FIG. 15.1 An example of an assistive device that is designed to facilitate correct placement of the distal limb.

stimulate joint proprioceptors. PROM exercises must be applied safely and effectively, with a relaxed patient and a secure handling technique. Several massage techniques can provide multiple benefits for the neurologically impaired patient. In addition to relieving pain and stress, enhancing blood circulation and lymphatic drainage, stimulating sensation, and improving hypotonicity, massage can reduce hypertonicity, with the relief of the signs associated with this.

Therapeutic exercise

There are several therapeutic exercises that can be tailored for patients with varying levels of mobility and strength. Regardless of whether the patient is ambulatory or nonambulatory, they should be constantly reviewed and adjusted as indicated. Targeted exercises, when completed daily, will minimize muscle atrophy as well as joint stiffness and fibrosis, optimize joint health, and enhance core and dynamic stability. These active exercises stimulate the transmission of nerve signals, joint proprioceptors, and motor pathways in addition to restoring the automatic response seen during activities such as standing, transitions from one position to another, and walking.[13]

For the very weak nonambulatory patient, one of the first exercise progression is aimed at the patient maintaining independent sternal recumbency. The importance of this exercise is twofold: to maintain and improve core control in a position with a large base of support and to optimize respiratory health and function. The patient may then progress to transitions from lying to half sternal and full sternal recumbency to varying levels of exercise in standing and sitting, which may be supported initially. The latter should be performed on a nonslip surface. When supporting the patient in these postures, appropriate limb placement to achieve a good spinal alignment and base of support and an even distribution of weight avoiding torsion, rotation, distraction, or compression of the spine is desired (Fig. 15.2).

For patients with an absent reflex arc (i.e., lower motor neuron signs), greater manual support is required in stance to prevent collapse of the affected limbs. Proprioceptive input can then be enhanced by adding in joint compressions while in this supported standing position.

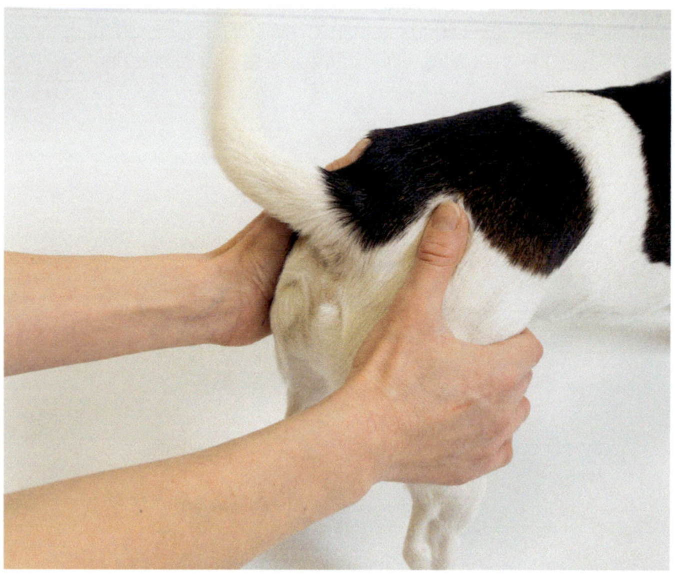

FIG. 15.2 Appropriate handling in order to perform joint compressions in supported standing.

Gait reeducation is a term used to describe the technique when restoring and optimizing motor function and normal movement patterns is the goal. This may be done on land with or without assistive devices, on a dry treadmill, or in an underwater treadmill. See above for more details on gait reeducation.

Performing assisted stands and gait reeducation in water is particularly beneficial for the painful and weak patient using the properties of water, buoyancy, and hydrostatic pressure to support them and thus optimize postural control and tidal volume. Walking in the controlled environment of an underwater treadmill, the water velocity creates resistance for the limbs to pass through, aiding core and dynamic strengthening. The treadmill speed can be adjusted to influence resistance but, at all levels, resistance will slow the movement and allow for a greater reaction time for correct placement of the limbs. For those patients that are not able to correctly place the limb themselves, the therapist may still need to facilitate correct limb placement, therefore enhancing proprioception and reinforcing a normal gait sequence.

Other benefits of underwater treadmill therapy include an increased range of motion in specific joints due to the water buoyancy and resistance and the reduction of edema and optimization of blood circulation and lymphatic drainage through hydrostatic pressure and a warm water temperature (28–32 °C).[14]

For a patient with an independent mobility status, exercises to enhance core and dynamic strength, balance, proprioception, and coordination are an important feature of the rehabilitation program. The frequency, type of exercise, number of exercise repetitions, and for some exercises, duration of hold, will vary for each individual patient. Quality of the position, movement, and/or gait, not quantity, is a common phrase heard in the rehabilitation setting following the Bobath principle in neurological rehabilitation.[15]

Neuromuscular electrical stimulation

NMES is an electrotherapy modality that provides an electrical impulse via electrodes positioned over specific skeletal muscles or motor points to produce a muscle contraction. It is used when voluntary motor function is weak or absent or as an adjunct to active exercises in order to optimize function. For many neurological conditions, we see a reduction in protein synthesis resulting in neurogenic muscle atrophy. NMES is used to minimize this reduction in protein synthesis, thus preserving muscle fiber mass and improving the performance of the affected skeletal muscles.[16] In the absence of voluntary motor function, NMES should be applied daily with a recurring contraction followed by a period of rest during each application.

Transcutaneous electrical nerve stimulation

Transcutaneous electrical nerve stimulation (TENS) is an electrotherapy modality used for the relief of pain. It is applied through electrodes positioned around the area of pain and/or inflammation. It can be applied as frequently as it is required to optimize pain relief.

Video 15.1

Gait reeducation on land and in the water treadmill.

Photobiomodulation therapy

Light amplification by stimulated emission of radiation (LASER) therapy or PBMT is the application of monochromatic light (visible or nonvisible), which is commonly used to accelerate wound healing, reduce pain, and optimize tissue healing including neural structures in the neurological patient. PBMT has a wide range of positive effects at a cellular and molecular level.[17]

A preliminary study[18] has highlighted a reduced time to ambulation in nonambulatory paraparetic or paraplegic dogs after PBMT had been applied daily for 5 days post hemilaminectomy.

Indications for physical rehabilitation

Intervertebral disc disease

The acute onset of neurological signs is typical for Hansen type 1 intervertebral disc extrusion (IVDE). Decompressive surgery may be indicated in some of these patients, but a combination of therapeutic interventions is strongly recommended post surgically or for conservative management. Physiotherapy immediately after injury or surgery will focus on pain management and supportive care before then using techniques to enhance the return to function.

Dogs with cervical IVDE who have severe neurological deficits or recurring neck pain are recommended to undergo surgery. Postsurgical rehabilitation can be implemented safely within the first 3 days; compared to dogs that do not undergo rehabilitation, those that do so show a significant improvement in neurological recovery.[19] The same is seen in postsurgical thoracolumbar IVDE patients.[20]

Determining a patient's prognosis for return to function will depend on progress within the first 2–4 weeks of recovery.[21] For those more severely affected, restoring deep pain sensation and recovering voluntary motor function is usually seen within this time period, although for some it can be as long as 9 months.

Intensive rehabilitation facilitates central nervous system reorganization and works on achieving a balance between the central pattern generators, spinal rhythm-generating circuits, the descending pathways, and sensory feedback. For thoracolumbar patients with severe acute IVDE (i.e., paraplegic and deep pain positive or negative), an intensive postsurgical rehabilitation protocol that includes gait training and functional and/or transcutaneous electrical stimulation can restore ambulation in up to 99.4% of dogs with deep pain perception and 58.5% of dogs with absent deep pain perception. For those patients who do not recover deep pain, up to 37.2% can achieve "spinal walking" within 3 months.[10]

Another retrospective study has looked at the effect of an intensive physiotherapy protocol on the development of an involuntary unassisted gait; 59% of patients with complete spinal cord injury and absent deep pain perception developed this gait.[22] This highlights the importance of physiotherapy for patients with absent deep pain perception for which a poor prognosis for recovering motor function would otherwise be considered.

Conversely, a prospective study has investigated the functional recovery rate post surgery for thoracolumbar intervertebral disc herniation in nonambulatory paraparetic or paraplegic with deep pain perception patients. Each group underwent a basic or intensive physiotherapy routine. There was no statistically significant difference between the two groups.[23]

In a case series of 16 dogs with chronic (after 3 months) postsurgical IVDE that scores 0 or 1 on the modified Frankel score (MFS), a rehabilitation protocol consisting of gait training, functional electrical stimulation, TENS, and 4-aminopyridine pharmacological management obtained ambulation in 88% of these patients,[24] suggesting that patients can still achieve a successful functional outcome during this later phase of their recovery.

Fibrocartilaginous embolic myelopathy

FCEM is a nonprogressive and noncompressive spinal cord pathology of a vascular nature. Fibrocartilaginous material histologically similar to the nucleus pulposus blocks the artery causing ischemia and death of the irrorated tissue (see Chapter 31).

Physiotherapy is similar to that recommended for intervertebral disc disease although, as always, it is patient-specific depending on the neurolocalization and clinical signs. Patients may have increased or decreased neuromuscular tone. Manual techniques, NMES, postural education, gait reeducation, and hydrotherapy are recommended. As the patient regains independent mobility, the rehabilitation activity will become more challenging.

A retrospective study by Gandini et al.[25] found that 73.4% of dogs that immediately underwent intensive rehabilitation following the diagnosis of FCEM regained independent mobility within 2 weeks. The remaining 26.6% regained independent mobility by 45 days.

Acute canine polyradiculoneuritis

ACP is a neuromuscular disease and is characterized by rapid generalized muscle weakness progressing to lower motor neuron tetraparesis or tetraplegia. The respiratory system can be affected in most severe cases. This condition is considered self-limiting, and the prognosis in most cases is good (see Chapter 37). Patients can experience a prolonged period of recovery that may last weeks to months and for which supportive care and intensive physiotherapy is essential.

In the early phase, the objectives are to optimize respiratory function, maintain range of motion preventing joint contractures, and delay neurogenic muscle atrophy. This may be done through positioning, manual techniques, NMES, and postural education, which may start in supported sternal recumbency and supported standing (Fig. 15.3). For dogs who display good head and neck control, standing and early gait reeducation, at a later stage, may be done in an underwater treadmill.

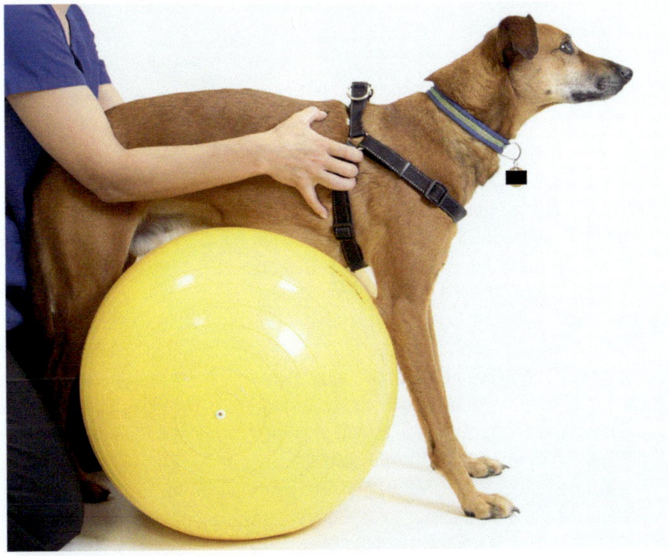

FIG. 15.3 Supported standing over a peanut ball.

The vast majority of patients will have a complete recovery, though a few will have some residual neurological deficits or recurrence. The author has observed rare cases that showed no clinical improvement.

Degenerative myelopathy

DM is a degenerative spinal cord disease in large dogs that has progressive clinical signs not dissimilar to motor neuron disease. It is characterized by proprioceptive ataxia, spastic paresis, and disuse muscle atrophy in the early phase, progressing to lower motor neuron paraplegia and neurogenic muscle atrophy in the later phase. Beyond this phase, signs will include progressive loss of spinal reflexes, paresis of the thoracic limbs, fecal and urinary incontinence, and dysphagia (see Chapter 35). Physiotherapy and hydrotherapy, preferably underwater treadmill therapy, are the mainstay of treatment, and daily intensive rehabilitation has proven to delay the time to loss of independent mobility and significantly increase survival time compared to no physiotherapy.[26] Physiotherapy activities can include soft tissue mobilization techniques, passive limb movements, postural and functional strengthening activities, and regular walks in addition to hydrotherapy.

Summary

Positive outcomes associated with veterinary physical therapy and rehabilitation have been documented in the literature, but more prospective, blinded, and controlled trials are needed particularly for FCEM, ACP, and DM.[27] In summary, a multimodal approach that should include gait reeducation, active and targeted exercises, and NMES is essential for optimum outcomes in the neurological patient.

KEY POINTS

- The goals for neurological physiotherapy and rehabilitation are to minimize pain and optimize function.
- A neurological patient's needs, motivation, and functional status all aid in the design of a personalized neurological rehabilitation program.
- Neuroplasticity is the fundamental property of the nervous system that allows it to change its activity in response to intrinsic or extrinsic stimuli by reorganizing its structure, functions, or connections.
- Endogenous neurotrophins enhance functional recovery of the neurological patient and are stimulated through physical activity and exercise.
- A multimodal neurological rehabilitation protocol that includes caregiver advice and education, supportive care, manual and exercise therapies, and the application of electrotherapeutic agents will optimize the patient's functional outcome.
- The most common neurological disorders for which physiotherapy is beneficial are intervertebral disc disease, degenerative myelopathy, fibrocartilaginous embolic myelopathy, and acute canine polyradiculoneuritis.

References

1. Olby NJ, De Risio L, Muñana KR, et al. Development of a functional scoring system in dogs with acute spinal cord injuries. *Am J Vet Res.* 2001 Oct;62(10):1624–1628.
2. Levine GJ, Levine JM, Budke CM, et al. Description and repeatability of a newly developed spinal cord injury scale for dogs. *Prev Vet Med.* 2009 May 1;89(1-2):121–127.
3. Boström AF, Hyytiäinen HK, Koho P, et al. Development of the Finnish neurological function testing battery for dogs and its intra-and inter-rater reliability. *Acta Vet Scand.* 2018 Dec;60(1):1–9.
4. Frank LR, Roynard PFP. Veterinary Neurologic Rehabilitation: The Rationale for a Comprehensive Approach. *Top Companion Anim Med.* 2018 Jun;33(2):49–57.
5. Fu J, Wang H, Deng L, Li J. Exercise Training Promotes Functional Recovery after Spinal Cord Injury. *Neural Plast.* 2016;2016:4039580.
6. Ilha J, Meireles A, de Freitas GR, et al. Overground gait training promotes functional recovery and cortical neuroplasticity in an incomplete spinal cord injury model. *Life Sci.* 2019 Sep 1;232:116627.
7. Han S, Wang B, Jin W, et al. The linear-ordered collagen scaffold-BDNF complex significantly promotes functional recovery after completely transected spinal cord injury in canine. *Biomaterials.* 2015 Feb;41:89–96.
8. Hutchinson KJ, Gómez-Pinilla F, Crowe MJ, et al. Three exercise paradigms differentially improve sensory recovery after spinal cord contusion in rats. *Brain.* 2004 Jun;127(Pt 6):1403–1414.
9. Mehrholz J, Kugler J, Pohl M. Locomotor training for walking after spinal cord injury. *Cochrane Database Syst Rev.* 2012 Nov 14;11:CD006676.
10. Martins Â, Gouveia D, Cardoso A, et al. A Controlled Clinical Study of Intensive Neurorehabilitation in Post-Surgical Dogs with Severe Acute Intervertebral Disc Extrusion. *Animals (Basel).* 2021 Oct 22;11(11):3034.
11. Spejo AB, Oliveira AL. Synaptic rearrangement following axonal injury: Old and new players. *Neuropharmacology.* 2015 Sep;96(Pt A):113–123.
12. Rood MS. Neurophysiological mechanisms utilized in the treatment of neuromuscular dysfunction. *Am J Occup Ther.* 1956;10:220–225.
13. Le Sant G, Lecharte T, Goreau V, et al. Motor performance, motor impairments, and quality of life

after eccentric resistance training in neurological populations: A systematic review and meta-analysis. *NeuroRehabilitation.* 2023;53(1):33–50.

14. Millis DL, Ciuperca IA. Evidence for canine rehabilitation and physical therapy. *Vet Clin North Am Small Anim Pract.* 2015 Jan;45(1):1–27.
15. Raine S, Meadows L, Lynch-Ellerington M (eds.). *Bobath Concept: Theory and Clinical Practice in Neurological Rehabilitation.* John Wiley & Sons; 2013.
16. Rahmati M, Gondin J, Malakoutinia F. Effects of Neuromuscular Electrical Stimulation on Quadriceps Muscle Strength and Mass in Healthy Young and Older Adults: A Scoping Review. *Phys Ther.* 2021 Sep 1;101(9):pzab144.
17. Watson T. *Laser therapy: Photobiomodulation.* Retrieved from: https://www.electrotherapy.org/laser. Accessed: June 2024.
18. Draper WE, Schubert TA, Clemmons RM, Miles SA. Low-level laser therapy reduces time to ambulation in dogs after hemilaminectomy: a preliminary study. *J Small Anim Pract.* 2012 Aug;53(8):465–469.
19. Gouveia D, Carvalho C, Cardoso A, et al. Early Locomotor Training in Tetraplegic Post-Surgical Dogs with Cervical Intervertebral Disc Disease. *Animals (Basel).* 2022 Sep 11;12(18):2369.
20. Hodgson MM, Bevan JM, Evans RB, Johnson TI. Influence of in-house rehabilitation on the postoperative outcome of dogs with intervertebral disk herniation. *Vet Surg.* 2017 May;46(4):566–573.
21. Olby N, Levine J, Harris T, et al. Long-term functional outcome of dogs with severe injuries of the thoracolumbar spinal cord: 87 cases (1996-2001). *J Am Vet Med Assoc.* 2003 Mar 15;222(6):762–729.
22. Gallucci A, Dragone L, Menchetti M, et al. Acquisition of Involuntary Spinal Locomotion (Spinal Walking) in Dogs with Irreversible Thoracolumbar Spinal Cord Lesion: 81 Dogs. *J Vet Intern Med.* 2017 Mar;31(2):492–497.
23. Zidan N, Sims C, Fenn J, et al. A randomized, blinded, prospective clinical trial of postoperative rehabilitation in dogs after surgical decompression of acute thoracolumbar intervertebral disc herniation. *J Vet Intern Med.* 2018 May;32(3):1133–1144.
24. Martins Â, Gouveia D, Cardoso A, et al. Functional neurorehabilitation in dogs with an incomplete recovery 3 months following intervertebral disc surgery: A case series. *Animals.* 2021 Aug 19;11(8):2442.
25. Gandini G, Cizinauskas S, Lang J, Fatzer R, Jaggy A. Fibrocartilaginous embolism in 75 dogs: clinical findings and factors influencing the recovery rate. *J Small Anim Pract.* 2003 Feb;44(2):76–80.
26. Kathmann I, Cizinauskas S, Doherr MG, Steffen F, Jaggy A. Daily controlled physiotherapy increases survival time in dogs with suspected degenerative myelopathy. *J Vet Intern Med.* 2006 Jul-Aug;20(4):927–932.
27. Spinella G, Bettella P, Riccio B, Okonji S. Overview of the Current Literature on the Most Common Neurological Diseases in Dogs with a Particular Focus on Rehabilitation. *Vet Sci.* 2022 Aug 13;9(8):429.

Canine idiopathic epilepsy

Sofie F. M. Bhatti
DVM, PhD

Canine idiopathic epilepsy (IE) is one of the most common chronic neurological diseases seen in veterinary practice, with an estimated prevalence of 0.6–0.75% in primary veterinary practice[1,2] and up to 1–5.6% in referral veterinary practice.[3] In referral hospitals, IE represents 53% of all epilepsy cases.[4] Epidemiological population prevalence studies have shown that the prevalence of IE can even be much higher in certain predisposed breeds (up to 17%) or specific breeding lines (up to 33%).[5]

The high disease prevalence has led to numerous research studies being carried out over the past decades. In 2015, the International Veterinary Epilepsy Task Force (IVETF) published a series of consensus statements on several aspects of epilepsy in dogs and cats.[6] A scientific and working clinical consensus statement on epileptic seizure management in dogs was also published by the American College of Veterinary Internal Medicine (ACVIM) panel in the same year.[7] This large amount of scientific information can thus be used as a framework to guide veterinary students, residents, primary care practitioners, and specialists in making certain decisions when faced with this often debilitating disease.

Disease definition, etiology, and semiology

Epilepsy is defined as a disease of the brain characterized by an enduring predisposition to generate epileptic seizures. In practice, this definition usually applies when at least two unprovoked epileptic seizures occur more than 24 hours apart.[8,9] An epileptic seizure is defined as "a transient occurrence of signs and/or symptoms due to abnormal excessive or synchronous neuronal activity in the brain".[9,10]

Etiology of idiopathic epilepsy

According to the IVETF guidelines, IE occurs in dogs aged between 6 months and 6 years at epileptic seizure onset and with an unremarkable interictal general physical and neurological examination and normal blood tests and urinalysis.[11] IE (with "idiopathic" defined as a disease in its own right) should be seen as an overarching and bridging term, which can be subclassified into three subgroups:[9]

- Genetic epilepsy, for which genetic analysis has identified a disease-causing variant (see dedicated section).
- Suspected genetic epilepsy, for which a genetic etiology is supported by a high breed prevalence (>2%), genealogical analysis, and/or familial accumulation of epileptic individuals. It is important to keep in mind that the epilepsy status within breeds may fluctuate over time and be influenced by differences between countries (e.g., due to preferences with respect to currently popular breeding lines).
- Epilepsy of unknown cause, for which the nature of the underlying cause remains unknown despite extensive diagnostic investigations and with no indication or suspicion of a structural cerebral pathology.

Epileptic seizure classification

The phenotypic classification system (semiology) described by the IVETF[9] distinguishes between generalized and focal epileptic seizures. Generalized epileptic seizures are characterized by the involvement of neuronal networks in both cerebral hemispheres. Focal epileptic seizures originate in a localized area of the brain, with abnormal electrical activity in a group of neurons or network within one cerebral hemisphere. IE in dogs can be characterized by the occurrence of both epilepsy types, and different epileptic seizure types can occur within the same dog. Focal epileptic seizures may become generalized with tonic-clonic activity. This is the most common seizure type observed in the dog; however, the focal onset might often remain unnoticed by the owner due to its brief nature.

This clinical classification requires a thorough observation of the onset of the epileptic seizure, its further course (with detection of any episodes of abnormal motor, behavioral, and autonomic signs), and the phase after the event.

Phases of an epileptic seizure

An epileptic seizure consists of three phases: the prodrome or preictal phase, the ictus or ictal phase, and the postictal phase (see also Chapter 2 and Box 2.1).[9]

The prodrome is a change in the dog's normal behavior, which can last hours to days. It is an indicator of a forthcoming epileptic seizure but is not always identified by the owner. In dogs, the most common prodromal signs described are restlessness, anxiousness, reluctance to perform normal activities, fearful behavior, attention seeking, withdrawal, irritation, or uncharacteristic aggression.[12] When prodromes are consistently noted by the owners, they can represent a potential and important therapeutic window for pulse therapy with fast-acting antiseizure medication (ASM) such as levetiracetam (LEV).

The ictus lasts seconds to minutes (if the seizure activity is self-limiting) and is characterized by alterations in consciousness, behavior, and motor activity and/or abnormal autonomic activity. The ictus may consist of a generalized or focal epileptic seizure or a generalized epileptic seizure with a focal onset.

The postictal phase, during which the brain restores its normal function, starts immediately after the ictus and may last seconds to days. Typically, the animal may show disorientation, repetitive vocalization, compulsive locomotion, inability to avoid obstacles, blindness, ataxia, hunger, thirst, fatigue, defecation, urination, deep sleep, and uncharacteristic aggression.

Epileptic seizures can occur as isolated seizures, cluster seizures, or status epilepticus.[9] Cluster seizures are defined clinically as two or more epileptic seizures within a 24-hour period, with complete recovery of consciousness between the seizures. Status epilepticus is defined as an isolated seizure lasting longer than 5 minutes, or two or more epileptic seizures without complete recovery of consciousness in between the seizures.

Diagnostic approach

The approach should be systematic, starting with the assessment of the dog's signalment (breed, age, and sex) before proceeding to a thorough and detailed medical history of the patient. In fact, the most fundamental step in this systematic approach is to determine if the events the dog is demonstrating truly represent epileptic seizures or if they are consistent with a different type of episodic paroxysmal disorder. Epileptic seizures will rarely happen when the dog is at the veterinary practice. Specific questions should therefore be asked about the paroxysmal or episodic event (via a standardized epilepsy questionnaire[11]) and about the period before and after the event. Owners should be instructed to record videos of any seizure their dog might experience, as these may provide crucial information to clarify the nature of the event and should thus be carefully reviewed.[13] Numerous disorders can result in episodic paroxysmal events that may mimic epileptic seizures (see chapters 2, 18, and 19).

IE is a diagnosis of exclusion, so the history should also aim to get insights into possible underlying causes for the epileptic seizures. Owners should be asked about the occurrence of IE in one of the family members, littermates, or ancestors of the dog, which might be an important clue. A complete general physical and neurological examination is the next step in the investigation of the seizure patient.

Finally, absolute confirmation of the epileptic nature of an event can only be obtained by simultaneously observing the characteristic electroencephalographic changes and the physical manifestations of the seizures.

Criteria for the diagnosis of idiopathic epilepsy

The IVETF has proposed recommendations for a stepwise diagnostic workup for IE.[11] A structured approach has been developed through tier levels of confidence (tiers I–III, Box 16.1) requiring progressively more advanced diagnostic confidence for the diagnosis of canine IE.

Tier I confidence level for the diagnosis of IE

This level describes the minimum requirements necessary for the diagnosis of IE. These include a history of two or more unprovoked epileptic seizures occurring at least 24 hours apart, an age at epileptic seizure onset between 6 months and 6 years, an unremarkable interictal physical and neurological examination (except postictal neurological deficits and ASM-induced neurological abnormalities, see dedicated section), and no clinically significant blood test and urinalysis abnormalities (Box 16.2). A family history of IE further supports the diagnosis.

Additional discretionary laboratory parameters depending on the index of disease suspicion should be measured (Box 16.3). In addition, imaging of the thorax and abdomen should be performed when metastatic neoplastic disease is a possibility. Ocular fundic examination and non-invasive blood pressure measurement should also be performed when hypertension is suspected.

Tier II confidence level for the diagnosis of IE

This level requires all the factors listed in tier I plus unremarkable fasting and postprandial bile acids, magnetic resonance imaging (MRI) of the brain, and cerebrospinal fluid (CSF) analysis (see dedicated section) (Boxes 16.2 and 16.3).

Box 16.1 Tier levels of diagnostic confidence for the diagnosis of idiopathic epilepsy in dogs as proposed by the International Veterinary Epilepsy Task Force.

Tier I confidence level

- A history of two or more unprovoked epileptic seizures occurring at least 24 hours apart.
- Age at epileptic seizure onset between 6 months and 6 years.
- Unremarkable interictal physical and neurological examination (except antiseizure medication–induced neurological abnormalities and postictal neurological deficits).
- No abnormalities (relevant for epileptogenesis) on blood tests and urinalysis (see Box 16.2).
- Additional diagnostic parameters should be investigated depending on the index of disease suspicion (see Box 16.3).

Tier II confidence level

- All the parameters listed in tier I.
- Unremarkable fasting and postprandial bile acid concentrations.
- No abnormalities (relevant to epileptogenesis) on magnetic resonance imaging of the brain and cerebrospinal fluid analysis.

Tier III confidence level

- All the parameters listed in tiers I and II.
- Ictal or interictal electroencephalographic abnormalities relevant to epileptogenesis.

Tier III confidence level for the diagnosis of IE

This level requires identification of ictal or interictal electroencephalographic abnormalities characteristic for epileptic seizure disorders (see dedicated section) according to the criteria validated in human medicine, in addition to the factors listed in tiers I and II (Boxes 16.2 and 16.3).

Neurological abnormalities in the postictal period and associated with antiseizure medications

The clinician should be aware of the presence of neurological deficits during the postictal period (e.g., obtundation, proprioceptive ataxia, delayed postural reactions, decreased menace response, blindness).[11] It is advised to repeat the exam after at least 1 week of seizure freedom to determine if the neurological deficits have resolved, improved, or worsened. The administration of ASMs can influence the neurological exam with the presence of obtundation, ataxia (mainly in the pelvic limbs), and decreased postural reactions.

Diagnostic imaging of the brain and cerebrospinal fluid examination

MRI

MRI is the diagnostic imaging modality of choice for evaluation of the brain, and it is regarded as an important diagnostic test to achieve a tier II level of confidence for IE diagnosis in dogs.[14] Brain MRI is also recommended in dogs with a presumptive tier I level diagnosis of IE that respond poorly to ASM therapy.

CSF examination

In dogs with epilepsy, CSF should be collected through a cervical puncture (cisterna magna or cerebellomedullary cistern) because of the fluid's craniocaudal circulation and closer proximity of the brain (compared to lumbar puncture). Results of routine CSF analysis (red blood cell count, total nucleated cell count [TNCC], total protein concentration and cytology) must always be interpreted in the context of the dog's signalment, medical history, neuroanatomical diagnosis, blood test results, and diagnostic imaging findings. CSF abnormalities are sensitive indicators of CNS disease; however, they are rarely specific for underlying etiologies.[11,14] The most important diagnostic value of CSF analysis in dogs presenting with a history of epileptic seizures is to determine the presence of inflammatory disease of the brain.

In dogs with (suspected) IE (based on the occurrence of recurrent seizures, a normal interictal physical and neurological exam, and normal blood tests and brain MRI), the likelihood of detecting an underlying cause was not increased when performing CSF analysis.[15] In these dogs,

Box 16.2 Blood and urine parameters to measure to fulfill tier I confidence level for the diagnosis of idiopathic epilepsy.

Tier I confidence level – Blood and urine tests

Blood	*Urine*
Hematology	Specific gravity
Serum biochemistry	Protein
Sodium (Na)	Glucose
Potassium (K)	pH
Chloride (Cl)	Sediment cytology
Calcium (Ca)	
Phosphorus (P)	
Alanine aminotransferase (ALT)	
Alkaline phosphatase (ALP)	
Total bilirubin	
Blood urea nitrogen	
Creatinine	
Total protein	
Albumin	
Glucose	
Cholesterol	
Triglycerides	
Fasting bile acids and/or ammonia	

Tier II confidence level – Blood and urine tests

- Blood and urine parameters see tier I + unremarkable fasting and postprandial bile acid concentrations

Box 16.3 Additional diagnostic examinations in case of suspicion of certain diseases.

Suspicion of	Additional diagnostics
Hepatic encephalopathy	Bile acid stimulation test (12-hour fasting and 2-hour postprandial bile acid concentration) and/or fasting ammonia
Thyroid disorder	Total thyroxin (TT4), free T4, thyroid-stimulating hormone (TSH)
Insulinoma	Fructosamine, insulin (if glucose <3.33 mmol/L or 60 mg/dL), glucose curve and or glucose:insulin ratio
Hypocalcemia	Ionized calcium
Cobalamin malabsorption	Vitamin D_{12}
Toxin exposure	Suspect feed or bait material, gastric content (vomitus or gastric lavage), blood or urine for toxicologic screening
Infectious disorders	Serology, PCR antigen testing
Inborn errors of metabolism	Quantification of amino acids and organic acids and determination of glycosaminoglycans, oligosaccharides, purines and pyrimidines in serum, CSF, and urine
Genetic epilepsy	DNA analysis (EDTA blood or buccal mucosa swab) Idiopathic: Lagotto Romagnolo (*LGI2*), Rhodesian Ridgeback (*DIRAS 1*), Structural: Wirehaired Dachshund (*EPM2b*), Staffordshire Bull Terrier (*L2HGA*)
Baseline function before initiating phenobarbital	Bile acid stimulation test (12-hour fasting and 2-hour postprandial bile acid concentration) and/or fasting ammonia, TT4, free T4, TSH
Metastatic neoplastic disease	Imaging thorax and abdomen
Hypertension	Ocular fundic examination and noninvasive blood pressure measurement

the diagnostic yield of CSF analysis is very low and the added value of collecting CSF, taking into account the increased risk (of anesthesia and the procedure itself), remains questionable.

Epileptic seizure-associated brain MRI and CSF changes

Epileptic seizure activity has been reported to cause intraparenchymal cerebral signal changes on MRI, which can be seen within 14 days of the last epileptic seizure.[16] These MRI signal changes are located in specific areas of the forebrain (most commonly the hippocampus, cingulate gyrus, and piriform lobes) and can be uni- or bilateral, local or remote to the epileptogenic focus, and partially or completely reversible. In canine IE, brain MRI signal changes due to epileptic seizures are T2-weighted hyperintense with no suppression of signal on fluid-attenuated inversion recovery (FLAIR) images and T1-weighted isointense or hypointense with contrast enhancement and a mass effect in some dogs.[16] These epileptic seizure-induced changes may resolve partly or completely on repeated MRI examination 2.5–4 months later; this indicates they are most likely due to cytotoxic and vasogenic edema induced by the epileptic seizures.[17] Histological examination of the affected temporal cortex, hippocampus, and piriform lobe revealed edema, neovascularization, reactive astrocytosis, and acute neuronal necrosis. In dogs with cerebral MRI signal changes suspected to be the result rather than the cause of the epileptic seizures, repeating the MRI, neurological examination, and if needed the CSF analysis after a period of seizure control may help to differentiate epileptic seizure-induced MRI changes from inflammatory or neoplastic epileptogenic structural lesions.

Epileptic seizure activity has also been reported to cause CSF abnormalities in dogs with IE,[18] which may consist of mild and transient postictal CSF pleocytosis and/or increased protein concentration. The pathophysiology of seizure-induced CSF pleocytosis remains unclear. These abnormalities may be the result of a transient disturbance of the blood–brain barrier function (which has been demonstrated after epileptic seizures in experimental animals) and release of chemotactic substances into the CSF during the epileptic seizures. The time to resolution of CSF abnormalities associated with the epileptic seizures is unknown.

Genetic testing

Genetic tests are currently available only for a few genetic IEs in single dog breeds. Most genetic epilepsies in dogs are very likely to have a polygenic (complex) inheritance and do not yet have a genetic test developed. In the past 10 years, a number of reviews have been published on canine genetic epilepsy.[19,20] The 2015 IVETF consensus paper[21] reviewed the evidence available for breeds that have been identified as being predisposed to IE with a proven or suspected genetic background, and highlighted different breed specific clinical features (e.g., age at onset, sex, seizure type), treatment response, prevalence rates, and proposed inheritance reported in the literature. Only two uncommon single-gene (monogenic) IEs have so far been identified in dogs:

- Lagotto Romagnolo dogs: a benign familial juvenile epilepsy syndrome has been described (*LGI2* autosomal recessive gene mutation).[22] The clinical characteristics of this form of epilepsy are different from those of most other (presumed genetic) IEs in dogs, in which the age of epileptic seizure onset is between 6 months and 6 years, and spontaneous remission rarely occurs. In Lagotto Romagnolo dogs, epileptic seizures start at 5–9 weeks of age and usually spontaneously resolve by 8–13 weeks (see also Chapter 12). The epileptic seizures are characterized by generalized (all body) tremors, ataxia, and stiffness. Most puppies appear conscious during the seizures. In adulthood, these dogs often present with behavioral changes characterized by inattention and hyperexcitability resembling attention deficit hyperactivity disorder in people.[23]
- Rhodesian Ridgebacks: a juvenile, generalized, and/or myoclonic epilepsy with photosensitivity has been described (*DIRAS1* mutation).[24] Epileptic seizure onset ranges between 6 weeks and 18 months. In these dogs, epileptic seizures are usually generalized and include myoclonic, generalized tonic-clonic, and absence epileptic seizures. Myoclonic epileptic seizures present as repetitive myoclonic twitches or violent myoclonic jerks that resemble electric shocks. A typical feature of this epilepsy is photosensitivity in approximately 35% of the dogs. Situations such as light flashes from cameras, the sudden appearance of light when opening the shutters in the morning, or sunlight interrupted by trees when walking through a forest were reported to induce myoclonic jerks. The myoclonic epileptic seizures appeared to respond best to LEV or potassium bromide.

Electroencephalography

Electroencephalography (EEG) is the study and recording of electrical activity from the brain via electrodes placed upon the head. Consequently, EEG is used to investigate cortical brain function. With EEG only, the often challenging question "is it an epileptic seizure?" can be answered, and the highest level of confidence in the diagnosis of IE (tier III) can be achieved objectively.[25] EEG can also assess whether ASM is efficacious and determine the presence of brain death. Simultaneous video recording provides visual information of the episodic event, thus allowing the physical manifestations of an episode to be characterized and correlated with the EEG data. Physiological artifacts (e.g., eye and tongue movement, muscle contractions, electrocardiogram) and physical factors (e.g., EEG instrumentation, electrode type and montage, methods of patient restraint) may affect the acquisition and interpretation of EEG tracings.[25,26]

The availability and use of EEG varies considerably between veterinary institutions, with a minority currently utilizing this technique on a daily or routine basis. Clinical barriers to the performance of EEG in dogs are mainly equipment availability, insufficient cases, and financial costs to clients. Correct recognition and interpretation of EEG abnormalities also requires training and experience. Nonspecific EEG abnormalities can be seen in multiple encephalopathies, in brain injury, and with the use of sedative medications. Detection of specific epileptogenic EEG abnormalities necessitates guidance and education. Efforts are currently in progress to further develop EEG recording in veterinary clinical practice, and a validated and standardized canine EEG protocol is hoped to improve the diagnosis and management of canine epilepsy. A normal interictal EEG does not rule out epilepsy and the percentage of normal dogs with EEG abnormalities is unknown.[26] EEG may become more widely used by veterinary neurologists for the investigation of selected cases in which a diagnosis of epilepsy is particularly challenging.

Management and outcome

ASMs play an important role in the management of IE. In most dogs, the goal of IE management is epileptic seizure control rather than cure, and this supportive approach is usually lifelong. Epileptic seizure eradication is often not likely in dogs with IE. More realistic goals are to decrease seizure frequency, duration, and severity and to avoid the occurrence of cluster seizures and status epilepticus, with limited and acceptable adverse effects (AEs) to optimize the dog's and owner's quality of life (QoL). Clinicians should consider the general health of the patient, as well as the owner's lifestyle, financial limitations, and comfort with the proposed management approach. Client education regarding the goals and expectations of management is an extremely important part of successful ASM administration and should be provided before any drug is chosen. A lifestyle adjustment might be required to ensure the dog receives its medication at the prescribed intervals each day. Owners should also be educated on the AEs associated with ASM administration.

Antiseizure medication

Administration of ASMs must be adjusted and tailored to the individual dog with some important principles to take into consideration regarding:

- When to start ASM.
- The most appropriate ASM and dose.
- How to develop a management plan and a follow-up.
  - How to adjust ASM dose.
  - When to add another ASM.
- How to assess therapeutic outcome.
- When a dog is drug resistant.
- When to stop with ASM, i.e., epilepsy remission.

When to start ASM?

It is recommended to initiate ASM in dogs with IE when any one of the following criteria is present:[7,27]

- Two or more isolated epileptic seizures within a 6-month period.
- Status epilepticus or cluster seizures.
- Postictal signs are considered especially severe (e.g., aggression, blindness) or last >24 hours.
- Epileptic seizure frequency and/or duration is increasing and/or seizure severity is deteriorating over three interictal periods.

Most appropriate ASM

There are no evidence-based guidelines regarding the choice of ASM in dogs. When choosing an ASM for the management of epilepsy in dogs, several factors need to be taken into account; these are drug-specific factors (e.g., mechanism of action, efficacy, safety and AEs, route of metabolism and possible drug interactions, ease of administration, cost, regulatory aspects), dog-related factors (e.g., seizure type, frequency and severity, underlying pathologies such as kidney/hepatic/gastrointestinal problems) and owner-related factors (e.g., lifestyle, financial circumstances). In the end, however, the choice of ASM is often made on a case-by-case basis.

In Europe, three ASMs have been licensed for the management of canine epilepsy. These drugs are phenobarbital (PB), potassium bromide (KBr), and imepitoin (IMP). Unfortunately, the range of mechanisms of action of these three drugs is rather similar and narrow, limited to an enhancement of GABAergic signaling and hyperpolarization. Other ASMs that have so far only been approved for human patients but can be used in dogs include LEV, zonisamide (ZNS), gabapentin, pregabalin, topiramate, and cannabidiol.[28–36]

It is important for clinicians to consider the quality and amount of evidence available when evaluating the efficacy of an ASM. Few randomized, blinded, controlled studies have evaluated the efficacy of ASMs in dogs. Trials are often nonblinded and do not involve a control or placebo group. The *ACVIM Consensus Statement on Seizure Management in Dogs*[7] and a systematic review by Charalambous et al.[37] critically evaluated the strength of published trials on ASM efficacy in order to make clear recommendations on their use.

Figures 16.1 and 16.2 illustrate the recommendations for ASM use as monotherapy or add-on therapy in dogs based on an assessment of published studies.[7,37]

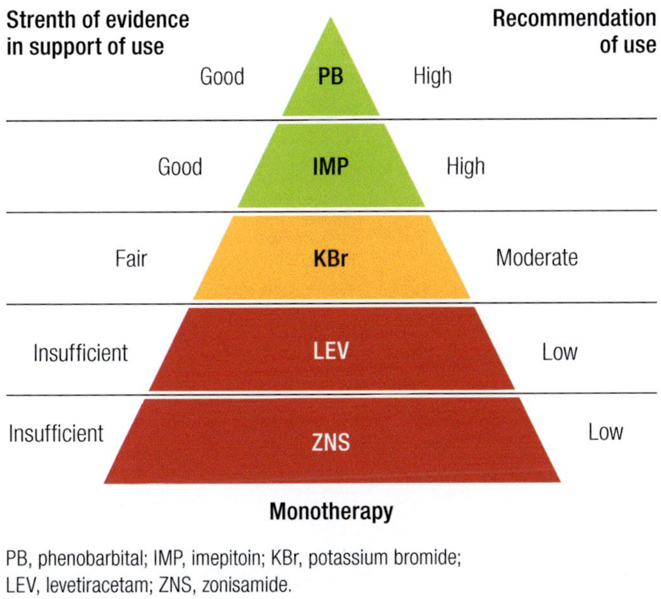

FIG. 16.1 Recommendations for antiseizure medication use as monotherapy in dogs based on assessment of published studies.[7,37]

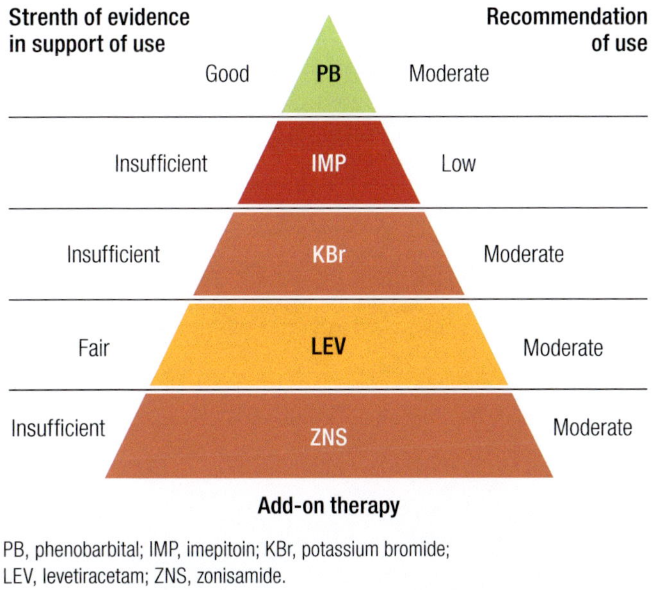

FIG. 16.2 Recommendations for antiseizure medication use as add-on therapy in dogs based on assessment of published studies.[7,37]

Safety is often a great concern for the owner of an epileptic dog. Clinicians should try to minimize the occurrence of AEs, as this impacts the QoL of the owner and dog significantly. The absence of AEs is almost impossible in most epileptic dogs, but efforts should be made to avoid serious effects. AEs can be categorized as type A (pharmacologically related) or type B (idiosyncratic reactions). Type A AEs are common, predictable, dose dependent, rarely life-threatening, and tend to be more severe at the onset of administration (mostly the first 2 weeks) or after a dose increase. Type A AEs are typically reversible upon dose adjustment and rarely require discontinuation of the drug. The most common reported type A AEs associated with ASMs are sedation and ataxia; these effects can occur with any ASM. Other frequent AEs in dogs include polyphagia, polyuria, and polydipsia and can be seen in association with PB, KBr, or IMP administration. In contrast, type B AEs occur unexpectedly and are not dose dependent. These idiosyncratic reactions are often more serious and include hepatotoxicity, blood dyscrasias, pancreatitis, dyskinesia, and superficial necrolytic dermatitis with PB; pancreatitis, panniculitis, and neuromyopathy with KBr; and hepatotoxicity and renal tubular necrosis with ZNS in dogs. As these idiosyncratic effects are mostly serious and sometimes life-threatening, discontinuation of the drug is necessary.

Charalambous et al.[38] conducted a meta-analysis of the safety of ASMs in dogs and concluded that LEV and IMP are the safest ASMs for use in this species, followed by PB and finally KBr, with a strong level of evidence supporting the safety profile of all these drugs.

TABLE 16.1 Adverse effects (type A and type B) of the most common antiseizure medications and possible changes in blood parameters.

Drug	Adverse effects (type A)	Idiosyncratic reactions (type B)	Changes in blood parameters
Phenobarbital	■ Sedation ■ Ataxia ■ Polyphagia ■ Polydipsia/polyuria	■ Hepatotoxicity ■ Bone marrow suppression ■ Superficial necrolytic dermatitis ■ Increased risk of pancreatitis ■ Dyskinesia ■ Anxiousness	■ Increase in ALP, ALT, GGT ■ Hypercholesterolemia and hypertriglyceridemia ■ Hypoalbuminemia ■ Anemia and/or thrombocytopenia and/or neutropenia ■ Decreased TT4 and fT4, slight increase in TSH
Potassium bromide	■ Sedation ■ Ataxia and pelvic limb weakness ■ Polyphagia ■ Polydipsia/polyuria ■ Nausea and/or vomiting and/or diarrhea	■ Aggression, irritability, hyperactivity ■ Erythematous dermatitis ■ Panniculitis ■ Persistent cough ■ Increased risk of pancreatitis	■ Hypercholesterolemia ■ Hypertriglyceridemia
Imepitoin	■ Polyphagia	■ Hyperactivity, restlessness, aggression, disorientation ■ Polydipsia/polyuria ■ Somnolence, lethargy, sedation ■ Hypersalivation ■ Emesis, diarrhea ■ Ataxia ■ Prolapsed nictitating membrane ■ Decreased vision and sensitivity to sound	
Levetiracetam	■ Sedation ■ Ataxia ■ Decreased appetite or anorexia ■ Vomiting ■ Behavioral changes		
Zonisamide	■ Sedation ■ Ataxia ■ Vomiting ■ Inappetence	■ Keratoconjunctivitis sicca ■ Polyarthropathy ■ Acute hepatopathy/hepatomegaly ■ Renal tubular acidosis	
Topiramate	■ Sedation, ataxia, and weight loss (as add-on) ■ No adverse effects in healthy Beagle dogs receiving an oral daily dose of 10–15 mg/kg for 15 days		
Gabapentin	■ Sedation ■ Ataxia		
Pregabalin	■ Sedation ■ Ataxia ■ Dizziness ■ Weakness		
Felbamate	■ Keratitis sicca		■ Thrombocytopenia ■ Lymphopenia and leucopenia

ALP, alkaline phosphatase; ALT, alanine aminotransferase; GGT, gamma-glutamyl transferase; TT4, total thyroxin; fT4, free thyroxin; TSH, thyroid-stimulating hormone.

Table 16.1 provides a list of AEs (type A and type B) and possible changes in blood parameters for the most common ASMs.

The choice of ASM should also take into account any concurrent systemic disease. PB, IMP, and ZNS (the most commonly used ASMs) undergo hepatic metabolism, and their use should be avoided in dogs with liver dysfunction. LEV is not metabolized by the liver and undergoes oxidation and hydrolysis in other tissues before being renally excreted. KBr is not metabolized and is excreted unchanged by the kidneys. As LEV and KBr are primarily excreted by the kidneys, dose adjustments may be needed in dogs with renal dysfunction.

Management plan and follow-up

Generally, administration of a single ASM rather than a combination of drugs is advised. This avoids drug–drug interactions and provides a simpler management plan that may improve owner compliance. Initiation should be done at the low end of the recommended maintenance dose range. A loading dose (see below) can be administered to achieve the desired serum concentrations more rapidly in dogs with frequent or severe epileptic seizures. This is mostly done for drugs with a long elimination half-life such as KBr.

Therapeutic drug monitoring is an important component of epilepsy management and involves the measurement of the drug's plasma or serum concentration. Blood concentrations are superior to dosage in assessing an ASM's clinical effectiveness and are strongly correlated with ASM concentrations in the brain. Monitoring should be routinely done for PB and KBr (and ZNS if the veterinary laboratory performs this analysis). Time points for the measurement of drug concentrations should be:

- After initiation of drug administration or dose adjustment once steady state concentration has been reached.
- When epileptic seizure control is not satisfactory despite an apparently adequate dose.
- When there are concerns about drug-related toxicity or drug–drug interactions.
- Every 6–12 months to screen for any changes over time.

Generally, trough samples (collected immediately before the next dose) are recommended when assessing seizure control, and peak samples (collected at the time maximum concentrations are expected based on the drug's pharmacokinetic properties) are recommended when assessing toxicity. In some cases, both trough and peak samples are useful to optimize the dosing schedule.[39] For drugs with long half-lives such as KBr, samples can be collected at any time during the day, as fluctuations in drug concentrations during a dosing interval are negligible. It is also good practice to be consistent in the timing of blood sample collection to allow for optimal direct comparison of multiple results.

Adding a second drug to the management plan should be done when success has not been achieved with the first ASM, i.e., when epileptic seizure control is insufficient despite using the maximum recommended dosage or achieving a blood concentration at the high-end of the reference range, or when unacceptable AEs occur. In most cases, the second ASM is added without stopping administration of the first, and polytherapy is continued. An abrupt switch (stopping one ASM and administering a second) is only recommended in case of serious adverse or idiosyncratic ASM-related reactions. To quickly reach blood concentrations within the desired reference range, the second ASM can be administered at a loading dose (see below), or a short-acting ASM (e.g., LEV) can be given for a short period of time to provide sufficient seizure control until the second ASM reaches the targeted blood concentrations. KBr can be administered at a loading dose when steady-state reference serum levels must be reached as rapidly as possible (e.g., dogs with frequent or severe seizures, or when PB must be discontinued rapidly because of severe AEs). Different protocols have been reported. Oral loading can be performed by administering KBr at 625 mg/

TABLE 16.2 Antiseizure medication dose recommendations, days to steady-state and elimination half-life, reference serum concentrations, and recommended diagnostics.

Drug	Initial recommended oral dose	Days to steady state* and elimination half-life	Reference serum concentration mg/L	Recommended diagnostics	Frequency
Phenobarbital	2.5–3 mg/kg BID	10–20 and 50 hours	25–35	CE, CBC, SB, bile acid stimulation test, SCM	Every 6–2 months
Potassium bromide	10–15 (add-on therapy) 15–20 (monotherapy) mg/kg BID	90–120 and 15–46 days	2000 (add-on)–3000 (mono)	CE, CBC, SB, urinalysis, SCM	Every 6–12 months
Imepitoin	10–30 mg/kg BID	1–2	†	CE, CBC, SB	Every 6–12 months
Levetiracetam	20–30 (when administered with PB) mg/kg TID	1 and 4 hours	5–46‡	CE, CBC, SB, Urinalysis	Every 6–12 months
Zonisamide	3–5 or 7–10 (when administered with PB) mg/kg BID	3–5 and 15 hours	10–40‡	CE, CBC, SB, SCM	Every 6–12 months
Topiramate	2–10 mg/kg BID	†	5–20‡		
Gabapentin	10–20 mg/kg TID–QID	1	2–20‡		
Pregabalin	2–4 mg/kg BID–TID	1–2	2.8–8.3‡		
Felbamate	20 mg/kg TID	1–2	30–60‡		

* Steady-state concentrations are reached after approximately five half-lives. † Not established in dogs. ‡ In people.
CE, clinical examination; CBC, complete blood count; SB, serum biochemistry; SCM, serum concentration monitoring; BID, twice a day; TID, 3 times a day; QID, 4 times a day.

TABLE 16.3 Reported antiseizure medication interactions in dogs.

1st ASM	Effect on 2nd ASM	Interaction	Dose adjustment necessary?
Phenobarbital	■ Levetiracetam ■ Zonisamide ■ Benzodiazepines ■ Topiramate ↓	■ Cytochrome P450 induction (ZNS, BZP, TPM) ■ Induction of nonhepatic oxidative enzymes (LEV)	■ Dose increase of 2nd ASM might be required
Clorazepate	■ Phenobarbital ↑	■ Presumed to inhibit drug metabolizing enzymes	■ Dose decrease of 2nd ASM might be required (based on PB serum concentration measurement before and after clorazepate administration)
Felbamate	■ Phenobarbital ↑	■ Inhibits hepatic microsomal cytochrome P450 enzymes	■ Dose decrease of 2nd ASM might be required (based on PB serum concentration measurement before and after felbamate administration)

ZNS, zonisamide; BZP, benzodiazepine; TPM, topiramate; LEV, levetiracetam; PB, phenobarbital; ASM, antiseizure medication.
The arrows indicate the effect on the blood concentration of the indicated drug.

kg divided in 8 or more doses over 48 hours, or 125 mg/kg/day divided in 3–4 daily administrations for 5 consecutive days. Loading is often associated with AEs (e.g., nausea, vomiting, diarrhea, sedation, ataxia and pelvic limb weakness, polydipsia, polyuria and polyphagia), and hospitalization of the animal is often recommended.[40]

Table 16.2 provides the dose recommendations, days to steady-state and elimination half-life, reference serum concentrations, and recommended diagnostic tests for ASMs.

When adding a second ASM, it is important to consider any potential pharmacokinetic interactions between both ASMs, as dose adjustments might be necessary (Table 16.3).

Therapeutic success and drug-resistance

In epilepsy management, ideally, the goal is seizure freedom. However, dogs with IE are often managed for life. Therapeutic success has been defined as seizure freedom for more than three times the longest pretreatment interseizure interval and at least 3 months (complete therapeutic success).[41] It is important to realize that a reduction in seizure frequency, seizure severity, seizure clusters, or status epilepticus may also be important for dogs and their owners and thus may be considered a partial therapeutic success.[41]

Drug resistance means that the appropriately selected drug or drug combination, administered at therapeutic and, if appropriate, maximally tolerated doses, fails to control epileptic seizure activity. In the context of an "appropriate drug selection", it is important to consider that limited data exist concerning the question of whether canine epileptic seizures respond differently to different drugs. In several studies, drug-resistant epilepsy is defined as failure to achieve a decrease in seizure frequency of ≥50% despite administration of at least two combined ASMs for a minimum of 6 months.[8,29,31,34]

Risk factors for drug-resistance have been described in canine IE. Certain dog breeds, a younger age of onset and sex (male) have been linked with a lower chance of therapeutic success. The fact that breed-specific IEs appear to differ in their therapeutic response seems to be in line with the intrinsic severity hypothesis of epilepsy. Published data on Australian Shepherds, Border Collies, Cane Corso dogs, Dogues de Bordeaux, Great Swiss Mountain Dogs, Rottweilers, and Italian Spinone dogs suggest an increased risk for cluster seizures and drug resistance in dogs adequately managed with PB and KBr.[42–47] A reduced life expectancy has been reported in Irish Wolfhounds, Border Collies, and Great Swiss Mountain Dogs.[43,47,48] However, in other breeds such as the Belgian Shepherd, Collie, Finnish Spitz, Labrador Retriever, and Poodle, the published data support an overall good response to GABAergic ASMs.[21]

Assessment of the therapeutic response is largely based on owner observations. Therefore, owners should be instructed to maintain a calendar of seizure frequency, to keep record of any observed AEs, and to note any deviations from the management regimen.

Epilepsy remission

An absence of epileptic seizures for at least 1 year is defined as seizure remission and is reported to occur in approximately 15% of dogs with IE.[41] This includes both dogs that experience seizure remission with ASM administration and those that experience spontaneous remission without ASM administration. A careful, slow, and systematic decrease in ASM dosage can be considered in dogs that are free of epileptic seizures for a minimum of 1–2 years. Reducing the dose by 25% every 2–4 weeks is advised. It is important to realize that seizures that recur with discontinuation of treatment can be more difficult to control.

Nondrug management options for epileptic seizure control

Considering the limited number of drugs licensed for dogs with epilepsy, efforts should be continued and intensified to identify and assess alternate nonpharmacological approaches, thus broadening the spectrum of management choices for drug-resistant canine patients. These non–drug management options currently include neurodietetics (particularly diets enriched with medium-chain triglycerides [MCTs]), lifestyle changes (e.g., ensuring a regular daily routine and sleep pattern, reducing stress, or avoiding individual epileptic seizure trigger factors), neurostimulation (mainly deep brain, vagal, or repetitive transcranial magnetic stimulation), and neurosurgery (especially disconnection or resection of the seizure focus), with the two latter options not being readily available in most veterinary practices or specialist centers.

Nutrition

The past decade has seen an increased interest in nutrition for the management of canine IE based on growing scientific evidence.[49,50] Diets can serve their functions through many pathways. One potential pathway includes the microbiota–gut–brain axis (MGBA), which highlights the relationship between the brain and the intestines. An important factor in this axis is the gastrointestinal microbiome (GIM), i.e., the collection of genomes from all the microorganisms present in the digestive tract.[51] The GIM is greatly influenced by nutrition.[52,53] Studies have shown the GIM plays an important role in the pathogenesis and management of epilepsy. Both human and canine studies have demonstrated that the gastrointestinal microbiota composition in epileptic patients was different to that of healthy controls, which supports a potential role for dysbiosis (i.e., disease-promoting imbalance in the gastrointestinal microbiota composition) in epileptogenesis.[54]

An MCT-enriched diet has been proposed for the management of IE. The antiseizure effect of MCTs might work through the MGBA.[55–57] A complete diet including MCTs seems to be superior to MCT supplementation to a basal diet. Approximately half of the dogs fed with a complete MCT-enriched diet showed a decrease in seizure frequency of at least 50%,[58–62] against only 18% of the dogs receiving MCTs as a supplement to their diet.[59] The available evidence is therefore satisfactory to support the use of MCT-enriched diets (which are commercially available) in canine IE, while it remains limited for most of the other nutritional interventions (e.g., gluten-free diet, elimination diet, nutraceuticals [e.g., coconut oil, fish oil, cannabis oil, milk thistle], omega-3 fatty acids). In dogs with IE receiving MCTs either as a component of a commercial diet or as a supplement to an adjusted diet for 3 months and showing no improvement of epileptic seizure control, it can be assumed that MCTs are unlikely to be helpful and could be discontinued.

Avoiding seizure-precipitating factors

Seizure-precipitating factors (SPFs) or triggers or provocative factors have been studied and reported in both humans and dogs with IE. In dogs, stress-related situations, hormonal factors, sleep deprivation, and the weather have been reported as SPFs.[63,64] The prevalence of SPFs in a study by Forsgård et al.[64] was 74%. Shell et al.[65] reported that common SPFs in dogs with IE were visits to veterinary and grooming facilities.

Mandigers and Santifort[66] described 6 unrelated Border Collies with IE in which several remarkable SPFs were identified; avoiding them improved the outcome of these dogs. It was hypothesized that although epilepsy in many breeds is most likely of genetic origin,[7] there are striking differences in possible SPFs for the different breeds. Dogs judged by breeders and breed clubs as more sensitive in nature, such as the Border Collie, Australian Shepherd, or Belgian Shepherd, may be more susceptible to SPFs than less sensitive breeds such as the Dutch Partridge Dog, Labrador Retriever, or Golden Retriever.

Veterinarians managing IE in dogs need to consider the dog's breed, its relationship with the owner, and the domestic situation or environment in which the dog is housed. Recognizing SPFs and taking measures with regard to management can lead to a reduction in epileptic seizure frequency and even seizure freedom.

Quality of life (QoL)

QoL is a very important outcome measure of chronic diseases such as IE, in which the likelihood of seizure freedom is low for many dogs. Canine IE not only has an effect on the perceived QoL of the affected dog, it is also significantly associated with the owner's perceived QoL.[67] Owners will choose euthanasia if the emotional stress, psychosocial challenges, and/or financial burden associated with having an epileptic dog in the household are worse than they expected. Dogs with epilepsy have been reported to have an increased risk of premature death as a result of euthanasia.[2,68] However, Fredso et al.[69] found that the median life span of dogs with IE was not decreased when compared with the median life span of dogs in general.[69] Hamers et al.[70] reported breed-specific differences in the perceived QoL of dogs with IE and their owners. In this study, Border Collies and their owners had statistically significantly lower QoL scores than dogs of other breeds and their owners. What influences the QoL score differs for each breed, although the age of seizure onset, the number of seizures, and their severity all had a negative influence on the perceived QoL. Owners of Labrador and Golden Retrievers reported a minimal impact of the epileptic seizures on their pet's QoL, and Chihuahua and Dachshund owners also reported an overall good QoL of their dogs. The tendency to develop cluster seizures or status epilepticus has also been found to negatively influence the outcome of dogs with IE.[71,72] Wessmann et al.[73] reported the creation of a disease-specific QoL questionnaire for dogs with IE and their owners (EpiQoL). The questionnaire design was based on the multidimensional aspects of QoL as defined by the World Health Organization; these were grouped into physical, social, and neurobehavioral (dog)/psychological health aspects (owner) and adapted for IE.[73] The questionnaire contains a limited number of key questions assessing the QoL in dogs with IE.

Greater awareness and empathy from veterinarians regarding the range and severity of comorbidities associated with this devastating disease is important and will improve communication between owner and vet, leading to better outcomes for both parties. Promoting continuity of care by assigning one veterinarian to each epilepsy case within a veterinary practice (if possible) will help veterinarians to build strong relationships with owners and understand the challenges they face.

KEY POINTS

- Canine idiopathic epilepsy (IE) is a common, chronic neurological disease.
- Differentiating an epileptic seizure from another nonepileptic paroxysmal event is a crucial step in the diagnosis but can sometimes be very challenging.
- The diagnosis of IE is one of exclusion and based on the tier levels of confidence recommended by the IVETF.
- Clinically, diagnosing IE relies on the occurrence of ≥2 epileptic seizures at least 24 hours apart, an age at seizure onset between 6 months and 6 years, a normal clinical/neurological exam, and no evidence of a toxic/metabolic cause or structural cerebral pathology.
- IE is an overarching term and encompasses genetic IE, suspected genetic IE, and IE of unknown etiology.
- Currently, there are only two uncommon, single-gene IEs identified in two dog breeds with an identified disease-causing variant (Rhodesian Ridgeback and Lagotto Romagnolo).
- Electroencephalography is not yet routinely used in (specialized) veterinary centers.
- Antiseizure medication (ASM) is essential in the management of IE, with phenobarbital (PB) or imepitoin (IMP) recommended as first-line medications in otherwise healthy dogs.
- There is moderate evidence to support the use of potassium bromide (KBr) as an add-on ASM.
- For ASMs with short half-lives (e.g., PB), trough and peak blood samples are recommended to assess seizure control and toxicity, respectively. For ASMs with long half-lives (e.g., KBr), samples can be collected at any time during the day.
- Nondrug options should also be considered in the management of IE.
- There is satisfactory scientific evidence supporting the use of MCT (medium-chain triglycerides)–triglycerides–enriched diets in canine IE.
- A severe epilepsy phenotype (high frequency of epileptic seizures, status epilepticus, cluster seizures) has a serious impact on the quality of life of the dog and owner.
- Seizure freedom is not often achieved in canine IE.

References

1. Kearsley-Fleet L, O'Neill DG, Volk HA, et al. Prevalence and risk factors for canine epilepsy of unknown origin in the UK. *Vet Rec.* 2013 Mar 30;172(13):338.
2. Heske L, Nødtvedt A, Jäderlund KH, et al. A cohort study of epilepsy among 665,000 insured dogs: incidence, mortality and survival after diagnosis. *Vet J.* 2014 Dec;202(3):471–476.
3. Oberbauer AM, Belanger JM, Bellumori T, et al. Ten inherited disorders in purebred dogs by functional breed groupings. *Canine Genet Epidemiol.* 2015,11;2:9.
4. Hall R, Labruyere J, Volk H, et al. Estimation of the prevalence of idiopathic epilepsy and structural epilepsy in a general population of 900 dogs undergoing MRI for epileptic seizures. *Vet Rec*, 2020,14;187(10):e89.
5. Berendt M, Gulløv CH, Fredholm M. Focal epilepsy in the Belgian shepherd: evidence for simple Mendelian inheritance. *J Small Anim Pract.* 2009 Dec;50(12):655–661.
6. Volk HA. International Veterinary Epilepsy Task Force consensus reports on epilepsy definition, classification and terminology, affected dog breeds, diagnosis, treatment, outcome measures of therapeutic trials, neuroimaging and neuropathology in companion animals. *BMC Vet Res.* 2015 Aug 28:11:174.
7. Podell M, Volk HA, Berendt M, et al. 2015 ACVIM Small Animal Consensus Statement on Seizure Management in Dogs. *J Vet Intern Med.* 2016 Mar-Apr;30(2):477–490.
8. Fisher RS, Acevedo C, Arzimanoglou A, et al. ILAE Official Report: A practical clinical definition of epilepsy. *Epilepsia.* 2014;55(4):475–482.
9. Berendt M, Farquhar RG, Mandigers PJ, et al. International veterinary epilepsy task force consensus report on epilepsy definition, classification and terminology in companion animals. *BMC Vet Res*, 2015,28;11:182.
10. Fisher RS, van Emde Boas W, Blume W, et al. Epileptic seizures and epilepsy: definitions proposed by the International League Against Epilepsy (ILAE) and the International Bureau for Epilepsy (IBE). *Epilepsia.* 2005 Apr;46(4):470–472.
11. De Risio L, Bhatti S, Muñana K, et al. International veterinary epilepsy task force consensus proposal: diagnostic approach to epilepsy in dogs. *BMC Vet Res.* 2015,11:148.
12. Finnegan SL, Volk HA, Asher L, et al. Investigating the potential for seizure prediction in dogs with idiopathic epilepsy: owner-reported prodromal changes and seizure triggers. *Vet Rec.* 2020 Aug 22;187(4):152.
13. Packer RMA, Berendt M, Bhatti S, et al. Inter-observer agreement of canine and feline paroxysmal event semiology and classification by veterinary neurology specialists and non-specialists. *BMC Vet Res.* 2015;11:39.
14. Rusbridge C, Long S, Jovanovik J, et al. International Veterinary Epilepsy Task Force recommendations for a veterinary epilepsy-specific MRI protocol. *BMC Vet Res.* MC Vet Res. 2015 Aug 28;11:194.
15. Gilbert SE, Cardy TJ, Bertram S, et al. Diagnostic utility of cerebrospinal fluid analysis in dogs with suspected idiopathic epilepsy. *Aust Vet J.* 2021 Jan;99(1-2):1–5.
16. Nagendran A, McConnell JF, De Risio, et al. Peri-ictal magnetic resonance imaging characteristics in dogs with suspected idiopathic epilepsy. *J Vet Intern Med.* 2021 Mar;35(2):1008–1017.
17. Mellema LM, Koblik PD, Kortz GD, et al. Reversible magnetic resonance imaging abnormalities in dogs following seizures. *Vet Radiol Ultrasound.* 1999 Nov-Dec;40(6):588–595.
18. Gonçalves R, Anderson TJ, Innocent G, et al. Effect of seizures on cerebrospinal fluid analysis

in dogs with idiopathic epilepsy. *Vet Rec.* 2010 Apr 17;166(16):497–498.
19. Ekenstedt KJ, Patterson EE, Mickelson JR. Canine epilepsy genetics. *Mamm Genome.* 2012 Feb;23(1-2):28–39.
20. Ekenstedt KJ, Oberbauer AM. Inherited epilepsy in dogs. *Top Companion Anim Med.* 2013;28:51–58.
21. Hülsmeyer VI, Fischer A, Mandigers PJ, et al. International Veterinary Epilepsy Task Force's current understanding of idiopathic epilepsy of genetic or suspected genetic origin in purebred dogs. *BMC Vet Res.* 2015 Aug 28;11:175.
22. Seppälä EH, Jokinen TS, Fukata M, et al. LGI2 truncation causes a remitting focal epilepsy in dogs. *PLoS Genet.* 2011 Jul;7(7):e1002194.
23. Jokinen TS, Tiira K, Metsähonkala L, et al. Behavioral Abnormalities in Lagotto Romagnolo Dogs with a History of Benign Familial Juvenile Epilepsy: A Long-Term Follow-Up Study. *J Vet Intern Med.* 2015;29(4):1081–1087.
24. Wielaender F, Sarviaho R, James F, et al. Generalized myoclonic epilepsy with photosensitivity in juvenile dogs caused by a defective DIRAS family GTPase 1. *Proc Natl Acad Sci U S A.* 2017;114(10):2669–2674.
25. James F. Introduction to electroencephalography. In: De Risio L, Platt S (eds). *Canine And Feline Epilepsy: Diagnosis and Management.* Wallingford:CABI; 2014. pp. 325–346.
26. James F. Electroencephalography. In: De Risio L, Munana K (eds.). *A Practical Guide to Seizure Disorders in Dogs and Cats.* Edra Publishing; 2021. pp. 153–181.
27. Bhatti SF, De Risio L, Muñana K, et al. International Veterinary Epilepsy Task Force consensus proposal: medical treatment of canine epilepsy in Europe. *BMC Vet Res.* 2015 Aug 28;11:176.
28. Volk HA, Matiasek LA, Luján Feliu-Pascual A, et al. The efficacy and tolerability of levetiracetam in pharmacoresistant epileptic dogs. *Vet J.* 2008 Jun;176(3):310–399.
29. Muñana KR, Thomas WB, Inzana KD, et al. Evaluation of levetiracetam as adjunctive treatment for refractory canine epilepsy: a randomized, placebo-controlled, crossover trial. *J Vet Intern Med.* 2012 Mar-Apr;26(2):341–348.
30. Fredsø N, Sabers A, Toft N, et al. A single-blinded phenobarbital-controlled trial of levetiracetam as mono-therapy in dogs with newly diagnosed epilepsy. *Vet J.* 2016 Feb:208:44–49.
31. von Klopmann T, Rambeck, Tipold A. Prospective study of zonisamide therapy for refractory idiopathic epilepsy in dogs. *J Small Anim Pract.* 2007 Mar;48(3):134–138.
32. Govendir M, Perkins M, Malik R. Improving seizure control in dogs with refractory epilepsy using gabapentin as an adjunctive agent. *Aust Vet J.* 2005 Oct;83(10):602–608.
33. Platt SR, Adams V, Garosi LS, et al. Treatment with gabapentin of 11 dogs with refractory idiopathic epilepsy. *Vet Rec.* 2006 Dec;159(26):881–884.
34. Dewey CW, Cerda-Gonzalez S, Levine JM, et al. Pregabalin as an adjunct to phenobarbital, potassium bromide, or a combination of phenobarbital and potassium bromide for treatment of dogs with suspected idiopathic epilepsy. *J Am Vet Med Assoc.* 2009 Dec 15;235(12):1442–1449.
35. Kiviranta AM, Laitinen-Vapaavuori O, Hielm-Björkman A, et al. Topiramate as an add-on antiepileptic drug in treating refractory canine idiopathic epilepsy. *J Small Anim Pract.* 2013 Oct;54(10):512–520.
36. McGrath S, Bartner LR, Rao S, et al. Randomized blinded controlled clinical trial to assess the effect of oral cannabidiol administration in addition to conventional antiepileptic treatment on seizure frequency in dogs with intractable idiopathic epilepsy. *J Am Vet Med Assoc.* 2019 Jun 1;254(11):1301–1308.
37. Charalambous M, Brodbelt D, Volk HA. Treatment in canine epilepsy--a systematic review. *BMC Vet Res.* 2014 Oct 22;10:257.
38. Charalambous M, Shivapour SK, Brodbelt DC, et al. Antiepileptic drugs' tolerability and safety--a systematic review and meta-analysis of adverse effects in dogs. *BMC Vet Res.* 2016 May 21;12:79.
39. Stabile F, Barnett CR, De Risio L. Phenobarbital administration every eight hours: improvement of seizure management in idiopathic epileptic dogs with decreased phenobarbital elimination half-life. *Vet Rec.* 2017 Feb 18;180(7):178.
40. Trepanier LA. Use of bromide as an anticonvulsant for dogs with epilepsy. *J Am Vet Med Assoc.* 1995 Jul 15;207(2):163–166.
41. Potschka H, Fischer A, Löscher W, et al. International veterinary epilepsy task force consensus proposal: outcome of therapeutic interventions in canine and feline epilepsy. *BMC Vet Res.* 2015 Aug 28;11:177.
42. Weissl, Hülsmeyer V, Brauer C, et al. Disease progression and treatment response of idiopathic epilepsy in Australian Shepherd dogs. *J Vet Intern Med.* 2012 Jan-Feb;26(1):116–125.
43. Hülsmeyer V, Zimmermann R, Brauer C, et al. Epilepsy in Border Collies: clinical manifestation, outcome, and mode of inheritance. *J Vet Intern Med.* 2010 Jan-Feb;24(1):171–178.
44. Erlen A, Potschka H, Volk HA, et al. Seizure occurrence in dogs under primary veterinary care in the UK: prevalence and risk factors. *J Vet Intern Med.* 2018 Sep;32(5):1665–1676.
45. Sauer-Delhées S, Steffen F, Reichler I, et al. Clinical characteristics of Idiopathic Epilepsy in Greater Swiss Mountain Dogs in Switzerland. *Schweiz Arch Tierheilkd.* 2020 Nov;162(11):697–706.
46. Heske L, Baranowska Körberg I, Nødtvedt A, et al. Clinical characteristics of epilepsy of unknown origin in the Rottweiler breed. *Acta Vet Scand.* 2015 Nov 6;57:75.
47. Ostermann TE, Nessler JN, Urankar H, et al. Phenotype of Idiopathic Epilepsy in Great Swiss Mountain Dogs in Germany-A Retrospective Study. *Front Vet Sci.* 2022 Jul 12;9:921134.
48. Casal ML, Munuve RM, Janis MA, et al. Epilepsy in Irish Wolfhounds. *J Vet Intern Med.* 2006 Jan-Feb;20(1):131–135.
49. Larsen JA, Owens TJ, Fascetti AJ. Nutritional management of idiopathic epilepsy in dogs. *J Am Vet Med Assoc.* 2014 Sep 1;245(5):504–508.
50. Han FY, Conboy-Schmidt L, Rybachuk G, et al. Dietary medium chain triglycerides for management of epilepsy: new data from human, dog, and rodent studies. *Epilepsia.* 2021 Aug;62(8):1790–1806.
51. O'Mahony SM, Clarke G, Borre YE, et al. Serotonin, tryptophan metabolism and the brain-gut-microbiome axis. *Behav Brain Res.* 2015 Jan 15;277:32–48.
52. Coelho LP, Kultima JR, Costea PI, et al. Similarity of the dog and human gut microbiomes in gene content and response to diet. *Microbiome.* 2018 Apr 19;6(1):72.
53. Muñana KR, Jacob ME, Callahan BJ. Evaluation of fecal Lactobacillus populations in dogs with idiopathic epilepsy: a pilot study. *Anim Microbiome.* 2020;2(1):19.
54. Weiss GA, Hennet T. 2017. Mechanisms and consequences of intestinal dysbiosis. *Cell Mol Life Sci.* 2017 Aug;74(16):2959–2977.
55. Bough KJ, Rho JM. Anticonvulsant mechanisms of the ketogenic diet. *Epilepsia.* 2007 Jan;48(1):43–58.
56. Owen OE, Morgan AP, Kemp HG, et al. Brain metabolism during fasting. *J Clin Invest.* 1967 Oct;46(10):1589–1595.
57. Olson CA, Vuong HE, Yano JM, et al. The gut microbiota mediates the anti-seizure effects of the ketogenic diet. *Cell.* 2018 Jun 14;173(7):1728-1741.e13.
58. Pilla R, Law TH, Pan Y, et al. The effects of a ketogenic medium-chain triglyceride diet on the feces in dogs with idiopathic epilepsy. *Front Vet Sci.* 2020 Dec 22;7:541547.
59. Berk BA, Packer RMA, Law TH, et al. Investigating owner use of dietary supplements in dogs with idiopathic epilepsy. *Res Vet Sci.* 2018 Aug;119:276–284.
60. Law TH, Volk HA, Pan Y, et al. Metabolic perturbations associated with the consumption of a ketogenic medium-chain TAG diet in dogs with idiopathic epilepsy. *Br J Nutr.* 2018 Sep;120(5):484–490.
61. Molina J, Jean-Philippe C, Conboy L, et al. Efficacy of medium chain triglyceride oil dietary supplementation in reducing seizure frequency in dogs with idiopathic epilepsy without cluster seizures: a non-blinded, prospective clinical trial. *Vet Rec.* 2020 Oct 31;187(9):356.
62. Verdoodt F, Watanangura A, Bhatti SFM, et al. The role of nutrition in canine idiopathic epilepsy management: Fact or fiction? *Vet J.* 2022 Dec;290:105917.
63. Finnegan SL, Volk HA, Asher L, et al. Investigating the potential for seizure prediction in dogs with idiopathic epilepsy: owner-reported prodromal changes and seizure triggers. *Vet Rec.* 2020 Aug 22;187(4):152.
64. Forsgård JA, Metsähonkala L, Kiviranta AM, et al. Seizure-precipitating factors in dogs with idiopathic epilepsy. *J Vet Intern Med.* 2019 Mar;33(2):701–707.

65. Shell L, Scariano R, Rishniw M. Features of stimulus-specific seizures in dogs with reflex epilepsy: 43 cases (2000-2014). *J Am Vet Med Assoc.* 2017 Jan 1;250(1):75–78.
66. Mandigers PJJ, Santifort KM. Remarkable anecdotes illustrating the nature and effect of seizure-precipitating factors in Border Collies with idiopathic epilepsy. *Front Vet Sci.* 2023 Sep 14;10:1254279.
67. Wessmann A, Volk HA, Packer RMA, et al. Quality-of-life aspects in idiopathic epilepsy in dogs. *Vet Rec.* 2016 Sep 3;179(9):229.
68. Berendt M, Gredal H, Ersbøll AK, et al. Premature death, risk factors, and life patterns in dogs with epilepsy. *J Vet Intern Med.* 2007 Jul-Aug;21(4):754–759.
69. Fredsø N, Koch BC, Toft N, et al. Risk factors for survival in a university hospital population of dogs with epilepsy. *J Vet Intern Med.* 2014 Nov-Dec;28(6):1782–1788.
70. Hamers MF, Plonek M, Bhatti SFM, et al. Quality of life in dogs with idiopathic epilepsy and their owners with an emphasis on breed-A pilot study. *Front Vet Sci.* 2023 Jan 11:9:1107315.
71. Saito M, Muñana KR, Sharp NJ, et al. Risk factors for development of status epilepticus in dogs with idiopathic epilepsy and effects of status epilepticus on outcome and survival time: 32 cases (1990-1996). *J Am Vet Med Assoc.* 2001 Sep 1;219(5):618–623.
72. Monteiro R, Adams V, Keys D, et al. Canine idiopathic epilepsy: prevalence, risk factors and outcome associated with cluster seizures and status epilepticus. *J Small Anim Pract.* 2012 Sep;53(9):526–530.
73. Wessmann A, Volk HA, Parkin T, et al. Evaluation of quality of life in dogs with idiopathic epilepsy. *J Vet Intern Med.* 2014 Mar-Apr;28(2):510–514.

CHAPTER 17

Management of status epilepticus and cluster seizures

Marios Charalambous
DVM, PhD, DACVIM (Neurology), DECVN, FHEA, MRCVS

Status epilepticus

Status epilepticus (SE) is defined clinically as prolonged seizure activity lasting >5 minutes or multiple seizures with incomplete recovery in between and remains a common neurological emergency.[1–3] Status epilepticus can occur in dogs with idiopathic epilepsy (IE), structural epilepsy (epilepsy due to brain pathology), and reactive seizures (seizures due to metabolic causes, such as liver dysfunction or electrolyte imbalances, or due to intoxication).[4–6] SE can lead to permanent brain damage and severe systemic complications; the occurrence and severity of SE-induced complications are proportionally related to the duration of seizure activity.[7–12] The overall mortality rate of dogs with SE is 25.3–38.5%.[4,13] Effective and quick first-line management at home and in the hospital is by far essential and life-saving.

The goals of therapy include cessation of seizure activity, prevention of additional seizures, and management of seizure complications and underlying etiologies.[12,14,15] It has been shown that the earlier seizure cessation is achieved, the better the overall outcome is (i.e., successful treatment of complications and response to antiseizure medications [ASMs]).[7,9,10,16–20] SE progresses to more refractory (drug-resistant) stages over time due to dysfunctional mechanisms at a molecular level. Although monotherapy is preferable to avoid drug interactions and minimize the incidence of drug-related adverse effects, polytherapy is usually necessary to reach the therapeutic aims. An early simultaneous polytherapy approach with first- and specific second-line agents, i.e., benzodiazepines and levetiracetam (LEV) (+/- phenobarbital [PB]), can be considered as a treatment approach in SE because it can:

1. Simultaneously address more than one of the main pathophysiological obstacles leading to initiation of SE and its self sustaining character.
2. Possibly increase the probability of early seizure activity termination.
3. Avert the development of refractory stages of SE.
4. Prevent complications related to continuous seizure activity, hospitalization, and adverse effects from multiple anesthetics.[12,15]

The focus should be placed not only on the pharmacotherapy of SE but also on the general management of neurological emergencies, which includes supportive therapy (e.g., patient stabilization, delivery of appropriate intravenous fluid and oxygen therapy, monitoring of the animal's clinical parameters, and correction of any deficits, hyperthermia, or metabolic complications, etc.) as well as a thorough diagnostic search for an underlying cause. Such measures are important for achieving seizure cessation and providing further neuroprotection.[12,15] Overall, SE can be subdivided into four stages, which differ in terms of treatment approach and response to the ASMs used;[7,9,10,12,14–20] the recommended treatment approach for each stage is provided in Figure 17.1. A summary of all the commonly used ASMs for seizure emergencies in dogs, including their doses and routes of administration, are provided in Table 17.1. The author also refers to the recent ACVIM Consensus Statement on the management of emergency seizure disorders for the official detailed therapeutic guidelines and treatment algorithms.[15]

First-line treatment

Benzodiazepines, in particular midazolam (MDZ) and diazepam (DZP), have been used for decades as first-line ASMs due to their high potency and rapid onset of action.[12,15,19,21,23] The adverse effects of benzodiazepines include respiratory and central nervous system (CNS) depression and hypotension.[7] In dogs, both DZP and MDZ can be effective in ceasing seizure activity, but MDZ might be more potent and safer than DZP.[12,15,19,23] A maximum of three benzodiazepine boluses at 2- to 5-minute intervals should be administered within a period of 24 hours. If seizures are not controlled, a second-line treatment should be initiated.[12,15] If seizures are controlled but relapse after 10–60 minutes from the last bolus, then an intravenous constant rate infusion (IV CRI) should be initiated.[15] DZP is diluted in a propylene glycol vehicle that can cause phlebitis and hypotension with rapid administration. The drug also adsorbs to plastic;[24] if a CRI is needed, it is useful to precoat the infusion line with DZP before administration. DZP is light sensitive,[25] and the infusion line should therefore be wrapped in a dense material. Chronic coadministration of PB[26] or LEV[27] might require administration of a higher or lower DZP dose, respectively.

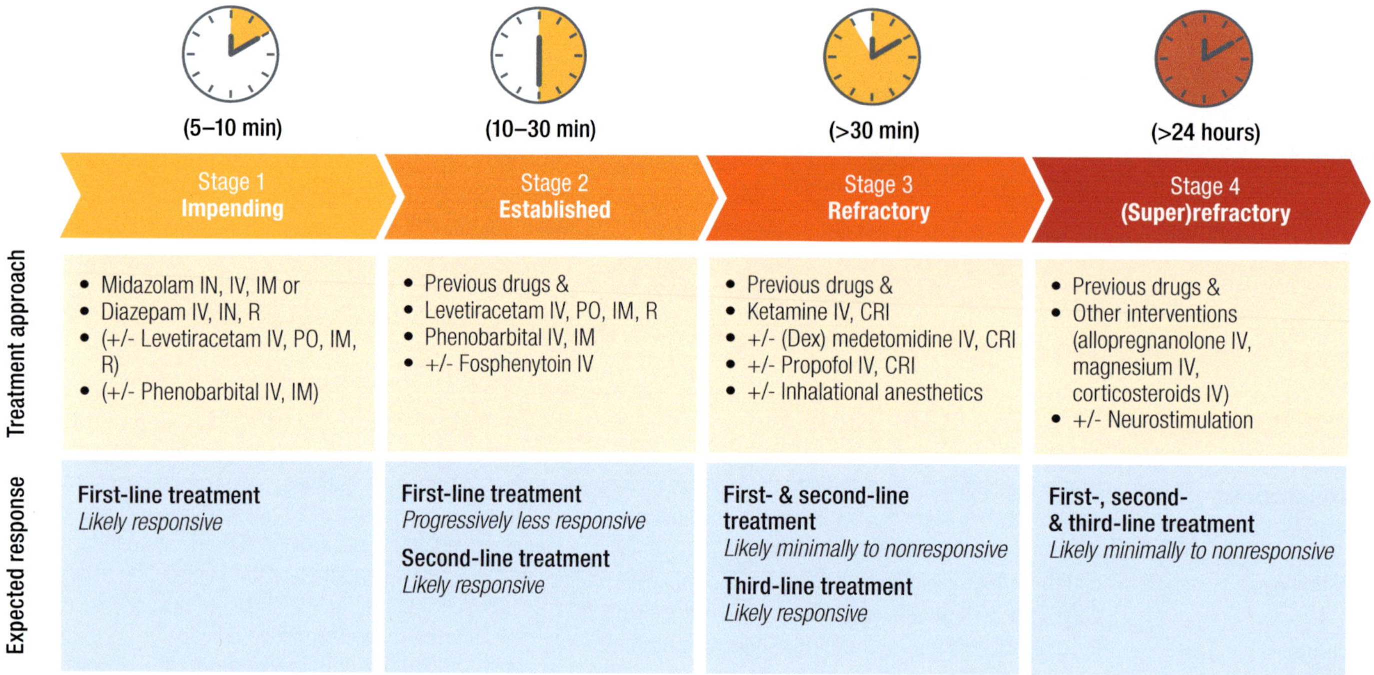

FIG. 17.1 Treatment approach and expected response to antiseizure medications (ASMs) per stage. As the stage of seizure epilepticus (SE) becomes more advanced, the responsiveness to ASMs, in particular first-line drugs (benzodiazepines) lessens. In more advanced stages of SE, further ASMs should be added in order to control the seizures. Early simultaneous polytherapy might be beneficial for ceasing as well as preventing refractory stages of SE. IN, intranasal; IV, intravenous; IM, intramuscular; R, rectal; PO, per os; CRI, constant rate infusion.

Propylene glycol toxicity (e.g., neurological abnormalities, metabolic acidosis, hyperosmolality, and organ dysfunction) is of vital concern, thus making DZP CRI less preferable, particularly in cats.[28]

Second-line treatment

Phenobarbital

PB is an effective and relatively safe ASM.[12,14,15,29–31] When the desired therapeutic concentrations need to be achieved more rapidly than 2–3 weeks from maintenance treatment initiation, a dose of 2.0–4.0 mg/kg can be administered multiple times (at least 20–30 minutes apart), up to a total dose of 15–24 mg/kg in 24–48 hours (loading dose). Respiratory suppression, ataxia, and sedation are common adverse effects. In dogs with preexisting hepatic disease, the use of PB is not recommended, and LEV may be used instead. If an animal is on maintenance PB therapy, a blood sample should be collected to assess serum PB concentrations before the drug is administered to treat SE, and/or before any adjustment in the maintenance dose of PB is performed.

Levetiracetam

LEV has a rapid onset of action and a favorable safety profile.[12,14,15,30–34] Intravenous LEV can be administered undiluted as a slow bolus over 5 minutes.[35] In dogs administered PB for 4 or more weeks, a higher LEV dose (within the reference range) might be needed, as PB increases the clearance of LEV.[36] The adverse effects of LEV are mild to moderate and dose-dependent (mainly sedation and ataxia).[30] LEV is excreted by the kidneys, which limits pharmacokinetic interactions with other ASMs, but its use can be problematic in animals with impaired kidney function.

Fosphenytoin

Fosphenytoin sodium is a phosphate ester and can be administered at a dose of 15 mg/kg IV in dogs only.[15,37] Even though the current evidence is limited, the efficacy rate for fosphenytoin has been shown to be 63%, compared to 22% for placebo treatment; vomiting might be the most significant drug-related adverse effect.[38]

Third-line treatment

Ketamine +/- dexmedetomidine

Ketamine is an anesthetic and analgesic drug with antiseizure and neuroprotective properties,[39] which is effective in refractory SE in humans[27,40–43] and animals.[12,15,44,45] Adverse effects that occur primarily with high dosages include cardiorespiratory depression, seizures, muscle tremors, and vomiting. Dexmedetomidine is an alpha-2 adrenoreceptor agonist that also exhibits antiseizure and neuroprotective properties with benefits in SE.[12,15,46,47] Adverse effects include decreased respiration, bradycardia, heart arrhythmias, and hypothermia.

Propofol

Propofol is an anesthetic medication with antiseizure properties that is recommended in SE.[12,15,48,49] The use of a CRI rather than repeat boluses is advised due to propofol's short duration of action. Adverse effects include cardiovascular and respiratory depression, pain at the injection site, and loss of gag reflex (predisposing animals to aspiration pneumonia).[50] Therefore, cardiovascular and respiratory function should be closely monitored, and endotracheal intubation should be anticipated. Propofol is usually formulated with 2% benzyl alcohol in order to prolong

TABLE 17.1 Recommended dosages of antiseizure medications used in dogs with seizure emergencies.

Antiseizure medication	Recommended dosages
Midazolam	■ 0.2–0.5 mg/kg IV, IN, IM bolus; can be repeated 2–3 times at 2- to 5-minute intervals ■ 0.2–0.5 mg/kg/hour IV CRI
Diazepam	■ 0.5–2.0 mg/kg IV, IN, rectal bolus; can be repeated 2–3 times at to 2- to 5-minute intervals ■ Dose at lower range when coadministered with levetiracetam ■ Dose at higher range when coadministered with phenobarbital ■ 0.1–0.5 mg/kg/hour IV CRI
Phenobarbital	■ 2–4 mg/kg IV, IM, PO every 12 hours (regular dose scheme) or every 20–30 mins with a maximum total dose of 24 mg/kg per day (loading dose scheme)
Levetiracetam	■ 20–60 mg/kg IV (administered over 5 mins), rectal, PO every 8 hours
Fosphenytoin	■ 15 mg/kg IV bolus
Ketamine	■ 3–5 mg/kg IV bolus followed by 0.1–0.5 mg/kg/hour IV CRI
Dexmedetomidine	■ 0.5 µg/kg IV bolus followed by 0.5–3 µg/kg/hour IV CRI
Propofol	■ 1–6 mg/kg IV bolus followed by 0.1–0.6 mg/kg/min IV CRI
Pentobarbital	■ 2.0–15.0 mg/kg IV bolus (slow; administered with caution) followed by 0.2–1.0 mg/kg/hour IV CRI

Cluster epilepsy (before occurrence of status epilepticus): twelve dogs (60%)
IV, intravenous; IN, intranasal; IM, intramuscular; CRI, constant rate infusion; PO, per os.

the drug's shelf life. This formulation is not labelled for CRI use, as it may cause neurological or cardiovascular adverse effects. In humans, a propofol-infusion syndrome (cardiac dysfunction, hyperkalemia, rhabdomyolysis, and acidosis) with high morbidity and mortality has been reported after prolonged anesthesia;[10] such an event has not been documented in veterinary medicine, except for one case report in a dog, which described a syndrome similar to the propofol infusion-syndrome in humans.[51]

Pentobarbital

Pentobarbital and sodium thiopental (thiopentone) are barbiturates used to terminate seizures in cases of refractory SE, but, due to safety issues, their use is recommended only after propofol, ketamine, and dexmedetomidine have failed to cease seizure activity.[12,15,52,53] Barbiturates can cause significant cardiovascular and respiratory depression, hypotension, and hypothermia; any patient receiving barbiturates should be closely monitored as an overdose can be fatal. Sodium thiopental administration in animals carries a higher risk of cardiac toxicity than pentobarbital administration.

Inhalation anesthetics

Inhalation anesthetics are usually reserved for refractory SE.[12,15,54–57] Isoflurane and desflurane are preferred over others because only a small percentage of drug is metabolized by the liver, resulting in a reduced risk of liver toxicity.[58] Inhalational anesthetics require ventilation and can cause hypotension as they decrease systemic vascular resistance.[52]

Other pharmacological and nonpharmacological interventions

Other interventions are reserved for animals that are refractory to all lines of treatment (refractory and super-refractory SE).[12,15] Continuation of intensive care, monitoring, and all previous medications is important; however, further adjunctive pharmacological and nonpharmacological interventions are required.[12,15] Even in human medicine, there is a lack of robust published data for such interventions, and in veterinary medicine, research evidence and clinical experience are quite limited to absent. Nonetheless, such interventions include (but are not limited to) IV magnesium, allopregnanolone, mild hypothermia, and neurostimulation.[15]

Cluster seizures

Cluster seizures (CS) are defined as the occurrence of ≥2 seizures over a 24-hour period, with complete recovery between seizure events.[3] CS can occur with either idiopathic or structural epilepsy or can be due to a metabolic cause or intoxication, similarly to SE. Approximately 38–77% of dogs with idiopathic epilepsy can experience CS at least once in their lifetime.[59,60]

The appropriate management of CS consists of a long-term plan and a short-term plan. The long-term treatment focuses mainly on the prevention of CS and is achieved with the appropriate implementation of antiseizure therapy of epilepsy, i.e., by optimizing, monitoring, and adjusting the doses and therapeutic schemes of the patient's long-term (maintenance) ASMs (e.g., PB, potassium bromide, zonisamide, LEV) (see Chapter 16 for more information on the long-term treatment of idiopathic epilepsy). Since this chapter focuses on emergency seizure disorders, only the short-term emergency treatment of CS is described. In general, the author recommends a three-step system for the short-term management of CS in dogs (Fig. 17.2). Treatment in the hospital setting for CS refractory to the three-step approach is similar to that for SE. First, a short-acting treatment can be administered during the event or immediately after the first seizure (if the animal is known to always exhibit CS when seizures occur) or usually after the second seizure within a time frame of 24 hours. Benzodiazepines are an ideal and potent short-acting treatment option and can be given at the same doses and routes as for SE. Overall, up to three benzodiazepine boluses can be administered in a 24-hour period. An IV CRI of MDZ can be initiated if there is inadequate seizure control or no response to boluses.[61] In parallel to the short-acting drugs (i.e., MDZ or DZP), longer-acting medication should be given with the aim of ceasing and preventing further seizures in the near future. LEV as a pulse therapy is recommended.[15] The pharmacokinetics of LEV are favorable for CS, even after oral administration.[36] LEV is most commonly administered orally to control CS in out-of-hospital settings. LEV pulse therapy includes an initial dose of 40–60 mg/kg after the first or second seizure, followed by 20 mg/kg every 6–8 hours until no seizures occur for 48 hours.[15,62] Pulse therapy has been recommended instead of long-term continuous therapy because it might reduce the development of

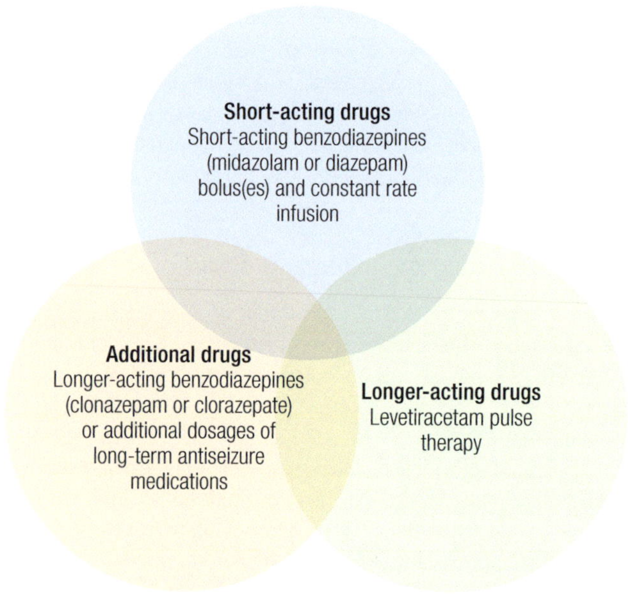

FIG. 17.2 Three-step short-term management of cluster seizures. Short-acting drugs such as midazolam or diazepam can be administered in parallel to longer-acting drugs such as levetiracetam pulse therapy. If these fail, then longer-acting benzodiazepines, such as clonazepam or clorazepate, or additional dosages of long-term antiseizure medications, such as phenobarbital, can be administered.

tolerance with the drug's chronic use.[62] In dogs on chronic PB therapy, a higher dose of LEV may be needed.[62] Rectal administration of LEV (suspension or parenteral solution) at a dose of 40 mg/kg has also been suggested as a successful alternative to oral dosing in dogs.[32,33,63] Within hospital settings, IV administration of LEV is recommended in dogs.[15] LEV is a safe drug, with sedation and ataxia as the main adverse effects. These occur more often with high doses (approximately 40% of dogs receiving 60 mg/kg PO can manifest ataxia and/or sedation).[62]

If these measures fail, then pulse therapy with longer-acting benzodiazepines such as clonazepam or clorazepate have also been utilized in the home treatment of CS in dogs, although there are no published studies evaluating their use. Clonazepam is administered orally at a dose of 0.5–2.0 mg/kg after the first seizures as soon as the dog can safely take oral medication, and then every 8–12 hours until the seizure cycle is broken. Clorazepate can be used in a similar manner, at an oral dose of 0.5 mg/kg PO every 8–12 hours. These drugs can be administered in conjunction with short-acting benzodiazepines and other prescribed ASMs, but they should not be used for more than a few days in dogs to prevent the development of tolerance.[15] In addition, in animals that already receive maintenance ASM therapy (e.g., phenobarbital), an additional dose can be administered after every seizure; these can be repeated at a minimum of 1-hour intervals and up to 3 times in a 24-hour period. In animals that do not receive any ASMs, initiation of a loading dose of PB can be considered.[15]

KEY POINTS

- Status epilepticus (SE) and cluster seizures (CS) are frequent neurological emergencies in dogs associated with high morbidity and mortality, if left untreated.
- Rapid intervention is vital because SE may cause severe brain and systemic complications and progress to more drug-resistant stages over time.
- Early simultaneous polytherapy, in particular during SE stage I, with a combination therapy of first- and specific second-line agents, i.e., benzodiazepines and levetiracetam (LEV; +/– phenobarbital [PB]), might be advantageous because it could:
  - Simultaneously address more than one of the main pathophysiological obstacles leading to the initiation of SE and its self-sustaining character.
  - Increase the probability of seizure activity termination.
  - Prevent the development of SE refractory stages III and IV.
  - Prevent complications related to continuous seizure activity, hospitalization, and adverse effects from multiple anesthetics.
- Benzodiazepines are first-line potent and fast-acting drugs that are crucial in successful SE management in dogs. The potency of benzodiazepines decreases over time; hence, second- and third-line interventions are needed in cases of prolonged seizure activity.
- Overall, the combined steps necessary for a successful outcome in SE include:
  - Early simultaneous polytherapy.
  - Supportive therapy.
  - Thorough diagnostic investigations (including laboratory tests on blood and urine).
  - Close monitoring of the animal's vital signs.
  - Treatment of any underlying conditions or complications.
- A combined approach is needed for successful cessation and prevention of CS in dogs including:
  - Administration of short-acting antiseizure medications (ASMs):
    - Benzodiazepines.
    - Midazolam or diazepam.
  - Administration of longer-acting ASMs:
    - LEV as a pulse therapy.
  - Administration of other ASMs:
    - When short- and longer-acting ASMs fail to break the CS cycle.
    - Long-term ASMs, such as PB, administered as additional doses (for animals already on ASMs) or loading doses (for drug-naïve animals).
    - Longer-acting benzodiazepines, such as clonazepam or clorazepate, as a pulse therapy.
  - Monitoring of serum concentration and dose adjustments of long-term ASMs (for animals already on ASMs).

References

1. Trinka E, Brigo F, Shorvon S. Recent advances in status epilepticus. *Curr Opin Neurol.* 2016;29(2):189–198.
2. Walker M. Status epilepticus: an evidence based guide. *BMJ.* 2005;331(7518):673–637.
3. Berendt M, Farquhar RG, Mandigers PJ, et al. International veterinary epilepsy task force consensus report on epilepsy definition, classification and terminology in companion animals. *BMC Vet Res.* 2015;11:182.
4. Bateman SW, Parent JM. Clinical findings, treatment, and outcome of dogs with status epilepticus or cluster seizures: 156 cases (1990-1995). *J Am Vet Med Assoc.* 1999;215(10):1463–1468.
5. Platt SR, Haag M. Canine status epilepticus: a retrospective study of 50 cases. *J Small Anim Pract.* 2002;43(4):151–153.
6. Saito M, Munana KR, Sharp NJ, Olby NJ. Risk factors for development of status epilepticus in dogs with idiopathic epilepsy and effects of status epilepticus on outcome and survival time: 32 cases (1990-1996). *J Am Vet Med Assoc.* 2001;219(5):618–623.
7. Costello DJ, Cole AJ. Treatment of acute seizures and status epilepticus. *J Intensive Care Med.* 2007;22(6):319–347.
8. Koestner A. Neuropathology of canine epilepsy. *Probl Vet Med.* 1989;1(4):516–534.
9. Lothman E. The biochemical basis and pathophysiology of status epilepticus. *Neurology.* 1990;40(5 Suppl 2):13–23.
10. Shorvon S, Ferlisi M. The treatment of super-refractory status epilepticus: a critical review of available therapies and a clinical treatment protocol. *Brain.* 2011;134(Pt 10):2802–2818.
11. Watson C. Status epilepticus. Clinical features, pathophysiology, and treatment. *West J Med.* 1991;155(6):626–631.
12. Charalambous M, Bhatti SFM, Volk HA, Platt S. Defining and overcoming the therapeutic obstacles in canine refractory status epilepticus. *Vet J.* 2022;283–284:105828.
13. Zimmermann R, Hulsmeyer V, Sauter-Louis C, Fischer A. Status epilepticus and epileptic seizures in dogs. *J Vet Intern Med.* 2009;23(5):970–976.
14. Charalambous M, Fischer A, Potschka H, et al. Translational veterinary epilepsy: A win-win situation for human and veterinary neurology. *Vet J.* 2023;293:105956.
15. Charalambous M, Muñana K, Patterson EE, et al. ACVIM Consensus Statement on the management of status epilepticus and cluster seizures in dogs and cats. *J Vet Intern Med.* 2024 Jan-Feb; 38(1):19–40.
16. Falco-Walter JJ, Bleck T. Treatment of Established Status Epilepticus. *J Clin Med.* 2016;5(5):49.
17. Gollwitzer S, Hamer HM. The Treatment and Prognosis of Refractory and Super-Refractory Status Epilepticus. *Aktuel Neurol.* 2017;44(9):662–668.
18. Podell M, Fenner WR, Powers JD. Seizure classification in dogs from a nonreferral-based population. *J Am Vet Med Assoc.* 1995;206(11):1721–1728.
19. Tesoro EP, Brophy GM. Pharmacological management of seizures and status epilepticus in critically ill patients. *J Pharm Pract.* 2010;23(5):441–454.
20. Zaccara G, Giannasi G, Oggioni R, Rosati E, Tramacere L, Palumbo P, et al. Challenges in the treatment of convulsive status epilepticus. *Seizure.* 2017;47:17–24.
21. Lowenstein DH, Alldredge BK. Status epilepticus. *N Engl J Med.* 1998;338(14):970–976.
22. Platt SR, Randell SC, Scott KC, et al. Comparison of plasma benzodiazepine concentrations following intranasal and intravenous administration of diazepam to dogs. *Am J Vet Res.* 2000;61(6):651–654.
23. Horikawa H, Tada T, Sakai M, et al. Effects of midazolam on the threshold of lidocaine-induced seizures in the dog--comparison with diazepam. *J Anesth.* 1990;4(3):265–269.
24. Winsnes M, Jeppsson R, Sjoberg B. Diazepam adsorption to infusion sets and plastic syringes. *Acta Anaesthesiol Scand.* 1981;25(2):93–96.
25. Calisto V, Domingues MR, Esteves VI. Photodegradation of psychiatric pharmaceuticals in aquatic environments--kinetics and photodegradation products. *Water Res.* 2011;45(18):6097–6106.
26. Aldawsari MF, Lau VW, Babu RJ, et al. Pharmacokinetic evaluation of novel midazolam gel formulations following buccal administration to healthy dogs. *Am J Vet Res.* 2018;79(1):73–82.
27. Mazarati AM, Baldwin R, Klitgaard H, et al. Anticonvulsant effects of levetiracetam and levetiracetam-diazepam combinations in experimental status epilepticus. *Epilepsy Res.* 2004;58(2-3):167 174.
28. Hansen BD. Analgesia and sedation in the critically ill. *J Vet Emerg Crit Car.* 2005;15:285.
29. Charalambous M, Brodbelt D, Volk HA. Treatment in canine epilepsy--a systematic review. *BMC Vet Res.* 2014;10:257.
30. Charalambous M, Shivapour SK, Brodbelt DC, Volk HA. Antiepileptic drugs' tolerability and safety--a systematic review and meta-analysis of adverse effects in dogs. *BMC Vet Res.* 2016;12:79.
31. Charalambous M, Pakozdy A, Bhatti SFM, Volk HA. Systematic review of antiepileptic drugs' safety and effectiveness in feline epilepsy. *BMC Vet Res.* 2018;14(1):64.
32. Peters RK, Schubert T, Clemmons R, Vickroy T. Levetiracetam rectal administration in healthy dogs. *J Vet Intern Med.* 2014;28(2):504–509.
33. Cagnotti G, Odore R, Gardini G, et al. Pharmacokinetics of rectal levetiracetam as add-on treatment in dogs affected by cluster seizures or status epilepticus. *BMC Vet Res.* 2018;14(1):189.
34. Patterson EE, Goel V, Cloyd JC, et al. Intramuscular, intravenous and oral levetiracetam in dogs: safety and pharmacokinetics. *J Vet Pharmacol Ther.* 2008;31(3):253–258.
35. Biddick AA, Bacek LM, Taylor AR. A serious adverse event secondary to rapid intravenous levetiracetam injection in a dog. *J Vet Emerg Crit Care.* 2018;28(2):157–162.
36. Moore SA, Muñana KR, Papich MG, Nettifee-Osborne JA. The pharmacokinetics of levetiracetam in healthy dogs concurrently receiving phenobarbital. *J Vet Pharmacol Ther.* 2011;34(1):31–34.
37. Coles LD, Leppik IE, Patterson EE, et al. Use of IV fosphenytoin pharmacokinetics to determine the loading dose for a clinical trial of canine status epilepticus. *Epilepsia.* 2015;56(6):888–894.
38. Patterson EE, Leppik IE, Coles LD, et al. Canine status epilepticus treated with fosphenytoin: A proof of principle study. *Epilepsia.* 2015;56(6):882–887.
39. Fujikawa DG. Starting ketamine for neuroprotection earlier than its current use as an anesthetic/antiepileptic drug late in refractory status epilepticus. *Epilepsia.* 2019;60(3):373–380.
40. Cohen SP, Bhatia A, Buvanendran A, et al. Consensus Guidelines on the Use of Intravenous Ketamine Infusions for Chronic Pain From the American Society of Regional Anesthesia and Pain Medicine, the American Academy of Pain Medicine, and the American Society of Anesthesiologists. *Region Anesth Pain M.* 2018;43(5):521–546.
41. Bertram EH, Lothman EW. NMDA receptor antagonists and limbic status epilepticus: a comparison with standard anticonvulsants. *Epilepsy Res.* 1990;5(3):177–184.
42. Borris DJ, Bertram EH, Kapur J. Ketamine controls prolonged status epilepticus. *Epilepsy Res.* 2000;42(2-3):117–122.
43. Williamson JM, Lothman EW. The Effect of Mk-801 on Kindled Seizures - Implications for Use and Limitations as an Antiepileptic Drug. *Ann Neurol.* 1989 Jul;26(1):85–90.
44. Serrano S, Hughes D, Chandler K. Use of ketamine for the management of refractory status epilepticus in a dog. *J Vet Intern Med.* 2006 Jan-Feb;20(1):194–197.
45. Gioeni D, Di Cesare F, D'Urso ES, et al. Ketamine-dexmedetomidine combination and controlled mild hypothermia for the treatment of long-lasting and super-refractory status epilepticus in 3 dogs suffering from idiopathic epilepsy. *J Vet Emerg Crit Care (San Antonio).* 2020;30(4):455–460.
46. Halonen T, Kotti T, Tuunanen J, et al. Alpha 2-adrenoceptor agonist, dexmedetomidine, protects against kainic acid-induced convulsions and neuronal damage. *Brain Res.* 1995;693(1-2):217–224.
47. Heidenreich DC, Giordano P, Kirby BM. Successful treatment of refractory seizures with phenobarbital, propofol, and medetomidine following congenital portosystemic shunt ligation

in a dog. *J Vet Emerg Crit Care (San Antonio).* 2016;26(6):831–836.
48. Rossetti AO, Reichhart MD, Schaller MD, et al. Propofol treatment of refractory status epilepticus: a study of 31 episodes. *Epilepsia.* 2004;45(7):757–763.
49. San-juan D, Chiappa KH, Cole AJ. Propofol and the electroencephalogram. *Clin Neurophysiol.* 2010;121(7):998–1006.
50. Hashim MA, Waterman AE. Effects of thiopentone, propofol, alphaxalone-alphadolone, ketamine and xylazine-ketamine on lower oesophageal sphincter pressure and barrier pressure in cats. *Vet Rec.* 1991;129(7):137–139.
51. Mallard JM, Rieser TM, Peterson NW. Propofol infusion-like syndrome in a dog. *Can Vet J.* 2018;59(11):1216–1222.
52. Platt SR, McDonnell JJ. Status epilepticus: Patient management and pharmacologic therapy. *Comp Cont Educ Pract.* 2000;22(8):722–729.
53. Raines A, Blake GJ, Richardson B, Gilbert MB. Differential selectivity of several barbiturates on experimental seizures and neurotoxicity in the mouse. *Epilepsia.* 1979;20(2):105–113.
54. Franks NP, Lieb WR. Molecular and cellular mechanisms of general anaesthesia. *Nature.* 1994;367(6464):607–614.
55. Ries CR, Puil E. Mechanism of anesthesia revealed by shunting actions of isoflurane on thalamocortical neurons. *J Neurophysiol.* 1999;81(4):1795-801.
56. Langmoen IA, Hegstad E, Berg-Johnsen J. An experimental study of the effect of isoflurane on epileptiform bursts. *Epilepsy Res.* 1992;11(3):153–157.
57. Sharpe MD, Young GB, Mirsattari S, Harris C. Prolonged desflurane administration for refractory status epilepticus. *Anesthesiology.* 2002;97(1):261–264.
58. Mirsattari SM, Sharpe MD, Young GB. Treatment of refractory status epilepticus with inhalational anesthetic agents isoflurane and desflurane. *Arch Neurol.* 2004;61(8):1254–1259.
59. Monteiro R, Adams V, Keys D, Platt SR. Canine idiopathic epilepsy: prevalence, risk factors and outcome associated with cluster seizures and status epilepticus. *J Small Anim Pract.* 2012 Sep;53(9):526–530.
60. Packer RM, Shihab NK, Torres BB, Volk HA. Risk factors for cluster seizures in canine idiopathic epilepsy. *Res Vet Sci.* 2016;105:136–138.
61. Bray KY, Mariani CL, Early PJ, et al. Continuous rate infusion of midazolam as emergent treatment for seizures in dogs. *J Vet Intern Med.* 2021 Jan;35(1):388–396.
62. Packer RM, Nye G, Porter SE, Volk HA. Assessment into the usage of levetiracetam in a canine epilepsy clinic. *BMC Vet Res.* 2015 Feb 7;11:25.
63. Cagnotti G, Odore R, Bertone I, et al. Open-label clinical trial of rectally administered levetiracetam as supplemental treatment in dogs with cluster seizures. *J Vet Intern Med.* 2019;33(4):1714–1718.

CHAPTER 18

Tremors and twitches

Mark Lowrie
MA, VetMB, MVM, DECVN, MRCVS, RCVS & EBVS® European Recognized Specialist in Veterinary Neurology

Tremors and twitches are a frequent concern for many dog owners. Determining the root of these involuntary contractions can be challenging and may require extensive diagnostic testing. At first, these two clinical signs may seem synonymous. However, the approach to a tremor or twitch syndrome can be very different, and differentiating one from the other is therefore paramount. The first step is to characterize what the involuntary contraction represents, and this in turn will give valuable information about which part of the nervous system is likely to be affected and the possible causes. This chapter will discuss tremors and twitches in turn.

Tremors

Tremor is one of the most common involuntary movement disorders in humans and can be surprisingly common as part of a clinical abnormality in dogs. However, there are no clear diagnostic guidelines described in veterinary patients, thus making evaluation difficult. Tremors can manifest in serious life-altering diseases or be part of a benign condition. They can be the result of any number of neuropathological changes or simply be a manifestation of normal behavior.

Identification

A tremor is a rhythmic, involuntary, oscillatory muscle contraction that causes shakiness in one or more parts of the body (Video 18.1). Tremors may affect the head, body, or legs in a focal manner or may be generalized affecting all parts of the body at once. They should only be observed when awake and disappear with sleep; if they persist, this is unlikely to be a true tremor.

Identification of tremors can be difficult. The keyword in identification is "rhythmicity", i.e., cycles of regular muscle contractions. Care should be taken not to mistake frequency and amplitude, as many tremors may have variable amplitude (e.g., intention tremors) despite a regular frequency. It is the rhythmical character that distinguishes tremors from other involuntary muscle contractions.

Video 18.1

Nine-year-old Greyhound with a high frequency tremor affecting the pelvic limbs but extending to involve the trunk and forelimbs.

Pathophysiology

A tremor is ultimately a movement disorder and as such the lesion could be anywhere within the central nervous system (CNS), peripheral nervous system or musculoskeletal system (the three systems responsible for normal movement). Therefore, localization of the lesion can be difficult when considering the clinical sign of tremor alone. Given neurological presentations in dogs require a neuroanatomical localization so the veterinarian can then appropriately proceed with targeted diagnostics; the inability to accurately localize the lesion leaves the clinician with a dilemma.

Tremors that occur or worsen when a patient is trying to perform purposeful movements (intention tremors) are most often associated with cerebellar disease. Fine tremors of low amplitude and high frequency appear to be more commonly associated with diffuse neuronal disease or muscle weakness. In many cases, other clinical signs may be present that reflect the location of the causative lesion (e.g., hypermetria, cerebellar ataxia, menace response deficit with normal vision, or vestibular signs associated with a cerebellar lesion).

In dogs, common sites of tremor origin include the cerebellum, diffuse neuronal cell bodies involved in segmental and supraspinal reflex mechanisms, components of the lower motor neuron, and the interconnecting pathways. Abnormalities of the mechanical apparatus of the limbs (e.g., bones, joints, tendons) may also result in tremor as a result of pain and weakness. However, in the absence of a clear neuroanatomical localization, classification of a tremor according to moment of occurrence remains the most optimal way of identifying the patient's problem.

Classification

Tremors can be classified according to whether they occur with rest or activity. A tremor occurring with activity is further classified according to its association with action or intention (Fig. 18.1).

Resting tremor

Resting tremors can be distinguished from other forms of tremor based on their occurrence when the tremoring body part is completely supported against gravity without

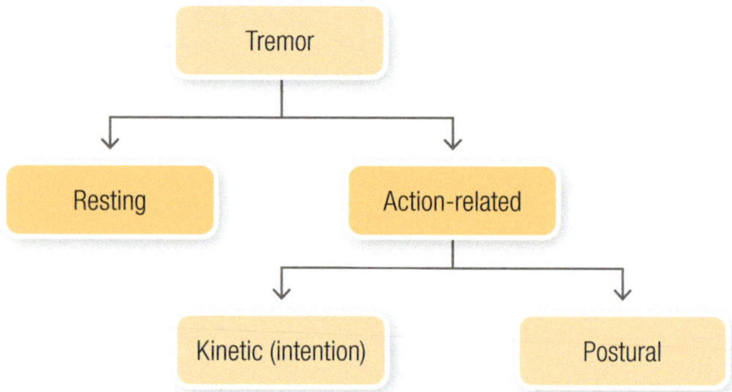

FIG. 18.1 Classification of tremors in veterinary patients.

voluntary muscle contraction. This form of tremor has not been reported in dogs. The best example of a resting tremor in people would be the tremor associated with Parkinson's disease.

Action-related tremor

As is inferred by the name, action tremors occur during movement and are absent at rest.

Postural tremor

Postural tremors occur during the voluntary maintenance of a position against gravity, for example, a tremor of the limbs when standing that dissipates on activity or when lying down.

- **ORTHOSTATIC TREMOR** Orthostatic tremor is a unique tremor syndrome, characterized by a pathognomonic high-frequency tremor, predominantly of the limbs, triggered exclusively by standing (Video 18.2). This disorder has been described in Great Danes and Scottish Deerhounds with an onset usually in the first 2 years of life. Affected dogs can appear reluctant to lie down and demonstrate a constant tremor when standing, which may involve the head and trunk. Dogs may be hesitant to sit or stand and consequently may appear weak. A characteristic feature is that the tremor disappears when walking, sitting and lying down. Neurological examination is normal.
- **IDIOPATHIC HEAD TREMOR SYNDROME** Canine idiopathic head tremor syndrome (IHTS) or intermittent head "bobbing" is a less understood type of postural tremor. It affects the postural muscles of the head and neck, resulting in a high frequency tremor in a vertical or horizontal plane. It typically disappears when the dog is distracted or lies down (Video 18.3). Dogs are completely normal in between these episodes. Bulldogs and Dobermans are commonly affected, with a suspected hereditary basis. However, any breed of dog may be affected, with a median age of onset of 3 years (range, 3 months to 12 years). The condition is benign and appears unresponsive to medication. Although it most commonly occurs as an idiopathic disorder, there are rare reports of similar clinical signs occurring in dogs with structural brain disease (especially with pathology affecting the thalamus).
- **BENIGN, IDIOPATHIC, RAPID POSTURAL TREMOR** Older dogs can develop a high frequency postural tremor of the pelvic limbs that is evident only when a dog is standing (Video 18.4). Movement can obliterate the tremor, suggesting a degree of tension in the pelvic limb muscles is required to elicit it. This suggests a role for the stretch reflex mechanism as also occurs in IHTS. The pathophysiology is unknown and a steady progression with age is often seen. These tremors fulfil many of the characteristics of essential tremor in people: they are bilaterally symmetrical, are unaccompanied by other neurological signs, and are postural in nature. However, they can involve features of kinetic tremor as well. The general recommendation is that this is benign and does not require treatment.
- **HYPOMYELINATION** Hypomyelination, or shaking puppy syndrome, is a congenital disorder affecting myelin production in the postnatal period in dogs, with any breed potentially being at risk. Clinical signs of a tremor are first evident at an early age (range, 2–8 weeks) but pups remain bright and responsive throughout (Video 18.5). The severity of the clinical signs varies between breeds, but generalized body tremors that subside or disappear at rest or sleep are a common clinical feature designating them as action-related postural tremors. Puppies may display a wide-based stance, exhibit ataxia due to hypomyelination of sensory fibers, and have postural reaction deficits on neurological examination. In several breeds, affected puppies can display a gradual improvement and are clinically normal by 12–18 months of age. The reason for this improvement is myelin production is merely delayed in some breeds and, therefore, affected puppies may show a gradual clinical improvement.

The etiology in dogs is unknown. Three mutations have been identified to date in dogs: in Springer Spaniels (*PLP*), Weimaraners (*FNIP2*), and

Video 18.2

Two-year, six-month old Great Dane demonstrating difficulty in sitting and standing. Notice the high frequency tremor that predominantly affects the limbs and is triggered by a change in position. This manifests as a reluctance to sit or stand. However, no problem is seen when the dog is walking, which designates this as an action-related, postural tremor.

Video 18.3

Three-year-old Staffordshire Bull Terrier with a high frequency tremor affecting the head. No other part of the body is affected, and this dog can be distracted from the tremor with food or by offering an activity such as exercise. This condition is benign and does not require medication.

Video 18.4

Eleven-year-old Border Terrier with a high frequency postural tremor of the pelvic limbs that is only seen when standing. This tremor disappears as the dog starts walking. Although this represents an obvious tremor, the condition is benign and does not affect strength or coordination and does not cause pain.

Video 18.5

Two 6-week-old Border Terrier littermates with generalized body tremors. These tremors are classified as action-related postural because they disappear when the dogs sleep and when they are not supported against gravity, e.g., when rolled on their back.

Australian Cattle and Shetland Sheepdogs (cytochrome *b*). PLP is the primary protein of CNS compact myelin and plays a critical role in the development and maturation of oligodendrocytes. FNIP2 is thought to play a similar role, but the reason for a mutation in cytochrome *b* causing hypomyelination is not understood. Toxic agents or an undefined in utero viral infection cannot be excluded in undefined causes of hypomyelination.

Definitive diagnosis can only be made postmortem. However, the potential for improvement in some breeds and the characteristic presentation mean a tentative diagnosis is reasonable. There is no known treatment for this condition. Nevertheless, the prognosis for a full clinical recovery can be favorable if clinical signs are not too severe. Some puppies display a gradual clinical improvement and by 1 year of age are clinically normal.

Kinetic (intention) tremor

Tremors that occur or worsen when performing a purposeful movement are defined as intention tremors. They are usually slow and coarse and disappear completely at rest. Their etiology is broad but despite the pathophysiology, the neuroanatomical localization is typically the cerebellum and its associated tracts. It is essential to stress that intention tremors are relatively uncommon in cerebellar disease. The main exceptions to this are diffuse disease processes such as inflammatory or degenerative conditions. Dogs with ischemic infarcts or neoplastic processes, for example, tend not to develop an intention tremor. Essentially, if an intention tremor is identified, then it is important to investigate causes for cerebellar disease.

Other signs of cerebellar disease that may accompany tremors include:

- Ataxia (incoordination, swaying from side to side)
- Hypermetria ("goose-stepping", overflexing of the limbs when walking)
- Menace deficits (with normal vision and pupillary light reflexes)
- Head tilt (can be paradoxical)
- Nystagmus (fast followed by slow movement of the eyes)
- Truncal sway
- Anisocoria (infrequent)

Cerebellar disease is best considered using the acronym DAMNITV or VITAMIN D referring to degenerative, anomalous, metabolic, neoplastic, nutritional, inflammatory, idiopathic, traumatic, and vascular disease processes. These different pathological processes are listed below with the important diseases causing them discussed.

- **DEGENERATIVE DISEASES**

  Hereditary ataxias. Hereditary ataxias are a group of degenerative diseases characterized by cerebellar ataxia, with or without intention tremors. The diseases are classified according to the location of their neuropathological abnormalities. There is no treatment, so classification is more an academic rather than clinically useful distinction. The classifications are summarized in Box 18.1, but for further information readers are directed to the article by Stee et al.[1]

  Storage diseases. Storage diseases can result in cerebellar degeneration. Cellular products accumulate, most commonly due to a malfunctioning enzyme, and affect neuronal cells either physiologically or mechanically, resulting in cellular dysfunction and the appearance of clinical signs. The clinical signs can include signs suggestive of a progressive cerebellar disease and are most commonly seen in young purebred dogs. Diagnosis is based upon the examination of biopsy or necropsy samples and/or genetic tests where available. No treatment is effective.

Box 18.1 Classification of hereditary ataxias in dogs.

- Cerebellar cortical degenerations
  - Primary Purkinje cell degeneration
  - Primary granule cell degeneration
- Spinocerebellar degenerations
- Cerebellar ataxias without substantial neurodegeneration
- Multifocal degenerations with predominant (spino)cerebellar degeneration
- Episodic ataxia
- Other neurodegenerative diseases causing cerebellar dysfunction as a core feature

Video 18.6

A 5-month-old crossbreed puppy demonstrating a marked intention tremor of the whole body involving the head, trunk, and limbs. The dog also has cerebellar signs, including cerebellar ataxia and hypermetria.These clinical signs are all attributable to a congenital, structural brain malformation affecting the cerebellum and associated tracts.

- **ANOMALOUS DISEASES**

  Congenital malformations. Congenital malformations of the cerebellum may potentially result in an intention tremor. These include aplasia (absence of cerebellar tissue) and partial agenesis or hypoplasia (partial or uniform lack of cerebellar tissue). Cerebellar hypoplasia has been associated with infection or toxin exposure during a critical stage of cerebellum development in utero. Caudal vermian hypoplasia is described in some dogs with associated ventricular dilatation (Dandy–Walker malformation; Video 18.6), with a causal genetic mutation (*VLDLR*) for this condition being identified in the Eurasier breed. This condition has been reported in many breeds, although no associated mutation has been identified.

  Neuroaxonal dystrophy. Neuroaxonal dystrophy (NAD) can be a congenital or acquired disorder. The congenital form represents a fatal, neurodegenerative cerebellar disorder affecting many different breeds and is considered hereditary in most cases. Those forms with a genetic mutation identified include the juvenile onset condition in Papillons (*PLA2G6*) and Spanish Water Dogs (*TECPR2*), the adult-onset condition in Rottweilers (*VPS11*), and the neonatal onset condition in the Giant Schnauzer-Beagle cross (*MFN2*). The acquired disorder is exceptionally rare and associated with vitamin E deficiency in Cocker Spaniels.

- **IDIOPATHIC GENERALIZED TREMOR SYNDROME** This is a condition in which a dog may develop a sudden marked intention tremor of the head and limbs, which worsens with exercise, stress, and excitement but disappears with sleep (Video 18.7). Although classified here as an intention tremor, this condition is unusual to other types in that it can also be seen as a tremor at rest, which makes it difficult to classify. The term "white shaker syndrome" was coined due to the high prevalence of this condition in young, mature (<2 years), small white-breed dogs, particularly the Maltese and West Highland White Terrier. However, since the early reports of this condition, it has become apparent that it is not breed specific and can occur in dogs of any color or breed. Subsequently, the terms "sporadic acquired tremors of adult dogs" and "idiopathic cerebellitis" have been used to describe this condition, although "idiopathic generalized tremor syndrome" is the most widely accepted term.

Other signs that may accompany the tremor are mild cerebellovestibular signs and an ocular tremor (opsoclonus). Signs are progressive over 1 to 3 days and then remain static until treatment is initiated. In a few cases there can be spontaneous clinical improvement months later. Early in the course of the disease, owners may interpret the tremor as the animal being "scared" or "cold". When the tremors become more persistent, owners may elect veterinary evaluation. Generalized tremor syndrome is often associated with a mild degree of CNS inflammation.

Video 18.7

A 2-year-old Maltese with a sudden onset intention tremor of the head and limbs, which worsens with exercise, stress, and excitement but disappears with sleep. Although classified as an intention tremor, this condition is unusual to other intention tremors in that it can also be seen as a tremor at rest, which makes it difficult to classify. With appropriate corticosteroid treatment this tremor can easily be treated.

Video 18.8

A 9-month-old Belgian Malinois with undulating muscle contractions of the left forelimb including the proximal and distal muscles. This dog would also get similar contractions in other parts of the body including the other limbs, neck, and trunk. This is a twitch known as myokymia and can be focal or generalized but is reminiscent of worms beneath the skin.

Video 18.9

A Jack Russell Terrier rescue dog of unknown age with generalized muscle stiffness following a period of activity. This dog would also experience mild episodes of myokymia that did not affect movement. This episode of muscle stiffness without relaxation can be life-threatening as it can create severe hyperthermia, so this dog was cooled by bathing with cold water to reduce the risk of this happening.

Video 18.10

A 10-year-old Weimaraner with episodic and irregular muscle contractions producing contraction of the forelimbs. This sustained muscle contraction is predominantly affecting the extensor muscles without relaxation. The problem is intermittent in that this dog experiences episodes of muscle contraction. It is therefore described as tetany rather than tetanus; the latter referring to a persistent state of contraction. This dog was found to have hypercalcemia and once the problem was managed these episodes disappeared.

Video 18.11

A 5-year-old Weimaraner with fasciculations and twitches of the whole body. These twitches can be seen here in the head and pelvic limb muscles but were visible throughout the body intermittently and at varying amplitudes. This dog had ingested metaldehyde shortly before this video was taken. Toxicities produce this variable amplitude of muscle contraction rather than a regular frequency tremor.

Diagnosis is based on the history, signalment, and phenomenology of the tremor in the absence of a structural brain lesion (by performing magnetic resonance imaging of the brain) and a normal to moderate lymphocytic pleocytosis on cerebrospinal fluid analysis. Differential diagnoses for this type of tremor include toxicities (e.g., pyrethrins, metaldehyde, mycotoxins, organophosphates, etc.) and metabolic (e.g., hypocalcemia) causes for twitches. However, toxicities tend to produce twitches rather than tremors and so can be clinically differentiated by their irregular frequency.

Corticosteroids (prednisolone at a dose of 1–2 mg/kg orally every 12 hours) and benzodiazepines (diazepam at a dose of 0.5–1 mg/kg orally every 8 hours) are both reported to manage this condition successfully, usually in combination.[2] If no response is seen with these medications, then propranolol (0.5–1.0 mg/kg orally every 8 hours) may be considered. The dose of corticosteroids is slowly tapered by 50% every 2–4 weeks to the lowest dose that maintains a remission of clinical signs. This tapering treatment can last 6 weeks to several months but a full remission off medication is anticipated in all cases without exception.

Twitch

Twitches are a recently described phenomenon that encompass a number of disorders that were previously considered to be tremors, such as metabolic and toxic insults resulting in involuntary muscle contractions.

Identification

A twitch is different from a tremor in that it has an irregular frequency of variable amplitude and therefore lacks the sinusoidal pattern of a tremor.[4] Tremors of metabolic and toxic origin are interesting to consider here as they have recently been reclassified as twitches given their irregular frequency and hence their deviation from the true definition of tremor. When presented with a dog that has suffered an intoxication, the involuntary contractions have an erratic rather than regular frequency, thus giving the appearance of twitches rather than tremors. A similar situation is observed in dogs with metabolic derangements of electrolytes and glucose. Twitching in response to metabolic and toxic insults is therefore considered to be a twitch rather than a tremor, and the common causes are considered below.

Some of the clinical signs that can manifest as twitches are as follows, from mild to most severe:

- Cramps are easily identified in people as a sudden, severe, and involuntary muscle contraction. The key identifying feature is that they can cause mild to excruciating pain and an immobility of the affected muscle(s). Onset is usually sudden, and it resolves on its own over a period of several seconds, minutes, or hours. The identification of pain is therefore much harder in veterinary practice, but when involuntary muscle contractions occur that appear painful, cramps should be considered.
- Fasciculations are brief spontaneous contractions affecting a small number of muscle fibers, often causing a flicker of movement under the skin.
- Myokymia refers to the presence of focal or generalized continuous muscle twitching, often exhibiting a rippling "bag of worms" appearance under the skin (Video 18.8).

- Neuromyotonia is a continuous muscle activity characterized by muscle stiffness (Video 18.9). It is distinguished from myokymia (involuntary rippling of muscles) in that it results in generalized muscle stiffness with delayed relaxation, often resulting in collapse. Both may occur simultaneously.
- Tetany and tetanus both refer to the clinical sign of sustained muscle contraction, usually the extensors, without relaxation. The degree of extensor rigidity can be variable. Tetanus defines a persistent state of contraction, whereas tetany refers to intermittent muscular contractions (Video 18.10). Additionally, the term "tetanus" is most commonly used to describe the disease caused by the production of the neurotoxin tetanospasmin, usually within an anaerobic wound, and "tetany" refers to increased neuronal excitability most commonly associated with hypocalcemia.

Pathophysiology

A twitch results from peripheral nerve hyperexcitability (PNH). The term PNH describes a motor neuron dysfunction causing clinical signs such as cramps, fasciculations, myokymia, neuromyotonia, tetany, and tetanus. These clinical signs share similar features and are clinically difficult to distinguish, with cramps and fasciculations representing a mild manifestation of PNH, while myokymia and neuromyotonia can be more severe. The origin of a twitch is the motor nerve manifesting PNH. The pathophysiology appears to center on the activity of voltage-gated potassium channels (VGKCs) within the motor nerve, with PNH resulting from autoimmunity, genetic factors, electrolyte abnormalities, or toxic compounds.

Classification

A veterinary classification has been proposed based on the pathophysiological mechanisms affecting the VGKCs in people (Table 18.1).

TABLE 18.1 Pathophysiological classification of generalized nerve hyperexcitability syndromes.

Classification	Mechanism
Hereditary channelopathies	VGKC mutation
Immune-mediated channelopathies	VGKC-complex antibodies
Paraneoplastic	VGKC-complex antibodies
Polyneuropathies	Demyelination leading to paranodal reorganization of VGKC and VGKC-complex proteins
Motor neuron disease	Ion channel dysfunction via various mechanisms
Neurodegenerative disease	VGKC dysfunction
Metabolic disease	Prolonged depolarization of the action potential relating to electrolyte disturbance or endocrinopathy
Benign	Stress, exercise

VGKC, voltage-gated potassium channel.

Metabolic diseases

Tetany is the most common clinical sign associated with metabolic derangements, with hypocalcemia being the most important in dogs. Decreased ionized calcium may increase axonal excitability and lead to tetany or myokymia. Another metabolic cause for PNH that has been reported in dogs is hypoadrenocorticism, which was responsible for painful episodic muscle cramps that reversed on treatment of the endocrine abnormality. There have also been some anecdotal reports of cramping in hypothyroid dogs. Muscle weakness or stiffness may be the first and only presenting clinical sign in dogs with endocrine disorders, and therefore the recognition of cramps should lead to a consideration of an electrolyte disturbance or endocrine disorder. Tetany and fasciculations occurring with metabolic conditions tend to be episodic and irregular in frequency. In addition, they are also more common with hypocalcemia than with hypercalcemia.

Toxicities

Some acute toxicities may result in PNH manifesting most commonly as generalized fasciculations or tetany (Video 18.11). PNH is possible with intoxications with a number of substances including pyrethrins, metaldehyde, mycotoxins, lead, avermectins, organophosphates, nicotine, bromethalin, organochlorines, strychnine, chocolate, amphetamines, caffeine, hexachlorophene, and methylxanthines.

The mechanism responsible for PNH with many of these toxic substances is not known. Toxins may lower the threshold for stimulation or directly stimulate muscles and nerves, resulting in fasciculations. Organophosphate intoxication potentiates the effect of acetylcholine at the neuromuscular junction and other synapses by binding with and inactivating acetylcholinesterase. This leads to increased acetylcholine concentrations at the neuromuscular junction, increased receptor stimulation, and fatigue. Pathological alterations in the nervous system (such as intramyelinic edema caused by hexachlorophene and bromethalin) could potentially alter nerve impulse conduction, leading to PNH. Other substances most likely result in imbalances in neurotransmitter concentrations. Avermectins increase the concentration and effect of the inhibitory neurotransmitter gamma-aminobutyric acid (GABA) in the CNS. Numerous drug therapies (e.g., fentanyl/droperidol, adrenaline, isoproterenol, and 5-fluorouracil) may cause fasciculations as a side effect, possibly through alterations in the normal function of the extrapyramidal system (part of the motor system causing involuntary actions) or in the balance of normal neurotransmitter levels.

Hereditary channelopathies

Terriers and Belgian Malinois dogs can develop myokymia and neuromyotonia associated with hereditary cerebellar ataxia (see Hereditary ataxias). Terriers with spinocerebellar ataxia, generalized myokymia, and neuromyotonia have been identified to have a missense mutation in *KCNJ10*, a gene that encodes for an inwardly rectifying potassium channel resulting in spinocerebellar ataxia with myokymia, seizures or both (SAMS). The same mutation has been found in Belgian Malinois dogs with myokymia and neuromyotonia. However, not all terriers with SAMS are homozygous for the *KCNJ10* mutation, which suggests other mutations are likely responsible for this presentation. Furthermore, a myokymia-like syndrome has been observed in Belgian Malinois dogs with spinocerebellar ataxia resulting from a mutation in *SLC12A6,* a gene encoding a potassium chloride cotransporter. The mechanisms by which this syndrome occurs are unknown.

Polyneuropathies

Congenital and acquired polyneuropathies have been associated with myokymia, neuromyotonia, fasciculations, and cramps in people, in particular demyelinating rather than axonal neuropathies. Demyelinating neuropathies have been shown to result in PNH. It is uncertain whether this is the result of an antibody-mediated channelopathy, reorganisation of VGKCs at the sites of demyelination, or nerve hyperexcitability in newly formed unmyelinated collaterals. This phenomenon has not been reported in small animals but may explain the presence of tremor-like signs in dogs with neuromuscular disease. However, fasciculations associated with these diseases are often of short duration, episodic, and present during attempts at muscle activity.

Motor neuron diseases

In dogs, motor neuron disease encompasses a group of rapidly progressive and universally fatal disorders that affect the cell bodies of the lower motor neuron, leading to degeneration of the cell in the ventral horns of the spinal cord and occasionally the cranial nerve nuclei. Muscle weakness and fasciculations are the main presenting signs. It is thought that potassium channels have reduced conductance in these conditions, potentially due to decreased expression of VGKCs, and this may contribute to the PNH.

This condition is suspected to be inherited in the Brittany Spaniel and Swedish Lapland Dog, but it has also been reported in many other breeds. Signs of motor neuropathies include fasciculations, progressive weakness, cervical ventroflexion, dysphagia, and muscle atrophy. CSF analysis is normal, as are imaging studies. Sadly, there is no known treatment.

Benign causes

Fasciculations and cramps without weakness or muscle atrophy are recognized as a benign syndrome in people. They occur in healthy individuals with no concurrent illness during strenuous exercise, pregnancy, or sleep. A similar phenomenon has not been described in dogs, but its benign and transient nature makes it likely to go unreported.

KEY POINTS

- Tremors are rhythmic oscillations of regular amplitude caused by intermittent muscle contractions.
- Tremors are classified according to whether they are present at rest or with activity.
- Twitches are arrhythmic contractions of varying frequency and amplitude.
- Metabolic and toxic diseases result in twitches rather than tremors.
- Computed tomographic evidence of heterogeneous pancreatic contrast enhancement and portal vein thrombosis indicate a more serious form of pancreatitis.

References

1. Stee K, Van Poucke M, Lowrie M, et al. Phenotypic and genetic aspects of hereditary ataxia in dogs. *J Vet Intern Med.* 2023 Jul-Aug; 37(4):1306–1322.
2. Parker AJ. How do I treat "Little white shakers"? *Prog Vet Neurol.* 1991; 2:151.
3. Kent M. Acute tremors and involuntary movements. In: Platt S, Garosi L (eds.). *Small Animal Neurological Emergencies*, 1st ed. London, UK: Manson publishing; 2012. p. 252.
4. Lowrie M, Garosi L. Classification of involuntary movements in dogs: Tremors and twitches. *Vet J.* 2016 Aug; 214:109–116.

CHAPTER 19

Paroxysmal dyskinesia

Mark Lowrie
MA, VetMB, MVM, DECVN, MRCVS, RCVS & EBVS® European Recognized Specialist in Veterinary Neurology

Paroxysmal dyskinesia is characterized by episodic attacks of involuntary muscle contractions and movements and abnormal postures occurring at rest, with sudden movements, or with exercise.[1] These abnormal episodes are not associated with altered consciousness or autonomic signs, which aids in differentiating them, in most cases, from epileptic seizures. Episodes last from minutes to hours; they might occur as frequently as several times each day or be interspersed by months or years. Dogs with this condition are normal most of the time, with a normal general clinical and neurological examination.

TABLE 19.1 Clinical signs associated with paroxysmal dyskinesia.

Terminology	Definition
Ballism	An abrupt contraction of the limb muscles, which results in a flailing movement of the limb that is often unilateral
Chorea	An abrupt, unsustained contraction of different muscle groups producing dance-like movements
Cramp	A sudden, severe, and involuntary muscle contraction or overshortening that is generally temporary and benign
Dystonia	A sustained, slow contraction of agonist and antagonist muscles of a body region producing a twisted posture of the limbs, trunk, or neck
Fasciculations	Involuntary, often irregular, contractions or twisting of groups of muscle fibers
Myoclonus	A sudden, brief, shock-like jerks due to sudden involuntary contraction or relaxation of one or more muscles
Myokymia	A focal or generalized continuous muscle contraction, often exhibiting an undulation of the skin overlying the affected muscle
Myotonia	Delayed muscle relaxation immediately following muscle contraction, usually preceded by a period of rest, and improving with continuous activity
Neuromyotonia	A continuous spontaneous muscle activity characterized by muscle rippling, muscle stiffness, and myotonia
Paradoxical (pseudo)myotonia	Delayed muscle relaxation that occurs and worsens only after repeated muscle contraction (exercise) and improves with rest
Pseudomyotonia	Delayed muscle relaxation following muscle contraction, characterized by continuous repetitive discharges that end abruptly on electromyography
Tetanus	Sustained muscle contraction, usually of the extensors, without relaxation
Tetany	Intermittent muscular contractions without relaxation
Tremor	Involuntary, rhythmic oscillatory movements of a body part

Terminology

There has been some confusion around the terminology related to paroxysmal dyskinesia. A recent consensus statement clarified the use of many of these terms.[2]
The first is the term paroxysmal dyskinesia itself. It is reserved to describe the overall disease manifesting as self-limiting, episodic, involuntary muscle contractions and movements, and abnormal posture in animals (Video 19.1). Therefore, in this chapter, the term paroxysmal dyskinesia will refer collectively to the different manifestations of the disease.
A second aspect to consider is that the disease can manifest with a number of clinical signs that may be present alone or in combination, but these all constitute typical features of paroxysmal dyskinesia. The taskforce advises against using these individual terms and recommends that the disorder is simply defined as a paroxysmal dyskinesia with a description of the movements using the terminology for the specific clinical signs observed. A summary of these clinical signs and their definitions is given in Table 19.1.

Pathophysiology

The basal nuclei are collections of gray matter located subcortically, in the white matter of the cerebral hemispheres (Fig. 19.1). There is no consensus in the literature about which brain nuclei make up the basal nuclei. In veterinary texts, the term basal nuclei generally includes the caudate nucleus (including the nucleus accumbens, which is a ventral extension of the head of the caudate), the putamen, the endopeduncular nucleus (a caudal extension of the globus pallidus projecting towards the subthalamus, which is termed the internal portion of the

Video 19.1
A black Labrador during an episode of paroxysmal dyskinesia. Clinical signs of dystonia, tremor, and chorea are evident.

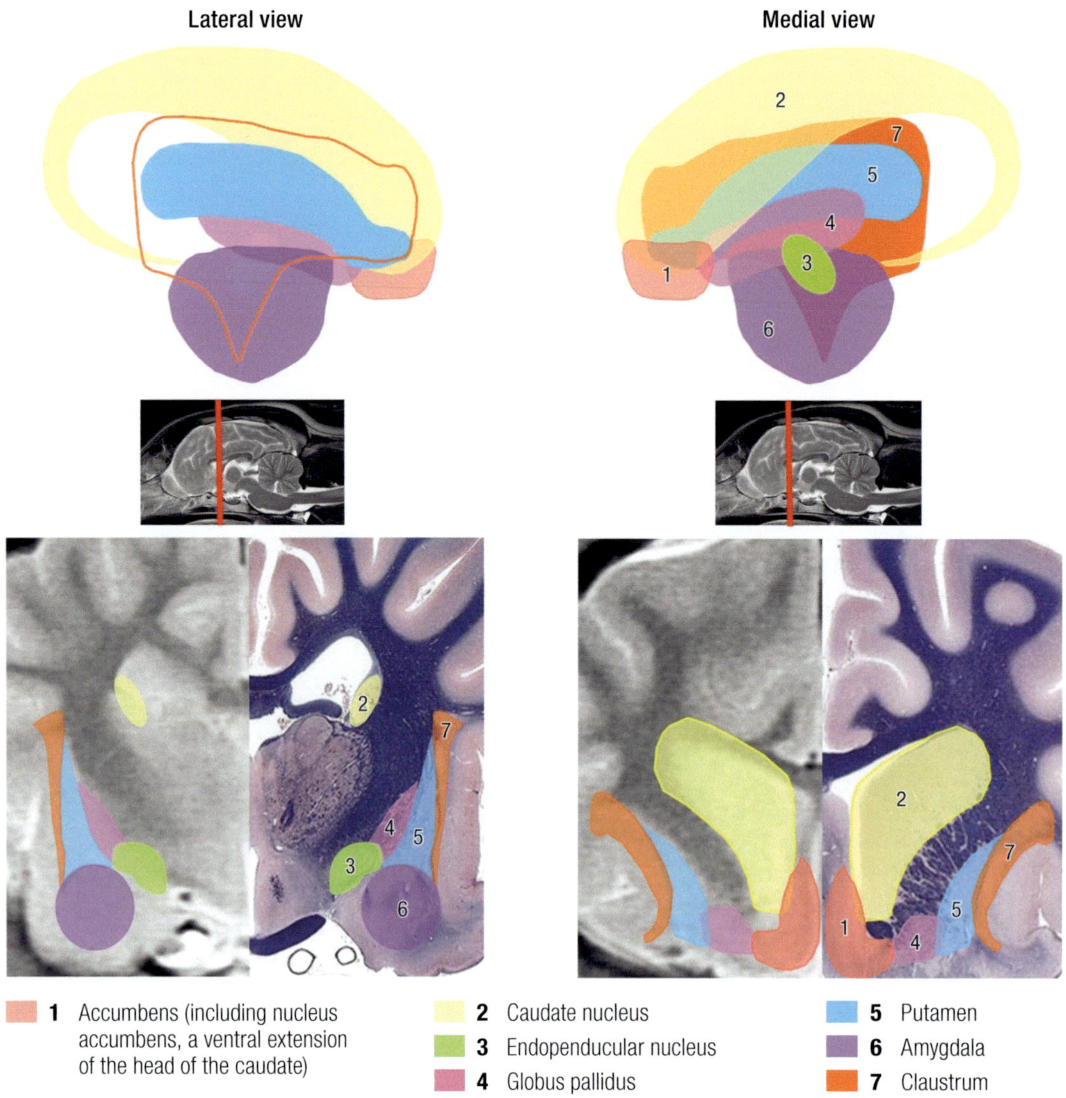

FIG. 19.1 Neuroanatomical location of the basal ganglia in dogs.

globus pallidus in people), the globus pallidus (or pallidum), the claustrum, and the amygdala.[3,4]

Other subcortical nuclei important in dyskinesia include the subthalamic nucleus, the pedunculopontine tegmental nucleus, the red nucleus, and the substantia nigra. In people and rodent models, they are sometimes considered as basal nuclei.[5] The substantia nigra is made up of two distinct regions: the substantia nigra pars compacta and the substantia nigra pars reticulata. Most of the dopamine-producing neurons of the brain are primarily found in the substantia nigra pars compacta, with the substantia nigra pars reticulata being more heavily populated with gamma-aminobutyric acid (GABA) neurons. The substantia nigra projects to two other structures of the basal ganglia, the caudate and the putamen (which together are referred to in some texts as the corpus striatum). These dopaminergic neural projections are referred to as the nigrostriatal pathway.[6] This pathway is critical in facilitating movement. In contrast, the GABAergic neurons of the substantia nigra pars reticulata can stimulate or inhibit motor activity. This therefore highlights the important role that the substantia nigra has in motor control.[6] A good example of this function is seen in patients with Parkinson's disease. This neurodegenerative condition that reduces the number of functioning dopamine neurons in the substantia nigra causes people to suffer from profound symptoms relating to movement such as a fine, coarse tremor, muscle stiffness, and impaired coordination.[7]

In the normal animal, the caudate and putamen receive afferents from the substantia nigra pars compacta and communicate through a direct inhibitory pathway or through a multisynaptic indirect pathway (Fig. 19.2).[6] The direct pathway projects from the caudate and putamen to the substantia nigra reticulata to initiate movement and the indirect pathway begins and ends in the same place but projects via the globus pallidus and the subthalamic nucleus to inhibit movement.

Dopamine is the neurotransmitter responsible for initiating movement and interacts with the direct and indirect pathways in a complex manner.

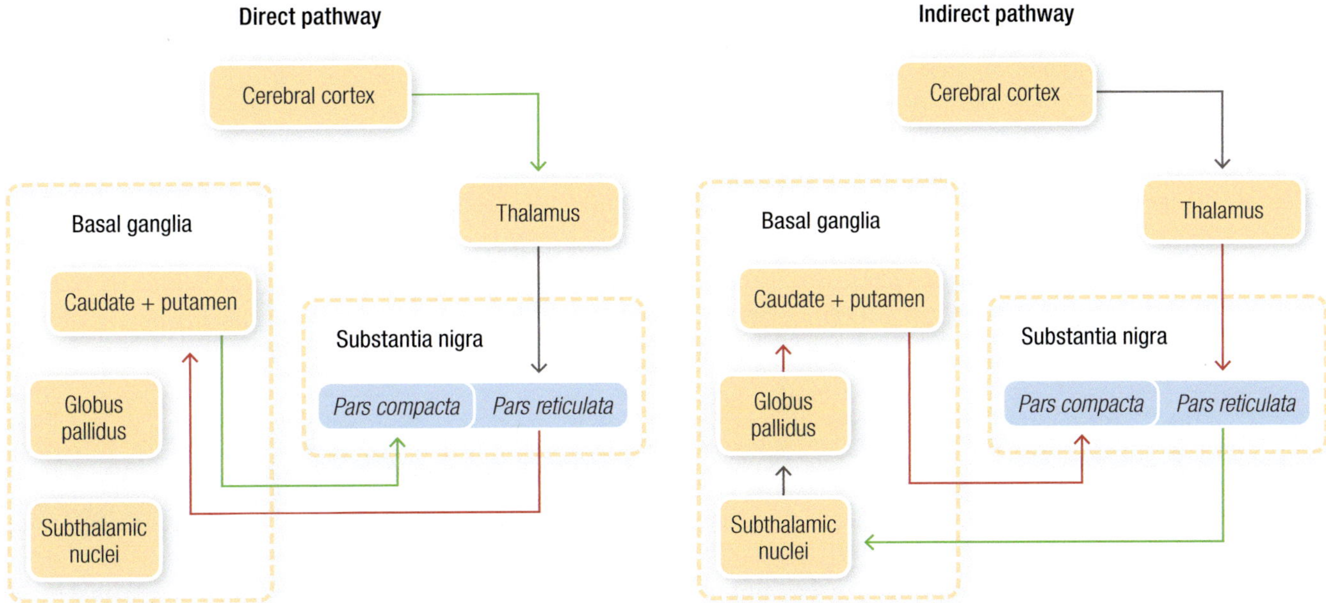

FIG. 19.2 Schematic diagram of the basal ganglia and their role in paroxysmal dyskinesia. Red depicts inhibitory pathways. Green depicts facilitatory pathways. Direct pathway: when a movement is initiated, the excitatory dopamine signal activates the caudate and putamen. This induces direct inhibition over the neurons of the pars reticulata causing disinhibition (inhibition of an inhibitor causes excitation) of the neurons of the thalamus over the cerebral cortex. This mechanism facilitates movement and allows the initiated movement to be maintained. Indirect pathway: the caudate and putamen are inhibited by D_2 receptors resulting in inhibition of the globus pallidus. This decreased activity within the globus pallidus causes disinhibition of the subthalamic nucleus and in turn increases activity in the pars reticulata, which inhibits the thalamus and suppresses movement.

The dopaminergic nigrostriatal input excites the direct pathway but inhibits the indirect pathway. These opposing effects of dopamine in the caudate and putamen are mediated by different dopamine receptors, with D_1 receptors exciting the direct system and D_2 receptors inhibiting the indirect pathway.[8] Therefore, a lack of dopamine, as seen in Parkinson's disease in people, results in a hypokinetic movement disorder, whereas disease affecting the indirect pathway leads to a hyperkinetic movement disorder.

Movement disorders were considered to originate from the basal ganglia. However, there is now evidence that the cerebellum and cerebral cortex may also be involved.[9,10] This suggests that it is more of a network disorder, although the pathogenesis remains unknown. The traditional view was that the basal ganglia and cerebellum communicated via the cortex. More recently, it was shown that the basal nuclei and cerebellum communicate directly via an interneuron forming a disynaptic pathway (Fig. 19.3).

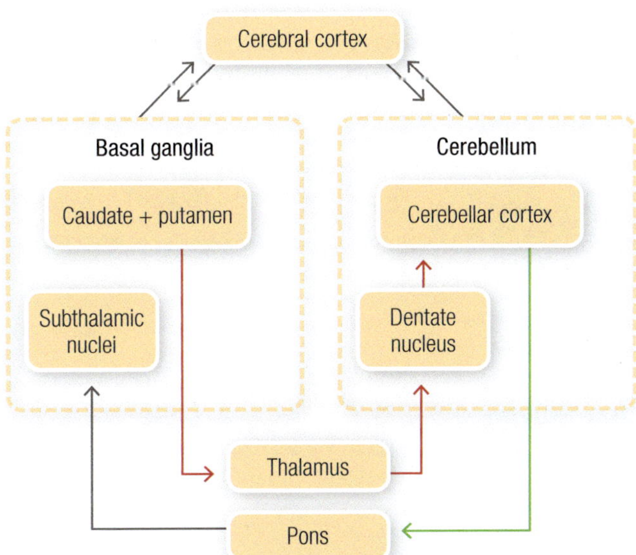

FIG. 19.3 Schematic diagram of the connections between the basal nuclei and the cerebellum. The dentate nucleus in the cerebellum projects via the thalamic nuclei to the corpus striatum and the subthalamic nucleus (functionally considered part of the basal ganglia although anatomically part of the subthalamus) projects via an interneuron in the pons onto the cerebellar cortex.

Etiology

Clinically, paroxysmal dyskinesias all look very similar and so cannot be separated by clinical signs alone. Most paroxysmal dyskinesias in animals are classified as primary in that they are believed to be hereditary.[1] Secondary or symptomatic dyskinesia occurs in dogs due to drug administration (e.g., propofol and phenobarbital) or structural intracranial lesions. Secondary paroxysmal dyskinesias are more readily identifiable because they tend to be accompanied by additional neurological signs that are persistent between attacks.

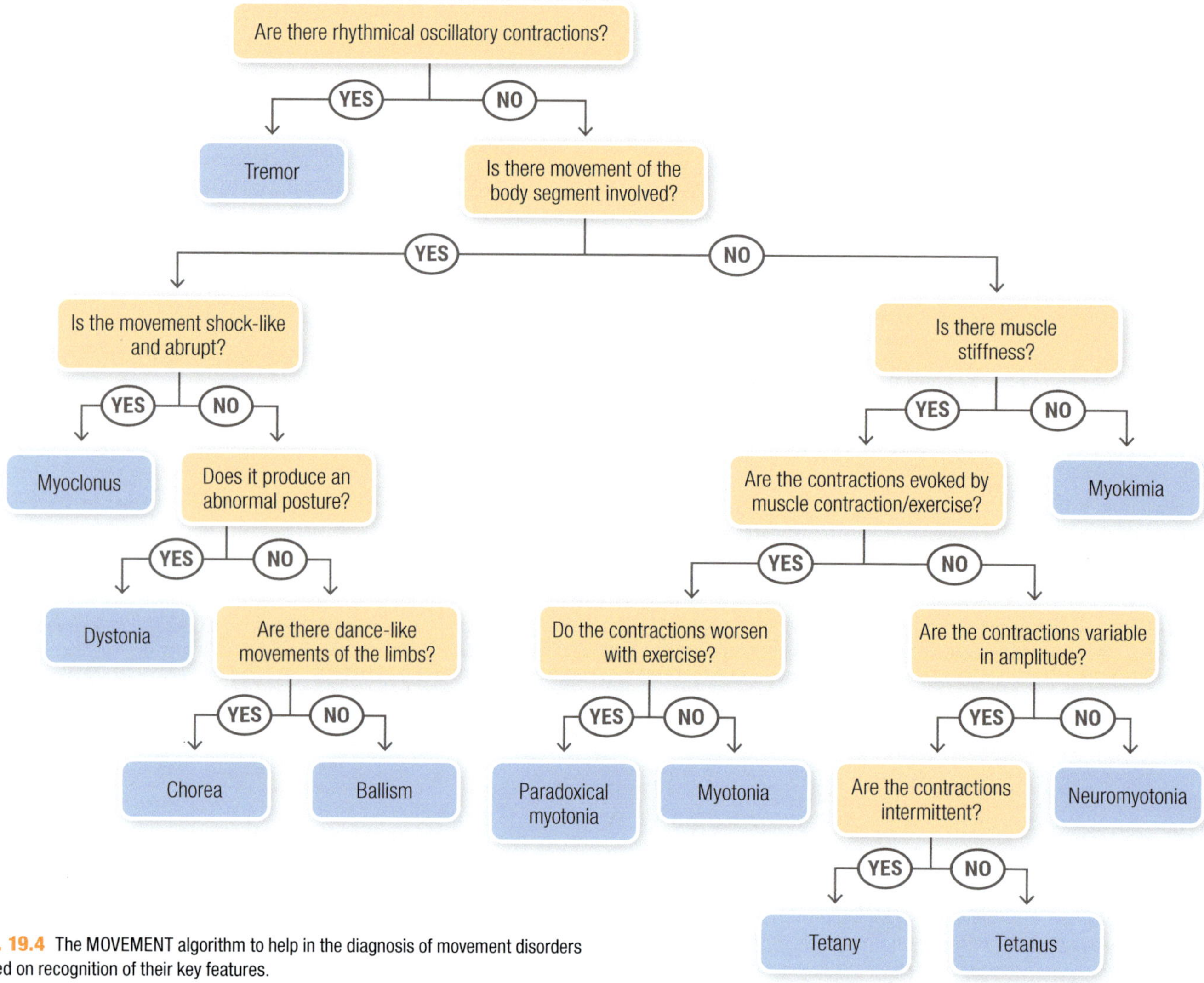

FIG. 19.4 The MOVEMENT algorithm to help in the diagnosis of movement disorders based on recognition of their key features.

Video 19.2

A chocolate Labrador with episodes of myoclonic contractions.

Video 19.3

Myokymia in the muscle of the forelimb resulting in undulating movements of the skin overlying the affected muscle.

Video 19.4

Dance-like movements seen in the pelvic limbs during an episode of paroxysmal dyskinesia. Note this dog also demonstrates dystonia manifesting as an abnormal posture.

Video 19.5

Ballism can be seen as a flailing movement of the left pelvic limb.

Video 19.6

Two cats demonstrating severe muscle stiffness immediately following muscle contraction as they land on the floor.

Video 19.7

A Spaniel with myotonic stiffness precipitated by exertion when trying to climb the stairs.

Clinical features

Table 19.1 gives a summary of all the clinical signs associated with paroxysmal dyskinesia. It can be difficult to differentiate some of these clinical signs when evaluating a dog with suspected paroxysmal dyskinesia. This may be because of inadequate descriptions of these clinical signs in the veterinary literature, but it may also be due to the presence of both elements. In order to distinguish these relevant clinical signs, a method has been developed from work at the author's referral practice (Movement Referrals: Independent Veterinary Specialists) to generate the MOVEMENT disorder algorithm (Fig. 19.4).

The first question on this algorithm asks if the contraction is rhythmical in nature. Rhythmicity is a hallmark of tremor and is discussed in detail in Chapter 18.

If the muscle contractions are not rhythmical, the next step is to ask if there is movement of the body segment involved. Contractions involving movement include ballism, chorea, dystonia, and myoclonus. If the contraction was shock-like and abrupt, then this would suggest the presence of myoclonus. Myoclonus is a sudden, brief, shock-like involuntary muscle jerk that can be focal, multifocal, or generalized (Video 19.2). Myoclonic muscle contractions are mostly accompanied by some movement of the affected body segment, in contrast to myokymia, for example, where the twitches remain within the affected body segment and movement is not observed (Video 19.3). Dystonia is differentiated by the adoption of an abnormal posture and is one of the few involuntary contractions that can be detected on a still photograph rather than in a video. If the contraction does not cause abnormal posture, then chorea (Video 19.4) or ballism (Video 19.5) is considered, with the former giving characteristic dance-like movements of the limbs (typically the pelvic limbs).

If the veterinarian determines there is no movement in the affected body segment, then they evaluate the involuntary contraction for muscle stiffness. A lack of stiffness would imply myokymia (Video 19.3). Myokymia refers to the presence of focal or generalized continuous muscle twitching, often described as vermicular or rippling muscle contractions (looking like a "bag of worms" under the skin; see Chapter 18).

If there is evidence of muscle stiffness, then other forms of peripheral nerve hyperexcitability (specifically neuromyotonia, tetany, and tetanus) or myotonia may be present (see Chapter 18). Contractions that worsen with muscle contraction include myotonia (Video 19.6) and paradoxical pseudomyotonia (Video 19.7). Both clinical signs result in stiffness following muscle contraction, with delayed relaxation. Myotonia occurs immediately after muscle contraction. In humans, a myotonic patient can be quickly identified by a simple handshake, as the patient is unable to relax and release their hand. Paradoxical pseudomyotonia, in contrast, results from repeated muscle contraction. Therefore, the dog may be normal when movement is initiated, but it can quickly worsen as exercise continues or becomes prolonged. In both cases the stiffness resolves with rest.

If there is no worsening from muscle contractions, then the veterinarian considers the amplitude of the contractions and whether they vary. If no variability is seen, then neuromyotonia should be considered (Video 19.8; see also Chapter 18). Neuromyotonia can be considered as a progressed form of myokymia. The main features are persistent muscle stiffness and delayed muscle relaxation. It is typical for neuromyotonia and myokymia to present simultaneously in the same patient. Any variability in the amplitude would suggest tetanus or tetany, the difference between these two clinical signs being their persistence. An intermittent muscle contraction of variable amplitude would likely denote tetany, whereas a persistent contraction is consistent with tetanus.

Differential diagnoses

Two important differential diagnoses for paroxysmal dyskinesia are epileptic seizures (specifically focal seizures; see Chapter 2 or 17, Video XXX) and tetany (due to hypocalcemia; see Video 19.9).

Focal epileptic seizures

In order to differentiate paroxysmal dyskinesia from epileptic seizures, several features should be considered:

- Maintaining a normal consciousness. A normal consciousness does not immediately rule out an epileptic seizure as focal seizures can occur with preservation of consciousness. However, if a dog is evaluated with motor activity in all four legs, then the consciousness would be expected to be abnormal in a generalized tonic-clonic seizure, and hence an unimpaired mentation would support a paroxysmal dyskinesia.
- No progression to a typical generalized tonic-clonic seizure. Many focal seizures will progress or evolve to become generalized tonic-clonic seizures, either during the initial event or during subsequent episodes. A lack of transformation to a generalized tonic-clonic seizure does not rule out epileptic seizure activity but should increase the suspicion of a paroxysmal dyskinesia.
- Lack of a postictal phase even after episodes lasting hours. Paroxysmal dyskinesia can last minutes to hours. Epileptic seizure activity tends to be much shorter, lasting only minutes. On the rare occasions on which seizure activity becomes prolonged, an obvious period of postictal behavior is observed consisting of mild forebrain signs, e.g., central blindness, pacing, and decreased awareness. Following a paroxysmal dyskinesia, regardless of duration, normal behavior and activity is immediately resumed. Therefore, a lack of postictal behavior following a prolonged episode should support a paroxysmal dyskinesia.
- No autonomic signs. Most epileptic seizures are accompanied by autonomic signs, specifically urination and salivation. In contrast, these are not features of paroxysmal dyskinesia. Therefore, observing autonomic signs during an episodic event is strongly supportive of an epileptic seizure.

Tetany (hypocalcemia)

Hypocalcemia is one of the main differential diagnoses that must be excluded when considering paroxysmal dyskinesia. Tetany is a clinical sign that results from hypocalcemia, but it may also be observed in paroxysmal dyskinesia. Decreased ionized calcium increases axonal excitability and leads to weakness, tetany, fasciculations, cramping, rigidity,

Video 19.8

A Jack Russell having an episode of neuromyotonia characterized by sustained muscle contraction resulting in extension of all four limbs and lateral recumbency. The video also shows an episode of myokimia of the left triceps and adjacent muscles.

Video 19.9

A hypocalcemic dog demonstrating evidence of tetany manifesting as an intermittent muscle stiffness with delayed muscle relaxation of varying amplitude.

and twitching. Signs can also include facial rubbing, seizures, weakness, or ataxia. More information on tetany resulting from hypocalcemia can be found in the article by Gagliardo et al.[11]

Classification

Across the many different breeds and individual dogs, episodes of paroxysmal dyskinesia share similar features without any distinguishing signs (Video 19.1). Given all types of paroxysmal dyskinesia have the potential to look the same, there is no specific characteristic that allows for differentiation on clinical grounds alone. Most paroxysmal dyskinesias in animals are classified as primary in that they are believed to be hereditary, with hematology, serum biochemistry, magnetic resonance imaging (MRI) of the brain, and cerebrospinal (CSF) analysis being normal.[1] Secondary or symptomatic dyskinesia occurs in dogs resulting from drug administration (e.g., propofol and phenobarbital) and structural intracranial lesions. Secondary paroxysmal dyskinesias are identifiable because they tend to be accompanied by additional neurological signs that are persistent between attacks. In view of the large number of breeds affected with this condition, it is important to say that any breed could be affected with paroxysmal dyskinesia, but reporting the breed specific conditions provides information on presentation, diagnosis, treatment, and prognosis.

Primary (presumed hereditary) paroxysmal dyskinesia

Paroxysmal gluten-sensitive dyskinesia in Border Terriers

Canine epileptoid cramping syndrome is the former name given to a paroxysmal dyskinesia in Border Terriers.[12] This term is a misnomer, and it now appears more appropriate to apply the name paroxysmal gluten-sensitive dyskinesia (PGSD).[13] Episodes are seen in dogs as young as 6 weeks up to 7 years of age.[12] PGSD consists of episodes of difficulty walking, ranging from ataxia to a complete inability to stand, tremors, and dystonia of the limbs, head, and neck. Episodes can last minutes or hours with dogs being normal in between. Mild to severe gastrointestinal signs such as borborygmi, vomiting, or diarrhea may be observed in between episodes.[14]

Gluten appears to trigger these episodes via a food sensitivity in genetically susceptible animals, although the exact mechanism of this is not understood. It is believed that there is an immune-mediated pathogenesis with cross-reactivity of gluten antibodies with antigenic epitopes on Purkinje cells in the cerebellum. Some dogs exhibit purely neurological signs in the form of paroxysmal dyskinesia, whilst others may have isolated gastrointestinal or dermatological signs. Gluten may be responsible for a much wider spectrum of clinical signs in this breed.[15]

Serology can be performed to test for antibodies against gluten and its associated enzymes (anti-gliadin and transglutamise-2 antibodies), although it is important to ensure the dog is not already receiving a gluten-free diet when this is done, as this can result in false negative results. Monitoring can also be performed to check for adherence to a gluten-free diet (i.e., to ensure the patient is not scavenging scraps of food containing gluten unobserved by the owner).

Strict adherence to a gluten-free diet can lead to complete remission of episodes of paroxysmal dyskinesia. It also seems to aid in managing some of the gastrointestinal and dermatological signs associated with this condition.[15] Prognosis is fair.

Episodic hypertonicity in Cavalier King Charles Spaniels

This condition, also known as episodic falling syndrome (EFS) in Cavalier King Charles Spaniels, was the first genetically mapped paroxysmal dyskinesia in companion animals.[16,17] Episodes are triggered by exercise, stress or excitement and characterized by progressive hypertonicity throughout the thoracic and pelvic limbs, resulting in a characteristic "deer-stalking" position or kyphosis. Onset of signs can be between 14 weeks and 4 years of age. As with most paroxysmal dyskinesias, dogs are normal in between episodes.

The mutation resulting in this condition has been characterized as a deletion affecting the brevican gene (*BCAN*), which encodes a brain-specific component of the extracellular matrix proteoglycan complex; it has an autosomal-recessive mode of inheritance. Brevican is thought to be involved in homeostasis, and mutations of this protein result in a disruption of axonal conduction and synaptic stability.[16,17] Diagnosis is by exclusion of other conditions, and correlation with an appropriate history and clinical signs are required. Genetic testing can confirm this specific condition of EFS. However, asymptomatic homozygous individuals have been reported.[17]

The carbonic anhydrase inhibitor acetazolamide (4–8 mg/kg PO every 8–12 h) works well in affected dogs. Acetazolamide promotes metabolic acidosis across the blood–brain barrier, thereby lowering the pH and reducing the conductance of potassium channels. This in turn alters the transmembrane potential and neuronal excitability, thus providing a therapeutic action. Prognosis is good, with many dogs achieving remission without treatment in later life.

Paroxysmal dyskinesia in Chinooks

A familial paroxysmal nonkinesigenic dyskinesia (PNKD) has been described in Chinooks; it is characterized by an inability to stand, head tremors, and involuntary flexion of one or more limbs.[18] In keeping with the characteristics of other paroxysmal dyskinesias, dogs have episodes lasting minutes or hours, demonstrate no autonomic signs, maintain normal awareness, and appear normal in between episodes. An interesting feature is that some dogs experience concurrent generalized tonic-clonic seizures. Based on pedigree analysis, the disorder is considered to be consistent with a partially penetrant autosomal recessive or polygenic trait.

Dancing Doberman disease

A condition causing intermittent flexion (chorea) of one or both pelvic limbs has been reported in Dobermans. Muscle atrophy, weakness, and postural reaction deficits may be seen in chronic cases. The underlying cause is not known.

Paroxysmal kinesigenic dyskinesia (PKD) in German Short-Haired Pointers

This is a paroxysmal dyskinesia that is induced by movement and sometimes can require significant exercise until an episode is precipitated. It is unusual to other paroxysmal dyskinesias in that it is responsive to phenobarbital (3 mg/kg every 12 h).[19] The condition shares many similarities with dancing Doberman disease.

Paroxysmal dyskinesia in Labradors and Jack Russell Terriers

These two breeds are among the most common breeds presented to referral neurology clinics for paroxysmal dyskinesia in the UK.[20] Paroxysmal dyskinesia in these breeds is triggered by startle or sudden movements and has a male bias (29/44 Labradors and 15/23 Jack Russell Terriers).

The median age at episode onset has been reported as 2 years 3 months (range, 9 months to 10 years 8 months) in Labradors and 4 years 8 months (range, 1 year to 8 years) in Jack Russell Terriers.[20] Labradors are more prone to have cluster episodes (i.e., more than one episode in a week) than Jack Russell Terriers (19/44 Labradors and 2/23 Jack Russell Terriers), but episode duration and frequency vary dramatically, even within an individual. The natural history was self-limiting, with 32% of affected dogs entering remission and an improvement in 75%. In Labradors, frequency and duration of episodes decreased in 25 out of 36 dogs, progressed in 5, and remained static in 6. Owners of Jack Russell Terriers reported an improvement in duration and frequency in 19 out of 23 dogs, a deterioration in 2 and a static course in 2. Episodes reduced in terms of frequency and duration, but remission was lower in dogs with cluster episodes than those without.

Paroxysmal dyskinesia in Norwich Terriers

In a study describing 26 affected Norwich Terrier dogs, the median age at the first observed episode of paroxysmal dyskinesia was 3 years.[21] All dogs were neurologically normal between episodes. The level of consciousness and awareness remained normal during the entire episode, which was characterized by sustained hypertonicity of the muscles in the pelvic limbs (100%), with many dogs exhibiting thoracic limb signs too, and some exhibiting kyphosis and an arched tail. Some dogs were unable to stand up during the entire episode, which lasted up to 30 minutes. The events in many dogs were associated with excitement, stress, anxiety, or exercise. Gluten-free, low-protein, beef-free, and hypoallergenic diets have been associated with a decrease in episode frequency.[21]

Scotty cramp

Scotty cramp describes a syndrome of intermittent exercise-, stress-, or excitement-induced paroxysmal dyskinesia in Scottish Terriers. Episode onset is between 6 weeks and 18 months, with the duration of signs being up to 20 minutes, although severe episodes can last hours.[22] Dogs may show changes in pelvic limb gait when running that progress to severe generalized cramp. However, a milder phenotype is described that is confined to the pelvic limbs and manifests as skipping, bunny hopping, and kicking while running, but without collapse and lasting no more than 20 minutes. It is possible that this phenotype is present in other small breed dogs, manifesting as a skipping lameness that is present during the trot phase of gait but disappears at walk and sprint speed.

This recessive, inherited, nonprogressive disorder is thought to be associated with relative deficiencies of the inhibitory neurotransmitter 5-hydroxytryptamine (serotonin). Its pathophysiology may therefore be different to that of other paroxysmal dyskinesias in that the administration of serotonin antagonists (e.g., methylsergide) can evoke episodes. A presumptive diagnosis is based on clinical signs and breed. All laboratory tests are within normal limits.

Treatment with the serotonin antagonist fluoxetine (0.5–1 mg/kg every 12 h) has been reported to be beneficial in some dogs.[23] Severe forms can be refractory to fluoxetine and show a better response to diazepam. Prognosis is good.

Paroxysmal dyskinesia in the Soft Coated Wheaton Terrier

Soft Coated Wheaten Terriers also suffer from a paroxysmal dyskinesia reminiscent of PNKD. This condition shares many of the features of other paroxysmal dyskinesias in dogs, though recently, a mutation in the *PIGN* gene has been identified that is associated with this condition.[24] The disease is inherited in an autosomal-recessive manner. The *PIGN* gene encodes glycosylphosphatidylinositol anchors, which attach many different proteins to cell surfaces. It is uncertain how this results in the condition in dogs.

Secondary paroxysmal dyskinesia

Drug-induced causes of secondary paroxysmal dyskinesia include phenobarbital, which has been reported to elicit PNKD in an epileptic Chow Chow.[25] The pathophysiology is unknown, but the signs were reversible on cessation of the medication. Propofol has also been reported to cause PNKD in a Golden Retriever.[26]

Clinicopathological findings

Identification of paroxysmal dyskinesia is based on clinical evaluation, including a thorough neurological examination, and careful questioning about the nature of the episodes with video footage.[12,15,27] There is no consensus on how best to investigate the underlying cause of suspected paroxysmal dyskinesia, but many clinicians use screening tests, including a complete blood count (CBC) with differential, serum biochemistry profile, bile acid stimulation testing, MRI of the brain, and CSF analysis. Ionized calcium and fasting glucose levels should be included in the biochemistry profile. Gluten sensitivity in Border Terriers and genetic testing in Cavalier King Charles Spaniels and Soft-Coated Wheaten Terriers should be considered in these specific breeds.

Video 19.10

A Border Terrier exhibiting an episode of muscle stiffness, dystonia, and tremors. These signs are consistent with paroxysmal gluten-sensitive dyskinesia.

Video 19.11

An episode of paroxysmal dyskinesia in a Cavalier King Charles Spaniel that carries the brevican mutation associated with episodic hypertonicity.

Video 19.12

A Jack Russell Terrier demonstrating an episode of chorea and hypertonicity affecting all four limbs. This is compatible with paroxysmal dyskinesia.

Video 19.13

A 2-year-old Labrador having an episode of paroxysmal dyskinesia.

Diagnostic imaging

Paroxysmal dyskinesia, with video correlation, normal interictal findings, and a normal neurological examination is unlikely to yield abnormal findings when performing screening diagnostic procedures. Whether a neuroimaging procedure should be done in every patient after suspecting paroxysmal dyskinesia is controversial. It is clear that these procedures will not increase the suspicion of dyskinesia, and their aim is simply to rule out structural intracranial disease. Despite this, the abandonment of screening diagnostic tests for all paroxysmal dyskinesia patients seems premature, and it is likely that secondary causes for canine paroxysmal movement disorders will be identified as knowledge and awareness of the condition increases.

Treatment

It is important to emphasize that, with the exception of secondary paroxysmal dyskinesia, primary or hereditary paroxysmal dyskinesia is not a life-threatening or life-limiting condition. Although episodes may be very disturbing and concerning to observe, death is not reported to occur during an episode of dyskinesia. However, these episodes clearly impinge on a patient's quality of life, so any treatment that can be offered is worth pursuing if episodes are frequent.

There are breed-specific incidences where treatment can be tailored. These are reported individually in the appropriate breed-specific conditions already mentioned. However, for the majority of paroxysmal dyskinesias the treatment is broadly similar.

In dogs, medications that have found individual success in treating dogs with paroxysmal dyskinesia include clonazepam (0.5 mg/kg PO every 8–12 h) and acetazolamide (4–8 mg/kg PO every 8–12 h). Fluoxetine (1 mg/kg PO every 24 h) is an alternative, but these patients are in the minority. Antiepileptic medication is rarely useful in paroxysmal dyskinesias. Given the erratic pattern of these episodes, careful and critical evaluation of the episodes over a long time frame (e.g., 2 to 3 months) is important to assess the need and, if required, the effect of any therapeutic trial.

Prognosis

Long-term follow-up of some paroxysmal dyskinesias has shown these to be benign and self-limiting.[17,20,22] The condition is certainly not considered to be life-limiting.

KEY POINTS

- Episodic movement disorders are best characterized by video footage.
- An algorithm can be used to diagnose the type of movement disorder present.
- Paroxysmal dyskinesias tend to look similar among different breeds.
- Paroxysmal dyskinesias are benign and can be self-limiting.
- Medication is often unwarranted in paroxysmal dyskinesia.

References

1. Lowrie M, Garosi L. Classification of involuntary movements in dogs: Paroxysmal dyskinesias. *Vet J.* 2017 Feb; 220:65–71.
2. Cerda-Gonzalez S, Packer RA, Garosi L et al. International veterinary canine dyskinesia task force ECVN consensus statement: Terminology and classification. *J Vet Intern Med.* 2021 May; 35(3):1218–1230.
3. de Lahunta A, Glass E. Nonolfactory rhinencephalon: limbic system. In: de Lahunta A, Glass E (eds.). *Veterinary Neuroanatomy and Clinical Neurology*, 3rd ed. St. Louis, MO: W.B. Saunders; 2009, p. 448–453.
4. Thomson C, Hahn C. *Veterinary Neuroanatomy: A Clinical Approach.* Edinburgh, UK: Saunders Elsevier; 2012.
5. Obeso JA, Rodríguez-Oroz MC, Rodríguez M et al. The basal ganglia and disorders of movement: pathophysiological mechanisms. *News Physiol Sci.* 2002 Apr;17:51–55.
6. Visser JE, Bloem BR. Role of the basal ganglia in balance control. *Neural Plast.* 2005; 12(2-3):161–174; discussion 263–272.
7. Damier P, Hirsch EC, Agid Y, Graybiel AM. The substantia nigra of the human brain. II. Patterns of loss of dopamine-containing neurons in Parkinson's disease. *Brain.* 1999 Aug; 122 (Pt 8):1437–48.
8. Gerfen CR. The neostriatal mosaic: multiple levels of compartmental organization. *Trends Neurosci.* 1992 Apr;15(4):133–139.
9. Tewari A, Fremont R, Khodakhah K. It's not just the basal ganglia: Cerebellum as a target for dystonia therapeutics. *Mov Disord.* 2017 Nov; 32(11):1537–1545.
10. Kaji R, Bhatia K, Graybiel AM. Pathogenesis of dystonia: is it of cerebellar or basal ganglia origin? *J Neurol Neurosurg Psychiatry.* 2018 May;89(5):488-492.
11. Gagliardo T, Ruggeri R, Di Paola A et al. Clinical features of muscle cramp in 14 dogs. *J Vet Intern Med.* 2021 Jan; 35(1):372–377.
12. Black V, Garosi L, Lowrie M et al. Phenotypic characterisation of canine epileptoid cramping syndrome in the Border terrier. *J Small Anim Pract.* 2014 Feb;55(2):102–107.
13. Lowrie M, Garden OA, Hadjivassiliou M et al. The Clinical and Serological Effect of a Gluten-Free Diet in Border Terriers with Epileptoid Cramping Syndrome. *J Vet Intern Med.* 2015 Nov-Dec; 29(6):1564–1568.
14. Lowrie M, Garden OA, Hadjivassiliou M et al. Characterization of Paroxysmal Gluten-Sensitive Dyskinesia in Border Terriers Using Serological Markers. *J Vet Intern Med.* 2018 Mar; 32(2):775–781.

15. Lowrie M, Hadjivassiliou M, Sanders DS, Garden OA. A presumptive case of gluten sensitivity in a border terrier: a multisystem disorder? *Vet Rec.* 2016 Dec 3;179(22):573.
16. Gill JL, Tsai KL, Krey C et al. A canine *BCAN* microdeletion associated with episodic falling syndrome. *Neurobiol Dis.* 2012 Jan;45(1):130–136.
17. Forman OP, De Risio L, Stewart J et al. Genome-wide mRNA sequencing of a single canine cerebellar cortical degeneration case leads to the identification of a disease associated *SPTBN2* mutation. *BMC Genet.* 2012 Jul 10; 13:55.
18. Packer RA, Patterson EE, Taylor JF et al. Characterization and mode of inheritance of a paroxysmal dyskinesia in Chinook dogs. *J Vet Intern Med.* 2010 Nov-Dec; 24(6):1305–1313.
19. Harcourt-Brown T. Anticonvulsant responsive, episodic movement disorder in a German shorthaired pointer. *J Small Anim Pract.* 2008 Aug; 49(8):405–407.
20. Lowrie M, Garosi L. Natural history of canine paroxysmal movement disorders in Labrador retrievers and Jack Russell terriers. *Vet J.* 2016 Jul; 213:33–37.
21. De Risio L, Forman OP, Mellersh CS, Freeman J. Paroxysmal Dyskinesia in Norwich Terrier Dogs. *Mov Disord Clin Pract.* 2016 May 19; 3(6):573–579.
22. Urkasemsin G, Olby NJ. Clinical characteristics of Scottie Cramp in 31 cases. *J Small Anim Pract.* 2015 Apr; 56(4):276–280.
23. Geiger KM, Klopp LS. Use of a selective serotonin reuptake inhibitor for treatment of episodes of hypertonia and kyphosis in a young adult Scottish Terrier. *J Am Vet Med Assoc.* 2009 Jul 15; 235(2):168–171.
24. Kolicheski AL, Johnson GS, Mhlanga-Mutangadura T et al. A homozygous PIGN missense mutation in Soft-Coated Wheaten Terriers with a canine paroxysmal dyskinesia. *Neurogenetics.* 2017 Jan;18(1):39–47.
25. Kube SA, Vernau KM, LeCouteur RA. Dyskinesia associated with oral phenobarbital administration in a dog. *J Vet Intern Med.* 2006 Sep-Oct; 20(5):1238–1240.
26. Mitek AE, Clark-Price SC, Boesch JM. Severe propofol-associated dystonia in a dog. *Can Vet J.* 2013 May; 54(5):471–474.
27. Packer RM, Berendt M, Bhatti S et al. Inter-observer agreement of canine and feline paroxysmal event semiology and classification by veterinary neurology specialists and non-specialists. *BMC Vet Res.* 2015 Feb 18; 11:39.

CHAPTER 20

Canine cognitive dysfunction syndrome

Natasha Olby
DVM, PhD, MRCVS,
DACVIM (Neurology)

Neurons, arguably the most important component of the central nervous system, are largely postmitotic, and there is gradual neuronal attrition with age across mammalian species.[1] Improvements in healthcare for both people and dogs have extended their lifespan, and as a result, the impact of age-related neuronal loss has increased in importance.[2] In both people and dogs, the neuronal loss is particularly prevalent in certain regions of the forebrain, leading to gradual age-associated cognitive decline and ultimately development of Alzheimer's disease (AD) in people and a syndrome of behavioral abnormalities known as canine cognitive dysfunction syndrome (CCDS) in dogs.[3] This canine syndrome has many similarities with AD and has been proposed as a model of this devastating human condition. There is an extensive body of high-quality work published on aging of cognitive function in Beagles that categorizes their decline into healthy aging, impaired, and severely impaired based on a memory task that also tests cognitive flexibility.[4] The severely impaired group suffer from CCDS. Using this model of canine cognitive aging, a research group has performed numerous studies on the underlying pathophysiology as well as clinical trials of a wide range of therapeutic agents.[5] Their work is now being extended into a clinical client-owned population. The information generated about Beagles is powerful because it is based on dogs that are extremely carefully monitored while living in a controlled environment and trained to perform a variety of tasks that test different cognitive domains. The data reported on clinical populations is by necessity rather different in nature. Much is being generated through remotely delivered questionnaires only, and so alternative diagnoses in this clinically complex population of aged dogs might be missed. Indeed, diagnostic standards have not yet been described for a clinical population. This is not meant to imply that the data do not have value, simply that cautious interpretation is needed.

TABLE 20.1 Pathophysiological events contributing to the development of canine cognitive dysfunction syndrome.

Event	Consequence
Amyloid deposition	Angiopathy, neurodegeneration, neuroinflammation
Hyperphosphorylated tau accumulation	Neurotoxicity
Cholinergic dysfunction	Memory loss
Oxidative damage	Mitochondrial dysfunction
Neuroinflammation	Neurodegeneration
Reduced rate of neurogenesis	Atrophy of dentate gyrus – memory loss
Dysbiosis of oral and gastrointestinal microbiota	Toxicity of gingipains, neuroinflammation

Etiology and pathophysiology

CCDS is characterized by atrophy of the cerebrum, first detectable in the frontal lobe and hippocampus, leading to narrowing of gyri, widening of sulci, and enlargement of the ventricles. Histopathologically, there is loss of cortical neurons, particularly in the prefrontal and frontal lobes and the hippocampus, and amyloid deposition in the prefrontal, frontal, parietal, occipital, and entorhinal cortices.[6] Amyloid is present in a fibrillar form in diffuse plaques, and immunohistochemical staining shows these plaques predominantly contain amyloid β_{42}. In addition, amyloid β_{40} and β_{42} are found in the walls of small-diameter blood vessels (cerebral amyloid angiopathy), within neurons, and within the dentate gyrus of the hippocampus. Other age-related changes include intraneuronal lipofuscin deposits (indicative of oxidative damage), Lafora bodies, astrogliosis and increased numbers of microglia (indicating neuroinflammation), microhemorrhages, and ubiquitin deposits within the white matter. These changes start to appear around 8–9 years of age and progressively worsen. A pathological threshold at which a histological diagnosis of CCDS is made has not been clearly defined.

The underlying etiology is likely multifactorial (Table 20.1), and it is important to note that in dogs, the greatest risk factor for CCDS is age. Indeed, there are data suggesting that chronological age, not life stage, is important in declining performance on cognitive tests in companion dogs.[7] Unlike in people, genetic risk factors in dogs have not been identified to date, and there is no clear breed predilection described at this time. All dogs carry the *APOE4* allele that is a risk factor in people. Human familial forms of early onset AD are associated with mutations that result in the generation of increased amounts of insoluble neurotoxic amyloid fragments, suggesting that amyloid accumulation is central to the pathology of AD. Much interest has been focused on preventing or removing amyloid deposits, with disappointing results and conflicting information emerging on the relationship between amyloid load and cognitive performance in humans. Similarly, several studies have shown an association between amyloid accumulation and cognition in dogs and have related cognitive performance on tasks testing specific brain regions (e.g., the prefrontal cortex) to amyloid load in that region of the brain.[8–10] Other studies in companion dogs have failed to show an association between amyloid pathology and CCDS clinical signs, but they assessed cognitive performance with owner questionnaires rather than performance on very specific tasks.[11,12] Neurofibrillary tangles composed of hyperphosphorylated tau protein are also an important feature of AD, and while not as prominent a feature of aging in dogs, hyperphosphorylated tau deposits, both intra- and extracellular, are found in the hippocampus and cortex.[13–15]

The cholinergic theory of AD proposes that dysfunction of the cholinergic system is associated with memory loss and cognitive decline. Antagonism of acetylcholine at muscarinic receptors using scopolamine results in deficits in working memory at low doses and more global deficits in cognition at higher doses. Aging dogs are more sensitive than younger dogs, implying decline in their cholinergic system, and treatment with an acetylcholinesterase inhibitor (e.g., phenserine) improves learning and memory.[16]

There is histopathological evidence of increasing oxidative damage with age, and importantly, this pathology is associated with amyloid deposits as well as cognitive decline.[17]

Inflammation manifesting as activation of astrocytes and microglia is also present and believed to play an important role in disease progression.[15]

There is an association between oral health and both AD and CCDS, leading to the proposal that pathology is induced by release of a toxic protease, lysine-gingipain, by *Porphyromonas* bacterial species found in the mouth. These bacteria have been detected within the brains of aged, cognitively impaired dogs, along with presence of the protease, and their prevalence increases with age.[18,19] The health of the gastrointestinal microbiome is likely also important.[20] Finally, while most neuronal populations are postsynaptic, neurogenesis does occur continually over life in certain niches, including the dentate gyrus of the hippocampus. The rate of neurogenesis in the hippocampus is age associated and does correlate with cognitive function.[21]

Clinical presentation

Dogs affected with CCDS have behavioral deficits relating to dysfunction in various cognitive domains that can be captured using the acronym DISHAAL. These deficits include a loss of spatial memory and awareness (Disorientation), changes in social (I)nteractions, disturbances in the (S)leep/wake cycle, (H)ouse soiling, (A)ctivity changes, (A)nxiety, and loss of (L)earning. The onset of signs is gradual, with owners initially reporting subtle changes. Changes in social interaction are typically reported first, followed by alterations in sleep/wake cycles.[22] Two different questionnaires that generate scores from a series of owner-answered questions have classified dogs as having normal, mild, moderate, or severe cognitive impairment or as belonging to normal, at risk, or CCDS groups.[22,23] Following dogs longitudinally using these questionnaires, there is gradual progression, with a high proportion of old dogs moving to a new category over a one-year period. The presence of a urinary tract infection or development of polyuria/polydipsia for a wide variety of reasons can of course complicate the interpretation of behaviors. Signs reported by owners can be complicated by hearing and vision loss, but sensory loss is known to accelerate dementia in people, and hearing loss has been shown to be related to worse cognitive performance in dogs.[24]

Video 20.1

This 15-year-old female spayed Labrador Retriever is unable to engage with the handler, in spite of being treat motivated until this point. She has a tendency to pace with no particular purpose evident, which can be seen when she walks away from the handler. A hands-on neurological examination is essentially normal apart from her affect and attention.

Diagnosis

There is currently no gold standard for antemortem and even postmortem diagnosis. The threshold at which the changes constitute a formal diagnosis of CCDS has yet to be established. The pillars of establishing a diagnosis include an appropriate signalment and history, owner-reported neurobehavioral abnormalities, the absence of alternative causes for the signs on physical examination (e.g., house soiling can be caused by polyuria/polydipsia, urinary tract infection, pain), a serum biochemistry panel, a complete blood cell count, and a urinalysis/culture. Blood pressure should always be measured. In elderly dogs, many different comorbidities could be present and should be considered as possible contributors to behavioral changes. For example, pain from multi-joint osteoarthritis could affect behaviors quite dramatically, and its influence should be gauged by careful treatment. Ideally, a full diagnostic workup would include magnetic resonance imaging (MRI) of the brain and cerebrospinal fluid analysis. Given the age of these dogs, thoracic radiographs should be taken prior to general anesthesia to investigate for possible comorbidities.

MRI findings include atrophy of the interthalamic adhesion, widening of the sulci, and enlargement of the lateral and third ventricles, all indicating cortical atrophy (Fig. 20.1). Other common findings include the presence of microhemorrhagic infarcts (of unknown significance in the pathology of CCDS) and leucoaraiosis (i.e., bilateral, symmetrical white matter lesions that are isointense to normal white matter on MRI T1-weighted pulse sequences, non-contrast-enhancing, and hyperintense on T2-weighted and fluid-attenuated inversion recovery [FLAIR] pulse sequences). If the hippocampus volume can be measured, it is reduced, and an absolute interthalamic adhesion thickness of <5 mm or a ratio of interthalamic adhesion thickness to brain height (at the same level) of $<13.6\%$ are strongly suggestive of CCDS, although diagnostic accuracy of these measures has not been established.[25,26]

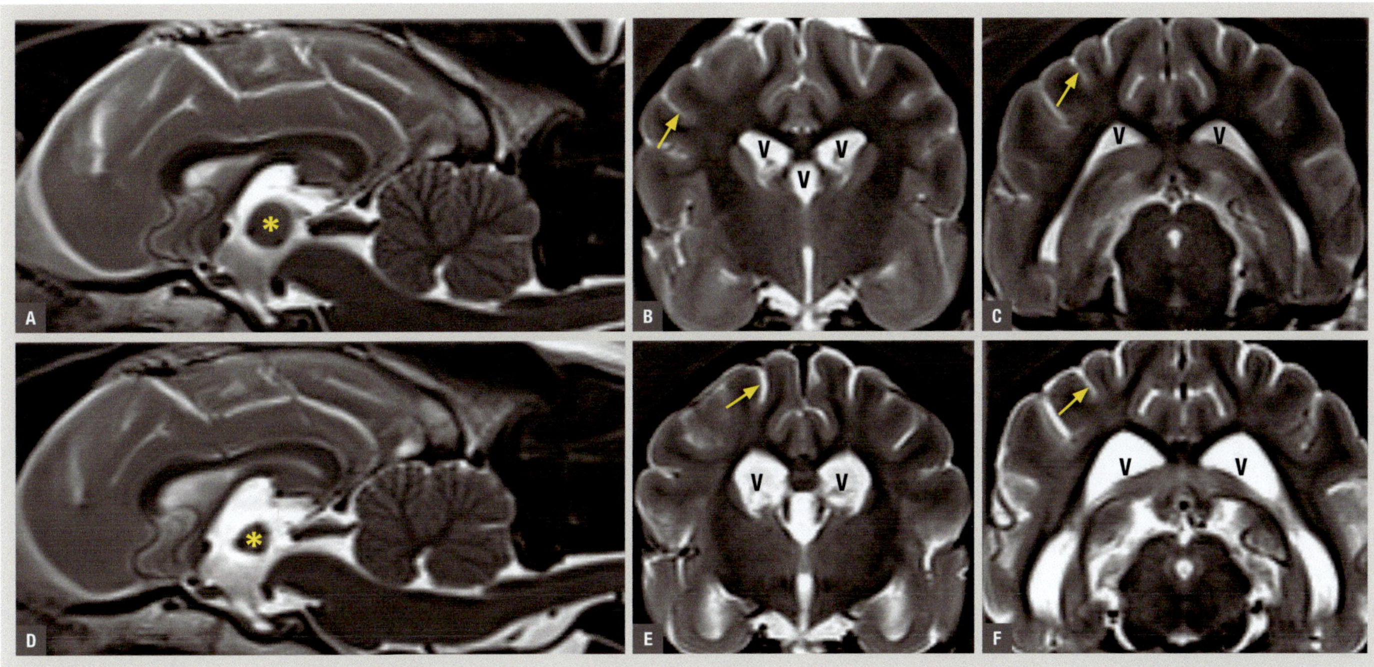

FIG 20.1 (A–C) Sagittal and transverse T2-weighted images of the brain of a 12-year-old mixed breed dog. (D–F) Sagittal and transverse T2-weighted images of the brain of the same dog 18 months later. On the midsagittal images, the interthalamic adhesion (*) is dramatically atrophied in D compared with A. On the transverse images at the level of the thalamus (B, E) and midbrain (C, F), the lateral ventricles (V) enlarge over time, and the sulci (arrows) widen due to cerebral atrophy.

Prognosis and treatment

Unfortunately, this insidious neurodegenerative process cannot be cured, so the focus is on prevention, slowing of deterioration and symptomatic treatment. Beyond age, frequency of feeding and activity levels are risk factors for the development of CCDS, with increased activity, a history of training, and once-daily feeding reducing the risk.[27–29] A wide range of therapies have been tested in laboratory-based aging Beagle colonies, open-label clinical studies and, in a smaller number of instances, placebo-controlled clinical trials. Some more novel therapies have undergone proof of principle trials. When reading these studies, it is important to note that owner questionnaires are associated with a large placebo effect in this type of trial.[30] These therapeutic approaches span dietary enrichment with antioxidants, flavonoids, and medium-chain fatty acids,[31,32] antiamyloid vaccination,[33] alteration in neurotransmitter levels,[34–36] exercise and environmental enrichment,[37,38] supplements containing a wide variety of different neuroactive, anti-inflammatory, neuroprotective and antiaging substances,[30,39–42] cellular transplants[43] and transcranial photobiomodulation[44] (Table 20.2). Some of these therapies are early in development or unavailable, so current advice is provided below.

Prevention/slowing progression

Understanding the risk factors for CCDS allows the identification of methods to delay deterioration. These include exercise, socialization, and perhaps reduced frequency of feeding. It is normal for activity levels in aging dogs to go down, but it is also important to both continue to interact with them and keep them as active as possible. Optimizing the environment to make the dog comfortable and confident is important. For example, most older dogs are prone to falling, and use of nonslip carpet runners can increase their willingness to exercise. Careful attention to pain levels is also merited. The factors that contribute to neurodegeneration can be targeted using diets or supplements that are rich in antioxidants and flavonoids, omega fatty acids, and medium chain triglycerides as well as other neuroactive or neuroprotective substances (Table 20.2). One randomized controlled trial identified a small benefit using a combination of a senolytic and an NAD (nicotinamide adenine dinucleotide) precursor. Use of owner questionnaires to document changes over time will also help to bring awareness of the condition to the fore for both owners and veterinarians. It is also important to note that urinary tract infections and endocrine disorders can dramatically change house soiling behaviors, and any change in answers on house soiling should trigger an appropriate investigation by the veterinarian. The role oral health plays in progressive cognitive decline is unclear, but there is an association between cognitive status and the oral microbiome. Owners should be encouraged to maintain dental cleanings and ideally brush their dog's teeth.

Symptomatic therapy

The only drug approved for treatment of CCDS is selegiline at a dose of 0.5–1 mg/kg orally once a day in the morning. Owners report alleviation of pacing, improved sleep patterns, and improved interactions. Sleep disturbances can be treated by establishing a routine; supplementation with melatonin will help some dogs (3–9 mg orally). If pain could be a contributor to lost sleep, carefully addressing comorbidities with anti-inflammatories is important, and addition of gabapentin just prior to sleep can help. Anxiety can be addressed using a benzodiazepine (e.g., lorazepam), trazodone, diphenhydramine, fluoxetine, buspirone, sertraline, or others, with the specific choice depending on the individual dog's comorbidities and the character of the anxiety. Caution around polypharmacy should be exercised given the advanced age of these dogs and frequency of comorbidities.

TABLE 20.2 Therapeutic trials for canine cognitive dysfunction syndrome.

Therapy	Mechanism	PB or CO	Trial design Outcome measure	N	Conclusion/comments
Neurotransmitters					
Selegiline[32,33]	Inhibition of MAO-B	PB	■ Placebo-controlled ■ Memory task	8	Aged dogs improved memory performance
		CO	■ Open-label trial ■ Questionnaire	641	77.2% dogs showed an improvement by 60 days. Good safety profile
Butyryl cholinesterase[34] *Not commercially available currently*	Acetylcholinesterase inhibition	CO	■ Controlled trial ■ 2 groups, 6 months ■ Questionnaire, cognitive tests	14	Improved questionnaires and cognitive testing
Dietary management					
Commercial diet 1[29]	Enriched with antioxidants, flavonoids, carotenoids, L-carnitine, omega-3 fatty acids, alpha-lipoic acid	PB	■ Several controlled trials ■ Cognitive tests		Improvement on cognitive testing
Commercial diet 2[30]	Enriched with MCTs	CO	■ Blinded, placebo-controlled ■ 3 groups ■ Questionnaire	87	Significant improvement in questionnaires for dogs in 6.5% MCT diet and control diet by 3 months No comparison between groups
Supplements					
Supplement 1[40]	Antioxidants, free radical scavengers, fatty acids, phosphatidyl serine	CO	■ Blinded, randomized, placebo-controlled ■ 2 groups, 6 weeks ■ Questionnaires	27	Note removed outliers Improvement in questionnaire scores in treatment group
Supplement 2[38,39]	Combination of vitamin E, *Ginkgo biloba*, pyridoxine, phosphatidylserine	PB	■ Blinded cross over design ■ 2 months each arm ■ Memory test	9	Improved memory as tested by the delayed non-matching to position task
		CO	■ Open-label trial ■ 3 months ■ Questionnaire	8	Improved questionnaire outcomes
Supplement 3[28]	Senolytic and NAD precursor	CO	■ Blinded, randomized, placebo-controlled ■ 3 groups, 3 months ■ Questionnaires, activity monitors, cognitive testing	70	Improved questionnaire outcomes in all groups – significant difference across groups, with full dose showing largest improvement
Supplement 4[37]	SAMe, phosphatidylserine, coenzyme Q10, vitamin E curcumin, zinc, blend of Chinese herbs, *Polygala tenuifolia*, *Salvia miltiorrhizae*	CO	■ Open label ■ 2 months ■ Questionnaire	10	Improved questionnaire outcomes
Miscellaneous approaches					
Aβ vaccination and behavioral enrichment[31]	Removal of amyloid plaques	PB	■ Controlled trial ■ 4 groups, 20 months ■ Cognitive testing, histopathology	34	Combined therapy resulted in stabilization of learning, reduced Aβ load, increased BDNF mRNA, increased microhemorrhages
Autologous skin derived neural precursor cells[41]	Preservation of hippocampal synaptic density	CO	■ Open-label ■ Questionnaire and cognitive tests, activity/spatial monitoring, histology	6	Majority of dogs improved on all outcomes
Photobiomodulation[42]	Multiple mechanisms proposed	CO	■ Open-label ■ 2 months ■ Questionnaire	5	Improved questionnaire outcomes
Crisdesalazine *Not published*	Antioxidant, microsomal PGE synthase-1 inhibitor	CO	■ Blinded, placebo-controlled, randomized ■ 2 groups, 2 months	48	Improved questionnaires

MAO-B, monoamine oxidase; NAD, nicotinamide adenine dinucleotide; Aβ, amyloid beta; SAMe, S-adenosyl-L-methionine; BDNF, brain-derived neurotrophic factor; PB, purpose bred; CO, client-owned; N, number of dogs; MCT, medium-chain triglyceride; PGE, prostaglandin E.

Conclusions

With advancing age, the prevalence of cognitive decline and ultimately CCDS increases exponentially. A diagnosis of CCDS is challenging to make without brain MRI, but the condition can be diagnosed presumptively in dogs with a consistent history of progressive DISHAAL signs, normal blood work, urinalysis, blood pressure, lack of serious comorbidity, and an absence of focal neurological deficits on neurological examination. While there are numerous supplements on the market, open-label trial results should be viewed with caution due to the large placebo effect in owner questionnaires on their dog's cognition. As for people, a good diet, activity, and socialization are important in slowing decline. Behavioral changes should be investigated carefully in elderly dogs, and comorbidities that could contribute to the DISHAAL phenotype displayed by dogs with CCDS should be addressed carefully and persistently.

KEY POINTS

- Canine cognitive dysfunction (CCDS) is an age-associated neurodegenerative disease characterized by cortical atrophy and amyloid deposition.
- The most important risk factor for CCDS is age.
- Diagnosis is made from history, clinical signs, and exclusion of other causes.
- Management is aimed at delaying progression with diets and supplements rich in antioxidants and antiaging substances and maintaining activity and socialization.
- Symptomatic therapy can be used to alleviate anxiety and sleeping issues.
- As new therapies emerge, the importance of randomized, blinded, placebo-controlled trials is emphasized due to the large placebo effect seen with client questionnaires.

References

1. Youssef SA, Capucchio MT, Rofina JE, et al. Pathology of the Aging Brain in Domestic and Laboratory Animals, and Animal Models of Human Neurodegenerative Diseases. *Vet Pathol.* 2016 Mar;53(2):327–348.
2. Lewis TW, Wiles BM, Llewellyn-Zaidi AM, et al. Longevity and mortality in Kennel Club registered dog breeds in the UK in 2014. *Canine Genet Epidemiol.* 2018 Oct 17;5:10.
3. Landsberg GM, Nichol J, Araujo JA. Cognitive dysfunction syndrome: a disease of canine and feline brain aging. *Vet Clin North Am Small Anim Pract.* 2012 Jul;42(4):749–768, vii.
4. Mongillo P, Araujo JA, Pitteri E, et al. Spatial reversal learning is impaired by age in pet dogs. *Age (Dordr).* 2013 Dec;35(6):2273–2282.
5. Cotman CW, Head E. The canine (dog) model of human aging and disease: dietary, environmental and immunotherapy approaches. *J Alzheimers Dis.* 2008 Dec;15(4):685–707.
6. Head E, McCleary R, Hahn FF, et al. Region-specific age at onset of β-amyloid in dogs. *Neurobiol Aging.* 2000;21:89–96.
7. Watowich MM, MacLean EL, Hare B, et al. Age influences domestic dog cognitive performance independent of average breed lifespan. *Anim Cogn.* 2020 Jul;23(4):795–805.
8. Head E, Pop V, Sarsoza F, et al. Amyloid-beta peptide and oligomers in the brain and cerebrospinal fluid of aged canines. *J Alzheimers Dis.* 2010;20(2):637–646.
9. Cummings BJ, Head E, Afagh AJ, et al. Beta-amyloid accumulation correlates with cognitive dysfunction in the aged canine. *Neurobiol Learn Mem.* 1996 Jul;66(1):11–23.
10. Tapp PD, Siwak CT, Gao FQ, et al. Frontal lobe volume, function, and beta-amyloid pathology in a canine model of aging. *J Neurosci.* 2004 Sep 22;24(38):8205–8213.
11. Ozawa M, Chambers JK, Uchida K, Nakayama H. The Relation between canine cognitive dysfunction and age-related brain lesions. *J Vet Med Sci.* 2016 Jul 1;78(6):997–1006.
12. Schütt T, Helboe L, Pedersen LØ, et al. Dogs with Cognitive Dysfunction as a Spontaneous Model for Early Alzheimer's Disease: A Translational Study of Neuropathological and Inflammatory Markers. *J Alzheimers Dis.* 2016 Mar 15;52(2):433–449.
13. Habiba U, Ozawa M, Chambers JK, et al. Neuronal Deposition of Amyloid-β Oligomers and Hyperphosphorylated Tau Is Closely Connected with Cognitive Dysfunction in Aged Dogs. *J Alzheimers Dis Rep.* 2021 Oct 6;5(1):749–760.
14. Papaioannou N, Tooten PC, van Ederen AM, et al. Immunohistochemical investigation of the brain of aged dogs. I. Detection of neurofibrillary tangles and of 4-hydroxynonenal protein, an oxidative damage product, in senile plaques. *Amyloid.* 2001 Mar;8(1):11–21.
15. Hines AD, McGrath S, Latham AS, et al. Activated gliosis, accumulation of amyloid β, and hyperphosphorylation of tau in aging canines with and without cognitive decline. *Front Aging Neurosci.* 2023 Apr 27;15:1128521.
16. Araujo JA, Studzinski CM, Milgram NW. Further evidence for the cholinergic hypothesis of aging and dementia from the canine model of aging. *Prog Neuropsychopharmacol Biol Psychiatry.* 2005 Mar;29(3):411–422.
17. Head E, Rofina J, Zicker S. Oxidative stress, aging, and central nervous system disease in the canine model of human brain aging. *Vet Clin North Am Small Anim Pract.* 2008 Jan;38(1):167–178, vi.
18. Arastu-Kapur S, Nguyen M, Raha D, et al. Treatment of Porphyromonas gulae infection and downstream pathology in the aged dog by lysine-gingipain inhibitor COR388. *Pharmacol Res Perspect.* 2020 Feb;8(1):e00562.
19. Templeton GB, Fefer G, Case BC et al. Longitudinal Analysis of Canine Oral Microbiome Using Whole

TABLE 21.1 Arterial blood supply and distribution to the dog's brain.

Rostral cerebral artery	Rostromedial surface of the cerebral cortex and dorsal surface along each side of the medial longitudinal fissure
Middle cerebral artery	Lateral surface of the cerebral cortex
Caudal cerebral artery	Caudomedial surface of the cerebral cortex and dorsal surface along each side of the medial longitudinal fissure
Rostral cerebellar artery	Rostral aspect of the cerebellar hemisphere, vermis, and dorsolateral aspect of the brainstem
Caudal cerebellar artery	Caudal and ventral aspects of the cerebellum, lateral aspect of the medulla
Striate arteries	Globus pallidus, putamen, internal capsule, claustrum, and part of the caudate nucleus
Proximal perforating artery arising from the caudal communicating artery	Rostromedial aspect of the thalamus
Distal perforating artery arising from the caudal communicating artery	Caudolateral aspect of the thalamus and subthalamus
Caudal perforating artery arising from the basilar bifurcation and paramedian branches arising from the proximal portion of the caudal cerebral artery	Median and paramedian region of the caudal portion of the thalamus, midbrain, and upper region of the pons

affected region.[2,6–7] For instance, a small ischemic infarct of the medulla can produce severe neurological deficits referable to a central vestibular syndrome, with potentially multiple cranial nerve deficits (Video 21.1).
Larger infarcts are more often located in the forebrain or cerebellum, secondary to involvement of the middle cerebral artery or rostral cerebellar artery respectively, while smaller infarcts tend to more commonly affect the thalamus.
Sometimes, dogs can experience neurological signs that closely mimic an ischemic infarct due to their acute onset and the typical location to a specific brain area of distribution of a well-known arterial blood vessel. However, these signs may spontaneously resolve within minutes or hours (usually no more than 24 hours). These signs are generally referred to as TIAs, and their diagnosis is presumptive, based on the acute onset and spontaneous regression of the focal neurological deficits without any changes in the magnetic resonance images in most cases. Vestibular syndrome is one of the most frequent clinical presentations of TIAs. Recurrences are not infrequent in dogs with TIA signs and, based on the experience in human medicine, it is also assumed that these patients may have a greater chance of developing a true CVA in the future.[1,6,8]

Video 21.1

Right-sided central vestibular syndrome due to an acute ischemic infarct, with right head tilt, severe nonambulatory tetraparesis, increased tone in the left-sided limbs, multiple proprioceptive deficits that are more pronounced in the right-sided limbs, positional ventral strabismus of the right eye, and a mild tendency to right rotatory nystagmus.

Pathophysiology

The pathophysiology of ischemic stroke is based on the principle that with limited energy stores, the brain relies on a constant supply of glucose and oxygen to maintain ionic pump function.[1,3,4] The brain accounts for less than 2% of the total body mass in humans, yet it utilizes approximately 20% of the total body energy intake due to its inherently high metabolic requirements. The brain's limited local glucose storage and minimal reserves of high-energy phosphates create a dependency on a consistent supply of glucose and oxygen. If cerebral perfusion fails to meet the energy demands and waste product removal requirements of the brain, a state of ischemia develops. Irreversible neuronal injury can start within minutes of the onset of ischemia, with adenosine triphosphate (ATP) depletion resulting in failure of Na^+/K^+ ATPase activity, intracellular sodium and water influx (cytotoxic edema), and neuronal depolarization.[1,3,4] If perfusion pressure is not quickly restored, then ischemia progresses to infarct. Secondary release of excitatory neurotransmitters (particularly glutamate) and inflammatory mediators contributes to progressive injury, along with mitochondrial dysfunction, lipid peroxidation, and vascular injury. The increased intracellular concentration of calcium activates programmed cell death pathways and their lysis. The disruption of the blood–brain barrier will then lead to vasogenic edema, which typically takes 4 to 6 hours to develop once blood flow decreases to ischemic levels, and may continue to progress for 24 to 48 hours; this can sometimes also be responsible for the progression of the clinical signs in the first 2–3 days after the acute onset.[1,3,4] Because neurons have the highest demand for oxygen, neuronal function is first affected; this is followed, in declining order of vulnerability, by the function of oligodendrocytes, astrocytes, mesodermal microglia, and fibrovascular elements. The infarct is therefore an area of severely compromised brain parenchyma, caused by a focal occlusion of one or more blood vessels. The obstruction can develop directly within the occluded vessels (thrombosis), or the obstructive material can originate from another vascular bed and travel to the brain (thromboembolism).
From a histological point of view, two regions can be distinguished in an ischemic infarct: the core, where ischemia is severe and infarction develops rapidly, and the surrounding penumbra, where the decrease in cerebral blood flow (CBF) is more moderate, thus allowing a longer period of ischemic stress to be tolerated. Over time, the penumbra decreases in favor of the core. The factors responsible for the evolution of the penumbra to irreversible injury are multiple and complex and include the degree of blood flow reduction, the region of the brain involved, and the individual patient's response to a pathological insult.[1,3,4] Tissue within the penumbra has the potential for recovery and therefore is the target for therapy in acute ischemic stroke.

Etiology

CVAs are very common in human medicine and in proportion are only rarely reported in dogs. The lower incidence of CVAs in dogs compared with humans could also be in part related to differences in cerebral blood supply. Specifically, dogs have a higher number of intra-extracranial arterial anastomoses. In humans, many predisposing factors and causes of ischemic CVAs have been extensively documented, with thromboembolism in association with cardiac diseases being relatively frequent among others.[1]
In a previous study in dogs with brain infarcts, a concurrent medical condition was detected in over 50% of dogs, the most common conditions being hyperadrenocorticism, chronic kidney disease, hypothyroidism, and hypertension.[1,7,9–11] Suspected underlying causes identified

in histopathologically confirmed cases include: septic thromboemboli associated with bacterial endocarditis or other sources of infection; atherosclerosis associated with primary hypothyroidism; hyperlipoproteinemia in Miniature Schnauzers; parasitic emboli (e.g., of *Dirofilaria immitis*); embolic metastatic tumor cells; intravascular lymphoma; and aortic or cardiac thromboembolism.[1,7,9] No age, sex, or breed predisposition was identified in that study, although Cavalier King Charles Spaniels and Greyhounds were overrepresented.

Clinicopathological findings

Routine blood test and urinalysis results are usually within normal limits, unless there is a predisposing underlying disease, such as hypothyroidism or renal failure, alone or in association with hypertension. However, further investigations—such as targeted testing for endocrine diseases, serial measurements of systemic blood pressure, a coagulation profile, an echocardiogram, and an abdominal ultrasound aimed at identifying a possible predisposing cause for ischemic CVAs—should usually be performed after confirmation of the ischemic vascular accident itself. Overall, it is estimated that almost half of the infarcts do not have an underlying cause in dogs.

Diagnostic imaging findings

Advanced imaging modalities are necessary to definitively confirm the diagnosis. Computed tomography (CT) images are often normal during ischemic CVAs and are more useful to rule out other causes of acute brain disorders that can mimic a stroke. However, on a few occasions and especially in severe ischemia, loss of gray/white matter differentiation and mild local mass effect can be identified.[15,17,18]

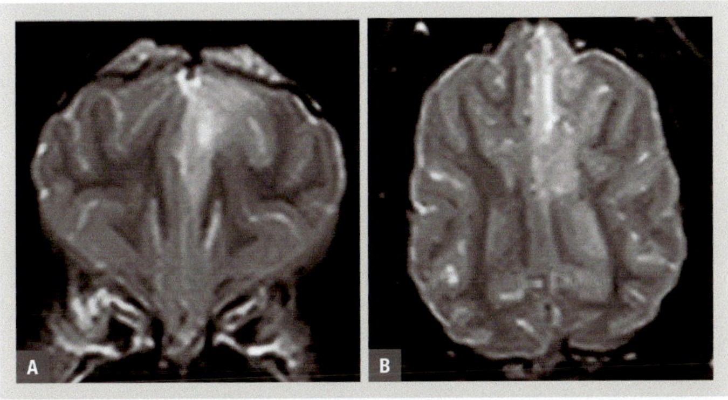

FIG. 21.2 Transverse (**A**) and dorsal (**B**) T2-weighted magnetic resonance images showing minimal mass effect of an acute ischemic infarct of the left cerebral hemisphere, with mild right shifting of the midline.

Magnetic resonance imaging (MRI) is the gold standard technique to diagnose CVAs, as soon as 12–24 hours after the onset of neurological signs. In the vast majority of cases, ischemic lesions affect the gray matter and, since they are caused by occlusion of a blood vessel, they conform to a vascular territory with a sharp demarcation from the surrounding normal brain tissue and minimal or no mass effect (Fig. 21.2). Depending on the blood vessel involved, as previously stated, they can be differentiated into lacunar and territorial infarcts. The first ones tend to generally affect the deepest arteries and are therefore commonly observed in the thalamus, the basal nuclei, or the cerebellum. Cerebellar infarcts frequently have a wedge shape, with the apex towards the innermost area. Ischemic CVAs are hyperintense on T2-weighted images and fluid-attenuated inversion recovery (FLAIR) images and isointense and, in more dramatic cases, mildly hypointense on T1-weighted images. After intravenous injections of a paramagnetic medium such as gadolinium, contrast enhancement can vary from none in the acute phase to mild and superficial, usually after the first week (Fig. 21.3). Brain inflammation and infiltrative tumors such as lymphoma or gliomas can sometimes be difficult to distinguish from infarcts. However, careful evaluation of the lesion, its distribution, and its appearance helps to rule out other similar-looking brain disorders. More advanced magnetic resonance techniques can also support the diagnosis of acute infarcts. Diffusion-weighted imaging (DWI) and apparent diffusion coefficient (ADC) mapping provide functional information about the behavior of water molecules in tissue, and they can definitely improve the sensitivity and specificity of the diagnosis of acute stroke. Even if this is not pathognomonic, acute ischemic infarcts appear hyperintense on DW images and hypointense on ADC maps (Fig. 21.4). Over time, however, this aspect disappears, and the infarcts becomes hyperintense in both, exactly as the most common brain inflammations might appear.

If the findings are very doubtful, the MRI scan can be repeated after a few weeks (2–4) for lesion follow-up and to establish the definitive diagnosis. In fact, subacute to chronic infarcts are smaller than acute infarcts and generally develop into necrotic areas that, depending on their severity, can be associated with overall brain atrophy and/or hydrocephalus ex-vacuo, due to the loss of brain parenchyma (Fig. 24.5).

Finally, even if not well developed and routinely used in veterinary neuroradiology, angiographic techniques such as time-of-flight (TOF)

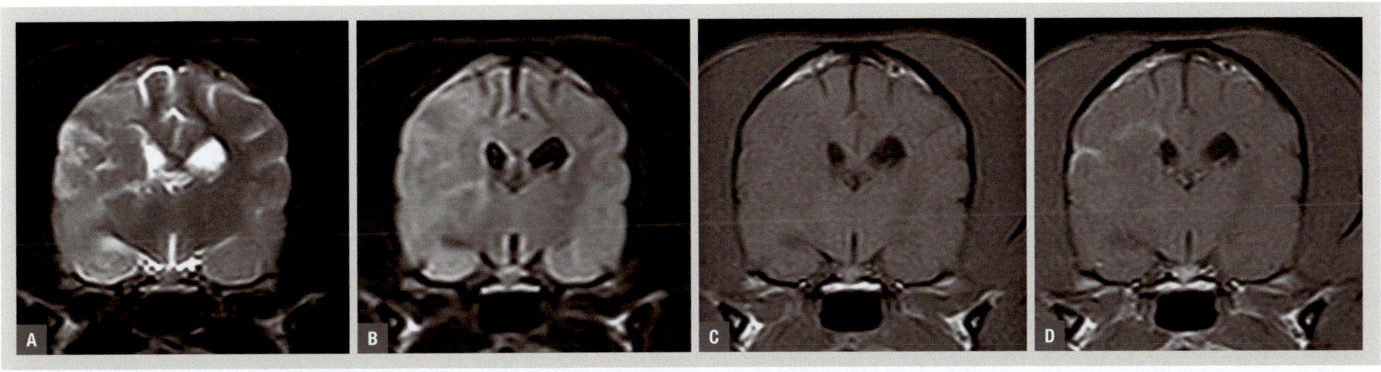

FIG. 21.3 Transverse T2-weighted (**A**), fluid-attenuated inversion recovery (FLAIR) (**B**), and T1-weighted pre- (**C**) and postgadolinium (**D**) magnetic resonance images of a subacute ischemic infarct in the right cerebral hemisphere, showing mild and especially superficial contrast enhancement.

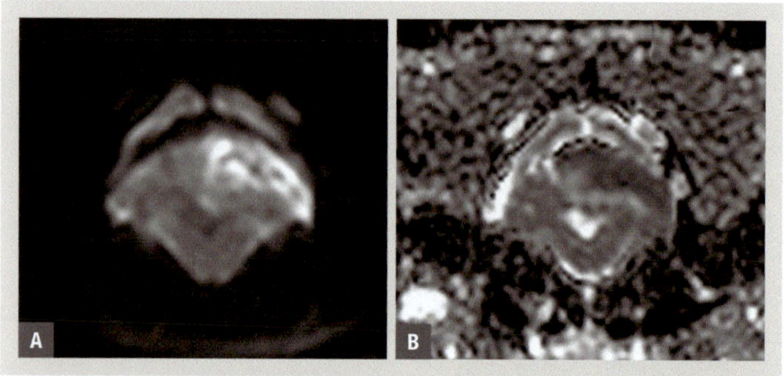

FIG. 21.4 Transverse diffusion weighted (DW) image (**A**) and apparent diffusion coefficient (ADC) map (**B**), showing the typical appearance of an acute ischemic infarct (hyperintense on the DW image and hypointense on the ADC map).

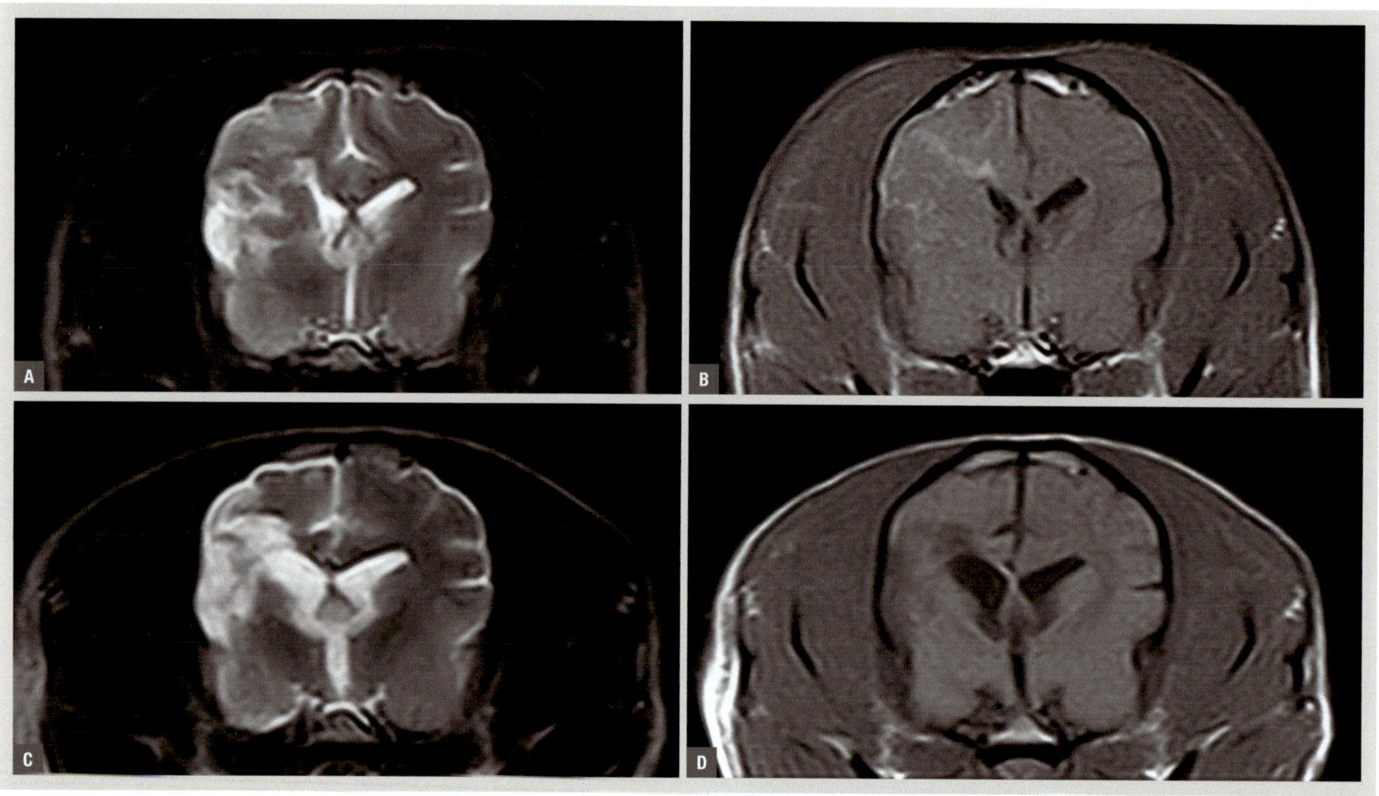

FIG. 21.5 Transverse T2-weighted (**A**) and T1-weighted postgadolinium magnetic resonance (MR) (**B**) images of an ischemic infarct in the right cerebral hemisphere. Transverse T2-weighted (**C**) and T1-weighted (**D**) postgadolinium MR images of the same dog 60 days later: note the right cerebral atrophy with ex-vacuo dilation of the ventricular system and midline shift towards the right side.

and contrast-enhanced magnetic resonance angiography may be used to look for arterial stenosis, vascular malformations, and aneurysms.[17]

Ancillary diagnostic tests

Cerebrospinal fluid (CSF) analysis might help in differentiating between disease categories and especially vascular diseases from inflammation. Although in many cases, CSF parameters in ischemic disease are within normal limits, mild to moderate changes may sometimes be observed both in cell and protein content. CSF analysis results should thus be interpreted cautiously. Most importantly, CSF analysis should be part of a thorough clinical diagnostic workup that also takes into account the patient's signalment, history, and particularly the onset and evolution of the neurological signs.

Treatment and prognosis

If the patient suffers from a predisposing condition, this should be treated whenever possible to prevent the occurrence of new ischemic episodes. Specific treatment is mostly supportive and consists in maintaining adequate tissue oxygenation in addition to managing neurological signs (e.g., seizures) and potentially other secondary complications such as decubital ulcers, aspiration pneumonia, and urine scald. Enteral nutrition may be required.[22] Physical therapy may speed up the recovery in patients with severe motor compromise.

To date, there is no evidence-based data demonstrating that more specific therapies are of benefit for dogs with ischemic CVAs. In humans, neuroprotective agents or antiplatelet and thrombolytic therapy are indicated in case of ischemic stroke.[1,22] Although these therapeutic strategies have led

to a reduction in the size of the ischemic lesion in experimental animal models, they have either failed to prove their efficacy in clinical trials or are awaiting further investigation.
Most patients suffering from ischemic cerebral infarction experience significant improvement only with supportive therapy, usually within a few weeks of the event. Obviously, the more extensive or important (e.g., brainstem) the brain area affected, the longer the recovery time may be and the higher the possibility of residual deficits. Dogs rarely die of CVAs, unless there are serious predisposing diseases.

Hemorrhagic cerebrovascular accidents

Hemorrhagic CVAs, also known as hemorrhagic strokes, are rarer than ischemic infarcts, especially if we exclude hemorrhages secondary to head trauma, which are also uncommon, except in small dogs due to their greater vulnerability and predisposition to serious cerebral sequelae resulting from trauma.

Clinical presentation

Clinical signs secondary to hemorrhagic CVAs are very similar to those mentioned for their ischemic counterparts, with an acute/peracute onset and rapid progression over the first 24–72 hours. Clinical signs usually reflect the involvement of a focal brain area and not uncommonly begin with epileptic seizures. The severity and evolution of the clinical signs depend on the size of the hematoma and the affected area, with potentially lethal cases due to the sudden increase in intracranial pressure (ICP) and possible cerebral herniation if the cerebral autoregulatory pressure mechanisms are unable to compensate. However, clinical signs usually tend to remain stable or regress within a few days, as the size of the hematoma decreases.

Pathophysiology and etiology

Hemorrhage occurs when blood flows directly into the brain parenchyma or, sometimes, into the subarachnoid space.[1] The hemorrhage is more rarely epidural, subdural, or intraventricular (Fig. 21.6). The clinical signs are a direct consequence of the destruction of the brain tissue and/or its compression by the hematoma. In addition, edema in the surrounding brain tissue contributes to an increased mass effect and ICP, which ultimately leads to worsening of the clinical signs. The brain has its own self-regulation mechanisms which, according to the Monro-Kellie doctrine, will initially lead to volume changes, particularly in the CSF and blood volumes, so that the total intracranial volume remains constant, also with respect to the volume of the brain parenchyma.[1] When the mass effect exceeds the pressure compensation mechanisms, then the ICP reaches critical values and brain herniation often develops, with potential lethal effects if not promptly treated.
Head trauma, such as that caused by road traffic accidents or falls from heights but also by penetrating injuries (e.g., secondary to bite wounds), can be associated with cerebral hemorrhages.[15]
Local brain diseases such as brain tumors (both primary and metastatic), congenital vascular malformations, and necrotizing vasculitis can be associated with intracranial hemorrhage.[7,13–16] Extracranial diseases leading to disseminated intravascular coagulopathy and other causes of spontaneous bleeding, such as infestation by *Angiostrongylus vasorum* or ingestion of anticoagulant rodenticide, can also result in spontaneous brain hemorrhage. Hypertension is very rarely the cause of a primary hemorrhagic strokes in dogs.[24] In older dogs, cerebral amyloid angiopathy resulting from amyloid deposits in cerebral arteries can lead to weakening of the arterial walls and then bleeding, typically at the gray/white matter junction.[13–16] It is not rare for these hemorrhages to be multiple and small in size, which is why they are often referred to as cerebral microbleeds.[26] Although uncommon, hemorrhage can also occur as a secondary effect of ischemic strokes following reperfusion.

Clinicopathological findings

Routine blood test and urinalysis results are usually within normal limits unless there is a predisposing underlying disease. A coagulation profile should be performed to rule out coagulopathies. Serial measurements of systemic blood pressure as well as an echocardiogram and abdominal ultrasound could also add valuable information to rule in or out other diseases potentially predisposing to systemic bleeding. Serological detection of circulating antigen of *Angiostrongylus vasorum* and/or fecal demonstration of the parasite's larvae are crucial for confirming the diagnosis of the infection. They are highly suggested in all endemic areas.[27]
The same considerations mentioned for CSF analysis in patients with ischemic infarction apply in cases of hemorrhagic CVAs.

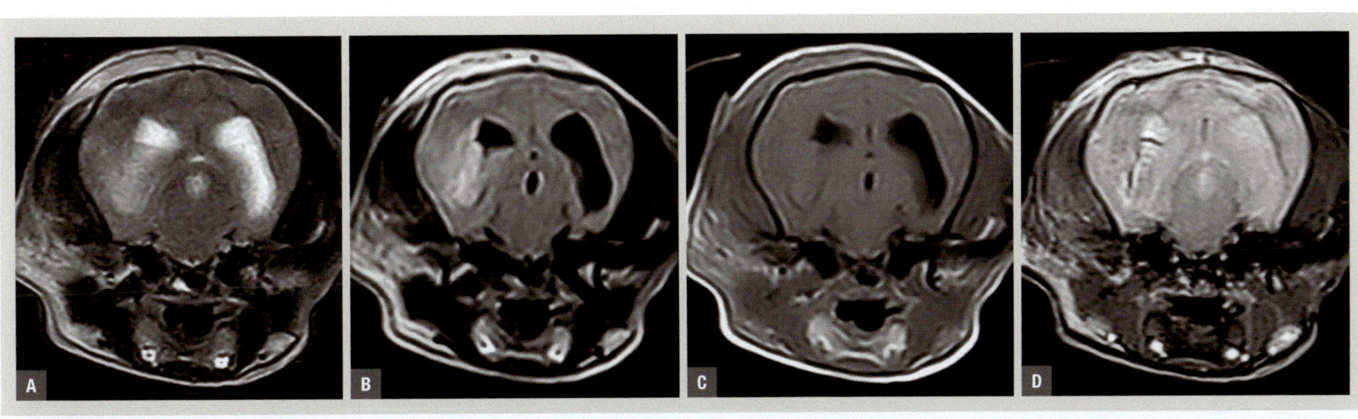

FIG. 21.6 From left to right, transverse T2-weighted, fluid-attenuated inversion recovery (FLAIR), T1-weighted, gradient-echo T2* magnetic resonance images of an intraventricular hemorrhage in the right lateral ventricle.

Diagnostic imaging findings

CT is very sensitive for acute hemorrhage and has the major advantage of being very quick to perform. It is strongly recommended in all cases of head trauma in which bleeding can be potentially life-threatening. Acute hemorrhage is generally seen as an area of increased attenuation, which tends to increase for the first 72 hours and remains visible for approximately 1 week, before slowly decreasing to isodensity about 1 month after the hemorrhage. On CT scans, the periphery of the lesion may enhance from approximately 6 days to 6 weeks after onset.[12]

MRI has good sensitivity for hemorrhagic strokes, although routine T1- and T2-weighted images lack specificity, especially in the acute phase. Hemorrhagic strokes can be more easily confirmed after some time because of the paramagnetic properties of blood breakdown products, which are responsible for an hyperintense signal on T1-weighted images and for the magnetic susceptibility artifact, which appears as a hypointense spot on gradient echo (GE) T2* images and susceptibility weighted (SW) sequences.[17,19,21] This finding is directly related to the field strength of the MRI machine; therefore, high-field units (>1 Tesla) are more suitable for the diagnosis of hemorrhage than low-field machines. Because blood breakdown products have different magnetic properties, five distinct stages of MRI appearance of intracranial hemorrhages have been defined based on the evolution of these products at the site of the hemorrhage (Table 21.2).[1,20] GE T2* and SW sequences can increase both the sensitivity and specificity for hemorrhagic strokes. On these sequences, a hemorrhage will appear as a signal void lesion (hypointense), which will be more evident at the periphery of the lesion due to the paramagnetic effect of hemosiderin. SW imaging has been shown to be even more reliable than GE T2* imaging for the detection of brain hemorrhage and particularly for cerebral microbleeds, which typically appear as multiple small, mostly roundish, hypointense lesions (Fig. 21.7). The most common differential diagnosis of hemorrhagic infarcts is neoplasia, which can sometimes coexist or even be the actual cause of the hemorrhage.[25] In addition to the aforementioned sequences, a repeat MRI scan can also help in differentiating between a tumor and a hematoma and in reaching a definitive diagnosis (Fig. 21.8).

Treatment and prognosis

The first therapeutic approach in dogs with brain hemorrhage is generally medical management.[1] Medical therapy should be guided by the clinical signs and imaging findings and is frequently aimed at controlling/reducing the increase in ICP. The risk of neurological deterioration and cardiovascular instability is highest during the first 24 hours, as the space-occupying hematoma slowly expands and surrounding vasogenic edema develops.[8,22] Careful monitoring of vital parameters and adequate intervention when relevant changes are observed are therefore essential in this period, during which it is essential for oxygen levels, blood pressure, fluid balance, and body temperature to be maintained within the reference values. Adequate ventilation and normovolemia should be guaranteed in all patients with increased ICP. Hyperventilation can temporarily be used to reduce the ICP. To avoid excessive hyperventilation and hypocapnic vasoconstriction, the $PaCO_2$ should be closely monitored with serial arterial blood gas analysis.[1,8,22]

Intravenous administration of mannitol (e.g., 18–20%) at a dose of 0.25–1.0 g/kg over 10 to 20 minutes and of a hypertonic solution (e.g., 7.5% saline) at a dose of 5–6 mL/kg over 5–10 minutes is crucial to treat

TABLE 21.2 Hemorrhage appearance on magnetic resonance T2- and T1- weighted images, based on the evolution of the hemorrhage over time and the products of hemoglobin degradation.

Hemorrhage stages	T2-weighted images	T1-weighted images	Hemoglobin degradation products
Hyperacute (12–24 hours)	Hyperintense	Isointense	Intracellular oxyhemoglobin
Acute (1–3 days)	Hypointense	Isointense	Intracellular deoxyhemoglobin
Early subacute (4–7 days)	Hypointense	Hyperintense	Intracellular methemoglobin
Late subacute (7–14 days)	Hyperintense	Hyperintense	Extracellular methemoglobin
Chronic (>14 days)	Hypointense	Hypointense	Ferritin hemosiderin

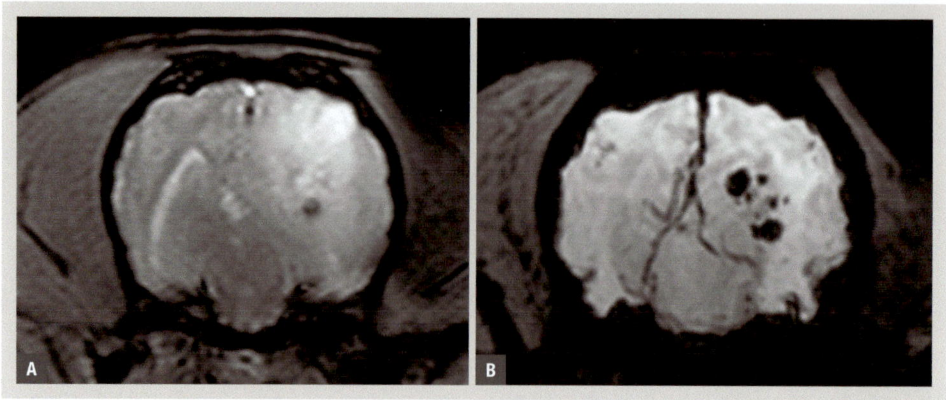

FIG. 21.7 Gradient echo T2* (A) and susceptibility weighted (SW) magnetic resonance (b) images of a left-sided cerebral hemorrhage, clearly visible on the SW image as multiple hypointense spot-like lesions.

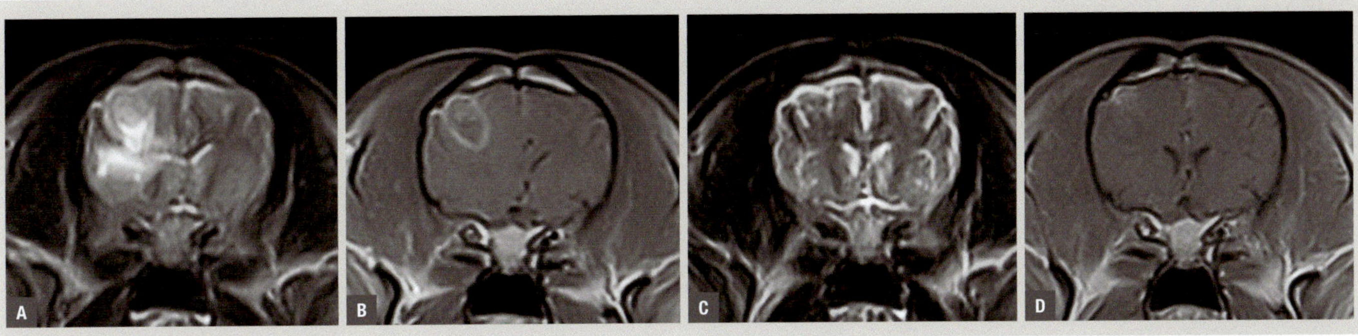

FIG. 21.8 Transverse T2- (**A**) and T1-weighted (**B**) postgadolinium magnetic resonance images of a hemorrhagic infarct of the right parietal lobe. The transverse T2- (**C**) and T1-weighted (**D**) postgadolinium magnetic resonance images of the same dog performed 60 days later confirm the non-neoplastic nature of the lesion, which was indeed a hematoma.

intracranial hypertension. To date, there is no evidence that mannitol or hypertonic solutions exacerbate intracranial hemorrhage, even in the event of their leakage through a ruptured blood vessel.[1,8] If epileptic seizures are part of the whole clinical spectrum, they should be treated according to their severity with the most common antiepileptic drugs. Steroids may also be used in case of cerebral edema and brain herniations. If a predisposing disease is diagnosed, it should also be treated accordingly. Close systemic and neurological monitoring is fundamental to determine the effectiveness of the treatment.

In the event of a continued deterioration of the neurological status despite various medical attempts, a surgical approach may be considered to remove the cerebral hematoma or, if in a relatively easily accessible area, drain a subarachnoid hemorrhage.[1,8]

Although the prognosis is fair in most cases, this strictly depends on the severity of the initial clinical presentation and, obviously, on the response to therapy. As a general rule, the more serious the clinical signs, the size of the hematoma and therefore the increase in ICP, the more guarded/poorer the prognosis.

KEY POINTS

- Cerebrovascular accidents (CVAs), also known as strokes or infarcts, are increasingly common in dogs.
- CVAs can be either ischemic or hemorrhagic, with the former being more common.
- Clinical signs usually have an acute/peracute onset, with potential progression for the first 24–72 hours.
- Hyperadrenocorticism, chronic kidney disease, hypothyroidism, and hypertension may be underlying causes of ischemic stroke.
- Hemorrhagic strokes are more often due to brain trauma, intravascular coagulopathy, brain tumors, *Angiostrongylus vasorum* infection, or ingestion of anticoagulant rodenticide.
- Definitive diagnosis is confirmed by CT (especially for hemorrhage) and, more importantly, by MRI.
- Therapy is mostly supportive/symptomatic and generally aimed at controlling the intracranial pressure (ICP). If a predisposing disease is present, it must be treated accordingly.
- The prognosis is usually fair/good but more guarded in patients with a hemorrhagic stroke, especially if it is associated with a severely increased ICP.

References

1. Garosi LS. Cerebrovascular disease. *Vet Clin North Am Small Anim Pract.* 2010 Jan;40(1):65–79.
2. Garosi LS, McConnell JF, Platt SR, et al. Clinical characteristics and topographical magnetic resonance of suspected brain infarction in 40 dogs. *J Vet Intern Med.* 2006;20:311–321.
3. Kogure T, Kogure K. Molecular and biochemical events within the brain subjected to cerebral ischaemia (targets for therapeutical intervention). *Clin Neurosci.* 1997;4:179–183.
4. Collins RC, Dobkin BH, Choi DW. Selective vulnerability of the brain: new insights into the pathophysiology of stroke. *Ann Intern Med.* 1989;110:992–1000.
5. Patterson J, Rusely M, Zachary J. Neurologic manifestations of cerebrovascular atherosclerosis associated with primary hypothyroidism in a dog. *J Am Vet Med Assoc.* 1985;186:499–503.
6. Platt SR, Garosi L. Canine cerebrovascular disease: do dogs have strokes? *J Am Anim Hosp Assoc.* 2003;39:337–342.
7. Garosi LS, McConnell JF, Platt SR, et al. Results of investigations and outcome of dog brain infarcts. *J Vet Intern Med.* 2005;19:725–731.
8. Hillock SM, Dewey CW, Stefanacci JD, et al. Vascular encephalopathies in dogs: risk factors, pathophysiology, and clinical signs. *Compend Contin Educ Pract Vet.* 2006;28:196–207.
9. Cook LB, Coates JR, Dewey CW, et al. Vascular encephalopathy associated with bacterial endocarditis in four dogs. *J Am Anim Hosp Assoc.* 2005;41:252–258.
10. Hess RS, Kass PH, Van Winkle TJV. Association between diabetes mellitus, hypothyroidism or hyperadrenocorticism, and atherosclerosis in dogs. *J Vet Intern Med.* 2003;17:489–494.
11. Thomas WB, Adams WH, McGavin MD, et al. Magnetic resonance imaging appearance of intracranial hemorrhage secondary to cerebral vascular malformation in a dog. *Vet Radiol Ultrasound.* 1997;38:371–375.
12. Tidwell AS, Mahony OM, Moore RP, et al. Computed tomography of an acute hemorrhagic cerebral infarct in a dog. *Vet Radiol Ultrasound.* 1994;35:290–296.
13. Dennler M, Lange EM, Schmied O, et al. Imaging diagnosis—metastatic hemangiosarcoma causing cerebral hemorrhage in a dog. *Vet Radiol Ultrasound.* 2007;48:138–140.
14. Packer RA, Bergman RL, Coates JR, et al. Intracranial subarachnoid hemorrhage following lumbar myelography in two dogs. *Vet Radiol Ultrasound.* 2007;48:323–327.
15. Dewey CW. Head-trauma management. In: Dewey CW (ed.). *A Practical Guide to Canine and Feline Neurology.* Ames (IA): Iowa State University Press; 2003. p. 179–192.
16. Wessmann A, Chandler K, Garosi LS. Ischaemic and haemorrhagic stroke in the dog. *Vet J.* 2009;180:290–303.
17. Arnold SA, Platt SR, Gendron KP, et al. Imaging Ischemic and Hemorrhagic Disease of the Brain in Dogs. *Front Vet Sci.* 2020;7:279.
18. Schriger DL, Kalafut M, Starkman S, et al. Cranial computed tomography interpretation in acute stroke: physician accuracy in determining eligibility for thrombolytic therapy. *J Am Med Assoc.* 1998;279:1293–1297.
19. Garosi LS, Platt SR, McConnell JF, et al. Intracranial haemorrhage associated with *Angiostrongylus vasorum* infection in three dogs. *J Small Anim Pract.* 2005; 46:93–99.
20. Tamura S, Tamura Y, Tsuka T, et al. Sequential magnetic resonance imaging of an intracranial hematoma in a dog. *Vet Radiol Ultrasound.* 2006;47:142–144.
21. Hodshon AW, Hecht S, Thomas WB. Use of the T2*-weighted gradient recalled echo sequence for magnetic resonance imaging of the canine and feline brain. *Vet Radiol Ultrasound.* 2014 Nov-Dec;55(6):599–606.
22. Garosi LS, Platt SR. Treatment of cerebrovascular disease. In: Bonagura JD, Twedt DC (eds). *Current Veterinary Therapy XIV.* St Louis (MO): Saunders Elsevier; 2009. pp. 1074–1047.
23. Acierno MJ, Labato MA. Hypertension in dogs and cats. *Compendium* 2004;26:336–345.
24. The National Institute of Neurological Disorders and Stroke rt-PA Stroke Study Group. Intracerebral haemorrhage after intravenous t-PA therapy for ischaemic stroke. *Stroke.* 1997;28:2109–2918.
25. Ródenas S, Pumarola M, Gaitero L, et al. Magnetic resonance imaging findings in 40 dogs with histologically confirmed intracranial tumours. *Vet J.* 2011 Jan;187(1):85–91.
26. Fulkerson CV, Young BD, Jackson ND, et al. MRI characteristics of cerebral microbleeds in four dogs. *Vet Radiol Ultrasound.* 2012 Jul-Aug; 53(4):389–393.
27. Lowrie M, De Risio L, Dennis R, et al. Concurrent medical conditions and long-term outcome in dogs with nontraumatic intracranial hemorrhage. *Vet Radiol Ultrasound.* 2012 Jul-Aug;53(4):381–318.

CHAPTER 22

Traumatic brain injury

Louise Clark
BVMS, Cert VA, DECVAA, MSc (Clinical Management of Pain), FRCVS

A traumatic brain injury (TBI) can result from a forceful blow or jolt to the head or body, or from an object that pierces the skull and enters the brain. Some types of TBI can cause temporary problems with normal brain function, including problems with cognition, movement, and general behavior. Serious TBI can lead to severe and permanent disability or death.

Some injuries are considered primary, meaning the damage is immediate. Secondary effects of TBI occur gradually over the course of hours to days or appear weeks later. These secondary brain injuries are the result of reactive processes that occur after the initial head trauma and contribute significantly to morbidity.

There are two broad types of head injuries: penetrating and nonpenetrating TBI.

- Penetrating TBI (also known as open TBI) happens when an object pierces the skull (e.g., a bullet, shrapnel, a bone fragment, or a weapon such as a hammer or knife) and enters the brain tissue. Penetrating TBI typically damages only part of the brain.
- Nonpenetrating TBI (also known as closed head injury or blunt TBI) is caused by an external force strong enough to move the brain within the skull. Causes include falls, motor vehicle crashes, blast injury, or being struck by an object.

Some accidents such as explosions or other extreme events can cause both penetrating and nonpenetrating TBI in the same individual.

How TBI affects the brain

Damage resultant to TBI can be confined to one area of the brain and is known as a focal injury, or it can occur over a more widespread area and is known as a diffuse injury. The type of injury also affects how the brain is damaged. Primary effects on the brain include bleeding and tearing forces that injure nerve fibers and cause inflammation, metabolic changes, and brain swelling. Secondary brain injury (SBI) occurs in the hours or days after TBI, providing a window for therapeutic interventions. TBI can lead to more chronic syndromes:

- **Diffuse axonal injury (DAI).** This is one of the most common types of brain injuries and is usually resultant to rotational forces or sudden forceful stopping that stretches or tears axon bundles (shear stress). It commonly occurs following motor vehicle accidents, falls, or sports injuries. DAI results in widespread damage to white matter and can disrupt and break down communication among neurons in the central nervous system. The primary insult leads to a secondary cytokine cascade. Damage may be temporary or permanent, and clinical recovery can be prolonged.
- **Concussion.** This is a type of mild TBI that may be considered temporary but could take minutes to several months to heal. There is either a sudden loss of consciousness or altered state of consciousness or awareness. A second concussion closely following the first one causes further damage to the brain—the so-called "second hit" phenomenon—and can lead to permanent damage or even death in some instances. Postconcussion syndrome involves clinical signs that last for weeks or longer. Concussion is not well described in the veterinary literature.
- **Hematomas.** A hematoma is bleeding in and around the brain caused by a ruptured blood vessel. Several types of hematomas exist depending on where the blood collects relative to the meninges, which are made up of three layers: dura mater (outermost), arachnoid mater (middle), and pia mater (innermost). Epidural hematomas involve bleeding between the skull and the dura mater and can occur within minutes to hours after damage to a vessel under the skull; they are particularly dangerous. Subdural hematomas involve bleeding between the dura and the arachnoid mater, and, like epidural hematomas, they exert pressure on the outside of the brain. Subarachnoid hemorrhage (SAH) is bleeding between the arachnoid mater and pia mater. Bleeding into the brain itself is called intracerebral hematoma/hemorrhage (ICH).
- **Contusions.** Contusions are bruising or swelling of the brain that occurs when small blood vessels bleed into brain tissue. They can occur directly under the impact site ("coup" injury) or, more often, on the complete opposite side of the brain from the impact (a "contrecoup" injury). These coup and contrecoup lesions occur when the head abruptly decelerates, which

causes the brain to bounce back and forth within the skull (such as in a high-speed car crash). Note that their appearance can be delayed.

- **Skull fractures.** Skull fractures are resultant to blunt force trauma and can cause damage to the membranes, blood vessels, and brain under the fracture. Thus, they are often associated with other types of brain injury.
- **Post-traumatic neuroendocrine disorders.** The pituitary gland is sensitive to acceleration and deceleration injuries and is vulnerable because of its location. Mechanisms of damage include interruption of fragile vascular supply and the systemic stress response. Although neuroendocrine abnormalities are rare in mild TBI, hypopituitarism after severe TBI has a prevalence of 50% to 80% in people and is reported in veterinary species.[1] In the acute postinjury phase, hyperprolactinemia was the highest reported complication, followed by diabetes insipidus, syndrome of inappropriate adrenocorticotropic hormone secretion, human growth hormone deficiency, and adrenocorticotropic hormone (ACTH) deficiency. Addressing these issues can assist both cognitive and physical recovery. In the absence of clinical suspicion, current guidelines do not suggest routine monitoring of growth hormone, ACTH, thyrotropin, and gonadal axes in the acute phase in people, except for those in an induced coma because treatable neuroendocrine disorders may impede emerging consciousness. There is no guidance for veterinary species.
- **Post-traumatic hydrocephalus (PTH).** PTH is important to identify because treatment can affect the functional outcome. Ventricle enlargement owing to brain tissue atrophy or ex vacuo dilation after craniectomy makes PTH difficult to distinguish on imaging. Considering the clinical signs is helpful in conjunction with imaging. Treatment may involve the placement of a ventriculoperitoneal shunt.

Secondary brain injury

SBI occurs in the hours or days after head trauma, providing a window for therapeutic interventions. It involves a cascade of interconnected biochemical, cellular, and molecular events. Hypoxia and ischemia underlie much of the SBI, leading to cell apoptosis, cerebral swelling, DAI, and inflammation. One example of SBI is hemorrhagic progression of a contusion. These injuries occur when an initial contusion from the primary injury continues to bleed in and around the parenchyma and to expand over time, thus creating a new or larger lesion. This increased exposure to blood, which is toxic to neurons, leads to swelling and further neuronal loss. A breakdown in the blood–brain barrier allows large molecules (e.g., red blood cells, plasma proteins) to leak into the space between neurons in the brain and to trigger a chain reaction that causes brain swelling. It also causes a profound inflammatory response and permits the uncontrolled release of neurotransmitters.

Intracranial pressure

Intracranial pressure (ICP) is defined as the pressure measured within the intracranial vault. This is a dynamic parameter consisting of the systolic, diastolic, and derived mean pressures; it may fluctuate physiologically. Normal ICP (measured as the mean) is typically 10 to 20 cm H20 or 7 to 14 mmHg. ICP is governed by the relationship between the volumes of brain tissue, cerebrospinal fluid (CSF), and intracranial blood in the arterial and venous compartments enclosed within the almost rigid cranial vault. The brain parenchymal volume takes into consideration extra- and intracellular compartments and contributes ~80% of the total volume. The blood volume (which includes both arterial and venous blood) and the CSF volume each contribute ~10% of the total volume.

The Monro–Kellie doctrine or hypothesis states that the sum of the volumes of the brain, cerebrospinal fluid (CSF), and intracerebral blood is constant. An increase in one of these elements should cause a reciprocal decrease in either one or both remaining two. It is fundamental to our understanding of the negative effect of raised intracranial pressure (ICP) on the brain. In the normal healthy cranium, an equilibrium between these three components is maintained to preserve a normal intracranial pressure. If the volume of one of the components within the cranium increases, the volume of a different component must decrease to maintain this equilibrium and sustain a normal ICP. A value above 20 mmHg usually signifies the point at which intervention may be required to avoid significant or life-threatening consequences. If a pathological condition affects any one of the three components, or a new component is introduced into the almost fixed volume of the cranium, then this equilibrium may be disrupted. For example, if a patient has a TBI and a hematoma forms, initially, as the hematoma is growing, its volume may be small enough that the skull volume can accommodate it, and compensatory mechanisms can be employed to maintain a normal ICP. The main compensatory mechanisms are increased drainage of blood or CSF from the cranial cavity, which allows for space to be created for this new lesion. This means that the ICP remains normal. However, if the hematoma continues to develop, it will reach a size where these compensatory mechanisms will become exhausted, and no further drainage of blood or CSF will be possible. At this point, the equilibrium becomes disrupted, and the intracranial pressure will begin to rise (Fig. 22.1). This pressure can cause neuronal damage hypoxia by decreasing cerebral perfusion

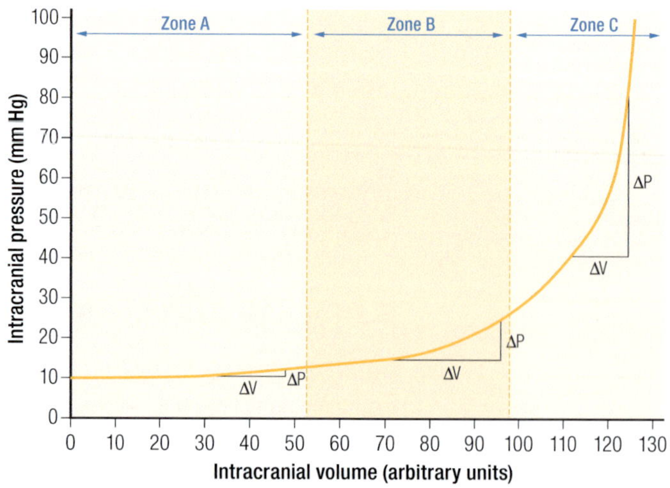

FIG. 22.1 Intracranial pressure-volume curve. Zone A: Compensatory and buffering mechanisms (decrease in cerebrospinal fluid and venous volumes) are intact and, therefore, large changes in volume cause little or no change in intrcranial pressure (ICP) (i.e., low elastance [ΔP/ΔV] with high compliance [ΔV/ΔP]). Zone B: As compensatory measures progressively reduce, the change in ICP for the same change in volume starts to increase (i.e., increasing elastance and decreasing compliance). Zone C: Once the threshold for compensatory and buffering capacity has been exceeded (the "decompensation point"), a small increase in volume results in a substantial and often exponential increase in ICP (i.e., high elastance with low to almost no compliance).

pressure (CPP) and cerebral blood flow (CBF). It can be exacerbated by arterial hypotension, hypertension, hypoxemia, edema, fever, seizures, hypo- and hyperglycemia, and hyper- and hypocapnia.

Pathophysiology after TBI. Cellular mechanisms

Figure 22.2 simplifies the pathophysiology at the cellular level after TBI.[2,3]

How to manage TBI in the acute phase

Initial physical assessment of a TBI case should focus on any imminently life-threatening abnormalities and evaluation of vital functions, all of which can influence not only the interpretation of the neurological examination but also the overall prognosis.

The aims of the neurological examination are to determine if the nervous system is affected, obtain an anatomic diagnosis (forebrain, brainstem, cerebellar, ± spinal cord involvement, or multifocal), and gain information about the prognosis.

Initial management should focus on extracranial stabilization (oxygen therapy, management of ventilation, fluid resuscitation, and support of mean arterial blood pressure), closely followed, if any of these interventions are indicated, by therapies directed towards intracranial stabilization (hyperosmolar therapy, hyperventilation) and surgical decompression.

Corticosteroids are not recommended for the treatment of TBI.

Tranexamic acid is not currently recommended for the initial treatment of TBI.

The most important consideration in TBI is maintenance of cerebral perfusion and oxygenation. Hypovolemia and hypoxemia must be recognized and treated immediately.

Brain imaging is recommended in patients with moderate to severe neurological deficits that are refractory to aggressive stabilization.[4,5]

Practical management of TBI

Initial patient assessment

Human studies have shown that up to 60% of head trauma (TBI) patients have concurrent systemic injuries involving the thorax, abdomen, spine, and/or long bones. Initial physical assessment of emergency cases should focus on any immediately life-threatening abnormalities and evaluation of vital functions, all of which can influence not only the interpretation of the neurological examination but also the prognosis for the patient. Upon arrival, the animal should be triaged, with immediate assessment of the ABCs (airway, breathing, circulation) to determine whether it is stable. Concurrent conditions, even if not critical, may require appropriate monitoring so that potential problems can be anticipated and prevented. Systemic stabilization must be prioritized to ensure CPP is maintained.

Initial neurological evaluation

Once the primary survey is complete and any conditions that are life-threatening have been identified and addressed, the specific neurological assessment can take place. Extensive blood loss, moderate or severe hypothermia, and hypoxemia should be addressed before drawing any conclusions about a patient's level of consciousness.

The aims at this stage are to:

- Determine whether the nervous system is indeed affected.
- Obtain an anatomic diagnosis (forebrain, brainstem, cerebellum, spinal cord, or multifocal).
- Gain information about the prognosis.

The neurological examination of a dog with TBI consists primarily in an evaluation of mental status, posture and gait, and cranial nerve function.

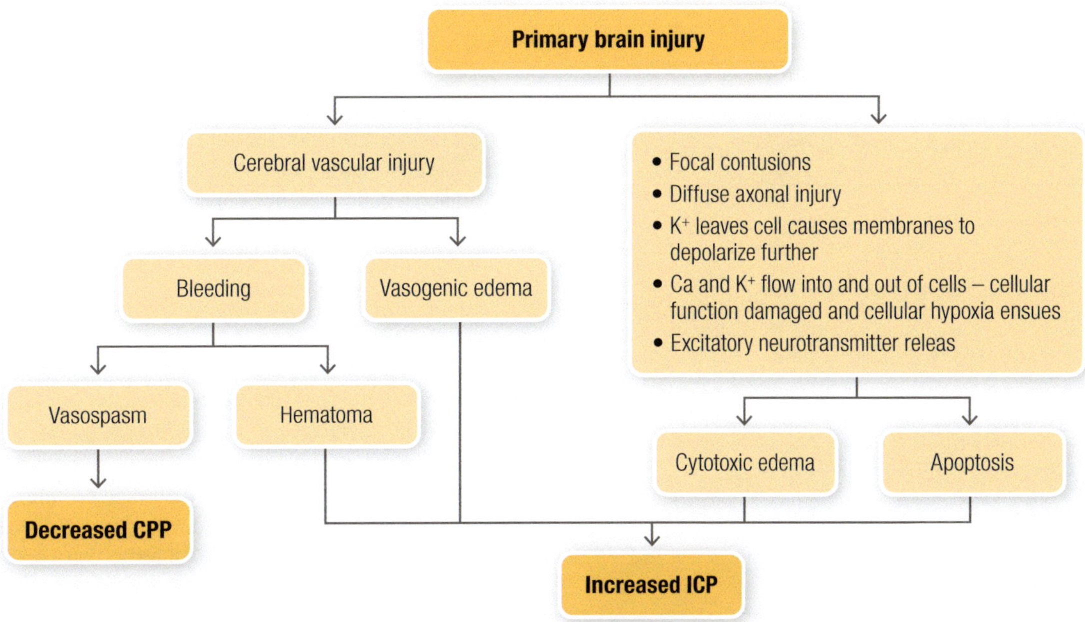

FIG. 22.2 Pathophysiology at the cellular level after traumatic brain injury. CPP, cerebral perfusion pressure; ICP, intracranial pressure.

Injuries involving the brainstem or causing increased ICP can result in severe alterations in mental status, leading to stupor or coma. Permanent lateral recumbency and severe motor changes indicate direct brainstem injury or severe increased ICP.

The primary goal of cranial nerve examination is to assess the integrity of the brainstem functions. Regular assessment of pupil size and the pupillary light reflex (PLR) is critical because of its ease of execution, its repeatability, and the importance of the prognostic information it provides.

In mild trauma, the pupils are isochoric and normoresponsive. In more severe trauma, the pupils are myotic and poorly responsive (or not at all) to light stimulation. More severe intracranial injuries associated with a poor short-term prognosis are characterized by mydriatic and unresponsive pupils.

The Modified Glasgow Coma Scale (MGCS) is a scoring system that plays an important role in the assessment of dogs with TBI and can be useful in triage and monitoring of patients over time. The MGCS covers three areas: 1) level of consciousness, 2) posture and limb motor function, 3) brainstem reflexes — with a score of 1–6 being assigned to each domain. The total score ranges from 3 to 18, with lower scores indicating more severe neurological deficits (Table 22.1).[4,7]

Readers are directed to references 4 and 6 as well as to Chapter 1, which discusses altered mentation in detail.

TABLE 22.1 Modified Glasgow Coma Scale.[7]

		Score
Motor activity	Normal gait, normal spinal reflexes	6
	Hemiparesis, tetraparesis, or decerebrate activity	5
	Recumbent, intermittent extensor rigidity	4
	Recumbent, constant extensor rigidity	3
	Recumbent, constant extensor rigidity with opisthotonus	2
	Recumbent, hypotonia of muscles, depressed or absent spinal reflexes	1
Brain stem reflexes	Normal pupillary light reflexes and oculocephalic reflexes	6
	Slow pupillary light reflexes and normal to reduced oculocephalic reflexes	5
	Bilateral unresponsive miosis with normal to reduced oculocephalic reflexes	4
	Pinpoint pupils with reduced to absent oculocephalic reflexes	3
	Unilateral, unresponsive mydriasis with reduced to absent oculocephalic reflexes	2
	Bilateral, unresponsive mydriasis with reduced to absent oculocephalic reflexes	1
Level of consciousness	Occasional periods of alertness and responsive to environment	6
	Depression or delirium, capable of responding but response may be inappropriate	5
	Semicomatose, responsive to visual stimuli	4
	Semicomatose, responsive to auditory stimuli	3
	Semicomatose, responsive only to repeated noxious stimuli	2
	Comatose, unresponsive to repeated noxious stimuli	1

It is important that the initial neurological examination is interpreted in the light of the cardiovascular and respiratory systems, as shock can have a significant effect on neurological status.

The neurological assessment should be repeated every 30–60 min in severe head injury to evaluate for deterioration and monitor the efficacy of any therapies administered.

Recent work[7] concludes that the MGCS score is a useful prognostic indicator in both dogs and cats. However, a single value in individual patients should not be used in isolation to prognosticate survival in patients with TBI. Although an almost linear correlation between the MGCS score on admission and the probability of survival over a 48-hour period exists in dogs, there is limited data assessing long-term outcome and functional outcome in dogs or cats with TBI. The impact of any sedation or other pharmacological intervention on the ability to perform an effective neurological assessment should always be considered.

Additional point-of-care testing

Because of the likelihood of multisystemic injury associated with head trauma, the initial emergency database should focus on the degree of blood loss (packed cell volume [PCV]/total solids); blood glucose; blood pressure; electrocardiography; and arterial blood gas analysis to assess perfusion, ventilation, oxygenation, and acid–base status.

Specific consideration should be given to serum glucose concentration since cats with head trauma may have hyperglycemia, and the degree of hyperglycemia is associated with the severity of head trauma. However, the degree of hyperglycemia does not appear to be associated with the outcome in cats but may be in dogs.[7] The development of hyperglycemia following head trauma is considered a component of the stress response to injury, which results in many metabolic alterations.

Point-of-care ultrasound (POCUS) of the thoracic and abdominal cavities may be indicated, as may thoracic radiography prior to consideration of any advanced imaging.

Advanced imaging

Brain imaging is recommended in cases with moderate to severe neurological deficits that are refractory to stabilization and in those with progressive neurological signs. Skull radiographs are usually of limited value but can sometimes identify fractures of the calvarium. The two modalities of choice are magnetic resonance imaging (MRI) and computed tomography (CT). Both have their advantages, although CT seems to be the most suitable for cases with head trauma (being faster, less expensive, and providing a better resolution of bone details and acute hemorrhage).

Brain Trauma Foundation guidance – how do we apply it?

There is very little species-specific evidence relating to the management of clinical TBI in cats and dogs. Readers can refer to the Brain Trauma Foundation (BTF) guidance for humans,[8] which can be modified based on the available resources and specific patient needs.

The initial approach should focus on systemic stabilization (oxygen therapy, management of ventilation, fluid resuscitation, and support of mean arterial blood pressure), closely followed, if any of these interventions are indicated, by therapies directed towards intracranial stabilization (hyperosmolar therapy, hyperventilation) and surgical decompression.

Other metrics, such as ICP (intracranial bolt), CPP, and brain oxygenation, are important in the acute hospitalization phase in people but are rarely available in veterinary medicine outside research facilities.

Monitoring

Patients with suspected TBI should be monitored for hypoxemia (<90% arterial hemoglobin saturation), hypotension (<100 mmHg systolic blood pressure [SBP]), hypertension (150 mmHg SBP or higher), hypoventilation (end-tidal CO2 >45 mmHg), hyperventilation (end-tidal CO_2 <35 mmHg) and hypo- or hyperthermia.

Oxygenation, blood pressure, ventilation

Blood oxygen saturation should be continuously measured with a pulse oximeter, and supplemental oxygen administered to maintain saturation above 90%.

Arterial blood pressure should be measured using the most accurate method available, and it should be measured frequently (every 5–10 min) or monitored continuously if possible.

Ventilation should be assessed for all patients with an altered level of consciousness. Continuous capnography (if available) can be used but has limited utility if the patient is panting. Arterial blood gas (ABG) analysis to assess $PaCO_2$ is preferable if available.

Temperature

The patient's temperature should be measured, and efforts undertaken to maintain euthermia. There is no benefit to hypothermia.

Managing airway, ventilation, and oxygenation

All patients with suspected severe TBI should be placed on continuous oxygen supplementation via a nasal cannula (with care) or face to minimize secondary insults related to hypoxia. Methods of oxygen supplementation that cause stress or induce coughing/sneezing should be avoided.

Patients with a decreased level of consciousness should be nursed and positioned to maintain a clear airway. A slight head-up positioning is preferable to maintain CPP and reduce CVP, but this must not exceed 30 degrees.

Hypoxemia (oxygen saturation [SpO_2] <90%) should be monitored using continuous pulse oximetry and corrected immediately by:

- Ensuring appropriate airway positioning (brachycephalic dogs and craniofacial trauma cases).
- Administering continuous, supplemental oxygen.
- If signs of hypoxia persist (central cyanosis and/or hypoxemia on pulse oximetry/ABG) despite increasing the flow and concentration of continuous supplemental oxygen, consider endotracheal intubation and mechanical ventilation if deemed ethical and appropriate.

Fluid therapy

Intravenous fluids should be administered. Hypotensive patients should be treated with blood products and/or isotonic fluids to target systolic blood pressure of approximately 100 mmHg.

No specific fluid has shown benefit. Albumin administration is associated with worse outcomes. Hypertonic fluid resuscitation may be administered to patients in whom increased ICP is suspected; CPP should be prioritized.

Hyperventilation and hyperosmolar therapy for suspected increased ICP

Persistent hyperventilation should be avoided. Ventilation strategies should target eucapnia and avoid hypocapnia (i.e., end-tidal CO_2 of 35 mmHg approx. to target a $PaCO_2$ of 4.5–5.0 Kpa, monitored using capnography). Confirmation of $PaCO_2$ by blood gas analysis is ideal (see guidance above). When used to address signs of active and imminent herniation, hyperventilation should target an end-tidal CO_2 of 30 mmHg using capnography. In veterinary patients, this is generally going to be in animals that are already anesthetized. Ethics of mechanical ventilation in TBI cases should be carefully considered.

Tranexamic acid

Administration of tranexamic acid (TXA) therapy is not generally and widely indicated for the prophylactic treatment of suspected ICH or elevated ICP.[9,10] TXA is a low-cost drug with minimal adverse effects; many centers will continue to administer this as an early treatment for all patients with isolated TBI despite a lack of comparative (human) evidence of benefit.

Hyperosmolar therapy

Although hyperosmolar therapy may lower ICP, there was insufficient evidence about its effects on clinical outcomes to support a specific recommendation in the current BTF guidance or the use of any specific hyperosmolar agent for patients with severe TBI. The following considerations can be taken into account:

- Osmotherapy can reduce intracranial pressure after TBI.
- Mannitol and hypertonic saline have distinct actions and adverse effects.
- There is currently no evidence to support the overall superiority of one agent.
- It is unknown whether osmotherapy improves neurological outcome or mortality in TBI.[11]
- Mannitol should not be used until CPP is restored, whereas hypertonic saline can be considered as part of the resuscitation process because it augments blood volume.

Steroids

The use of steroids acutely in TBI is not recommended for improving outcome or reducing ICP.[9] In patients with severe TBI, high-dose methylprednisolone was associated with increased mortality and is contraindicated.

Seizure management

Seizures can occur following TBI and may worsen SBI. Current practice tends to be to manage seizures initially as they occur (often with benzodiazepines), and if they are frequent, longer-acting antiseizure medications are initiated. Levetiracetam is a novel antiepileptic drug that has become increasingly popular due to its low incidence of adverse effects.

Decompressive craniectomy

While there is extensive data in people, including the recent RESCUEicp (Randomized Evaluation of Surgery with Craniectomy for Uncontrollable Elevation of Intracranial Pressure) trial, decisions in veterinary medicine tend to be made on a case-by-case basis, depending upon finances, pathology, prognosis, and the availability of skilled neurosurgeons and anesthetists. Outcome must be carefully considered.

Analgesia and sedation

Rationale and indications for sedation

Sedation may be part of clinical care in the management of TBI and is used for its direct and indirect neuroprotective effects, reducing further SBI. Sedation lowers cellular metabolism in the brain, potentially reducing tissue hypoxia and ischemia. It reduces ICP and mitigates the ICP elevation caused by agitation, anxiety, and coughing/crying. Sedation may also aid in the prevention of seizures. While sedatives have the potential to improve outcomes, they can be challenging to administer and are associated with potentially dangerous complications, which must be considered when choosing and using sedative drugs.

Veterinary hospitals do not have specialized neurointensive care units or high dependency units. Monitoring of these patients may be limited, consisting of intermittent measurement of vital signs. Continuous monitoring of vital signs, invasive blood pressure, and particularly ICP monitoring is often not possible. Therapeutic options such as continuous infusions, vasoactive medications, mechanical ventilation, and other advanced organ support modalities may not be available or ethically appropriate. Evidence-based guidelines for sedation in veterinary patients are not readily available.

Choice of sedative drugs and other aspects of patient care

Sedation should be effective, safe, affordable, and feasible. The ideal sedative drug should have neurophysiological benefits, including lowering ICP and cerebral blood flow and improving cerebral perfusion; it should not produce active metabolites; and it should be easy to titrate and with a low risk of side-effects and complications. Sedatives that are complex to use or require advanced devices for administration are less appropriate, and intermittent provision rather than infusion may need to be considered in some settings. There is little evidence favoring one drug over another in veterinary TBI patients.

Hypotension and hemodynamic instability can result from sedation, and treatment with IV fluids should always be available. Vasopressors, such as noradrenaline given continuously using a syringe driver, are very useful for treating sedation-induced hypotension if available and should be given through a central venous catheter if possible.

Other important aspects of patient care must always be considered. These include overall nursing care and physiotherapy management (e.g., standing and turning). Bladder management (including urinary catheterization) to aid urine output monitoring is helpful. Adequate nutrition should be established early and in accordance with the degree of pathology, especially in animals with craniofacial trauma.

KEY POINTS

When managing a traumatic brain injury (TBI) case, it is essential to bear the following in mind:

- Prioritize systemic assessment. Cerebral perfusion and oxygenation are dependent upon systemic blood pressure and oxygenation.
- The initial neurological examination can provide information about the prognosis. Neurological assessment should be repeated every 30–60 minutes.
- Initial management should focus on extracranial stabilization through the following:
  - Oxygen therapy
  - Fluid resuscitation
  - Support of arterial blood pressure
- Extracranial stabilization should be closely followed by therapies directed towards intracranial stabilization (hyperosmolar therapy, hyperventilation) and surgical decompression if any of these interventions are indicated.
- Corticosteroids are not recommended for the treatment of TBI.
- Tranexamic acid is not currently recommended for the initial treatment of TBI.
- Brain imaging is recommended in patients with moderate to severe neurological deficits that are refractory to aggressive stabilization.[4,5]

References

1. Platt SR, Chrisman CL, Graham J, Clemmons RM. Secondary hypoadrenocorticism associated with craniocerebral trauma in a dog. *Am Anim Hosp Assoc.* 1999 Mar-Apr;35(2):117–122.
2. Capizzi A, Woo J, Verduzco-Gutierrez M. Traumatic Brain Injury: An Overview of Epidemiology, Pathophysiology, and Medical Management. *Med Clin North Am.* 2020;104(2):213–238.
3. Flavin K, Morkane C, Marsh S. In: *Questions for the Final FFICM Structured Oral Examination.* Cambridge University Press; 2018:i-ii.
4. Garosi L, Adamantos S. Head trauma in the cat: 2. assessment and management of traumatic brain injury. *J Fel Med Surg.* 2011;13(11):815–823.
5. Fletcher D, Syring R. Traumatic brain injury. In: Silverstein D, Hopper K (eds.). *Small Animal Critical Care Medicine.* St Louis: Elsevier Saunders, 2009. pp. 658–662.
6. Platt SR, Radaelli ST, McDonnell JJ. The prognostic value of the modified Glasgow Coma Scale in head trauma in dogs. *J Vet Intern Med.* 2001;15(6):581–584.
7. Cameron S, Weltman JG, Fletcher DJ. The prognostic value of admission point-of-care testing and modified Glasgow Coma Scale score in dogs and cats with traumatic brain injuries (2007–2010): 212 cases. *J Vet Emerg Crit Care (San Antonio).* 2022;32(1):75–82.
8. Carney N, Totten AM, O'Reilly C, et al. Guidelines for the Management of Severe Traumatic Brain Injury, 4th ed. [Internet]. Brain Trauma Foundation; 2016 Sep [cited 17 Oct 2024]. Available from: https://braintrauma.org/coma/guidelines/guidelines-for-the-management-of-severe-tbi-4th-ed
9. Wiles MD. Management of traumatic brain injury: a narrative review of current evidence. Anaesthesia. 2022 Jan;77 Suppl 1:102–112.
10. Siebers NW, Steiner LA. Anesthesia for traumatic brain injury. Curr Opin Anaesthesiol. 2024 Oct 1;37(5):486–492.
11. Freeman N, Welbourne J. Osmotherapy. science and evidence-based practice. *BJA Education.* 2018;18(9):284–290.

CHAPTER 23

Idiopathic peripheral vestibular disease

Marika Menchetti
DVM, PhD, DECVN

Gualtiero Gandini
DVM, PhD, DECVN

The vestibular system is primarily responsible for maintaining balance in the body, a function accomplished through integration with the visual system and the general proprioceptive system. The vestibular system also plays a key role in maintaining a correct posture and coordinating eye movements with the position and movement of the head.[1,2] Dysfunction of the vestibular system produces a complex of clinical signs referred to as vestibular syndrome, which is characterized by varying degrees of loss of balance and results in postural instability, gait incoordination, and altered eye movements.[3]

Vestibular disorders are one of the most common reasons for neurological consultations in primary care veterinary practices. Of these, idiopathic peripheral vestibular disease (IPVD) is certainly one of the most common.[3–5]

The vestibular apparatus is anatomically divided into a peripheral and a central part. The peripheral part consists of structures located in the inner ear, the vestibule and semicircular canals, and the vestibular component of the 8th pair of cranial nerves. The central part consists of the four vestibular nuclei located in the brainstem and the flocculonodular lobule and fastigial nucleus located in the cerebellum (Fig. 23.1).[1–3]

The clinician must always keep this anatomical division in mind when approaching an animal with vestibular signs, since the etiology, treatment, and, above all, the prognosis, are very different depending on whether the dysfunction involves the peripheral or the central part of the vestibular system.[3]

The reader is encouraged to read Chapter 3 of this book for information on the functional anatomy of the vestibular apparatus and the clinical signs associated with vestibular dysfunction.

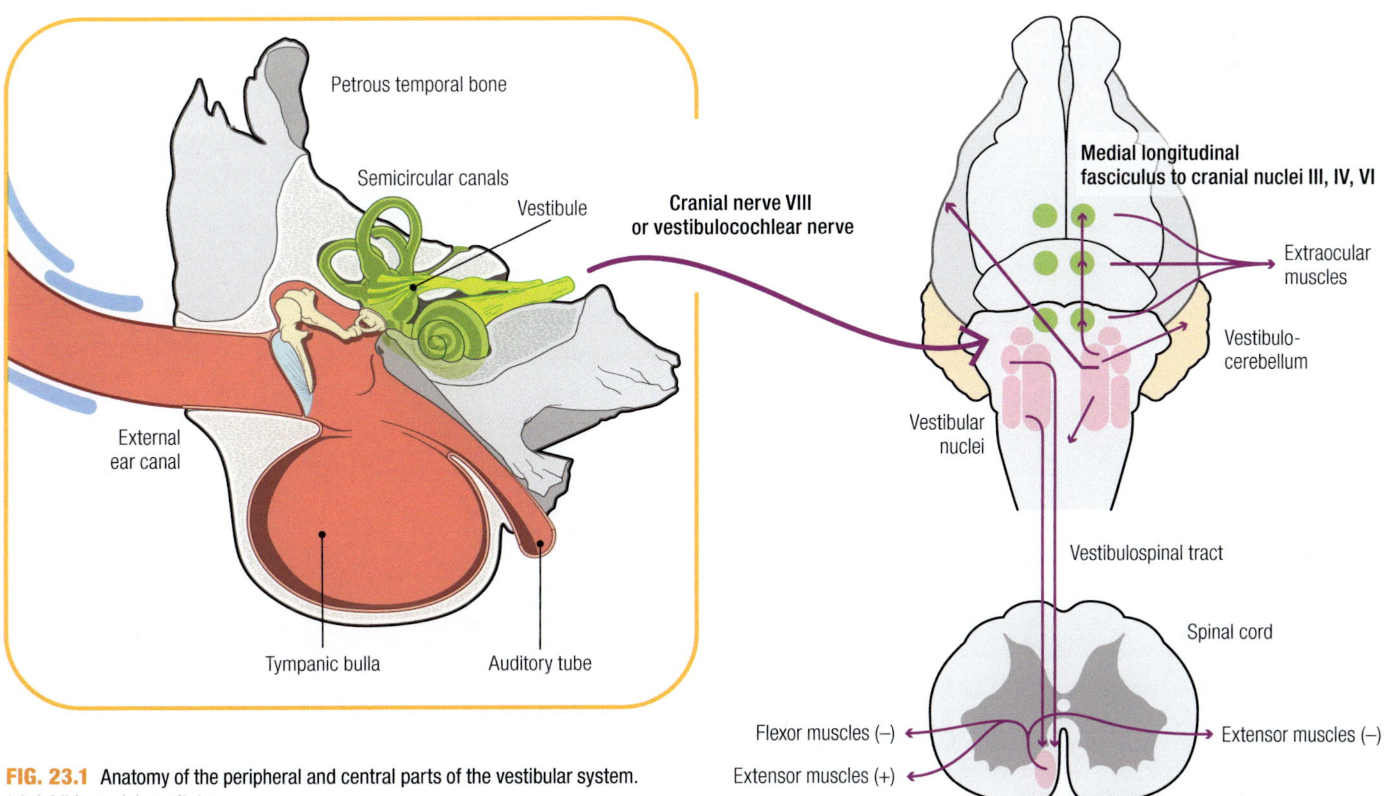

FIG. 23.1 Anatomy of the peripheral and central parts of the vestibular system. (–), Inhibitory; (+), excitatory.

Etiology

IPVD is one of the most common causes of peripheral vestibular dysfunction in dogs, and it is considered the most common presumptive clinical diagnosis in older dogs with acute signs of unilateral peripheral vestibular dysfunction.[1–5]

Over time, IPVD has been named in different ways, including benign idiopathic vestibular disease[1,4] and idiopathic vestibular syndrome (IVS).[2,4–6] The term "facial and vestibular neuropathy of unknown origin" (FVNUO) has been used in some papers to refer to those cases with clinical signs consistent with facial and vestibular neuropathy.[7,8]

Despite its frequency, IPVD still lacks a specific definition. A 2023 survey among veterinary neurologists showed that IPVD could be defined as a condition with a peripheral vestibular localization that is acute or peracute in onset and improves spontaneously and quickly.[6]

The lack of a specific definition is at the basis of possible controversies. In a large case series published in 1983, IPVD was considered the second most common cause of peripheral vestibular disease (PVD).[4] A 2020 retrospective study in 188 dogs concluded that IPVD is the most common cause of PVD and is associated with advanced age.[5] In their study, the authors diagnosed IPVD "when the MRI [magnetic resonance imaging] was unremarkable or identified facial and/or vestibulocochlear nerve changes in the absence of other abnormalities", which, strictly speaking, is not completely compliant with the definition of an idiopathic disease.

The etiology of IPVD is still debated and not yet clear. Because IPVD has a spontaneous benign course, pathology studies of the inner ear of affected dogs are lacking. Furthermore, the postmortem examination of the inner ear is not a routine procedure, as it requires decalcification of the petrous part of the temporal bone, making it difficult or impossible to detect possible abnormalities.[1]

It is possible that IPVD represents a functional disorder associated with a dysfunction of the membranous labyrinth, as proposed for Ménière's disease in humans.[1–3,6]

As in dogs, there are some PVDs in humans of unknown etiology. The most common cause of dizziness/vertigo worldwide is paroxysmal benign positional vertigo, which is characterized by paroxysmal vertigo and nystagmus occurring when the head is in a particular position. It is explained by migration of degenerated otoconia into the semicircular canals, rendering them sensitive to head motion.[9]

Ménière's disease is characterized by recurrent attacks of vertigo. The most acknowledged theory is that the paroxysmal attacks are related to the distension (endolymphatic hydrops) and rupture of the membranous labyrinth, which disrupts the homeostasis of inner ear fluids and leads to episodes of vertigo, tinnitus, hearing loss, and a feeling of "stuffed ears".[2,10]

Vestibular neuritis has been described in humans as a paroxysmal and prolonged single attack of vertigo. The cause is still uncertain, but there is increased evidence suggesting a reactivation of latent type 1 herpes simplex virus.[11]

Clinical presentation

IVPD can be seen at any age but is considered atypical in dogs under 5 years of age. Older, large breed dogs appear to be overrepresented, with an average age of 9–13 years.[2,3,12,13] For this reason, the syndrome is sometimes referred to as "geriatric vestibular disease".[2–5,14] In a 2021 study, an older age and higher bodyweight were significantly associated with a diagnosis of IVPD.[14]

The onset of clinical signs is typically peracute to acute. Affected dogs show clinical signs of acute unilateral vestibular dysfunction that may vary widely according to the severity of the disease. They include ipsilateral head tilt, vestibular ataxia, pathological horizontal or rotatory nystagmus with the fast phase directed away from the side of the head tilt, and vestibular strabismus (Figs. 23.2 and 23.3, Video 23.1).[2–4]

Vomiting may accompany or anticipate the onset of neurological vestibular signs.[3]

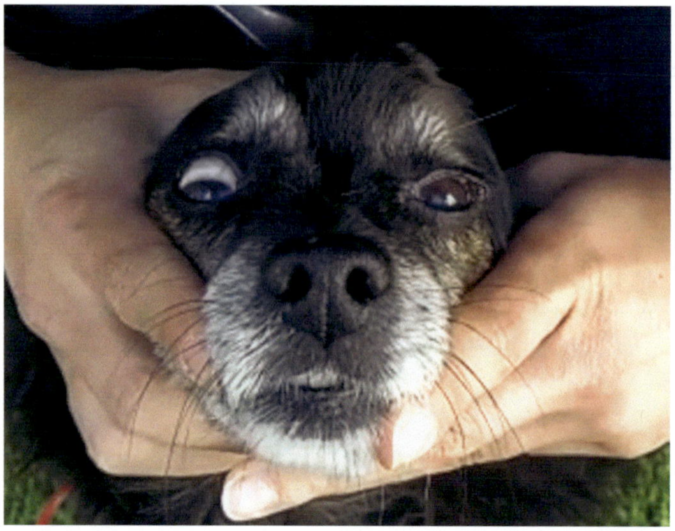

FIG. 23.2 Twelve-year-old mixed breed spayed female dog with idiopathic peripheral vestibular disease. Vestibular strabismus of the right eye is present. Vestibular strabismus is a ventral/ventrolateral strabismus observed when the head is in certain positions, e.g., elevated as in the picture or when the dog is kept lying on its back. The strabismus is ipsilateral to the site of the vestibular lesion.

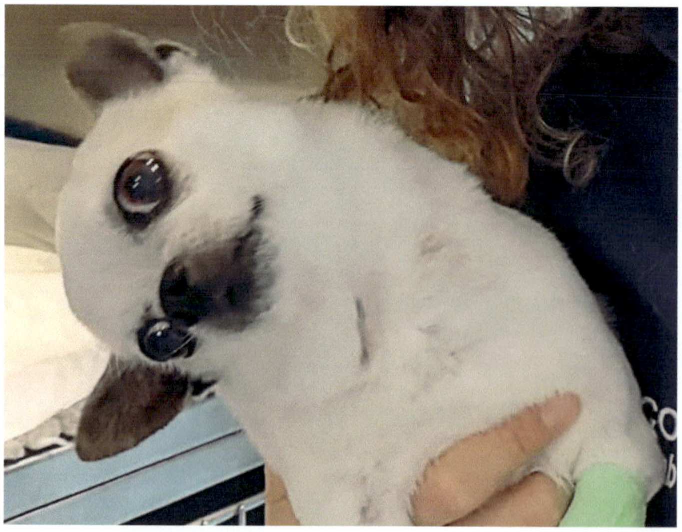

FIG. 23.3 Eleven-year-old male Chihuahua dog affected by idiopathic peripheral vestibular disease. A marked right-sided head tilt can be observed. The head tilt reflects the loss of coordination between the head and the neck, trunk, and limbs and is ipsilateral to the vestibular lesion. The side of the head tilt is defined according to the side on which the ear is held lower.

In milder cases, patients are ambulatory and vestibular ataxia is characterized by a tendency to lean and drift to the affected side, whereas in the most severe cases, the dog is unable to stand and will fall to the side of the lesion at any attempt to walk. In extreme cases, rolling may be observed, although it is not common in IPVD. In severe cases, caregivers can be overwhelmed by the severity of the acute presentation. They should be aware that, in general, the severity of the clinical signs is not correlated with the outcome of the disease, which improves rapidly within a few days (Video 23.2).[14]

In the past, acute IPVD was misdiagnosed as a stroke and often resulted in the unnecessary euthanasia of the dog.[1] A recent study in dogs with vestibular disease (VD) in primary care in the United Kingdom showed that 11.6% of the dogs were euthanized on first veterinary presentation with VD.[12]

According to most authors, dogs affected by IPVD should not have concurrent neurological signs,[3,14] although facial nerve neuropathy has been reported to be associated with IPVD in retrospective studies, in which it has been described in up to 50% of dogs.[1,2,5]

A condition called "facial and vestibular neuropathy of unknown origin" (FVNUO) has been described in dogs with facial paralysis and vestibular signs.[7] In these cases, MRI demonstrated involvement of the facial nerve more easily than vestibular involvement.[7,15] The presence of vestibular signs along with facial nerve dysfunction is probably related to their common pathway, as these nerves enter the petrous part of the temporal bone through the internal acoustic meatus and are enclosed in a common dural sheath.[7,15]

Based on the results of the most recent publications, it seems likely that IPVD is an umbrella term that encompasses more than one underlying cause, explaining the possible involvement of the facial nerve, the different MRI findings, and the outcome and recurrence of the clinical signs.[5] This leads to the consideration of whether the term IVPD is still appropriate to define this complex of signs or whether, based on new studies, the nomenclature should be reconsidered to define something that produces similar vestibular dysfunction with a benign outcome and is not probably due to a single etiology.

Differential diagnosis

It is crucial for the veterinarian to differentiate between peripheral and central vestibular syndrome. Evaluation of the mental status, cranial nerves, and, mainly, postural reactions is critical to making the correct anatomical diagnosis. Unfortunately, especially in the most severe cases, the neurological examination is not easy to perform and interpret due to the patient's difficulty in maintaining balance and the possible dysphoric/hyperexcited behavior. For this reason, it is always recommendable that the neurological examination is followed by appropriate advanced diagnostic imaging. In a retrospective study in 93 dogs with VD, the consistency between the neurological examination and the MRI findings was greater for central than for peripheral VD.[13] MRI results confirmed the lesion localization in 61 of the 62 (98.4%) dogs diagnosed with a central vestibular lesion on neurological examination, while 24 of the 31 dogs (77.4%) diagnosed with PVD on neurological examination had a lesion consistent with this diagnosis on their MRI scans.[13]

IPVD is diagnosed by ruling out other diseases that result in similar clinical signs and, more specifically, causes of peripheral vestibular dysfunction. Otitis media/interna (OMI) is considered one of the most common causes of PVD. Other less common causes include hypothyroidism, neoplasia of the ear and tympanic bulla, trauma, and ototoxicity. Most of these causes require diagnostic imaging to be ruled out. Trauma and ototoxicity may be suspected based on the patient's history.

OMI may be accompanied by discomfort or pain at palpation of the area and when opening the mouth. Facial nerve paralysis is a common clinical finding associated with OMI that results in absent ipsilateral blinking, an ipsilateral widened palpebral fissure, and an inability to move the ipsilateral ear and lips, which are flaccid. The absent tone of the inferior lip may provoke drooling.[16] Enophthalmos, third eyelid protrusion, and miosis of the ipsilateral pupil (Horner's syndrome) can also be commonly observed in case of OMI.

Otoscopy should always be performed in a patient displaying vestibular signs. In case of OMI, otoscopy may result in tympanic rupture or bulging and/or loss of translucence of the tympanic membrane. It is worth noting that the presence of an intact tympanic membrane does not rule out the occurrence of OMI.[2]

Clinicopathological findings

The minimum database should always include a complete blood count, biochemistry profile, and urinalysis, also due to the necessity to perform general anesthesia for advanced diagnostic imaging. As for many other neurological disorders, clinicopathological findings are often normal and not very helpful in discriminating the possible causes of the vestibular signs. An exception is hypothyroidism, which may produce increased

Video 23.1

Neurological examination of a 12-year-old mixed breed spayed female dog with idiopathic peripheral vestibular disease. The dog shows vestibular ataxia, right-sided head tilt, circling towards the right, right vestibular strabismus, pathological nystagmus with the fast phase directed to the left, normal postural and proprioceptive reactions, and normal spinal reflexes. Video by Marika Menchetti.

Video 23.2

Neurological examination of a 16-year-old mixed breed spayed female dog with idiopathic peripheral vestibular disease. The video shows the extreme difficulty in maintaining posture and walking unassisted immediately after onset. One week later, the dog has greatly improved but still shows signs of vestibular ataxia (drifting to the right) and a marked right head tilt. After 4 weeks, the ataxia had disappeared, and the head tilt was still present but had significantly improved. No treatment was administered. Video by Gualtiero Gandini.

cholesterol and triglyceride levels and a mild regenerative anemia. Confirmation of hypothyroidism requires evaluation of thyroid function through specific blood exams.

Cerebrospinal fluid analysis in dogs with IPVD, except in rare cases of mild pleocytosis or albuminocytological dissociation, appears to be within the normal limits.[5,17] This test can be of value in excluding other disorders, including diseases affecting the central part of the vestibular system.

Diagnostic imaging findings

Because the clinical signs of a peripheral or central lesion are often similar, advanced imaging is required to assess whether the peripheral or central part of the vestibular system is affected.

Imaging studies of the peripheral vestibular system should be normal in animals with IPVD.

Radiographs of the tympanic bullae and petrous part of the temporal bone are of limited value in the diagnostic workup of VD, as they are difficult to obtain and interpret and lack sensitivity.[18] For these reasons, conventional radiography should not be used when investigating vestibular disorders. Computed tomography (CT) offers advantages over conventional radiographs, especially when bone lesions are suspected, but MRI is the gold standard technique for evaluating the middle and inner ear due to its greater resolution of soft tissues, including the membranous labyrinth and its associated neural elements.[18] MRI scans are generally described as normal in patients with IPVD.[5,8,13,14,18]

As previously mentioned, several recent studies have documented MRI facial and vestibular nerve abnormalities in patients with IVPD.[5,7,14,15] In a study in dogs with FVNUO, high-field MRI studies showed contrast medium enhancement of the facial nerve, while low-field MRI examination yielded variable results, including an inability to detect the facial nerve, most probably due to technical limitations.[7] Another MRI study demonstrated the superior ability to visualize the facial nerve using thin-slice sequences.[15] These findings show that the use of high-field MRI in the diagnostic approach of PVD is producing new information and may lead in the future to a change in the current nomenclature.

A recent study that used high-field MRI showed a significant difference in the utricle asymmetricity ratio (UAR) between dogs with IPVD and unaffected dogs, suggesting a possible correlation between a structural atrophy of the vestibular system and IPVD.[8]

Treatment

Treatment of IPVD, considering its spontaneous benign course, is mainly supportive and symptomatic. Initial signs of improvement can be seen within 3 to 5 days, and most cases of IPVD resolve completely over 3–4 weeks.[2,3] In some dogs, a residual head tilt may be observed.[2,3] There is no evidence that medical treatment with corticosteroids or nonsteroidal anti-inflammatory drugs accelerates or influences recovery in IPVD-affected dogs.[3]

In the first 24 to 48 hours, if the clinical signs are severe, treatment with benzodiazepines or acepromazine may reduce the intensity of the clinical signs.[1]

Nausea and vomiting associated with vestibular disease can be treated symptomatically, although failure to control nausea can sometimes occur. A 2023 study collecting the opinion of experts on the diagnosis and treatment of IVS showed that maropitant at a dosage of 1 mg/kg once daily was the most commonly selected antiemetic. Metoclopramide and ondansetron were more rarely chosen.[6] Nausea can occur separately and should not be considered only as a sign preceding vomiting. Recently, two studies suggested a good efficacy of ondansetron, a 5-HT3-receptor antagonists against nausea in dogs with vestibular syndrome.[19,20]

Propentofylline at the dosage of 3 mg/kg twice daily was considered by European specialists.[6]

Prognosis

IPVD is considered a benign disorder with a good prognosis, with spontaneous resolution of the clinical signs within 1–3 weeks, although some dogs may require more time for a complete resolution of the signs.[1–5,14] A large retrospective study on PVD showed that the most common persistent sign was head tilt, affecting approximately one third of the patients. The same study on long-term follow-up showed relapse of vestibular signs in 17.6% of the dogs affected by IVPD.[5]

KEY POINTS

- Idiopathic peripheral vestibular disease (IPVD) is one of the most common causes of peripheral vestibular dysfunction.
- IPVD is a benign disorder of unknown etiology affecting adult and older dogs.
- Vestibular neurological signs are typically peracute/acute in onset and may appear very severe despite the benign course of the disease.
- Nausea and vomiting may precede or accompany the vestibular signs.
- Diagnosis of IPVD is made by ruling out other vestibular diseases, and MRI plays a crucial role in the diagnostic process.
- Therapy is symptomatic and supportive and includes antiemetic and antinausea treatment.
- The prognosis is good, and clinical signs usually resolve spontaneously within 1–3 weeks, but some dogs may take longer to fully recover.
- A few dogs may experience a relapse or a persistent head tilt.

References

1. Vestibular System: Special Proprioception. In: de Lahunta A, Glass E, Kent M, (eds.) *De Lahunta's Veterinary Neuroanatomy and Clinical Neurology*, 5th ed. Philadelphia, USA: Elsevier; 2021. pp. 345–373.
2. Kent M, Platt SR, Schatzberg SJ. The neurology of balance: function and dysfunction of the vestibular system in dogs and cats. *Vet J.* 2010 Sep;185(3):247–258.
3. Rossmeisl JH Jr. Vestibular disease in dogs and cats. *Vet Clin North Am Small Anim Pract.* 2010 Jan;40(1):81–100.
4. Schunk KL, Averill DR Jr. Peripheral vestibular syndrome in the dog: a review of 83 cases. *J Am Vet Med Assoc.* 1983 Jun 15;182(12):1354–1357.
5. Orlandi R, Gutierrez-Quintana R, Carletti B, et al. Clinical signs, MRI findings and outcome in dogs with peripheral vestibular disease: a retrospective study. *BMC Vet Res.* 2020 May 25;16(1):159.
6. Mertens AM, Schenk HC, Volk HA. Current definition, diagnosis, and treatment of canine and feline idiopathic vestibular syndrome. *Front Vet Sci.* 2023 Sep 22;10:1263976.
7. Jeandel A, Thibaud JL, Blot S. Facial and vestibular neuropathy of unknown origin in 16 dogs. *J Small Anim Pract.* 2016 Feb;57(2):74–78.
8. Won S, Yoon J. MRI utricle diameter asymmetry is significantly greater in dogs with idiopathic vestibular syndrome compared with unaffected dogs. *Vet Radiol Ultrasound.* 2020 Sep;61(5):540–544.
9. Kim HJ, Park J, Kim JS. Update on benign paroxysmal positional vertigo. *J Neurol.* 2021 May;268(5):1995–2000. Erratum in: *J Neurol.* 2021 May;268(5):2001.
10. Wright T. Menière's disease. *BMJ Clin Evid.* 2015; Nov 5:2015:0505.
11. Jeong SH, Kim HJ, Kim JS. Vestibular neuritis. *Semin Neurol.* 2013 Jul;33(3):185–194.
12. Radulescu SM, Humm K, Eramanis LM, et al. Vestibular disease in dogs under UK primary veterinary care: Epidemiology and clinical management. *J Vet Intern Med.* 2020 Sep;34(5):1993–2004.
13. Bongartz U, Nessler J, Maiolini A, et al. Vestibular disease in dogs: association between neurological examination, MRI lesion localisation and outcome. *J Small Anim Pract.* 2020 Jan;61(1):57–63.
14. Harrison E, Grapes NJ, Volk HA, et al. Clinical reasoning in canine vestibular syndrome: Which presenting factors are important? *Vet Rec.* 2021 Mar;188(6):e61.
15. Smith PM, Gonçalves R, McConnell JF. Sensitivity and specificity of MRI for detecting facial nerve abnormalities in dogs with facial neuropathy. *Vet Rec.* 2012 Oct 6;171(14):349.
16. Garosi LS, Lowrie ML, Swinbourne NF. Neurological manifestations of ear disease in dogs and cats. *Vet Clin North Am Small Anim Pract.* 2012 Nov;42(6):1143–1160.
17. Danciu CG, Szladovits B, Crawford AH, et al. Cerebrospinal fluid analysis lacks diagnostic specificity in dogs with vestibular disease. *Vet Rec.* 2021 Nov;189(10):e557.
18. Garosi LS, Dennis R, Schwarz T. Review of diagnostic imaging of ear diseases in the dog and cat. *Vet Radiol Ultrasound.* 2003 Mar-Apr;44(2):137–146.
19. Foth S, Meller S, Kenward H, et al. The use of ondansetron for the treatment of nausea in dogs with vestibular syndrome. *BMC Vet Res.* 2021 Jun 21;17(1):222.
20. Henze L, Foth S, Meller S, et al. Ondansetron in dogs with nausea associated with vestibular disease: A double-blinded, randomized placebo-controlled crossover study. *J Vet Intern Med.* 2022 Sep;36(5):1726–1732.

CHAPTER 24

Neoplasms affecting the central nervous system

John H. Rossmeisl
DVM, MS, DACVIM
(SAIM and Neurology)

Definition and etiology

A neoplasm, or tumor, is a "new growth", an abnormal proliferation of tissue, the growth of which exceeds and is uncoordinated with the surrounding normal parent tissue and persists after cessation of the stimuli that initiated the change. Neoplasms affecting the central nervous system (CNS) are a common etiology of morbidity and death in middle-aged to geriatric dogs and are classified as primary or secondary tumors.[1–3] Primary tumors (PTs) arise from the constitutive tissues of the brain and spinal cord, namely the meninges, glia, and neurons. Secondary tumors (STs) represent those cancers that spread hematogenously to the CNS from a distant, non-neural organ or compromise the neural parenchyma via direct local extension from a neighboring tissue, as may occur with nasal or vertebral tumors.

The incidence of brain tumors in necropsy-based studies ranges from 2–4.5% in dogs.[1] Tumors of the CNS can be seen in animals of any age; however, approximately 90% of these tumors have been reported in dogs >5 years old.[1,4] The proportions of PTs and STs affecting the canine CNS are nearly equal.[3] There are well-documented breed predilections for some CNS tumors, with >50% of all gliomas occurring in specific brachycephalic breeds (Boxers, Boston Terriers, English and French Bulldogs). This predisposition has been associated with a genetic susceptibility locus on canine chromosome 26.[4] The incidence of meningiomas is higher in Golden Retrievers and Boxers than in other breeds, and Golden Retrievers are also predisposed to choroid plexus tumors (CPTs).[4] Corgis and Shetland Sheepdogs are predisposed to developing primary CNS histiocytic sarcoma.[4]

Although histomorphological and immunohistochemical investigations have resulted in the description of dozens of neuropathologically distinct CNS tumor entities, a limited number of tumors account for most of those seen in clinical practice (Table 24.1). Meningiomas, gliomas, and CPTs account for 90% of PTs in the canine brain.[2,4] Hemangiosarcomas, pituitary tumors, lymphomas, and metastatic carcinomas account for most STs affecting the brain.[3]

The incidences of vertebral and spinal cord tumors in dogs are unknown, but overall, these tumors appear to occur less frequently than intracranial neoplasms.[2] Tumors affecting the vertebral column and spinal cord are commonly classified based on the circumferential tumor location relative to the neuraxis (Table 24.1).[2,5] Extradurally located tumors frequently arise from the vertebra and account for 50% of tumors affecting the vertebral column and spinal cord, while intradural-extramedullary tumors account for 35%, and intramedullary tumors for 15%.[2,5] Osteosarcoma is the most common extradural tumor arising from the vertebra, and meningiomas are the most common PT of the spinal cord and most common tumor found in the intradural-extramedullary location.

Large-breed, older dogs are predisposed to the development of vertebral tumors, and Boxers are overrepresented among dog breeds with spinal cord meningiomas.[2] Spinal cord PTs, such as ependymomas and gliomas, are more commonly seen in dogs <6 years old, and young German Shepherds and Golden Retrievers (<3 years of age) are predisposed to nephroblastoma.[2,5]

Clinical features

General clinical features and pathophysiology

The clinical signs manifested in most animals with CNS tumors reflect the disease location in the neuraxis rather than the disease etiology. Since most PTs and locally invasive STs manifest as solitary mass lesions, they are classically associated with chronic and progressive signs of focal brain or spinal cord dysfunction referable to the neuroanatomical location of the tumor.[2,4] Notably, the clinical presentation of dogs with a functional pituitary ST is often predominated by the presence of polysystemic clinical signs referable to hypercortisolism, without any observed neurological dysfunction. There may be visible or palpable mass lesions in dogs with tumors of the skull or vertebrae secondarily compromising the brain or spinal cord, respectively.

TABLE 24.1 Tumors frequently affecting the central nervous system (CNS) of dogs.

Brain tumors			
Primary tumors	**Proportion of CNS primary tumor diagnoses**	**Frequency of specific tumor type/grade**	
Meningioma	40–50%	Grade I (benign)	56%
		Grade II (atypical)	43%
		Grade III (malignant)	1%
Glioma	30–35%	Astrocytoma	20–25%
		High-grade	60–95%
		Low-grade	5–40%
		Oligodendroglioma	60–70%
		High-grade	75–83%
		Low-grade	15–25%
		Undefined glioma	5–13%
Choroid plexus tumors	6–10%	Grade I (papilloma)	36%
		Grade II (atypical)	2%
		Grade III (carcinoma)	62%

Secondary tumors	Proportion of CNS secondary tumor diagnoses	Comments
Pituitary tumors	10–25%	Majority are corticotroph adenomas
Lymphoma	12–20%	Also rarely occurs as primary tumor
Hemangiosarcoma	30–35%	Can also affect spinal cord
Various carcinomas	10–20%	Mammary, urothelial, pulmonary

Tumors of the axial skeleton and spinal cord		
Extradural	**Intradural-extramedullary**	**Intramedullary**
Primary bone tumors ■ Osteosarcoma ■ Chondrosarcoma ■ Multilobular tumors of bone	Meningioma	Glioma ■ Astrocytoma ■ Oligodendroglioma
Metastatic carcinomas	Nerve sheath tumors	Ependymoma
Multiple myeloma	Nephroblastoma	Hemangiosarcoma
Lymphoma	Lymphoma	Lymphoma
Fibrosarcoma		Metastatic carcinomas
Histiocytic sarcoma		Histiocytic sarcoma

Video 24.1

Paradoxical central vestibular signs in a dog with a right 4th ventricular choroid plexus tumor, depicted in the magnetic resonance image at the end of the video.

CNS tumors are space-occupying mass lesions that compress or invade the brain or spinal cord parenchyma by their growth and subsequently induce a cascade of secondary detrimental changes in the adjacent neuropil. Tumors variably cause edema, hemorrhage, necrosis, and inflammation in neural tissues, each of which can exacerbate the clinical manifestations of disease beyond those associated with the presence of a mass lesion.[2,4] Depending on the size and location of the tumor, cerebrospinal fluid (CSF) flow can also become obstructed, resulting in secondary hydrocephalus or syringohydromyelia.[2,4,5] As brain tumors and peritumoral changes progress within the closed confines of the calvarium, autoregulatory mechanisms that normally maintain intracranial pressure homeostasis are eventually overwhelmed, and intracranial hypertension develops and subsequently compromises brain perfusion. Brain herniations represent the terminal effects of mass lesions and intracranial hypertension and are often associated with acute and catastrophic clinical deterioration.[4]

Tumors of the nervous system, and particularly those affecting the vertebral column or spinal cord, may also result in clinical signs of pain.[2,5] Pain may arise from compression, stretching, inflammation, or invasion of the meninges, nerve roots, periosteum, or surrounding musculature, or from alterations in the processing of painful stimuli in the case of animals with syringohydromyelia.[5]

Clinical features of brain tumors

Tumors involving rostrotentorial brain structures occur more frequently than those arising infratentorially.[2,4] Epileptic seizures are a very common clinical presentation, occurring in 50–70% of dogs with forebrain tumors.[2,4] The presence of a brain tumor should be highly suspected in dogs that experience a new onset seizure after 5 years of age, especially in breeds with known brain tumor predispositions. Dogs with tumors involving the frontal lobe, associated with falcine or subtentorial brain herniations, and demonstrating marked contrast enhancement on magnetic resonance imaging (MRI) have been identified as having an increased risk for developing epileptic seizures.[6] Depressed levels of consciousness and abnormal behaviors are also common clinical complaints, and an acute and rapidly progressive decline in the level of consciousness with postural abnormalities (decerebrate or decerebellate postures) are hallmark signs of intracranial hypertension and brain herniations.[2,4] Central vestibular dysfunction (Video 24.1) is the most common clinical manifestation of brainstem tumors. Approximately 10% of dogs with brain tumors will also demonstrate signs of pain referable to the head or neck.

Although CNS tumors are usually associated with focal clinical signs of brain dysfunction, multifocal clinical signs can be observed. Multifocal signs can occur due to: a large tumor volume involving multiple brain regions; extensive peritumoral brain edema; a tumor-associated mass effect that compromises adjacent brain structures; multiple, discrete tumor foci (occurs in some meningiomas, with subarachnoid dissemination of CPT, or hematogenous ST); or diffuse brain involvement (gliomatosis cerebri, lymphoma).[2,4]

Clinical features of vertebral and spinal cord tumors

Dogs with vertebral and spinal cord tumors commonly present with progressive myelopathic signs, often with concurrent evidence of pain, referable to the neuroanatomical location of the tumor.[2,5] In cases with primary or metastatic vertebral tumors, pain may be the only clinical sign present and can be unrelenting and severe. Acute clinical deterioration with marked exacerbation of neurological deficits may occur secondary to a pathological fracture of neoplastic vertebrae or to hemorrhage in or around the spinal cord.

Clinicopathological findings

Routine clinical pathological tests, such as hemograms, biochemical profiles, and urinalyses, rarely provide data that are specific for the underlying cause of the neurological signs observed in dogs with CNS tumors.[4] However, as CNS tumors typically affect middle-aged to older dogs that may have significant concurrent disease, these tests are generally indicated to evaluate the animal's systemic health status, prior to the performance of higher-yield diagnostics that require general anesthesia (e.g., MRI, CSF analysis, tumor biopsy).

Diagnostic imaging findings

Radiography, myelography, and ultrasonography

Skull radiography is not usually helpful for the diagnosis of PTs of the brain, although radiographs can be useful when evaluating cases with locally invasive STs, especially for those with abnormalities of the head on clinical examination. In dogs with paraspinal hyperpathia or myelopathic signs, vertebral column radiographs may identify primary vertebral body tumors, pathological fractures, osseous metastases, as well as evidence of concurrent malignancy or disease, but are frequently normal in dogs with spinal cord tumors.[2]

Although it is very rare for CNS PTs to metastasize to extraneural organs, concurrent and unrelated neoplasms have been observed in up to 23% of dogs with PTs, the majority of which involved the thoracic or abdominal cavities.[7] Thus, imaging of the thorax and abdomen by means of thoracic radiography, abdominal ultrasonography, or thoracic and abdominal computed tomography (CT) should be considered in an attempt to identify related or unrelated neoplasms or other significant comorbidities, particularly prior to undertaking treatment of CNS tumors.[2]

Myelography has been used to diagnose vertebral and spinal cord tumors and assists in longitudinal and circumferential localization of the lesions in these cases. However, considering the invasiveness, potential adverse effects, and relatively nonspecific features of tumors on myelography, these studies have largely been supplanted by MRI examinations for the evaluation of dogs with spinal cord disease.

Cross-sectional imaging of the neuraxis

Cross-sectional imaging techniques, including CT and MRI, have revolutionized the antemortem diagnosis and management of CNS tumors.[2,4] MRI is the preferred modality for the evaluation of animals with neurological disease, due to its superior sensitivity and specificity compared to CT. The specificity of MRI is high (~95%) for CNS tumors, although its sensitivity is generally lower (50–90%) across all types of tumors.[8] Imaging-derived data, such as tumor number (solitary vs. multiple), origin within the neuraxis (extra-axial, intra-axial, or intraventricular in the brain; extradural, intradural-extramedullary, or intramedullary in the vertebral column), and intrinsic signal appearances collectively provide characteristic features that allow for refinement of the list of differential diagnoses and of the presumptive diagnosis of the most frequently observed CNS tumors (Table 24.2, Fig. 24.1).[4,5,9] A normal MRI examination does not exclude the possibility of a CNS tumor; normal imaging studies are a notable feature of diffuse tumors such as lymphoma and gliomatosis cerebri.

Meningiomas are the most frequently diagnosed extra-axial brain tumors and intradural-extramedullary spinal cord tumors in dogs. MRI features of meningiomas (Table 24.2, Figs. 24.1A-24.1C) typically include a broad base of attachment, well-defined tumor margination, dural tail sign, and marked and often uniform contrast enhancement. Meningiomas may also contain intratumoral fluid, cysts, or mineralization, and can be associated with calvarial hyperostosis.[4,9] The specific grades and histological subtypes of meningioma cannot be distinguished using standard MRI sequences.

Gliomas originate within the neuropil and thus appear as expansile intra-axial or IM mass lesions that may displace or invade the neural parenchyma of the brain or spinal cord.[4,5,9] Gliomas can appear well or poorly marginated and may or may not demonstrate enhancement following intravenous contrast administration.[4,9] The imaging appearances of the various types of gliomas have substantial overlap, and it is very difficult to accurately predict glioma type or grade using conventional MRI techniques (Table 24.2). However, high-grade tumors are more likely to demonstrate contrast enhancement (Figs. 24.1D and 24.1E). Compared to astrocytomas, oligodendrogliomas are also more likely to be T1 hypointense, contact or distort the ventricles, and demonstrate the T2-FLAIR (fluid-attenuation inversion recovery) mismatch sign, which is characterized by a homogeneous hyperintense T2-weighted signal and a hypointense signal with a hyperintense peripheral rim on FLAIR sequences.[10] The imaging features of gliomas, cerebrovascular accidents, and inflammatory lesions can be quite similar, and these categories of intra-axial lesions are frequently misclassified.[8,10]

CPTs are the most common intraventricular tumors, and these tumors often uniformly contrast enhance or are associated with ventriculomegaly or obstructive hydrocephalus (Figs. 24.1F and 24.1G).[4] Approximately 50% of CPTs are found in association with the 4th ventricle, 33% in the 3rd ventricle, and the remainder in the lateral ventricles. Choroid plexus carcinomas can be discriminated from choroid plexus papillomas if intraventricular or subarachnoid metastatic tumor foci are identified on MRI exams.

The imaging appearances of some STs (Table 24.2), such as pituitary tumors (Figs. 24.1H and 24.1I), osteosarcoma (Fig. 24.1J), lymphoma (Fig. 24.1K), multilobular tumors of bone, and hemangiosarcoma (Figs. 24.1L and 24.1M) have been described elsewhere, and each of these tumors is associated with some specific imaging features.[2,5,9] There are also imaging characteristics of the numerous types of extradural vertebral tumors that can assist with prioritization of differential diagnoses. For example, mesenchymal tumors are more likely to demonstrate substantial alteration of vertebral shape, cortical bone lysis (Fig. 24.1J), and heterogenous contrast enhancement, while round cell tumors of the vertebral column tend to spare cortical bone and have homogenous contrast enhancement (Fig. 24.1K).[11]

TABLE 24.2 Magnetic resonance imaging features of canine central nervous system (CNS) tumors.

Primary tumors

Imaging features	Meningioma	Astrocytoma	Oligodendroglioma	Choroid plexus tumor
Mass location	■ Extra-axial or extradural	■ Intra-axial or intramedullary	■ Extra-axial or extradural	■ Intra- or juxtaventricular (4th ventricle)
Lesion number	■ Usually solitary	■ Solitary	■ Usually solitary	■ Solitary or multiple (carcinoma)
T1-weighted signal intensity	■ Iso- to hypointense	■ Iso- to hyperintense	■ Iso- to hypointense	■ Hyper-, iso-, or hypointense
T2-weighted signal intensity	■ Hyper- to isointense	■ Hyperintense, often heterogeneous	■ Hyperintense, often heterogeneous	■ Hyperintense in 90%
Contrast-enhancement pattern and severity	■ Uniform, moderate to marked	■ Partial or ring, mild to severe* ■ No enhancement in 20%	■ Partial or ring, mild to severe* ■ No enhancement in 25%	■ Homogenous, marked
Peritumoral edema	■ Present in 90%	■ Any degree	■ Usually minimal to moderate	■ Present in >50%
Other features	■ Dural tail in 35% ■ Cystic regions in 20%	■ Cystic regions ■ Intratumoral hemorrhage	■ Ventricular distortion ■ Cystic regions ■ Intratumoral hemorrhage ■ T2-FLAIR mismatch sign	■ Often multilobular ■ Ventriculomegaly in 75%
Imaging differential diagnoses	■ Histiocytic sarcoma ■ Granular cell tumor ■ Inflammatory granuloma ■ Neuroblastoma	■ Oligodendroglioma ■ Cerebrovascular accident ■ Inflammatory granuloma ■ Hematogenous metastasis	■ Astrocytoma ■ Cerebrovascular accident ■ Inflammatory granuloma ■ Hematogenous metastasis	■ Ependymoma ■ Intraventricular meningioma ■ Cholesterol granuloma ■ Epidermoid cyst

Secondary tumors

Imaging features	Pituitary tumor	Osteosarcoma	Hemangiosarcoma	Lymphoma
Mass location	■ Extra-axial (sellar region)	■ Extra-axial or extradural	■ Intra-axial or intramedullary	■ Any location or combination of locations
Lesion number	■ Solitary	■ Solitary	■ Usually multiple	■ Usually multiple
T1-weighted signal intensity	■ Isointense	■ Mixed (iso-, hypo-, and hyperintense)	■ Mixed (iso-, hypo-, and hyperintense)	■ Iso- to hypointense
T2-weighted signal intensity	■ Hyperintense (mild)	■ Mixed (iso-, hypo-, and hyperintense)	■ Mixed (hypo- to hyperintense)	■ Majority hyperintense
Contrast-enhancement pattern and severity	■ Homogenous, marked	■ Usually moderate to severe, heterogenous	■ Often peripheral or ring type	■ Usually moderate to severe
Peritumoral edema	■ Variably present in large tumors	■ Variably present	■ Often marked	■ Variably present
Other features	■ Compression of thalamus/3rd ventricle ■ Intratumoral hemorrhage	■ Cortical lysis in majority ■ Changes in adjacent soft tissues ■ Alteration of vertebral shape	■ Intratumoral hemorrhage common	■ +/- Features of infarction or hemorrhage ■ Preservation of vertebral shape
Imaging differential diagnosis	■ Meningioma ■ Germ cell tumor ■ Craniopharyngioma	■ Undifferentiated sarcoma ■ Chondrosarcoma ■ Multilobular tumor of bone ■ Fibrosarcoma	■ Hematogenous metastases ■ Cerebrovascular accidents	■ Meningoencephalitis ■ Cerebrovascular accidents

* Features more commonly noted in high-grade tumors. FLAIR, fluid-attenuation inversion recovery.

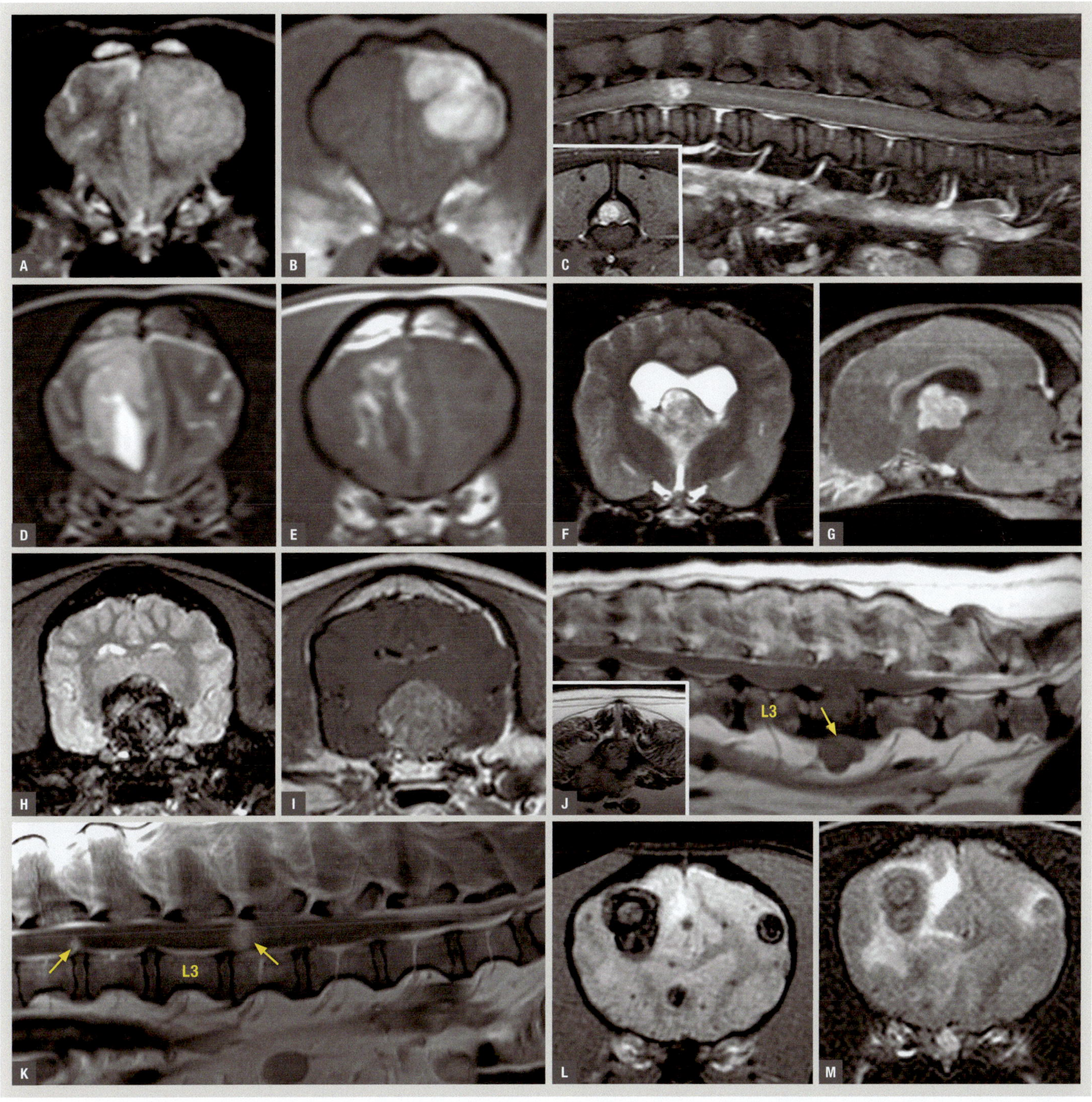

FIG. 24.1 Magnetic resonance imaging features of primary (**A-G**) and secondary (**H-M**) tumors affecting the canine central nervous system. Intracranial (**A, B**) and intraspinal (**C**) meningiomas characterized by well-defined masses with broad base of attachment, T2 hyperintensity (**A**), marked and uniform contrast enhancement (**B, C**), and dural tail sign (**B**). High-grade astrocytoma (**D, E**) demonstrating a heterogenous T2 signal (**D**) associated with an intratumoral cyst and partial ring enhancement (**E**). Multilobular 3rd ventricular choroid plexus tumor (**F, G**) associated with ventriculomegaly, with mixed T2 signal (**F**) and uniform contrast enhancement (**G**). Pituitary macrotumor (**H, I**) with marked intratumoral hemorrhage on T2* (**H**) and marked contrast enhancement (**I**). Osteosarcoma (**J**) manifesting as a multilobular, T2 iso- to hypointense mass that effaces the 4th lumbar vertebra, with marked extension of the mass into the paraspinal musculature (arrow). Spinal lymphoma (**K**) appearing as multiple, contrast-enhancing intramedullary nodules (arrows). Metastatic intracranial hemangiosarcoma characterized by multiple, variably sized T2* (**L**) and T2 hypointense (**M**) hemorrhagic lesions surrounded by perilesional edema.

Other diagnostic procedures

Tumor biopsy

Despite the utility and common clinical use of MRI for the presumptive antemortem diagnosis of CNS tumors, histopathological examination of representative tissue is required for the definitive diagnosis.[2,4] Tumors are histologically classified and graded using morphological criteria modeled after the World Health Organization criteria applied to human tumors. The grade reflects the biological behavior of the tumor, with lower grades tumor representing well-differentiated neoplasms with low proliferative potential and higher grades indicating increasing tendency towards anaplastic, mitotically active, and rapidly progressive cancers.[4] Excisional biopsy performed during surgical treatment of CNS tumors is the most frequent biopsy technique currently performed in veterinary practice. In cases in which the tumor may not be amenable to surgical resection, image-guided stereotactic biopsy or fine-needle aspiration of the brain, vertebra, or spinal cord can provide an alternative means for safely and effectively sampling the lesion for diagnosis.[2,4]

Cerebrospinal fluid analysis

CSF abnormalities are extremely sensitive indicators of CNS disease, and CSF is often abnormal in patients with CNS tumors.[4] However, the severity of elevated CSF total protein concentrations and types of pleocytoses that can be observed are highly variable and often nonspecific for neoplastic disease or tumor type. CSF analysis can assist with discrimination of choroid plexus carcinomas from papillomas, as a CSF total protein concentration >80 mg/dL was exclusively associated with a carcinoma diagnosis. Dogs with CNS lymphoma, histiocytic sarcoma (Fig. 24.2), and choroid plexus tumors also frequently exfoliate neoplastic cells into the CSF; these can be identified on cytological examination.[2]

Electroencephalography

Electroencephalography (EEG) examinations can provide information that supports the existence of a focal pathological process in dogs with brain tumors, but the EEG abnormalities identified are not specific for the presence of neoplasia or tumor type. The main diagnostic utility of EEG recordings is to confirm the presence of epileptic seizure activity in dogs presenting with paroxysmal events or unusual or stereotypical behavioral abnormalities.

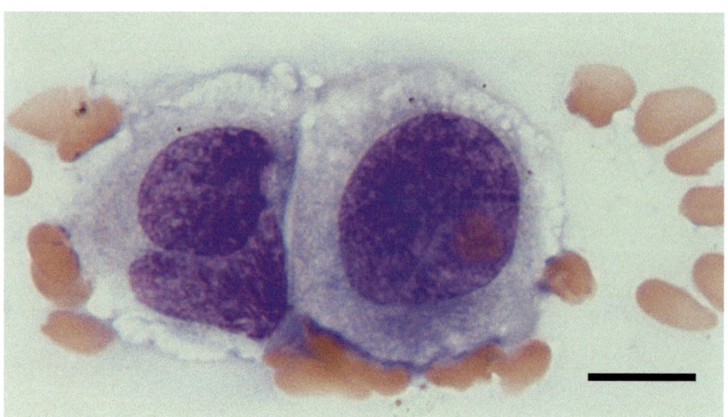

FIG. 24.2 Cerebrospinal fluid cytospin preparation from a dog with histiocytic sarcoma. Note the large, neoplastic, round cells with multiple and atypical nuclei admixed with numerous red blood cells. Wright's–Giemsa stain, bar = 12 µm.

Treatment and prognosis

General approaches to and current limitations of treatment

There are two basic approaches to the treatment of CNS tumors:

1. Administering palliative treatments with the goal of mitigating tumor- and patient-specific clinical signs to transiently improve quality of life by alleviating tumor-induced mechanisms of brain and spinal cord injury.
2. Using therapies with known direct or indirect antitumor effects with the intent of improving the quantity and quality of life by reducing the tumor burden or proliferative capacity of the neoplasm. Antitumor modalities used to treat CNS cancers include cytoreductive surgery, radiation treatment, and chemotherapeutics. These modalities are frequently used in various combinations, as well as in conjunction with palliative therapies.

The types of drugs primarily used for palliative care include: antiseizure drugs (ASDs) for tumor-associated structural epilepsy; corticosteroids (prednisone 0.5–1.0 mg/kg per os [PO] every 12–24 h) targeting peritumoral vasogenic edema and neuroinflammation; and analgesics for signs consistent with somatic, visceral, or neuropathic cancer pain.[4] Although epileptic seizures are a very common clinical sign associated with brain tumors, optimal ASD treatments of tumor-associated epilepsy are currently unknown.[4] Phenobarbital (2.5–3 mg/kg PO every 12 h), levetiracetam (20–30 mg/kg PO every 8 h), and zonisamide (5–10 mg/kg PO every 12 h) are frequently used ASDs. Further details on ASDs can be found in Chapter 16. Multiple ASDs are often required to control epileptic seizures in dogs with brain tumors, and poor seizure control is a frequent cause of euthanasia in dogs undergoing any kind of treatment for brain tumors.[4,12] Because dogs with CNS neoplasms are frequently receiving corticosteroids, non-NSAID analgesics are often prescribed (e.g., codeine 1 mg/kg PO every 8 h, gabapentin 10 mg/kg PO every 8–24 h, amantadine 3 mg/kg PO every 24 h).[2]

There is currently a considerable lack of evidence-based data regarding tumor type-specific therapeutic outcomes for many tumors affecting the CNS, as well as a lack of controlled trials comparing efficacies of treatment modalities.[4,12] Studies evaluating the treatment of CNS tumors in dogs frequently contain substantial limitations, such as the inclusion of small case numbers with no histopathological diagnoses or control groups, variable treatment protocols and endpoints, or a lack of inclusion of quantitative outcome metrics of therapeutic efficacy.[4,12] However, among studies that have included comparisons of dogs with CNS tumors receiving palliative versus antitumor treatments, most have demonstrated a significant survival benefit in those dogs receiving at least one antineoplastic treatment, regardless of tumor type.[4,5,12]

Treatment of brain tumors

Palliative care

The prognosis of dogs with PTs of the brain treated palliatively is poor, with median survival times (MSTs) in the 1- to 3-month range, with nearly one-third of deaths or euthanasias occurring within 2 weeks of diagnosis.[4] Palliative care of functional pituitary tumors is associated with more favorable outcomes, with a MST of nearly 12 months.[4,12]

Surgery

Surgical resection of brain tumors is associated with several advantages; these include the ability to establish a definitive histopathological diagnosis and the rapid reduction of ICP by reducing or eliminating the tumor burden, which often leads to a rapid postoperative clinical improvement in clinical signs. However, as excision of tumor-free histological margins is generally not achievable in brain tumor cases, surgery is rarely curative for canine PTs, with local recurrence occurring commonly.[2,4,12–14]

Surgical treatment of superficially located cerebral and cerebellar convexity, olfactory, parasagittal, and falcine meningiomas results in a MST of ~12 months. Surgery for meningiomas located on the floor of the skull or ventral brainstem is technically challenging and has not been frequently reported.

The currently available evidence indicates that management of canine gliomas using surgery as a sole modality is associated with a poor prognosis, with a MST of 2–3 months, which can improve to 6–9 months when surgery is combined with adjuvant radiation therapy, chemotherapy, or investigational therapeutics.[4,14] Surgical removal of intra-axial tumors is technically challenging, as these tumor types are poorly delineated and infiltrative, and it is thus more difficult to discriminate tumor margins from normal brain tissue.

Surgery can also be effective for the management of some STs. When performed by experienced surgeons, transsphenoidal hypophysectomy is capable of producing rapid and durable endocrinological and clinical remissions (77% 24-month disease free fraction) in cases of pituitary-dependent hypercortisolism, particularly when performed in cases without significant enlargement of the pituitary gland.[15] STs of the skull, such as multilobular tumors of bone, can also be managed surgically with good long-term outcomes, depending on the tumor grade.

Recent studies indicate that >94% of dogs with brain tumors treated surgically will survive to hospital discharge.[4,12–14] Adverse events associated with surgical treatment include a transient decline in neurological status, aspiration pneumonia, intracranial hemorrhage or infarction, provoked seizures, and electrolyte and osmotic disturbances.[4,12–13]

Radiation therapy

Radiation therapy (RT) has been demonstrated to be beneficial for extending the life and improving clinical signs in dogs with PTs and STs when used as a primary or adjunctive modality.[4,12] Inferring tumor-specific outcomes from the RT literature is confounded by a lack of histologically diagnosed tumors in most studies, grouping of heterogeneous intracranial masses into study designs, and significant variability in the RT protocols used.[2,4,15]

When studies with multiple types of presumptively diagnosed masses and treatment protocols are included, MSTs ranging from are reported in dogs treated with RT as a sole treatment modality for a PT.[2,15] MSTs associated with RT of extra-axial masses (mostly presumptive meningiomas) range from 9–19 months.[2,15] RT is also a useful adjuvant therapy for meningiomas, with combined surgical and RT producing MSTs of 16–30 months.[4] The reported MST for intra-axial tumors (presumptive gliomas) treated with RT ranges from 9–23 months.[4,15] Retreatment of brain tumors with RT upon recurrence has also been associated with a survival advantage. It is currently unclear if RT with adjuvant chemotherapy offers any clinically relevant benefits over RT alone.[4,12]

RT is effective at reducing tumor size, improving neurological signs, and providing a survival benefit in dogs with pituitary tumors, although it does not induce endocrinological remission as readily or completely as transsphenoidal hypophysectomy.[2,15] RT may be the preferred therapy for large pituitary tumors that cannot be safely treated with surgery.[4,12,15]

Adverse effects of RT are observed in approximately 10% of brain tumor cases and include aspiration pneumonia, pulmonary thromboembolism, acute CNS toxicity (deterioration in consciousness), and damage to at-risk organs in the treatment field.[4,12] Most RT-associated adverse events can be successfully managed with symptomatic treatment, and acute CNS toxicity is often responsive to treatment with corticosteroids.

Chemotherapy

There is very little evidence-based data evaluating the efficacy of chemotherapies for the management of brain tumors, with many of the limitations being the same as those described for RT.[4,12,16] Lomustine, temozolomide, and hydroxyurea are chemotherapy drugs often used for brain tumors, as they can all penetrate the blood–brain barrier.[4,16] When chemotherapy is used as a monotherapy in the setting of gross disease, results in dogs with presumptive brain tumors indicate that such a treatment provides modest or no survival benefits, with one study reporting that lomustine treatment had no impact on survival compared to palliative care, and another indicating that dogs receiving lomustine lived significantly longer (MST, 4 months) than those that received only supportive care (MST, 1 month).[12,16] At the doses prescribed to dogs, lomustine, temozolomide, and hydroxyurea are well tolerated, with discontinuation of treatment rarely necessary.[12,16]

Treatment of tumors of the vertebral column and spinal cord

The outcomes associated with many types of vertebral or spinal cord tumors are unknown due to very limited numbers of reported cases that received treatment, and highly variable treatment protocols.

Palliative care

Palliative treatment for vertebral and spinal cord tumors involves treating peritumoral edema with corticosteroids, multimodal pain relief protocols, and urinary bladder management plans as indicated by clinical signs. In addition to the analgesics described for use for brain tumors, dogs with bone pain from vertebral tumors may also experience pain relief from treatment with bisphosphonates (e.g., alendronate, pamidronate) or palliative courses of RT. Palliative treatment rarely results in extended survivals or prolonged improvements in myelopathic signs, with the MST typically <2 months.[2,5,17–18] As for brain tumors, regardless of the treatments administered, many dogs with spinal cord tumors die due to recurrence or progression of the neurological signs.[2,5,17–20]

Surgery and radiotherapy

In addition to providing a histopathological diagnosis, cytoreductive surgery often imparts a significant acute clinical benefit to the patient as it leads to decompression of the spinal cord regardless of the tumor type. As a sole treatment modality, surgery is the most efficacious for PTs of the spinal cord. The average MST for intraspinal meningiomas treated with surgery alone is approximately 15 months. Use of postoperative RT in dogs with intraspinal meningiomas increased the MST to approximately 45 months, and neurological decline was significantly slower in dogs receiving adjuvant RT than in dogs that did not.[18] Dogs with nephroblastoma treated with cytoreductive surgery and/or RT survived longer (MST, 12 months) than dogs treated palliatively (MST, 2 months).[19]

The long-term prognosis associated with vertebral tumors is guarded to poor, with an overall MST of 4.5 months (range, 0.5–10 months) in dogs with a variety of tumor types; an initial nonambulatory clinical status is associated with a shorter survival.[20] Vertebral tumors are often treated with multimodal therapy with surgery, RT, and/or chemotherapy. Dogs with vertebral osteosarcoma receiving multimodal treatment had a MST of 8.5 months compared to 1.5 months with surgery alone.[17] Commonly used contemporary neurosurgical techniques are largely insufficient to attain the goal of en bloc surgical excision of vertebral tumors, and more aggressive approaches including vertebrectomy with vertebral stabilization will likely be fundamental to improving surgical outcomes.[2]

Chemotherapy

Chemotherapy may be used as a primary treatment modality in cases of vertebral plasma cell tumors, multiple myeloma, or lymphoma, although chemotherapeutic protocols vary widely.[2] Platinum-based chemotherapeutic agents are often used as an adjunctive treatment in cases of vertebral osteosarcoma or other mesenchymal tumors.[17] Dogs with vertebral plasmacytomas and multiple myeloma may have favorable and durable responses to melphalan and prednisone chemotherapy, even in the face of multiple or diffuse vertebral lesions and signs of moderate spinal cord dysfunction.

KEY POINTS

- Tumors of the brain and spinal cord are a common cause of neurological problems in middle-aged to older dogs.
- The region of the nervous system causing the observed clinical signs is identified via the medical history and neurological examination.
- The diagnosis and treatment of tumors of the nervous system usually requires referral to a veterinary neurologist or other specialist.
- Diagnosis of brain and spinal cord tumors is most readily achieved by performing magnetic resonance imaging examinations of the affected area of the nervous system and tumor biopsy.
- Dogs with nervous system tumors should also have thoracic and abdominal imaging examinations performed to identify significant concurrent disease before undergoing any antitumor treatments.
- Treatment of brain and spinal cord tumors often involves surgery, radiation, or chemotherapy, and each of these treatments can extend the longevity and quality of life of affected dogs.

References

1. Song RB, Vite CH, Bradley CW, Cross JR. Postmortem evaluation of 435 cases of intracranial neoplasia in dogs and relationship of neoplasm with breed, age, and body weight. *J Vet Intern Med.* 2013 Sep-Oct; 27(5):1143–1152.
2. Rossmeisl Jr JH, Pancotto TE. Tumors of the nervous system. In: Vail DM, Thamm DH, Liptak JM. (eds.). *Withrow & MacEwen's Small Animal Clinical Oncology,* 6th edition. Philadelphia, PA, USA: Saunders; 2019. pp. 657–674.
3. Snyder JM, Lipitz L, Skorupski KA, Shofer FS, Van Winkle TJ. Secondary intracranial neoplasia in the dog: 177 cases (1986-2003). *J Vet Intern Med.* 2008 Jan-Feb; 22(1):172–177.
4. Miller AD, Miller CR, Rossmeisl JH. Canine Primary Intracranial Cancer: A Clinicopathologic and Comparative Review of Glioma, Meningioma, and Choroid Plexus Tumors. *Front Oncol.* 2019 Nov 8; 9:1151.
5. Pancotto TE, Rossmeisl JH Jr, Zimmerman K, et al. Intramedullary spinal cord neoplasia in 53 dogs (1990-2010): distribution, clinicopathologic characteristics, and clinical behavior. *J Vet Intern Med.* 2013 Nov-Dec; 27(6):1500–1508.
6. Schwartz M, Lamb CR, Brodbelt DC, Volk HA. Canine intracranial neoplasia: clinical risk factors for development of epileptic seizures. *J Small Anim Pract.* 2011 Dec; 52(12):632–637.
7. Snyder JM, Shofer FS, Van Winkle TJ, Massicotte C. Canine intracranial primary neoplasia: 173 cases (1986-2003). *J Vet Intern Med.* 2006 May-Jun; 20(3):669–675.
8. Wolff CA, Holmes SP, Young BD, et al. Magnetic resonance imaging for the differentiation of neoplastic, inflammatory, and cerebrovascular brain disease in dogs. *J Vet Intern Med.* 2012 May-Jun; 26(3):589–597.
9. Bentley RT. Magnetic resonance imaging diagnosis of brain tumors in dogs. *Vet J.* 2015 Aug; 205(2):204–216.
10. Garcia-Mora J, Parker RL, Cecere T, et al. The T2-FLAIR mismatch sign as an imaging biomarker for oligodendrogliomas in dogs. *J Vet Intern Med.* 2023 Jul-Aug; 37(4):1447–1454.
11. Auger M, Hecht S, Springer CM. Magnetic Resonance Imaging Features of Extradural Spinal Neoplasia in 60 Dogs and Seven Cats. *Front Vet Sci.* 2021 Jan 7; 7:610490.
12. Hu H, Barker A, Harcourt-Brown T, Jeffery N. Systematic Review of Brain Tumor Treatment in Dogs. *J Vet Intern Med.* 2015 Nov-Dec; 29(6):1456–1463.
13. Forward AK, Volk HA, Cherubini GB, et al. Clinical presentation, diagnostic findings and outcome of dogs undergoing surgical resection for intracranial meningioma: 101 dogs. *BMC Vet Res.* 2022 Mar 7; 18(1):88.
14. Hidalgo Crespo E, Farré Mariné A, Pumarola i Battle M, et al. Survival Time after Surgical Debulking and Temozolomide Adjuvant Chemotherapy in Canine Intracranial Gliomas. *Vet Sci.* 2022 Aug 12; 9(8):427.
15. Hanson JM, van't HM, Voorhout G, et al. Efficacy of transsphenoidal hypophysectomy in treatment of dogs with pituitary-dependent hyperadrenocorticism. *J Vet Intern Med.* 2005 Sep-Oct;19(5):687–694.
16. Moirano SJ, Dewey CW, Wright KZ, Cohen PW. Survival times in dogs with presumptive intracranial gliomas treated with oral lomustine: A comparative retrospective study (2008-2017). *Vet Comp Oncol.* 2018 Dec; 16(4):459–466.
17. Dixon A, Chen A, Rossmeisl JH Jr, Sturges B, et al. Surgical decompression, with or without adjunctive therapy, for palliative treatment of primary vertebral osteosarcoma in dogs. *Vet Comp Oncol.* 2019 Dec; 17(4):472–478.
18. Petersen SA, Sturges BK, Dickinson PJ, et al. Canine intraspinal meningiomas: imaging features, histopathologic classification, and long-term outcome in 34 dogs. *J Vet Intern Med.* 2008 Jul-Aug; 22(4):946–953.
19. Liebel FX, Rossmeisl JH Jr, Lanz OI, Robertson JL. Canine spinal nephroblastoma: long-term outcomes associated with treatment of 10 cases (1996-2009). *Vet Surg.* 2011 Feb; 40(2):244–252.
20. Dernell WS, Van Vechten BJ, Straw RC, et al. Outcome following treatment of vertebral tumors in 20 dogs (1986-1995). *J Am Anim Hosp Assoc.* 2000 May-Jun; 36(3):245–251.

CHAPTER 25

Infectious central nervous system disorders and discospondylitis

Renee Barber
DVM, PhD, DACVIM

Central nervous system (CNS) infections are important to consider in the diagnostic workup of dogs with signs of intracranial disease and/or a myelopathy. Additionally, bacterial or fungal infections leading to discospondylitis are an important rule-out for neck and back pain in the dog. Infectious agents are either neurotrophic, resulting directly in inflammation of the brain (encephalitis) and/or spinal cord (myelitis) parenchyma (e.g., rabies, canine distemper virus, protozoal infections), or cause primary vasculitis and/or meningitis with secondary parenchymal injury (e.g., *Rickettsia rickettsii*).

Infectious disease of the CNS should be more strongly considered in young or immunocompromised dogs. Although concurrent systemic signs (e.g., fever, weight loss, cough) or bloodwork changes (e.g., neutrophilia, eosinophilia) can increase suspicion for an infectious etiology, these findings are often lacking in dogs with CNS infection. Neurological deficits are typically progressive and multifocal and include any combination of signs referable to the prosencephalon, brainstem, cerebellum, or spinal cord (Fig. 25.1). It is important to remember that noninfectious inflammation, known as meningoencephalitis of unknown origin (MUO), is a key differential for young dogs older than 6 months of age exhibiting progressive multifocal CNS signs. Although many CNS infections occur worldwide, some are limited to certain geographic regions, making a thorough travel history important (Table 25.1).

Magnetic resonance imaging (MRI) is the most sensitive imaging method for evaluating the CNS for evidence of infection, but there can be an overlap of imaging features with other diseases such as MUO and neoplasia. Routine analysis of cerebrospinal fluid (CSF) is critical as it can allow differentiation between inflammatory disease and other etiologies, and certain cell types (e.g., neutrophils, eosinophils) may support an infectious etiology. Specific infectious disease testing should be researched for each suspected organism to ensure collection of appropriate fluid/tissue and maximize the sensitivity and specificity of the chosen tests.

This chapter covers the most common or important organisms that result in CNS infections in dogs. Less commonly reported organisms and their geographic distribution are listed in Table 25.1.

Viral infections

Rabies

Rabies virus is a lyssavirus responsible for a progressive, fatal polioencephalitis. It is zoonotic and fatal in people. Rabies is found worldwide with some notable exceptions, including Antarctica, Australia, Hawaii, Japan, New Zealand, and many islands in the Pacific Ocean and Caribbean Sea. All countries in the European Union except Hungary, Poland, Romania, and Slovakia are also considered rabies-free (Table 25.1). Bats, raccoons, skunks, foxes, mongooses, jackals, and domestic dogs are the primary reservoirs for rabies. Rabies is transmitted by the bite of an infected animal or via exposure of mucous membranes to infected saliva. Exposure may also occur during necropsy. The virus is not readily spread by fomites or other routes. Rabies has a variable incubation period of 3–24 weeks in dogs, after which the virus travels via

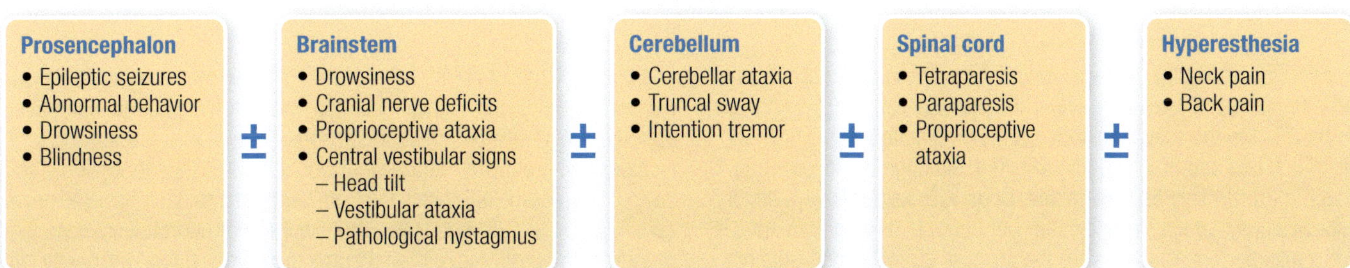

FIG. 25.1 Dogs with central nervous system infection typically present with progressive, multifocal neurological deficits.

TABLE 25.1 Geographic distribution of infectious agents affecting the canine central nervous system (CNS).

Pathogen		CNS disease	Geographic distribution
Viruses	Rabies virus	Fatal polioencephalitis	Worldwide except Antarctica, Australia, Hawaii, Japan, New Zealand, most countries in the European Union, and some islands in the Pacific Ocean and Caribbean Sea
	Canine distemper virus	Encephalitis/myelitis	Worldwide
	Tick-borne encephalitis virus	Encephalitis/myelitis	Central Europe, Sweden, Norway, Italy, Greece
	Eastern equine encephalitis virus	Necrotizing neutrophilic, lymphoplasmacytic meningoencephalitis in young puppies	North and South America
	La Crosse virus	Necrotizing panencephalitis in puppies	Eastern United States
	Pseudorabies virus	Encephalitis	Worldwide except Australia, Canada, Finland, Greenland, Norway, and Switzerland
	West Nile virus	Encephalitis	Africa, Asia, Europe, Oceania, North and South America
Parasites	*Angiostrongylus vasorum*	Hemorrhagic lesions in CNS more likely than aberrant parasite migration	Eastern Canadian provinces, United Kingdom, Northern Europe, South America, Uganda
	Baylisascaris procyonis	Eosinophilic meningoencephalitis	Asia, Europe, North America
	Cuterebra spp.	Encephalitis	North and South America
	Dirofilaria immitis	Aberrant parasite migration	Australia, Europe, Japan, North and South America
	Entamoeba histolytica	Granulomatous amebic meningoencephalitis	Worldwide
	Toxoplasma gondii	Meningoencephalitis/myelitis	Worldwide
	Neospora caninum	Meningoencephalitis (cerebellum)/myelitis	Worldwide
	Prototheca spp.	Eosinophilic meningoencephalitis/myelitis	Worldwide
Fungi	*Aspergillus* spp.	Sinonasal extension into cranial cavity/granulomatous meningoencephalitis/myelitis	Worldwide
	Blastomyces dermatidis	Sinonasal extension into cranial cavity/granulomatous meningoencephalitis/myelitis	Africa, Central America, North America (Mississippi; Missouri; Ohio River Valley; mid-Atlantic states; Canadian provinces of Alberta, Quebec, Manitoba, Ontario)
	Cladophialophora bantiana	Granulomatous meningoencephalitis/myelitis	Worldwide
	Coccidioides spp.	Granulomatous meningoencephalitis/myelitis	Central America, Mexico, South America, Southwestern United States
	Cryptococcus spp.	Sinonasal extension into cranial cavity/granulomatous meningoencephalitis/myelitis	Worldwide
	Histoplasma spp.	Granulomatous meningoencephalitis/myelitis	Worldwide
Bacteria	*Rickettsia rickettsii*	Meningoencephalitis/myelitis	North and South America
	Ehrlichia spp.	Meningoencephalitis/myelitis	Worldwide
	Anaplasma phagocytophilum	Meningoencephalitis/myelitis	Worldwide
	Non-arthropod-borne bacteria (e.g., *Staphylococcus* and *Streptococcus* spp.)	Meningitis/encephalitis/myelitis/abscess/empyema	Worldwide

the peripheral nerves to the CNS, where it multiplies and disseminates rapidly. In species known to transmit the disease, rabies virus spreads from the CNS to the salivary glands via the cranial nerves.[1]

Dogs of any age and breed can be affected, although those less than 4 weeks old are unlikely to have rabies. Dogs with rabies have a history of clinical signs that have progressed over hours to days, and death will occur a minimum of 10 days after the onset of clinical signs. Obtaining a thorough travel history over the previous 6 months is important as rabies can be imported.

The clinical signs of rabies are variable.[2] The disease can initially present with nonspecific signs, including fever, lethargy, and decreased appetite. There are two described forms. The furious (excitatory) form includes hyperactivity, aggression, vocalization, and generalized seizures. The dumb (paralytic) form includes drowsiness, cranial nerve deficits such as a dropped jaw, and lower motor neuron weakness that progresses to paralysis.[2] Often, neurological signs do not fall neatly into one of these two forms. For example, a dog could be presented with lameness of a single limb that is confused with orthopedic disease but ultimately represents a lower motor neuron weakness that will progress to CNS signs.

Recognizing when rabies should be high on the differential diagnosis list (warranting patient isolation) can be challenging (Video 25.1). Factors that should increase suspicion include an unvaccinated status, travel to or from a country with enzootic rabies in the 6 months prior to the onset of clinical signs, exposure to wild animals or animals suspected to have rabies, and clinical signs that have been progressing over hours to days for less than 10 days in total.

Unfortunately, there are no validated diagnostic tests to confirm a diagnosis of rabies antemortem. MRI findings of naturally infected dogs can reveal bilateral, non-contrast-enhancing T2-weighted (T2W) hyperintensities in the temporal lobes, hippocampus, hypothalamus, brainstem, cerebellum, and cervical spinal cord. There is limited information about CSF findings in clinical rabies, but a lymphocytic pleocytosis has been reported.[3,4]

Direct fluorescent antibody testing of fresh brain tissue is the gold standard for the diagnosis of rabies. Only vaccinated, trained personnel should prepare these samples for shipping, and the laboratory should be contacted ahead of time to ensure the samples are collected and shipped properly.

There is no treatment for rabies. Patients highly suspected of being rabid can be euthanized or will die within 10 days of the onset of clinical signs. Rabies is a major public health concern. Veterinary personnel should be vaccinated against rabies, and rabies suspects should be isolated and managed by designated, trained personnel. Local public health officials must be notified. Owners should be guided to consult with their physician about health risks.

Canine distemper virus

Canine distemper is a highly contagious multisystemic disease caused by a morbillivirus (canine distemper virus [CDV]). It has a worldwide distribution (Table 25.1). Transmission typically occurs via inhalation of virus particles that replicate in lymphoid tissue before moving to epithelial tissues, such as the respiratory and gastrointestinal tracts, conjunctiva/eyes, foot pads, and nose (leading to hyperkeratosis), as well as to the CNS. In the CNS, CDV replicates in neurons and glial cells of the gray matter and leads to demyelination of white matter.[5]

CDV can infect dogs of any age and breed, but more than half of cases occur in dogs less than 1 year of age. The duration of the neurological signs prior to diagnosis ranges from a few days to more than a month. CNS signs are uncommon in fully vaccinated dogs, but rare breakthrough cases have been reported. Classically, dogs are thought to have respiratory and gastrointestinal signs, which are followed by neurological signs several weeks to months later. However, neurological signs can occur concurrently with respiratory and gastrointestinal signs, and, in a report of 100 dogs with CDV infection, one third of the dogs had no extraneural signs.[6,7] Neurological signs in cases of canine distemper are highly variable and depend on the immune status of the affected dog. Acute CNS signs include generalized or focal epileptic seizures (Video 25.2), central vestibular or cerebellar signs (Video 25.3), and unilateral or bilateral blindness with an abnormal pupillary light reflex secondary to involvement of the optic nerves. Rhythmic muscle contraction, known as myoclonus, can occur in the head, limbs, or jaw in up to 40% of cases with neurological disease (Video 25.4). More chronic cases may show spinal cord signs such as paresis and proprioceptive ataxia (Video 25.5).

Diagnosis of CDV often relies on clinical suspicion and supportive diagnostic testing. During the viremic phase, severe lymphopenia is the most common finding on bloodwork. Magnetic resonance (MR) images can be normal or reveal multifocal T2W hyperintensities of the gray and white matter, with or without mild meningeal enhancement. CSF analysis can be normal or show a mononuclear pleocytosis. Elevated CSF anti-CDV antibodies are diagnostic as they are produced locally and not found secondary to vaccination, and there are several reverse transcription polymerase chain reaction (RT-PCR) assays based on field strains of CDV or quantitation of viral load that will not be affected by vaccination. Recent studies have shown that RT-PCR testing of urine has a high sensitivity for detection of CDV, but using two different body fluids such as urine and CSF can further increase the sensitivity of RT-PCR.[5,8–10]

Treatment of canine distemper consists of supportive care. Antiseizure medications should be administered as needed but are variably efficacious. Myoclonus can be treated with procainamide and clonazepam but is often irreversible and does not respond to treatment. Botulism toxin had a positive clinical effect in one dog with myoclonus secondary to CDV

Video 25.1

Video of an apparently normal young dog. The dog is interacting with other dogs and people. Notice, at the end of the video, the unjustified attack to another dog and the bite. The dog tested positive for rabies and developed clinical signs soon after. The video shows how difficult it is to recognize and prevent rabies. Video courtesy of Dr. Davide de Lorenzi.

Video 25.2

Two-month-old female Labrador Retriever with acute distemper encephalitis suffering a focal epileptic seizure. Note the abnormal mentation, motor activity of the masticatory muscles, and autonomic signs (hypersalivation). This type of seizure is considered quite typical for distemper encephalitis and was in the past referred to as "chewing gum fits". Video courtesy of Dr. Gualtiero Gandini.

Video 25.3

Four-month-old male dog with acute distemper encephalitis showing cerebellar signs. Note the cerebellar ataxia, characterized by hypermetria of the four limbs and the intention tremors. Video courtesy of Dr. Gualtiero Gandini.

Video 25.4

Four dogs with distemper encephalomyelitis and myoclonus affecting different parts of the body: the limb(s), the head, and the whole body. Video courtesy of Dr. Gualtiero Gandini.

Video 25.5

Young dog with a subacute form of distemper. Note the proprioceptive ataxia and truncal myoclonus. During the neurological examination, the tactile test on the front limbs is clearly abnormal. Video courtesy of Dr. Gualtiero Gandini.

infection. Usually, once the virus has reached the CNS, the prognosis is poor, and the disease progresses until death. In very rare cases, especially in dogs that showed a good immune response, stabilization of the clinical signs has been documented.

Tick-borne encephalitis

Tick-borne encephalitis (TBE) is caused by a flavivirus transmitted by *Ixodes* and *Dermacentor* spp. ticks, which produces mononuclear inflammation of the meninges and gray matter of the brain and spinal cord. TBE is endemic in central Europe, Sweden, Norway, northern Italy, and Greece (Table 25.1).[11]

Dogs of any age or breed can be affected by TBE, but Rottweilers, Newfoundlands, and Labrador Retrievers may be overrepresented. Clinical signs are often acute in onset and progress over days to weeks, starting with nonspecific signs; fever is present in up to two-thirds of patients. Neurological deficits are multifocal, affecting the prosencephalon, brainstem, and spinal cord (Fig. 25.1).[11,12]

Definitive antemortem diagnosis of TBE is not possible. Routine bloodwork may show nonregenerative anemia, neutrophilic leukocytosis, lymphopenia, and elevated liver enzymes. MR images may be normal or show bilaterally symmetrical T2W hyperintensities in the thalamus, basal nuclei, hippocampus, pons, medulla, and spinal cord gray matter. CSF analysis reveals a mononuclear pleocytosis. Serum and CSF antibodies can be measured but are difficult to interpret as subclinical dogs in endemic regions will have high antibody titers. Ultimately, a presumptive diagnosis is made based on the patient's geographic location and a consistent clinical picture. Definitive diagnosis is made via postmortem histopathology.[11,12]

Treatment of TBE predominantly consists of supportive care. Anti-inflammatory glucocorticoids may be beneficial. Historically, TBE has been considered a fatal disease, with death occurring within 4–7 days from the onset of signs. However, in a recent retrospective study of 54 dogs, 90% of the dogs were treated with glucocorticoids, and the mortality rate was 33%.[12]

Parasitic infections

Angiostrongyliasis

Migration of the nematode *Angiostrongylus vasorum* in the CNS has been documented, but neurological disease typically results from hemorrhage in the CNS secondary to a parasite-induced hemostatic disorder. Although neurological sequelae are uncommon, it is an important differential diagnosis in endemic regions, including the eastern Canadian provinces, United Kingdom, northern Europe, South America, and Uganda (Table 25.1).[13,14]

CNS angiostrongyliasis is more common in dogs less than 2 years of age, and several breeds are overrepresented in the literature, including the Cavalier King Charles Spaniel, Labrador Retriever, Staffordshire Bull Terrier, and hunting dogs. Infected dogs may or may not have concurrent signs of systemic illness affecting the lungs, heart, gastrointestinal tract, and hemostasis. CNS signs are referable to the location of the hemorrhage in the brain and/or spinal cord (Fig. 25.1).

Common diagnostic findings consistent with systemic disease include evidence of pulmonary disease, hypertension, and elevated prothrombin time (PT), activated partial thromboplastin time (aPTT), and d-dimers. MRI reveals focal or multifocal hemorrhage in the brain, spinal cord, or subarachnoid space. CSF may contain a high total protein concentration and show evidence of erythrophagia. Diagnosis can be achieved using the Baermann method to identify first-stage larvae in feces. A new rapid in-clinic assay has been shown to have a low to moderate sensitivity and high specificity in comparison with the Baermann method.[15]

Affected dogs should be treated supportively with antiseizure medications as needed. For definitive treatment, fenbendazole at 25 mg/kg for 20 days has an efficacy of 91.3%, milbemycin oxime at 0.5 mg/kg once a week for 4 weeks has an efficacy of 84.8%, and single treatment with a spot-on formulation of 10% imidacloprid and 2.5% moxidectin has an efficacy of 85.25%. Additionally, the spot-on treatment stops larval shedding with the first treatment. The prognosis is variable, but one study of dogs with intracranial hemorrhage reported a good outcome in 14 out of 16 dogs.[16–18]

Neosporosis

Neospora caninum is a coccidial protozoan parasite that is found worldwide (Table 25.1). Dogs and other canids are the definitive host. Dogs, as well as many other species (including bovids), can also act as intermediate hosts. *N. caninum* can be transmitted transplacentally or via ingestion of infected tissues or sporulated oocysts in the environment. Disease is caused by asexual reproduction to produce tachyzoites as well as cyst-forming bradyzoites, which are found in the nervous system.[19]

N. caninum can cause neurological disease in any age or breed of dog. There are three major clinical presentations:

1. Puppies with transplacental transmission develop clinical signs of polyradiculoneuritis and myositis from 4 weeks to 6 months of age. They will initially present with lower motor neuron paresis or paralysis of the pelvic limbs and then develop severe muscle atrophy and muscle and joint contracture (see Video 35.2, Chapter 35). Not all puppies in the litter will develop clinical signs, but titers should be checked in unaffected littermates so they can be preemptively treated.
2. Adult dogs can develop meningoencephalomyelitis with focal or multifocal lesions in the brain and/or spinal cord (Video 25.6). The cerebellum is most commonly affected. Signs of cerebellar dysfunction can be acute (days to weeks) or chronic (up to a year) and are typically progressive.
3. Polymyositis can occur concurrently with meningoencephalomyelitis or, rarely, be the primary reason for presentation. Signs include reluctance to walk with a stiff, short-strided gait.[20,21]

There are no specific hematological or biochemistry abnormalities consistently identified in cases of neosporosis, but elevated creatine kinase or aspartate aminotransferase levels in a dog with CNS signs should increase suspicion. The most common MRI finding in cases of meningoencephalomyelitis is severe bilateral cerebellar atrophy. Focal or multifocal T2W hyperintensities with variable contrast enhancement have

Video 25.6

Part of the neurological examination of a 2-year-old female mixed-breed dog affected by central nervous system neosporosis. The dog, found and given to an animal rescue center, had been displaying progressive signs, including seizures, for 2 months. Note the nonambulatory tetraparesis, left-sided head tilt, and pathological nystagmus. Video courtesy of Gualtiero Gandini.

also been reported. Evidence of changes in the muscles of mastication, including muscle atrophy, should raise suspicion of a protozoal parasite. CSF analysis may reveal a mononuclear or mixed cell pleocytosis. Tachyzoites may rarely be found in CSF and must be differentiated from *Toxoplasma gondii* tachyzoites.[19–21]

Immunofluorescent antibody and enzyme-linked immunosorbent assays are commonly used to test for exposure to *N. caninum*. Seropositivity without clinical disease is possible and more common in dogs living in rural areas or with exposure to cattle. Rising serum titers may be useful in acutely affected dogs, particularly in an area of high seroprevalence. In chronically affected dogs, a serum titer greater than 1:800 is used for diagnosis. PCR testing can be performed on CSF, but results should be interpreted with caution; sensitivity varies among laboratories, and positive PCR results can be found in tissues from healthy animals.[19]

Numerous treatment protocols have been reported. Clindamycin at 10–12 mg/kg twice daily and trimethoprim-sulfa at 15 mg/kg twice daily have a microbiostatic effect on *N. caninum*. Pyrimethamine at 1 mg/kg once daily and ponazuril at 20 mg/kg once daily have a microbicidal effect and should be considered in patients with CNS disease. Treatment should continue for a minimum of 4–8 weeks but may be necessary for up to 6 months. The prognosis for puppies with muscle and joint contracture is poor. There are variable reports on the prognosis for dogs with meningoencephalomyelitis, which ranges from grave to excellent.[19]

Toxoplasmosis

Toxoplasma gondii is an obligate intracellular coccidial protozoan parasite that is found worldwide, with a seroprevalence ranging from 20–91% depending on the geographic region (Table 25.1). Felids are obligate hosts; all the other hosts are intermediate. Transmission can be congenital or occur secondary to ingestion of infected tissue or sporulated oocysts. Clinical disease is caused by tachyzoites that invade cells and replicate intracellularly, leading to cell necrosis.[22]

Dogs of any age or breed can be infected, although toxoplasmosis is commonly linked with immunosuppression. Concurrent systemic disease is common as tachyzoites often spread to the skeletal muscles, liver, lungs, heart, skin, and eyes. Nonspecific signs such as fever and lethargy may be noted.[22] Although it is reported in many books as an important differential diagnosis, CNS toxoplasmosis is infrequently diagnosed in canine patients. Only a few reports have confirmed canine CNS toxoplasmosis, and serology in dogs with meningoencephalitis has demonstrated a low prevalence.[23] As with other infectious diseases, CNS signs depend on the location of tachyzoites.

For all dogs in which toxoplasmosis is suspected as a cause of CNS signs, clinicians must rule out infection with other protozoal parasites, including *Neospora caninum*. Routine bloodwork may be normal or demonstrate eosinophilia and elevation of hepatobiliary enzymes. An elevated creatine kinase may be seen with concurrent muscle disease. MRI and CSF findings in dogs with CNS toxoplasmosis are not well reported. A few reports suggest CSF will show a mixed cell pleocytosis and elevated total protein. Occasionally, tachyzoites can be identified in CSF, but additional testing is needed to differentiate them from *N. caninum* tachyzoites.

There is no single serological assay that can definitively confirm a diagnosis of toxoplasmosis. Typically, an elevated immunoglobulin M (IgM) titer (>1:64) without a concurrently elevated IgG titer is consistent with toxoplasmosis. This can be supported by a 4-fold rise in IgG titers over 2–5 weeks. PCR of serum, CSF, and other tissues should be interpreted with caution as positive results can be found in healthy animals. PCR of muscle biopsies may be useful in cases with an elevated creatine kinase.[22] Numerous treatments have been reported, including azithromycin 10 mg/kg once daily, clindamycin 10–12 mg/kg twice daily, ponazuril 20 mg/kg once daily, and trimethoprim-sulfa 15 mg/kg twice daily. Treatment should be administered for a minimum of 4–8 weeks. Clindamycin is an appropriate treatment for myositis, but trimethoprim-sulfa may be more appropriate in cases of CNS disease because it has better CNS penetration. Ponazuril should be considered as an additional therapy because it has been reported to be microbicidal in the treatment of tachyzoites. The prognosis is variable. There are reports of cases with CNS involvement and myositis that have responded to treatment, with resolution of the clinical signs.[22]

Fungal

Aspergillosis

Aspergillosis is caused by saprophytic, hyaline molds of the genus *Aspergillus*. These organisms are associated with opportunistic infections worldwide, particularly in dogs with inadequate immune responses (Table 25.1). Spores are inhaled from the environment and can germinate locally, leading to sinonasal disease, or disseminate to the CNS through the cribriform plate. Alternatively, spores can deposit in the bronchioles or alveolar spaces prior to hematogenous systemic spread, sometimes affecting the CNS. *Aspergillus fumigatus* is most commonly associated with sinonasal disease, and *Aspergillus terreus* is most commonly associated with systemic and CNS aspergillosis.[24]

Aspergillosis can affect dogs of any breed and age. Middle-aged German Shepherd dogs are overrepresented. Clinical signs are often slowly progressive and present for less than 2 months. Sinonasal disease is associated with nasal discharge, sneezing, epistaxis, mandibular lymphadenopathy, depigmentation or ulceration of the nares, and facial discomfort. Dogs with systemic disease may have weight loss, inappetence, cough, or vomiting (Table 25.2).[25]

Dogs with invasive sinonasal disease will display neurological signs referable to the prosencephalon; epileptic seizures and abnormal mentation are most commonly reported. When systemic spread occurs and

TABLE 25.2 Common extraneural sites and cytologic morphology of canine central nervous system mycotic infections.

	Common extraneural sites	Cytologic morphology
Aspergillosis	Lungs, bones, lymph nodes, kidney, spleen, pancreas, liver	Septate hyphae with dichotomous branching and parallel walls (2–3 μm)
Blastomycosis	Lungs, lymph nodes, skin, bones, eyes	Biconcave, thick-walled, broad-based budding yeast (8–15 μm)
Coccidiomycosis	Lungs, perihilar lymph nodes, bones, heart, pericardium, skin, eyes	Thick-walled spherules (100 μm) containing numerous 5–30 μm endospores
Cryptococcosis	Eyes, lymph nodes, skin	Round to oval yeast with a thick, clear capsule (4–10 μm); +/– thin-based budding

involves the CNS, the animal will commonly show multifocal neurological signs affecting the prosencephalon, brainstem, cerebellum, and/or spinal cord (Fig. 25.1). Aspergillosis can also result in mycotic discospondylitis. Routine bloodwork may be normal or reveal a nonregenerative anemia, mature neutrophilia, hyperglobulinemia, hypoalbuminemia, azotemia, or hypercalcemia. Fungal hyphae may be identified on urinalysis. Thoracic and abdominal imaging may show disease of extraneural organs. MRI features are similar to those of other inflammatory CNS diseases, with multifocal, contrast-enhancing T2W hyperintensities in the brain and/or spinal cord (Fig. 25.2). Evidence of sinonasal involvement and extension through the cribriform plate should always prompt further evaluation for *Aspergillus* organisms. On occasion, MR images are normal. A neutrophilic pleocytosis is found in the CSF.[26]

Diagnosis of sinonasal and systemic aspergillosis often comes from the identification of *Aspergillus* organisms via culture, cytology, or histopathology of affected sites (Table 25.2). Antibody tests should be interpreted with caution since they can have a low to moderate sensitivity and produce false-negative results. The galactomannan antigen test has a low sensitivity and should not be used in cases with suspected sinonasal extension. Galactomannan is useful in systemic aspergillosis without CNS involvement and has a high sensitivity and specificity in serum and urine samples, but its utility in CNS disease is unknown. It is important to note that the assay manufacturer recommends a galactomannan index ≥ 0.5 to be interpreted as positive; however, this can lead to false positives, so some have suggested a higher cutoff value (≥ 1.5). Additionally, with the galactomannan assay, there can be a cross reaction with other fungal species, and, importantly, administration of beta-lactam antibiotics or gluconate-containing fluids can lead to false-positive results.[27] PCR assays on blood have low sensitivity in detecting sinonasal disease and have not been validated for use in systemic disease.

Historically, nasal infusion of clotrimazole has not been recommended when sinonasal disease has extended through the cribriform plate. However, successful treatment using minimally invasive debridement and clotrimazole has been reported in 3 dogs and led to minimal side effects.[28] Numerous antifungal treatments have been used for systemic aspergillosis (Table 25.3). Fluconazole, voriconazole, and posaconazole have good CNS penetration, and voriconazole and posaconazole avoid concerns of antifungal resistance with fluconazole. Amphotericin B, echinocandins, and terbinafine can be used concurrently with azole drugs in an attempt to improve outcomes. Liposomal or lipid complex amphotericin B formulations may improve CNS penetration and reduce nephrotoxicity. Prolonged treatment is indicated, and lifelong treatment may be necessary. A short-term course of anti-inflammatory glucocorticoids may be indicated in certain cases, especially if the patients deteriorate clinically after beginning antifungal therapy.[27]

The prognosis of systemic aspergillosis with CNS involvement is not well established, but it is associated with a grave outcome. There are several case reports of dogs doing well up to 1–3 years after initiation of treatment.

Blastomycosis

Blastomyces dermatidis is a dimorphic fungus found in moist, acidic soil in Africa, Central America, and North America (Table 25.1). Infective spores enter the body through inhalation and convert to yeast in tissues. A primary pulmonary infection is established before the fungus spreads to other organs, where it causes pyogranulomatous inflammation. The lymphatic tissues, eyes, bones, and skin are most commonly affected (Table 25.2). The CNS is affected in 4–6% of cases. Rarely, yeast form a nasal mass that can extend into the cranial cavity.

CNS blastomycosis most commonly affects young, large breed dogs. It typically presents with acute, progressive signs. Concurrent lymphadenopathy occurs in up to 70% of cases, and pulmonary disease in up to 88% of cases. Blastomycosis can affect any part of the CNS, including the prosencephalon, brainstem, cerebellum, and/or spinal cord (Fig. 25.1). Visual deficits can be the result of CNS or ocular disease. Exophthalmos has been reported in several cases of CNS blastomycosis. Routine bloodwork is often normal; leukocytosis and elevated hepatobiliary enzymes have been reported. MRI findings either involve mass-like lesions with variable meningeal enhancement or ventriculitis. A mixed cell or mononuclear pleocytosis is seen on CSF analysis.[27,29,30]

Definitive diagnosis of blastomycosis relies on obtaining samples for culture, and less commonly histopathology, from affected extraneural sites (Table 25.2). Variable sensitivities have been reported for blastomycosis antigen and antibody tests. *Blastomyces* galactomannan antigen detection is 94% and 87% sensitive in urine and serum,

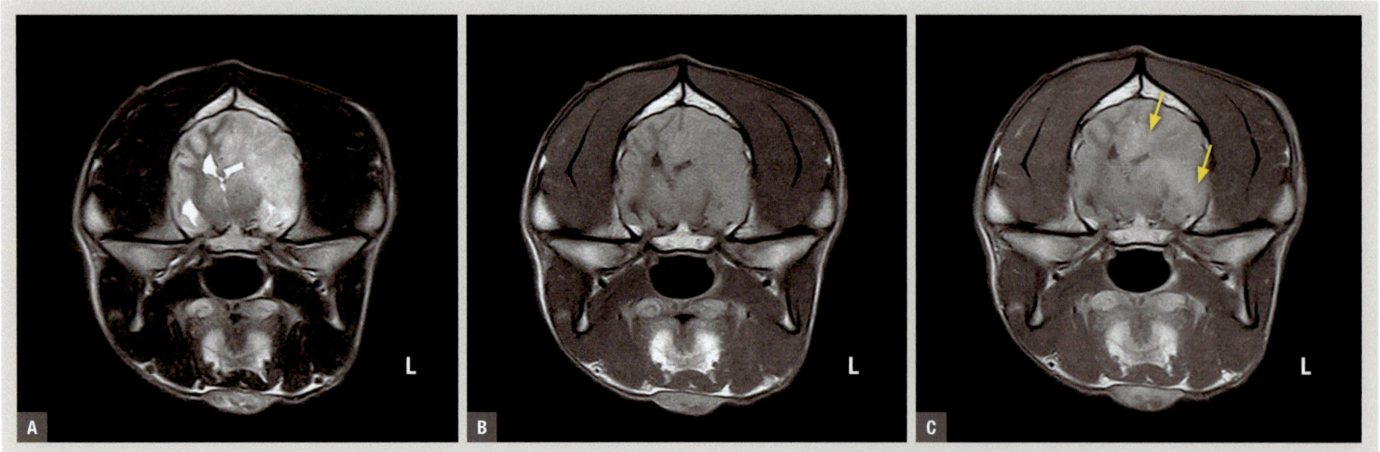

FIG. 25.2 Magnetic resonance imaging study of the brain of a dog with aspergillosis that was confirmed histologically. **(A)** Transverse T2-weighted image; **(B)** transverse T1-weighted image; **(C)** transverse T1W post contrast. Note the severe lesion in the left cerebral hemisphere, characterized by severe mass effect and displacement of the left lateral ventricle, which is hyperintense in A, isointense in B, and with diffuse contrast enhancement in C. L, left. Pictures courtesy of Dr. Massimo Baroni.

TABLE 25.3 Potential therapies for central nervous system fungal infections.

Drug	Dosage	Interval	Route	Notes
Amphotericin B	Varies depending on formulation	Varies depending on formulation	Varies depending on formulation	■ Numerous formulations ■ Effective against all common organisms causing canine fungal infections ■ Limited penetration of CNS ■ Close monitoring required to prevent nephrotoxicity
Fluconazole	5–10 mg/kg	Every 12 h	PO	■ Good CNS penetration ■ Poor activity against *Aspergillus* spp. ■ May be effective for blastomycosis, coccidiomycosis, cryptococcosis (but some *Cryptococcus* spp. can be resistant) ■ Monitor hepatic enzymes during treatment
Itraconazole	5 mg/kg	Every 12 h	PO	■ Poor CNS penetration ■ Used to treat aspergillosis, blastomycosis, coccidiomycosis, cryptococcosis ■ Monitor hepatic enzymes during treatment
	10 mg/kg	Every 24 h	PO	
Posaconazole	5 mg/kg	Every 48 h	PO	■ Dose is for delayed-release tablets, which have better bioavailability in dogs ■ Effective for aspergillosis, blastomycosis, coccidiomycosis, cryptococcosis ■ CNS penetration not known but appears effective for CNS cryptococcosis ■ Therapeutic drug monitoring recommended
Voriconazole	4–5 mg/kg	Every 12 h	PO	■ Known to be active against *Aspergillus* and *Cryptococcus* spp. ■ Good CNS penetration ■ Monitor hepatic enzymes during treatment ■ Therapeutic drug monitoring recommended
Capsofungin (echinocandin)	1 mg/kg	Every 24 h	IV Dilute in NaCl Give slowly (e.g., over 1 h)	■ Fungistatic against *Aspergillus* spp. ■ Effective in a mouse model of coccidiomycosis ■ Ineffective against *Cryptococcus* spp.
Terbinafine	30–35 mg/kg	Every 24h	PO	■ Efficacy in invasive fungal disease not known ■ May be synergistic when administered with other antifungal drugs ■ Ineffective against some human *Aspergillus* spp. infections

CNS, central nervous system; IV, intravenous; PO, per os (orally).

respectively. Antibody sensitivity using an enzyme immunoassay for the BAD-1 protein is 95%.[27] PCR assays are not commonly used to diagnose blastomycosis in dogs.

Treatment protocols and outcomes have been reported in 3 dogs with CNS blastomycosis (Table 25.3). Two dogs were treated with fluconazole as the sole antifungal agent, and one was treated with fluconazole and amphotericin B lipid complex. All dogs were alive at the time of publication, 13–36 months after initiation of treatment.[29,30]

Coccidiomycosis

Coccidioides immitis and *Coccidioides posadasii* are dimorphic fungi found in soil in the Southwestern United States and parts of Mexico, Central America, and South America (Table 25.1). Spores are inhaled and lead to pulmonary infection. Osteomyelitis is the second most common clinical sign after dissemination of disease systemically (Table 25.2). A minority of dogs develop CNS disease. Animals can develop clinical signs of infection up to 6 years after leaving an endemic region.

CNS coccidiomycosis can occur in dogs of any age or breed; the median reported age at CNS coccidiomycosis diagnosis is 7.5 years. Dogs with CNS coccidiomycosis may or may not present with evidence of systemic illness; fever and bone pain secondary to osteomyelitis have been reported. As occurs in other CNS infections, neurological deficits are often multifocal, but they can also be focal. Reported neuroanatomic localizations include the prosencephalon, brainstem, and cerebellum (Fig. 25.1); clinical signs of C6–T2 myelopathy and T3–L3 myelopathy have been described.

The bloodwork of dogs with coccidiomycosis may be normal, although neutrophilia and hyperglobulinemia have been reported. Pulmonary parenchymal lesions and/or tracheobronchial lymphadenopathy are commonly identified on radiographs. Usually, intra- or extraparenchymal masses are found in the brain and/or spinal cord on MRI and can be T2W hyper- or hypointense, with variable contrast enhancement. These masses can be difficult to distinguish from neoplasia. CSF can be normal or show a neutrophilic, lymphocytic, or large mononuclear pleocytosis; total protein was elevated in 71% of reported cases.[31]

Histological or cytological demonstration of the organism is required to establish a definitive diagnosis (Table 25.2). Serum for antibodies (not antigen) can be used to assess for exposure to *C. immitis*. Tube precipitation for IgM is typically positive within 2 weeks of exposure, and complement fixation for IgG is typically positive within 4–6 weeks of exposure. However, healthy dogs in endemic regions often have high antibody titers.[27] PCR assays have not been validated for clinical use in the diagnosis of canine coccidiomycosis infections.

Therapy with itraconazole and fluconazole has been reported with positive outcomes (Table 25.3).[27,31]

Cryptococcosis

Cryptococcosis is caused by dimorphic basidiomycetous fungi of the genus *Cryptococcus*, most commonly *Cryptococcus neoformans* in dogs. *C. neoformans* is found worldwide (Table 25.1). Clinical disease occurs when basidiospores are inhaled, which leads to infection in the nasal cavity or lungs, followed by secondary invasion of the cranial cavity or hematogenous systemic spread. The lymph nodes, eyes, skin, and CNS are most commonly affected (Table 25.2).[32]

Dogs of any age or breed can be affected. Doberman Pinschers, German Shepherd dogs, Great Danes and American Cocker Spaniels appear predisposed. CNS cryptococcosis can present with an acute or prolonged, progressive history. The most common concurrent clinical signs are related to ocular lesions or rhinosinusitis. Neurological signs are typically multifocal or referable to the prosencephalon, with epileptic seizures and central vestibular signs being commonly reported.[32] Some dogs may show focal/multifocal myelopathy signs.

Bloodwork and thoracic radiographs are typically normal. The most common MRI finding is multifocal T2W intraparenchymal hyperintensities with ill-defined contrast enhancement in the prosencephalon, cerebellum, and cervical spinal cord. Diffuse meningeal enhancement is common and is often the only finding. CSF pleocytosis is common and can be eosinophilic, neutrophilic, mononuclear, or mixed. Cryptococcal organisms are identified in CSF in up to 80% of cases.

Definitive diagnosis requires identification of the organism via cytology or histopathology (Table 25.2). Detection of the polysaccharide capsular antigen via latex agglutination is commonly used, but clinicians should be aware that false positives and false negatives can occur. PCR assays can be used to diagnose cryptococcosis but often are not necessary because infection can be diagnosed by cytology or antigen testing; false positives can occur.

Initial treatment with amphotericin B and fluconazole is recommended for dogs with CNS cryptococcosis (Table 25.3). Amphotericin B is continued for 2–4 weeks unless azotemia develops. Fluconazole is continued long term, which may be 12 months or more. If it is discontinued due to resolution of clinical signs and a negative antigen titer, antigen titers should be monitored every 6 months to allow early detection of a relapse. There are anecdotal reports that terbinafine may be beneficial. The prognosis is guarded, with reported success rates ranging from 30–55%.[27,33,34]

Bacterial

Rocky Mountain spotted fever

Rocky Mountain spotted fever (RMSF) is caused by the vector-borne, obligate intracellular bacteria *Rickettsia ricketsii*. It is found in North and South America and is transmitted by *Dermacentor andersoni* in the western United States and *Dermacentor variabilis* in the eastern United States (Table 25.1). *R. rickettsii* enters the body through the bite of an infected tick and is disseminated via the circulatory system, where it replicates within the endothelial cells of small arteries and venules leading to a necrotizing vasculitis that can affect many organs, including the CNS. In endemic regions, RMSF encephalitis must be ruled out prior to immunosuppression in dogs with suspected MUO.[35]

RMSF can infect dogs of any age and breed. However, purebred dogs are more commonly affected, and German Shepherd dogs are overrepresented. Clinical signs are acute and progressive. Fever is a common initial finding, and some dogs will develop petechial and ecchymotic hemorrhages. A retrospective study of 30 dogs with RMSF identified neurological signs in 50% of cases.[35] Neurological CNS signs are typically multifocal but can also be focal (Fig. 25.1); central vestibular signs are most common.[36]

Routine bloodwork can be normal or have nonspecific findings, including moderate to severe leukocytosis, thrombocytopenia, hypoalbuminemia, and hypercholesterolemia. MRI findings of RMSF encephalitis have not been reported. CSF analysis may reveal a neutrophilic, mononuclear, or mixed cell pleocytosis with a concurrent elevated in total protein. Diagnosis of RMSF is achieved by measurement of serum antibodies via an indirect fluorescent antibody assay. Definitive diagnosis requires a four-fold or greater increase in serum IgG antibodies because of the high seroprevalence in endemic regions. A single high titer greater than 1:1024 can be used if the sample was obtained 1 or more weeks after the onset of clinical signs. Negative results are possible early in disease.[32]

Doxycycline (5 mg/kg twice daily or 10 mg/kg once daily for a minimum of 7 days) is the treatment of choice. Dogs typically respond and have a successful clinical outcome.[32]

Ehrlichiosis

Ehrlichiosis in dogs is most commonly caused by *Ehrlichia canis*, which is found worldwide and transmitted by the brown dog tick, *Rhipicephalus sanguineus* (Table 25.1). *E. canis* is an obligate intracellular bacterium that multiplies in mononuclear cells and spreads throughout organ systems, including the CNS, causing vasculitis and inflammation.[37]

There is no age or breed predilection. The course of clinical disease can range from days to months. Clinical signs of ehrlichiosis can be nonspecific, including fever, lethargy, anorexia, weight loss, and lymphadenopathy. Petechial and ecchymotic hemorrhages or epistaxis may be seen. Dogs may develop signs secondary to inflammation and/or hemorrhage affecting one or more regions of the CNS (Fig. 25.1). Two case series reported neurological signs in 8–16% of dogs with ehrlichiosis.[38,39]

The most common bloodwork abnormalities are anemia, thrombocytopenia, leukopenia, and hypergammaglobulinemia. MRI findings have been reported in one dog with multifocal, punctate T2W hyperintensities in the brain and cervical spinal cord with parenchymal and leptomeningeal enhancement. CSF analysis reveals a mononuclear pleocytosis and increased total protein. Serology via indirect fluorescent antibody testing is the gold standard for diagnosis and may cross react with other *Ehrlichia, Anaplasma, Rickettsia, and Neorickettsia* spp. The presence of antibodies can represent exposure, so documenting a rising titer is ideal. Available point-of-care tests can also confirm exposure to *E. canis* in a rapid, affordable manner. PCR of blood or available tissues can be utilized; it is a highly specific test, but false negatives are common.[37]

Serology and PCR findings should be combined with the patient's history findings (e.g., prior residence in or travel to an endemic area or history of tick infestation).

The American College of Veterinary Internal Medicine (ACVIM) consensus statement on ehrlichial disease in small animals recommends treatment with doxycycline at 10 mg/kg once daily for 28 days for natural infection.[40] Serum titers will decrease and become negative after treatment. The response to therapy in dogs with CNS ehrlichiosis has not been documented. Recovery is variable in dogs with systemic ehrlichiosis with or without neurological signs; reported clinical remission rates are 45–84%.[38,39] Persistent neurological deficits are possible even in dogs with response to treatment.

Bacterial meningitis, abscess, empyema

A wide variety of aerobic and anerobic bacterial agents have been reported to cause CNS infections (Table 25.4). In dogs, bacterial organisms can spread into or around the CNS in a variety of ways:

- Contiguous spread from the nasal cavity or nasal sinuses
- Contiguous spread from the petrous temporal bone (otitis media and interna)
- Hematogenous spread
- Direct penetration (trauma, bite wound, foreign body)

The origin of bacterial CNS infections is not always identified.

Dogs with bacterial CNS infection may or may not have concurrent systemic signs such as fever, anorexia, lethargy, a neutrophilic leukocytosis, heart murmur from infectious endocarditis, or urinary tract infection.

Otogenic meningoencephalitis can occur in dogs of any age or breed but is most common in brachycephalic dogs.[41] A history of otitis externa is common but not always present. Neurological signs include progressive central vestibular or cerebellar signs, epileptic seizures, oral pain, and neck pain. MR images show evidence of otitis media with extension into the meninges and/or brain parenchyma of the temporal lobe (cerebrum), brainstem, and cerebellum. A neutrophilic or mixed cell CSF pleocytosis is seen in acute cases, while a mononuclear pleocytosis may be seen in chronic cases. Treatment can include medical management with a prolonged course of antibiotics that penetrate bone. Surgery (bulla osteotomy +/– total ear canal ablation) may be necessary in some cases. Ideally, antibiotic therapy should be guided by culture of CSF, middle ear fluid obtained by myringotomy, or surgical samples. External ear cultures may not be representative of the organisms in the middle ear and CNS.

TABLE 25.4 Aerobic and anaerobic organisms reported to cause bacterial central nervous system infection in dogs and cats.

Aerobic	Anaerobic
Staphylococcus spp.	*Listeria monocytogenes*
Streptococcus spp.	*Prevotella oralis*
Escherichia coli	*Fusobacterium* spp.
Pasteurella spp.	*Bacteroides* spp.
Klebsiella spp.	*Peptostreptococcus* spp.
Proteus spp.	*Eubacterium* spp.
Salmonella spp.	*Flavobacterium breve*
Actinomyces spp.	*Propionibacterium* spp.
Nocardia spp.	

Video 25.7

Ten-year-old male Italian Spinone with bacterial meningoencephalitis. Note the severe right-sided rolling reflecting central vestibular involvement. The dog was treated with an immunosuppressive dosage of prednisolone one month before the onset of the neurological signs and recovered completely after antibiotic treatment. Video courtesy of Dr. Gualtiero Gandini.

Cases of nonotogenic meningitis/meningoencephalitis,[42] CNS abscesses, and intracranial empyema[43] do not have an age, breed, or sex predilection. Acute presentation of clinical signs is common. Any region of the CNS can be affected (Video 25.7) (Fig. 25.1). With meningitis/meningoencephalitis, pyrexia is reported in 40% of cases, and neck pain is reported in up to 30% of cases. With intracranial empyema, a local source of infection is often identified and can be associated with exophthalmos/retrobulbar swelling, intraoral lesion, or trauma. MRI of meningitis/meningoencephalitis typically reveals meningeal contrast enhancement with or without concurrent T2W hyperintensities within the brain parenchyma. Abscesses will have ring contrast enhancement on MRI (Fig. 25.3). MRI findings for intracranial subdural empyema consist of a unilateral crescent-shaped T2W hyperintensity in the epidural space that does not suppress on fluid attenuation inversion recovery (FLAIR) sequences and exhibits ring contrast enhancement. A neutrophilic CSF pleocytosis is most common, but a mononuclear or eosinophilic pleocytosis has also been reported. Ideally, antibiotic selection will be based on culture results from blood, CSF, or other infected tissues/fluids such as urine. Surgery may be warranted for extraparenchymal abscesses or intracranial empyema.

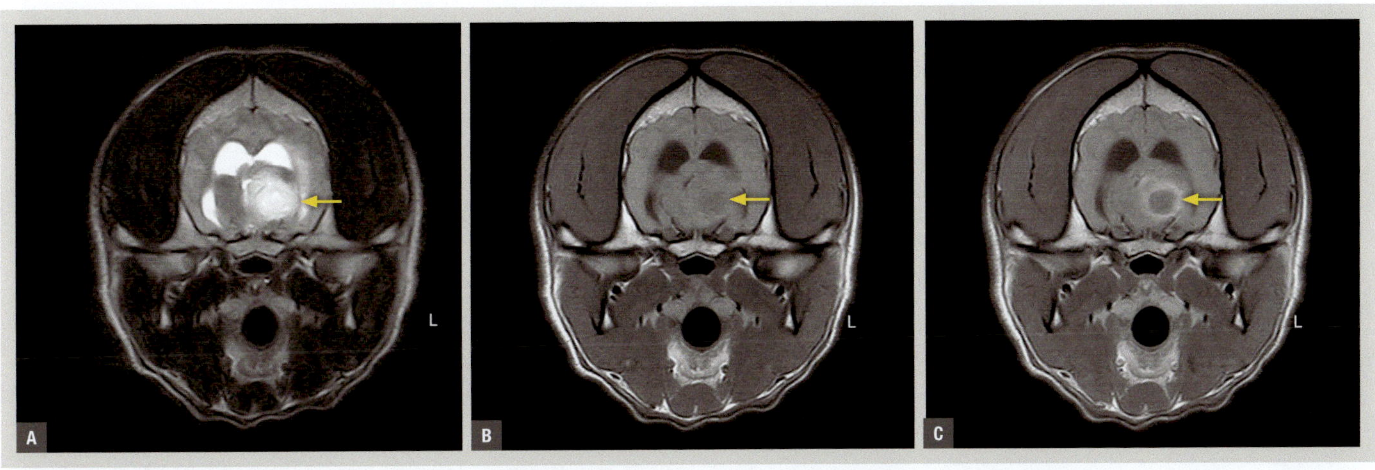

FIG. 25.3 Magnetic resonance imaging study of the brain of a dog affected by a left thalamic abscess. (A) Tranverse T2-weighted image; (B) transverse T1-weighted image; (C) transverse T1-weighted image post constrast. Note the severe space-occupying lesion of the left cerebral thalamus (arrows), hyperintense in A, isointense with a hypointense center in B, and with diffuse ring-pattern contrast enhancement in C. L, left. Pictures courtesy of Dr. Massimo Baroni.

Spinal empyema is more commonly reported in medium to large breed dogs but can affect dogs of any breed and age. Clinical signs include back or neck pain and myelopathy. The thoracic, lumbar, and sacral regions are more commonly affected than the cervical region. Concurrent discospondylitis and other infections such as urinary tract infections, prostatitis, dermatitis, penetrating wounds, and pyothorax are common. MRI reveals epidural mass-like lesions that are T2W hyperintense or of mixed signal intensity with peripheral or uniform contrast enhancement. CSF typically shows a neutrophilic pleocytosis. Both surgical and medical management have been reported with good outcomes.[6]

Ideally, treatment for bacterial infections is chosen based on the results of culture and antibacterial sensitivity panels. Alternatively, broad-spectrum antibiotics can be utilized. Clinicians should remember that cultures obtained from extraneural infections may or may not represent the organisms present in the CNS. The ideal duration of treatment is unknown, but prolonged treatment (minimum 8 weeks) should be considered. Generally, glucocorticoids should be avoided in bacterial infections, but in a severely affected patient, a low anti-inflammatory dosage administered in the short-term could be beneficial.[44,45]

The prognosis is generally good. Exceptions may include cases with multidrug-resistant organisms or severe neurological deficits on presentation. Dogs with otogenic meningoencephalitis, abscesses, or empyema that do not respond to medical management can have a good prognosis after surgical intervention.

Discospondylitis

Infection of the vertebrae in dogs most commonly involves primary infection of the cartilaginous endplates with secondary infection of the intervertebral disc, which is known as discospondylitis.[46] In dogs less than 2 years of age, the infection may be limited to the vertebral physis and not involve the disc space (physitis). Infectious organisms spread hematogenously from a distant site and establish infection in the endplates secondary to reduced blood flow through the capillary beds in that location. Commonly reported organisms include *Staphylococcus* spp., *Streptococcus* spp., *Escherichia coli,* and *Pasteurella* spp. Some studies have reported *Brucella canis* as a common causative agent, which is important because of its zoonotic potential.[47,40] Discospondylitis is less commonly caused by fungal organisms, but this should be considered if clinical signs do not improve despite appropriate antimicrobial therapy. The German Shepherd breed is overrepresented for fungal discospondylitis (Video 25.8).

Discospondylitis is most commonly seen in young to middle-aged medium and large breed dogs. Males and Boxers, Doberman Pinschers, English Bulldogs, German Shepherd dogs, Great Danes, Rhodesian Ridgebacks, and Rottweilers are overrepresented. Clinical signs are often progressive over weeks but can also occur acutely, especially if there is a secondary fracture or subluxation. The most common clinical sign is neck or back pain. Dogs may also present with fever, lethargy, and anorexia. Less commonly, dogs can present with signs of a myelopathy or nerve root signature.[46]

In cases with neck or back pain and no neurological deficits, radiographs can be used to screen for discospondylitis. Common radiographic findings include symmetrical lysis of the endplates at the affected disc space, often with secondary collapse of the intervertebral disc space. With chronicity, there will be sclerosis of the endplates, and spondylosis may develop ventrally and laterally (Fig. 25.4). Commonly affected sites are the lumbosacral junction, caudal cervical region, and mid-thoracic region, but any site in the vertebral column can be affected. Multiple sites may be affected. Importantly, radiographic evidence of discospondylitis may lag behind clinical signs by several weeks, necessitating repeat radiographs or referral for cross-sectional imaging if clinical signs persist. In dogs with no radiographic evidence of discospondylitis, computed tomography (CT) is more sensitive in 33% of cases, and MRI is more sensitive in 63% of cases.[48] CT will show multiple punctate areas of osteolysis surrounding the endplates. MRI will show evidence of endplate lysis, often with T2W hyperintensity of the intervertebral disc as well as contrast enhancement of the endplates and paravertebral soft tissues. MRI is the most sensitive diagnostic imaging procedure to detect discospondylitis and is recommended in dogs with neurological deficits to diagnose spinal cord compression secondary to tissue proliferation, empyema (Fig. 25.5), and/or subluxation, as this will help determine if surgical decompression or stabilization is warranted.

Urine culture should be performed for all dogs diagnosed with discospondylitis. In endemic regions, screening tests for *B. canis* should be performed. Blood cultures may also be of value. Ultrasound- or fluoroscopy-guided percutaneous fine-needle aspiration may provide a sample for culture. Alternatively, in patients not responding to antibiotic therapy or patients suspected to have fungal discospondylitis, surgical culture may be necessary.

Video 25.8

Ten-year-old female spayed German Shepherd dog with C5–C6 mycotic discospondylitis. Note the antalgic posture (low head carriage) due to the severe pain. Note also the short-strided gait in the front limbs and the reluctance to move. Magnetic resonance imaging confirmed the presence of the discospondylitis and adjacent empyema. Video courtesy of Dr. Gualtiero Gandini.

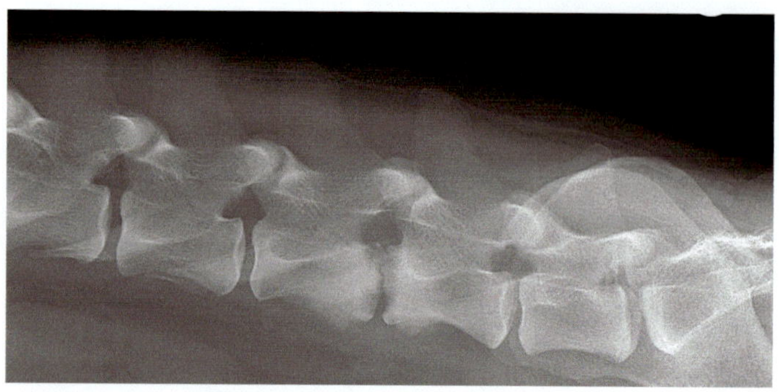

FIG. 25.4 Lateral radiograph of the lumbar vertebral column. At L5–L6, there is well-defined lysis of the endplates with adjacent sclerosis and collapse of the intervertebral disc space. Mild thickening and irregularity of the retroperitoneal soft tissues can be seen along the ventral aspect of this intervertebral disc space.

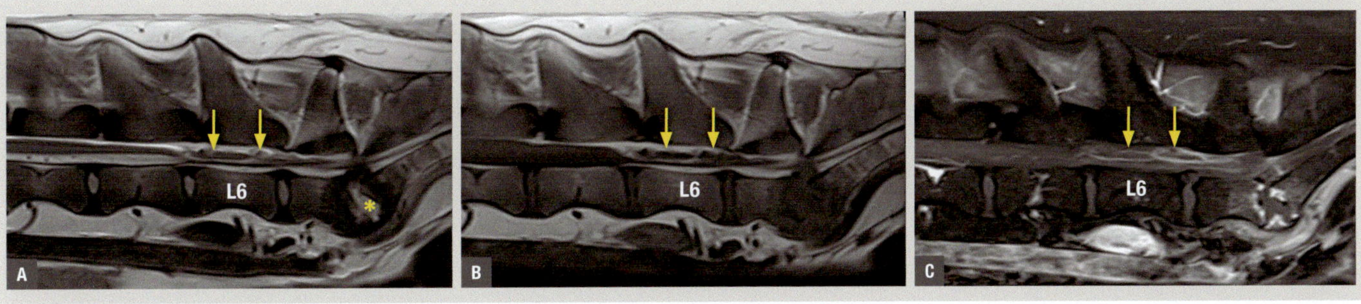

FIG. 25.5 Sagittal magnetic resonance images of the lumbosacral vertebral column: **(A)** T2-weighted (T2W) image, **(B)** T1-weighted image (TW1), and **(C)** T1W image post contrast administration with fat saturation. There is evidence of discospondylitis at the L7–S1 disc space. The disc space is widened. The endplates are severely irregular and lytic, with strong heterogeneous contrast enhancement. The adjacent vertebral medullary cavities are T2W and T1W hypointense, which is consistent with sclerosis. The disc space contains a moderate amount of heterogenous, amorphously shaped material that is T2W hyperintense centrally (*) and strongly and heterogeneously contrast-enhancing at the periphery. There is evidence of empyema dorsally, from the L5–L6 disc space to the L7–S1 disc space. This appears as amorphous material that is T2W hypointense and T1W isointense, and with strong peripheral contrast enhancement (arrows). Moderate spondylosis deformans can be seen along the ventral aspect L7–S1. The ventral paravertebral soft tissues at the level of L7–S1 are moderately enlarged, heterogenous, and contrast enhancing. There is moderate bilateral homogeneous contrast enhancement of the epaxial musculature.

Ideally, treatment should be guided by culture results. Historically, first-generation cephalosporins have been an excellent empiric therapy; however, they may become less efficacious as numbers of multi-drug-resistant infections keep rising. When an effective antibiotic has been chosen, dogs should become comfortable without additional pain medications in 3–5 days. There is no defined standard for the duration of treatment, although most neurologists treat for a minimum of 3–6 months and do not discontinue medications unless there is complete resolution of the clinical signs. Surgical decompression or stabilization may be needed in some patients.

Infection with *B. canis* is a public health concern, and infected dogs should be considered infected for life. Owners should be referred to their physician to discuss testing and treatment.

KEY POINTS

- Geographic region and travel history are key to prioritize infectious disease differentials.
- Central nervous system (CNS) infections occur most commonly in young or immunocompromised patients.
- Patients with CNS infection typically present with multifocal, progressive CNS signs.
- Antemortem diagnosis requires MRI, CSF analysis, and appropriate infectious disease testing.
- Infectious disease tests and tissues for sample acquisition must be chosen to maximize sensitivity and specificity.
- Viral CNS infections are treated symptomatically, while other CNS infections are treated with targeted antimicrobial therapy.
- The prognosis for recovery from CNS infection varies depending on the organism and patient situation.
- Rabies and *Brucella canis* are important public health concerns.

References

1. Chomel BB, Sykes JE. Rabies. In: Sykes, JE (ed.). *Greene's Infectious Diseases of the Dog and Cat*, 5th ed. Missouri: Elsevier Saunders; 2022. pp. 260–270.
2. Eng TR, Fishbein DB. Epidemiologic Factors, Clinical Findings, and Vaccination Status of Rabies in Cats and Dogs in the United States in 1988. *J Am Vet Med Assoc.* 1990;197:201–209.
3. Laothamatas J, Wacharapluesadee S, Lumlertdacha B, et al. Furious and Paralytic Rabies of Canine Origin: Neuroimaging with Virological and Cytokine Studies. *J Neurovirol.* 2008;14:119–129.
4. Barnes HL, Chrisman CL, Farina L, Detrisac CJ. Clinical Evaluation of Rabies Virus Meningoencephalomyelitis in a Dog. *J Am Anim Hosp Assoc.* 2003;39:547–550.
5. Sykes JE, Vandevelde M. Canine Distemper Virus Infection. In: Sykes, JE (ed.). *Greene's Infectious Diseases of the Dog and Cat*, 5th ed. Missouri: Elsevier Saunders; 2022. pp. 271–288.
6. Laws EJ, Sánchez L, Beltran E, et al. Multicenter Study of Clinical Presentation, Treatment, and Outcome in 41 Dogs With Spinal Epidural Empyema. *Front Vet Sci.* 2022 Mar 7;9:813316.
7. Tipold A, Vandevelde M, Jaggy A. Neurological Manifestations of Canine Distemper Virus Infection. *J Small Anim Pract.* 1992;33:466–470.
8. Amude AM, Alfieri AA, Alfieri AF. Antemortem Diagnosis of CDV Infection by RT-PCR in Distemper Dogs with Neurological Deficits without the

Typical Clinical Presentation. *Vet Res Commun.* 2006;30:679–687.
9. Sui P, Sun Y, Shi Y, et al. Establishment and Evaluation of a Multiplex Real-Time RT-PCR for Quantitative and Differential Detection of Wild-Type Canine Distemper Virus from Vaccine Strains. *Heliyon.* 2023;9:e19344.
10. Wilkes RP, Sanchez E, Riley MC, Kennedy MA. Real-Time Reverse Transcription Polymerase Chain Reaction Method for Detection of Canine Distemper Virus Modified Live Vaccine Shedding for Differentiation from Infection with Wild-Type Strains. *J Vet Diagn Invest.* 2014;26:27–34.
11. Sykes JE, Tipold A. Arthropod-Borne Viral Infections In: Sykes, JE (ed.). *Greene's Infectious Diseases of the Dog and Cat*, 5th ed. Missouri: Elsevier Saunders; 2022. pp. 489–500.
12. Kleeb C, Golini L, Beckmann K, et al. Canine Tick-Borne Encephalitis: Clinical Features, Survival Rate and Neurological Sequelae: A Retrospective Study of 54 Cases (1999-2016). *Front Vet Sci.* 2021 Nov 10;8:782044.
13. Wessmann A, Lu D, Lamb CR, et al. Brain and spinal cord haemorrhages associated with Angiostrongylus vasorum infection in four dogs. *Vet Rec.* 2006 Jun 24;158(25):858–863.
14. Di Cesare A, Traversa D. Canine Angiostrongylosis: Recent Advances in Diagnosis, Prevention, and Treatment. *Vet Med (Auckl).* 2014;5:181–192.
15. Liu J, Schnyder M, Willesen JL, et al. Performance of the Angio Detect™ in-Clinic Test Kit for Detection of Angiostrongylus Vasorum Infection in Dog Samples from Europe. *Vet Parasitol Reg Stud Reports.* 2017;7:45–47.
16. Lowrie M, De Risio L, Dennis R, et al. Concurrent Medical Conditions and Long-Term Outcome in Dogs with Nontraumatic Intracranial Hemorrhage. *Vet Radiol Ultrasound.* 2012;53:381–388.
17. Schnyder M, Fahrion A, Ossent P, et al. Larvicidal Effect of Imidacloprid/Moxidectin Spot-on Solution in Dogs Experimentally Inoculated with Angiostrongylus Vasorum. *Vet Parasitol.* 2009;166:326–332.
18. Conboy G. Natural infections of Crenosoma vulpis and Angiostrongylus vasorum in dogs in Atlantic Canada and their treatment with milbemycin oxime. *Vet Rec.* 2004 Jul 3;155(1):16–18.
19. Sykes JE, Lappin MR, Dubey JP. Neosporosis. In: Sykes, JE (ed.). *Greene's Infectious Diseases of the Dog and Cat*, 5th ed. Missouri: Elsevier Saunders; 2022. pp. 1163–1171.
20. Garosi L, Dawson A, Couturier J, et al. Necrotizing Cerebellitis and Cerebellar Atrophy Caused by Neospora Caninum Infection: Magnetic Resonance Imaging and Clinicopathologic Findings in Seven Dogs. *J Vet Intern Med.* 2010;24:571–578.
21. Fisher C, Seferidis N, Zilli J, et al. Insights into the Clinical Presentation, Diagnostics and Outcome in Dogs Presenting with Neurological Signs Secondary to Infection with Neospora Caninum: 41 Cases (2014-2023). *J Small Anim Pract.* 2024;65:582–588.
22. Lappin MR, Dubey JP. Toxoplasmosis. In: Sykes, JE (ed.). *Greene's Infectious Diseases of the Dog and Cat*, 5th ed. Missouri: Elsevier Saunders; 2022. pp. 1151–1162.
23. Coelho AM, Cherubini G, De Stefani A, et al. Serological Prevalence of Toxoplasmosis and Neosporosis in Dogs Diagnosed with Suspected Meningoencephalitis in the UK. *J Small Anim Pract.* 2019;60:44–50.
24. Barrs VR, Dear JD. Aspergillosis and Penicilliosis. In: Sykes, JE (ed.). *Greene's Infectious Diseases of the Dog and Cat*, 5th ed. Missouri: Elsevier Saunders; 2022. pp. 1069–1093.
25. Schultz RM, Johnson EG, Wisner ER, et al. Clinicopathologic and Diagnostic Imaging Characteristics of Systemic Aspergillosis in 30 Dogs. *J Vet Intern Med.* 2008 Jul-Aug;22(4):851–859.
26. Taylor AR, Young BD, Levine GJ, et al. Clinical Features and Magnetic Resonance Imaging Findings in 7 Dogs with Central Nervous System Aspergillosis. *J Vet Intern Med.* 2015;29:1556–1563.
27. Bentley RT, Taylor AR, Thomovsky SA. Fungal Infections of the Central Nervous System in Small Animals: Clinical Features, Diagnosis, and Management. *Vet Clin North Am Small Anim Pract.* 2018 Jan;48(1):63–83.
28. Ballber C, Hill TL, Bommer NX. Minimally Invasive Treatment of Sino-Nasal Aspergillosis in Dogs. *J Vet Intern Med.* 2018;32:2069–2073.
29. Hecht S, Adams WH, Smith JR, Thomas WB. Clinical and Imaging Findings in Five Dogs with Intracranial Blastomycosis (Blastomyces Dermatiditis). *J Am Anim Hosp Assoc.* 2011;47:241–249.
30. Lipitz L, Rylander H, Forrest LJ, Foy DS. Clinical and magnetic resonance imaging features of central nervous system blastomycosis in 4 dogs. *J Vet Intern Med.* 2010 Nov-Dec;24(6):1509–514.
31. Kelley AJ, Stainback LB, Knowles KE, et al. Clinical Characteristics, Magnetic Resonance Imaging Features, Treatment, and Outcome for Presumed Intracranial Coccidioidomycosis in 45 Dogs (2009-2019). *J Vet Intern Med.* 2021;35:2222–2231.
32. Reagan KL, Krockenberger M, Sykes JE. Cryptococcosis. In: Sykes, JE (ed.). *Greene's Infectious Diseases of the Dog and Cat*, 5th ed. Missouri: Elsevier Saunders; 2022. pp. 1014–1029.
33. Sykes JE, Sturges BK, Cannon MS, et al. Clinical Signs, Imaging Features, Neuropathology, and Outcome in Cats and Dogs with Central Nervous System Cryptococcosis from California. *J Vet Intern Med.* 2010;24:1427–1438.
34. Jacobson E, Morton JM, Woerde DJ, et al. Clinical Features, Outcomes, and Long-Term Survival Times of Cats and Dogs with Central Nervous System Cryptococcosis in Australia: 50 Cases (2000–2020). *J Am Vet Med Assoc.* 2023;261:246–257.
35. Gasser AM, Birkenheuer AJ, Breitschwerdt EB. Canine Rocky Mountain Spotted Fever: A Retrospective Study of 30 Cases. *J Am Anim Hosp Assoc.* 2001;37:41–48.
36. Mikszewski JS, Vite CH. Central Nervous System Dysfunction Associated with Rocky Mountain Spotted Fever Infection in Five Dogs. *J Am Anim Hosp Assoc.* 2005;41:259–266.
37. Harrus S, Waner T, Mylonakis ME, et al. Ehrlichiosis. In: Sykes, JE (ed.). *Greene's Infectious Diseases of the Dog and Cat*, 5th ed. Missouri: Elsevier Saunders. pp. 522–541.
38. Frank JR, Breitschwerdt EB. A retrospective study of ehrlichiosis in 62 dogs from North Carolina and Virginia. *J Vet Intern Med.* 1999 May-Jun;13(3):194–201.
39. Silvestrini P, Lloyd-Bradley B, Glanemann B, et al. Clinical Presentation, Diagnostic Investigations, Treatment Protocols and Outcomes of Dogs Diagnosed with Tick-Borne Diseases Living in the United Kingdom: 76 Cases (2005-2019). *J Small Anim Pract.* 2023;64:392–400.
40. Neer TM, Breitschwerdt EB, Greene RT, Lappin MR. Consensus statement on ehrlichial disease of small animals from the infectious disease study group of the ACVIM. American College of Veterinary Internal Medicine. *J Vet Intern Med.* 2002 May-Jun;16(3):309–315.
41. Butterfield S, Whittaker D, Tabanez J, et al. Bacterial Meningitis Secondary to Otogenic Infection in 10 French Bulldogs: A Retrospective Case Series. *Vet Rec Open.* 2023;10:e263.
42. Radaelli ST, Platt SR. Bacterial meningoencephalomyelitis in dogs: a retrospective study of 23 cases (1990-1999). *J Vet Intern Med.* 2002 Mar-Apr;16(2):159–163.
43. Forward AK, Plessas IN, Guilherme S, De Decker S. Retrospective evaluation of the clinical presentation, magnetic resonance imaging findings, and outcome of dogs diagnosed with intracranial empyema (2008-2015): 9 cases. *J Vet Emerg Crit Care (San Antonio).* 2019 Jul;29(4):431–438.
44. Lu C, Chang W, Lui C. Strategies for the Management of Bacterial Brain Abscess. *J Clin Neurosci.* 2006;13:979–985.
45. Tipold A, Vandevelde M, Barber R, Sykes JE. Miscellaneous Infections and Inflammatory Disorders of the Central Nervous System. In: Sykes, JE (ed.). *Greene's Infectious Diseases of the Dog and Cat*, 5th ed. Missouri: Elsevier Saunders. pp. 1710–1727.
46. Van Hoof C, Davis NA, Carrera-Justiz S, et al. Clinical Features, Comparative Imaging Findings, Treatment, and Outcome in Dogs with Discospondylitis: A Multi-Institutional Retrospective Study. *J Vet Intern Med.* 2023;37:1438–1446.
47. Burkert BA, Kerwin SC, Hosgood GL, et al. Signalment and Clinical Features of Diskospondylitis in Dogs: 513 Cases (1980–2001). *J Am Vet Med Assoc.* 2005;227:268–275.
48. Van Hoof C, Davis NA, Carrera-Justiz S, et al. Clinical Features, Comparative Imaging Findings, Treatment, and Outcome in Dogs with Discospondylitis: A Multi-Institutional Retrospective Study. *J Vet Intern Med.* 2023;37:1438–1446.

CHAPTER 26

Meningoencephalomyelitis of unknown origin

Renee Barber
DVM, PhD, DACVIM (Neurology)

Meningoencephalomyelitis of unknown origin (MUO) is a presumptive diagnosis of noninfectious, nonsuppurative inflammation of the brain, spinal cord, and/or leptomeninges in dogs. It is one of many noninfectious inflammatory disorders described in dogs (Fig. 26.1). The term meningoencephalitis may be used if there is thought to be no spinal cord involvement, and the term meningomyelitis may be used if there is thought to be no brain involvement. More commonly, the inclusive term meningoencephalomyelitis is used to describe the presence of inflammation affecting the meninges and one or more areas of the central nervous system (CNS). Although the prevalence of MUO is not known, it is one of the most commonly diagnosed disorders in neurology specialty practice. A recent retrospective study identified 633 dogs diagnosed with MUO at two referral hospitals between 2010 and 2022.

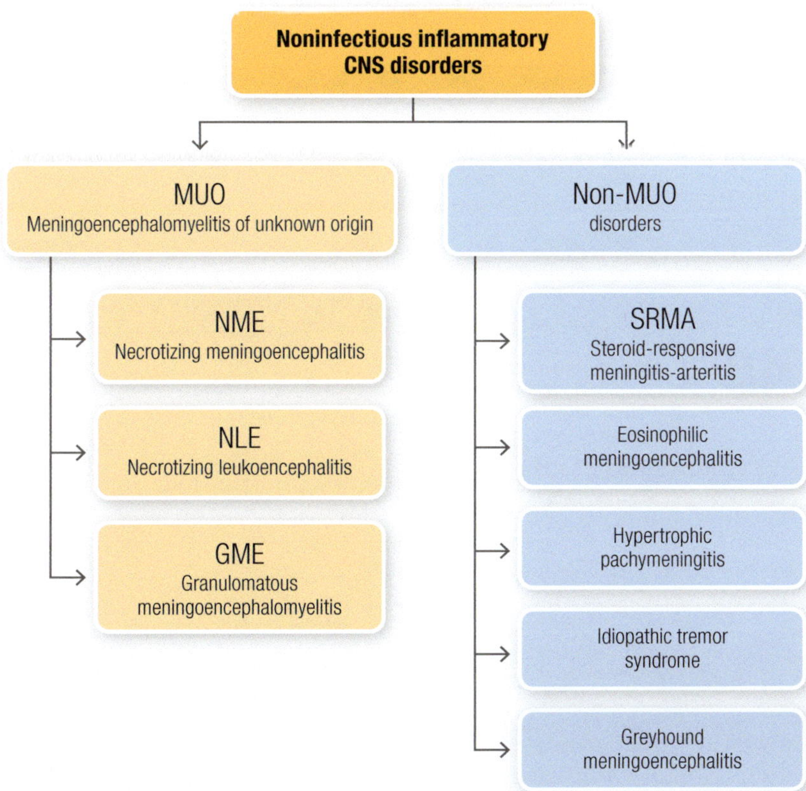

FIG. 26.1 Categorization of noninfectious inflammatory central nervous system (CNS) disease in dogs.

Technically, the diagnosis of MUO is intended to represent a presumptive clinical diagnosis of three specific, histological variants of CNS inflammation that were initially described in the 1970s–1990s: necrotizing meningoencephalitis (NME), necrotizing leukoencephalitis (NLE), and granulomatous meningoencephalomyelitis (GME).[1] Each of these variants has a slightly different distribution of inflammation, and, although the inflammation is always mononuclear, the distribution of cell types differs among the three variants. Additionally, as the names suggest, necrosis is found in NME and NLE but not in GME. Initially, NME and NLE were identified in the Pug and Yorkshire Terrier, respectively. This led them to be described as *Pug dog encephalitis* or *Yorkshire Terrier encephalitis*. These disorders have now been described in numerous breeds; to avoid confusing breed-specific terminology, they are now termed NME and NLE regardless of the breed in which they are diagnosed.

Brain biopsy and/or necropsy are not always possible, so many dogs diagnosed with MUO lack histological confirmation to determine whether they have NME, NLE, or GME. Because of this, the terminology *meningoencephalomyelitis of unknown etiology* was proposed for dogs with a consistent clinical diagnosis based on history, signalment, magnetic resonance imaging, cerebrospinal fluid (CSF) analysis, and negative infectious disease testing appropriate to the geographic region.[2] More recently, a switch to *meningoencephalomyelitis of unknown origin* (MUO) has been suggested to avoid confusion since the spelling of *etiology* varies depending on the geographic region.[1]

Etiology

The specific components of the etiopathogenesis of MUO are not well understood. Initial investigations tried to identify an infectious cause for the inflammatory lesions seen in MUO, but to date, no causative infectious agents have been identified.[1] Currently, most of the information suggests MUO is an autoimmune disease. Patients respond favorably, at least initially, to treatment with immunosuppressive medications. In people, the association of human leukocyte antigen class II alleles with autoimmune disease has been well documented for decades, and in NME, several toy breeds have been shown to share genetic risk associated with dog leukocyte antigen class II.[3] Evaluation of T cell phenotypes in dogs with MUO also supports an autoimmune pathogenesis. Alterations in T helper 1 and T helper 17 cells and cytokines have been identified in peripheral blood and brain lesions from dogs with MUO.[4,5] Autoantibodies to glial fibrillary acidic protein (GFAP) and transglutaminase 2 have also been documented in dogs with GME and NME, although it is unclear if these autoantibodies support the presence of a humoral autoimmune reaction or are the result of tissue damage secondary to already present inflammation.

Clinical features

Overview

MUO typically affects young to middle-aged dogs, with most cases occurring in dogs between 1–8 years. It typically does not affect dogs younger than 6 months or older than 12 years. Toy and small breed dogs are overrepresented, with dogs less than 15 kg representing greater than 75% of reported cases (Table 26.1). MUO typically has an acute onset with a progressive clinical course, although chronic cases progressing over several months have been reported. Clinical signs of MUO reflect the region of the CNS affected by inflammation, which most often results in multifocal and asymmetrical neurological signs. Dogs can be presented with epileptic seizures, neck pain, or back pain with no other neurological deficits. More commonly, the following neuroanatomical localizations have been reported: multifocal, prosencephalon, central vestibular, brainstem, cerebellum, optic nerves/chiasm.[6–9] Extraneural signs are typically lacking, but pyrexia has been reported in a small number of GME cases. A list of clinical signs most often seen in cases of MUO is presented in Table 26.2. It is also important to remember that specific features of the MUO variants (NME, NLE, and GME) can affect how dogs present clinically. In addition, MUO occasionally presents as a myelopathy with no signs of intracranial involvement.

TABLE 26.1 Breeds overrepresented in several large studies and systematic reviews of meningoencephalomyelitis of unknown origin.[6–9,13]

Small breeds (<15 kg)	Large breeds (> 15kg)
Boston Terrier	English Springer Spaniel
Cavalier King Charles Spaniel	Labrador Retriever
Chihuahua	
Dachshund	
French Bulldog	
Jack Russell Terrier	
Lhasa Apso	
Maltese	
Miniature Pinscher	
Poodle	
Pomeranian	
Prague Ratter	
Pug	
Shih Tzu	
West Highland White Terrier	
Yorkshire Terrier	

Necrotizing meningoencephalitis

NME has a median age of onset of 18 months and typically occurs in dogs aged 6 months to 7 years. The most commonly affected breeds are the Pug, Maltese, and Chihuahua, but it has been reported in other small breeds including the Boston Terrier, Brussels Griffon, Coton de Tulear, Lhasa Apso, Papillion, Pekingese, Pomeranian, Shih Tzu, West Highland White Terrier, and Yorkshire Terrier. NME typically has an acute onset with rapid progression of the neurological signs, or, less commonly, a chronic progression of 4–6 months. Inflammatory lesions affect the cerebral hemispheres, resulting in altered mentation and epileptic seizures. Affected dogs have also been reported to have circling and visual deficits. Cervical hyperesthesia can be seen if there is extensive involvement of the leptomeninges.

Necrotizing leukoencephalitis

NLE has an age of onset ranging from 1–12 years, but it is most often seen between 6 months to 5 years. To date, NLE has been described in the Yorkshire Terrier and French Bulldog, but it is known to affect other toy breeds as well. Dogs with NLE can have an acute or chronic (several months) progression of signs. NLE has a predilection for the white matter of the cerebrum but can also extend into brainstem and spinal cord. Mentation change, epileptic seizures, and visual deficits result from prosencephalic lesions, and dogs with brainstem involvement often have central vestibular signs. As in NME, neck pain has been reported and is thought to be due to leptomeningeal involvement.

TABLE 26.2 Summary of the clinical signs and percentage of dogs affected from a combined total of 937 dogs reported in several large studies and systematic reviews of meningoencephalomyelitis of unknown origin.[6–9]

		Percentage of dogs affected
Neurological deficits	Ataxia[b]	49
	Obtundation	45
	Paresis[a]	34
	Epileptic seizures	32
	Cranial nerve deficits	32
	Signs of increased intracranial pressure[c]	12
Neuroanatomical localization	Multifocal	50
	Prosencephalon	38
	Brainstem	16
	Central vestibular	12
	Myelopathy	7
	Cerebellum	4
	Optic nerves/chiasm	4
	Pain only	2

[a] Including tetraparesis and paraparesis. [b] Including general proprioceptive, vestibular, and cerebellar. [c] Altered mentation (obtundation, stupor, coma), decerebrate or decerebellate posture, changes in pupil size, abnormal physiological nystagmus.

Granulomatous meningoencephalomyelitis

All ages and breeds can be affected by GME, but it is most commonly seen in middle-aged toy and terrier breeds. GME lesion distribution has been reported to be focal, presenting as a single mass lesion mimicking neoplasia, but multifocal or ocular presentations are more common. Clinical signs of multifocal GME often reflect involvement of the brainstem with mentation change, central vestibular signs, and cervical hyperesthesia being more common than epileptic seizures. Anatomically, the optic nerves are an extension of the CNS surrounded by meninges and CSF, and GME has been reported to affect one or both optic nerves. Dogs with ocular GME typically present with an acute onset of visual impairment but can develop additional CNS signs as the disease progresses.

Meningomyelitis

Spinal cord involvement has been described in both NLE and GME, but this usually occurs with concurrent intracranial signs. GME has been histopathologically confirmed to only affect the spinal cord in some dogs. Meningomyelitis of unknown origin has been described in dogs from 10 months old to 11 years old. Although large breed dogs can be affected, dogs <15 kg are overrepresented, as occurs with intracranial cases of MUO. As with other forms of MUO, meningomyelitis is always progressive but can have an acute or chronic course. Dogs with meningomyelitis can have pain without neurological deficits or have a myelopathy. The most commonly reported localizations are the C1–C5 and T3–L3 spinal cord segments, and most dogs have paraspinal hyperesthesia. Rarely, multifocal spinal cord localizations are reported.[9,10] Although uncommon, it is possible for dogs to be so severely affected that paraplegia with loss of pain perception can occur with a thoracolumbar lesion localization, and hypoventilation can occur with a cervical lesion localization.

Clinicopathological findings

Overview

A definitive diagnosis of MUO requires histological evaluation of tissue via a brain biopsy. This is often impossible, so a clinical diagnosis of MUO is made based on a typical history and signalment, compatible magnetic resonance imaging (MRI) and CSF findings, and negative infectious disease testing appropriate for the geographic region (Fig. 26.2). The complete blood count and serum biochemistry results are typically normal.

Cerebrospinal fluid

A mononuclear pleocytosis and elevated protein are consistent with a diagnosis of MUO. However, cell counts and total protein levels show great variability and are occasionally normal in cases of histopathologically confirmed disease. In NME and NLE, a moderate to severe lymphocytic pleocytosis is most common, but mixed cell pleocytosis can also be seen. In GME, a lymphocytic, large mononuclear, or mixed cell pleocytosis are characteristic, but a neutrophilic pleocytosis is possible.

Diagnostic imaging findings

Overview

MRI is recommended to evaluate the brain and/or spinal cord parenchyma when making a diagnosis of MUO. MRI typically reveals focal, multifocal, or diffuse intraparenchymal lesions in the brain and/or spinal cord. The lesions are ill-defined, and multifocal lesions tend to be asymmetrical. Compared to the normal brain parenchyma, inflammatory lesions are hyperintense on T2-weighted (T2W) and T2W fluid attenuation inversion recovery sequences and iso- to hypointense on T1-weighted sequences. There is variable, nonuniform enhancement after administration of a gadolinium-based paramagnetic contrast agent. Evidence of mass effect and increased intracranial pressure can be identified in some cases of NME and GME. Although GME, NME, and NLE have certain characteristic findings on MRI, they cannot be distinguished from each other based on advanced imaging.

Necrotizing meningoencephalitis

In NME, lesions are found in the prosencephalon and are asymmetrical with focal or multifocal T2W hyperintensity that affects both the gray and white matter, making it challenging to identify the boundaries of gray versus white matter (Fig. 26.3). There may be focal or multifocal

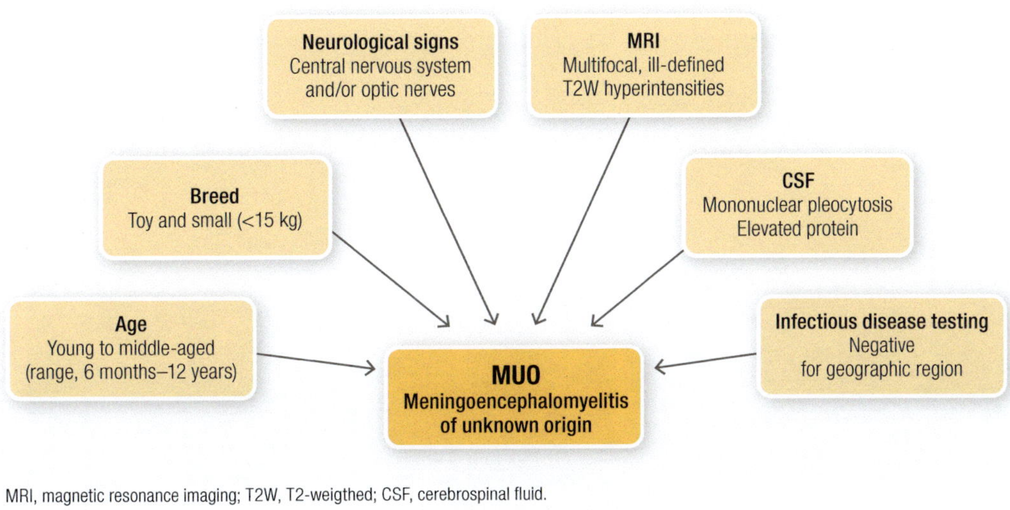

FIG. 26.2 Diagnostic variables utilized for a presumptive, antemortem diagnosis of meningoencephalomyelitis of unknown origin.

cavitation secondary to necrosis. Contrast enhancement of parenchymal lesions is inconsistent; it is patchy and inhomogeneous when present. There can be varying degrees of meningeal contrast enhancement, ventriculomegaly, mass effect, and brain herniation. Midline shift can occur secondary to mass effect with severe lesions, and transtentorial is the most common form of brain herniation identified.

Necrotizing leukoencephalitis

NLE lesions predominate in the subcortical white matter and have a multifocal distribution (Fig. 26.3). They occur less frequently in the brainstem, and spinal cord lesions are rarely identified on MRI. Multifocal areas of cavitation can occur secondary to necrosis. Contrast enhancement of parenchymal lesions is variable and, when present, is patchy and inhomogeneous. Ring enhancement can occur around cavitary lesions. Meningeal contrast enhancement and mass effect have not been reported. Ventriculomegaly is variably present and often of unknown clinical significance.

Granulomatous meningoencephalomyelitis

In GME, lesions typically are multifocal or diffuse with indistinct margins and found in both gray and white matter. They are often found in the brainstem, cerebellum, prosencephalon, and cervical spinal cord with meningeal involvement rarely noted (Fig. 26.4). Large lesions can mimic a solitary neoplastic lesion and cause a mass effect. In cases of optic neuritis, the optic nerves and/or chiasm can be T2W hyperintense, and there is often swelling of the nerves accompanied by loss of surrounding CSF.

Meningomyelitis

In cases with spinal cord involvement only, single diffuse lesions are the most common, but multifocal lesions have also been observed. The lesions are ill-defined and intramedullary. There typically is a loss of CSF and epidural fat observed adjacent to the lesion(s). Most lesions have parenchymal and meningeal contrast enhancement (Fig. 26.5).

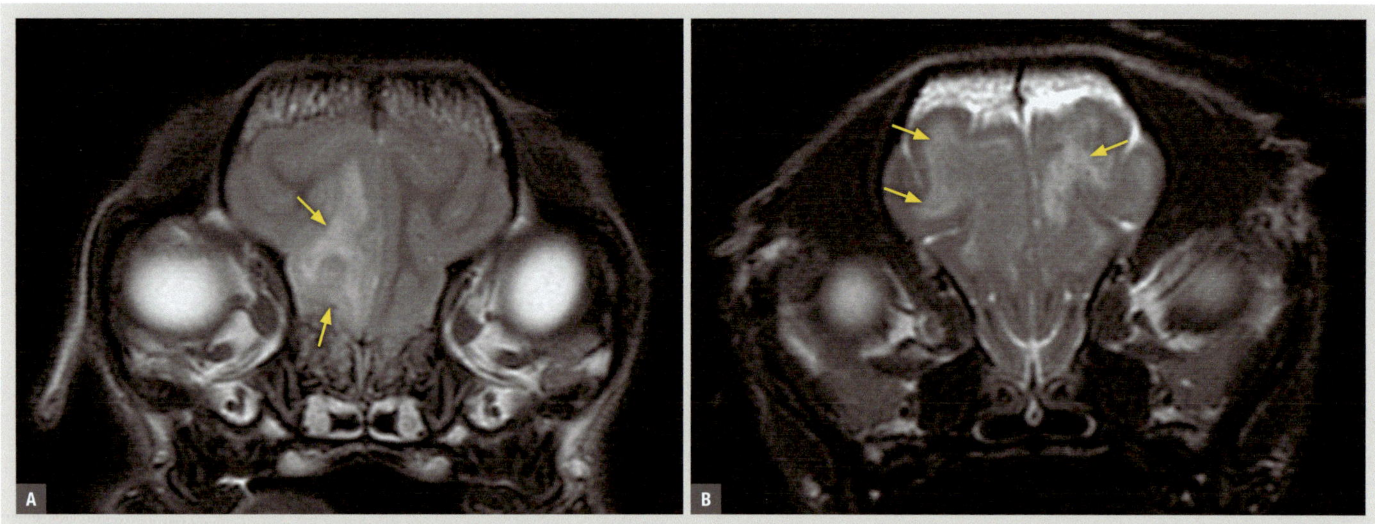

FIG. 26.3 Transverse, T2-weighted (T2W) magnetic resonance images at the level of the cerebral hemispheres (frontal/olfactory region). (A) Necrotizing meningoencephalitis in a 9-month-old Pug. There is an intraparenchymal T2W hyperintensity affecting the superficial gray matter and adjacent white matter (arrows). (B) Necrotizing leukoencephalitis in a 2-year-old Maltese dog. There is an intraparenchymal T2W hyperintensity multifocally affecting the white matter (arrows).

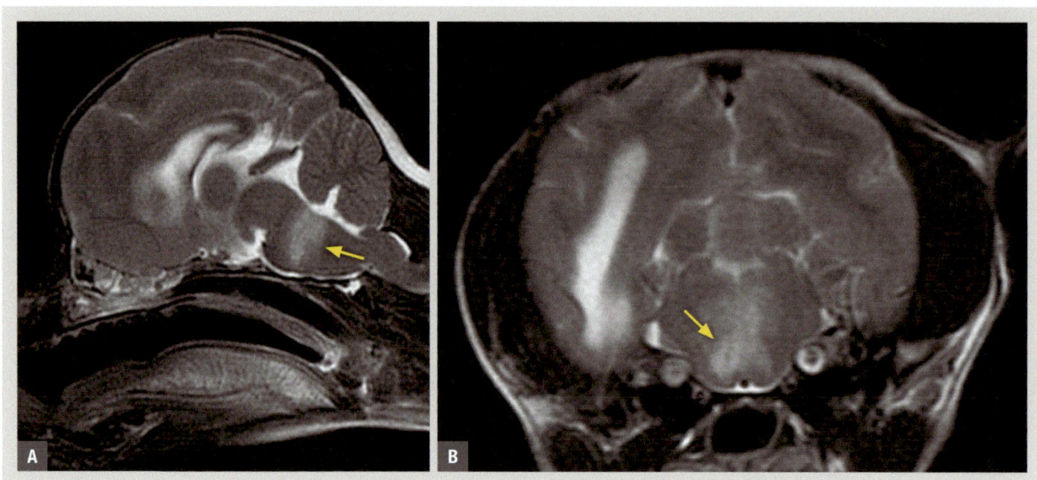

FIG. 26.4 Three-year-old Chihuahua with granulomatous meningoencephalomyelitis. (A) Midline sagittal T2-weighted (T2W) magnetic resonance (MR) image of the brain. (B) Transverse T2W MR image at the level of the cochlea. There is an ill-defined intraparenchymal T2W hyperintensity in the pons and rostral medulla (arrows).

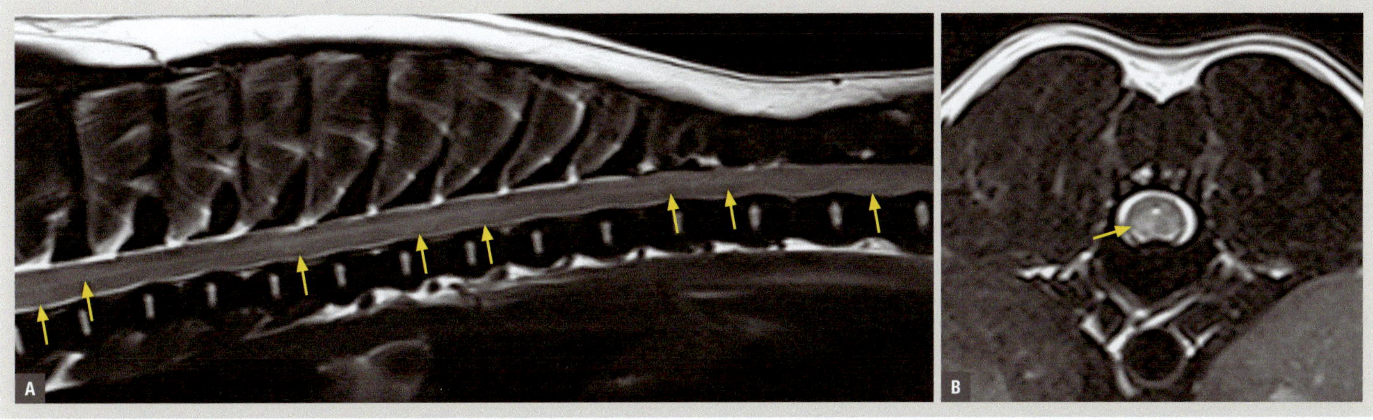

FIG. 26.5 Three-year-old Rat Terrier dog with meningomyelitis. **(A)** Midline sagittal T2-weighted (T2W) magnetic resonance (MR) image of the thoracic vertebral column. **(B)** Transverse T2W MR image at the level of the T13 vertebral body. There are multiple ill-defined T2W hyperintensities throughout the spinal cord (arrows).

Other diagnostic procedures

Brain biopsy

Brain biopsy has been suggested to allow antemortem diagnosis and treatment guidance in cases of MUO, although it is often not pursued due to inaccessibility of lesions, cost, and potential risk of morbidity. Free-hand, image-guided, stereotactic, and endoscopic techniques have all been described, and diagnostic accuracy is reported to range from 82% to 100%. It is possible with small biopsies that the pathologist is unable to differentiate MUO from infection or neoplasia based on the cell population; they may also not be able to distinguish between NME, NLE, and GME. A morbidity rate of 29% has been reported; these cases developed neurological signs that were transient and resolved in 3–14 days. An indirect fatality rate of 6% has been reported.[12]

Histopathology

Ultimately, histological evaluation of the entire brain is needed to truly confirm a diagnosis of NME, NLE, or GME. Pathologists need to evaluate the location and pattern of inflammation as well as the specific cell types present.

In NME, perivascular infiltrates of mononuclear cells with a predominance of lymphocytes occur in the leptomeninges and extend into the superficial cerebral cortex with varying degrees of accompanying necrosis. Although gray matter is affected, inflammation and tissue necrosis often extend into and predominate in the white matter. Reactive astrogliosis is also present and extensive. The brainstem, cerebellum, are not commonly affected. Spinal cord lesions have not been reported.

Histopathologically, NLE is characterized by nonsuppurative, predominately lymphocytic inflammation with concurrent necrosis and astrogliosis in the white matter of the cerebrum and, less commonly, the brainstem and spinal cord. Unlike in NME, leptomeningeal involvement is usual minimal.

GME is defined by three distinct patterns of CNS inflammation that can have a multifocal, focal, or ocular distribution. In multifocal GME, perivascular cuffs of mononuclear cells are present in the brainstem and frequently extend into the cerebrum, cerebellum, and spinal cord. Cerebral lesions most often affect the white matter and less commonly the gray matter and leptomeninges. Epithelioid differentiation of macrophages results in discrete nests of cells within the perivascular cuffs. In focal GME, a mass lesion in the cerebrum, cerebellum, brainstem, spinal cord, or some combination of these forms as the result of similar, coalescing perivascular infiltrates. The same perivascular infiltrates occur in ocular GME but are primarily located in the retinal and postretinal portions of the optic nerve and chiasm. Ocular GME is sometimes present in cases of multifocal GME.

Biomarkers

To date, numerous biomarkers have been investigated for their utility in the diagnosis, prognosis, and assessment of response to treatment, but none are currently used routinely in a clinical setting.

Genetic testing

Genetic testing for confirmation of GME, NME, and NLE does not yet exist, as specific, testable genetic mutations have not been identified in these diseases. The University of California, Davis began offering a test of genetic risk for NME in Pugs (also known as Pug dog encephalitis) over a decade ago. This test was intended for breeders to use in planning and is now offered by numerous laboratories. This test is not and should not be used as a diagnostic test. It can only be used in the Pug breed. Risk assessment is obtained by sequencing the *DQB1* gene in the DLA II region. Dogs with two "S" (i.e., susceptible) haplotypes are considered 12.75 times more likely to develop NME in their lifetime than dogs without susceptible haplotypes. Breeders are advised against attempts to breed out the "S" haplotype as it is present in 40% of the Pug population and is necessary for genetic diversity. It also is important to note that this test is just a guide as it is possible for Pugs to test negative for susceptible haplotypes (i.e., N/N) and still develop disease.

Treatment

Immunosuppression is the mainstay treatment of MUO. However, depending on the severity of the neurological signs, stabilization with oxygen (for hypoxemia), crystalloids, or colloids (to maintain cerebral perfusion and control hypertension), and/or osmotic therapy with mannitol or hypertonic saline (to reduce the elevated intracranial pressure) may be indicated. Additionally, antiseizure medications are required in the event the patient has one or more epileptic seizures.

Anti-inflammatory dosages of glucocorticoids are often utilized until negative infectious disease test results have been obtained. Glucocorticoids are then increased to immunosuppressive dosages (typically 1–2 mg/kg/day) and then tapered by 25% every 4–6 weeks until the lowest dosage that maintains remission is found or the drug can be discontinued. Although glucocorticoids can be used as a monotherapy, a second agent is often started to maintain immunosuppression while the glucocorticoids are being tapered. This can be helpful to minimize the adverse effects of glucocorticoids. A number of second agents have been used in the treatment of MUO, including azathioprine, cytosine arabinoside, cyclosporine, leflunomide, and mycophenolate mofetil (Table 26.3).[13–20] Radiation therapy has also been utilized.[21] Unfortunately, there is a lack of studies directly comparing treatment protocols, and many reports have low case numbers. At this time, there is no evidence for a superior treatment. Selection of the secondary agent often depends on the clinician's preference/experience, the patient's clinical status, and the owner's financial considerations.

Monitoring for response to treatment typically involves evaluation for clinical response and improvement, or ideally resolution, of neurological deficits. Repeat MRI and CSF analysis have been described for monitoring. It was found that abnormal CSF at the 3-month reexamination was associated with relapse, as was discontinuation of treatment before resolution of MRI abnormalities.[22] Although many of the secondary immunosuppressive agents used have a wide safety margin, several have the potential for serious risks, including hepatotoxicity and myelosuppression. It is important to routinely perform a complete blood count and serum biochemistry while patients are receiving these medications.

TABLE 26.3 Summary of immunomodulatory agents used in the treatment of meningoencephalomyelitis of unknown origin.

Drug	Dosages	Side effects	Reported median survival times in days and range
Azathioprine	■ 2 mg/kg PO every 24 h for 2 weeks, then decrease to 2 mg/kg every 48 h indefinitely	■ Myelosuppression, gastrointestinal upset, poor hair growth, acute pancreatitis, and hepatotoxicity ■ Do not use in cats	1,834 (50–2,469)
Cyclosporine	■ 6–10 mg/kg per day given PO every 24 h or divided every 12 h	■ Anorexia, vomiting, diarrhea, gingival hyperplasia, papillomatosis, rarely nephro- and hepatotoxicity	240 (30–365)
			423 (6–840)
			620 (8–870)
			930 (60–1,290)
			1,345 (487–unknown)
Cytosine arabinoside	■ Starting every 3 weeks then progressing to longer intervals: ■ 50 mg/m² SC, every 12 h for 2 consecutive days ■ Alternatively, 200 mg/m² IV over 8 h at the same dosing interval ■ Alternatively, 100 mg/m² IV over 24 h	■ Myelosuppression is an uncommon side effect ■ Rare side effects include anorexia, vomiting, diarrhea, conjunctivitis, oral ulceration, hepatotoxicity, fever, anaphylaxis	26 (0–2,250)
			384 (78–603)
			519 (120–900)
			531 (46–1025)
Leflunomide	■ 3–4 mg/kg PO once daily	■ Hyporexia, vomiting, diarrhea, myelosuppression, ulcerative skin lesions	365
Mycophenolate mofetil	■ 10 mg/kg PO every 12 h; 20 mg/kg PO every 12 h is associated with gastrointestinal signs	■ Hyporexia, vomiting, diarrhea, lethargy, lymphopenia, susceptibility to secondary infections	118 (10–240)
			250 (6 to >1,679)
			558 (3–2,634)
			731 (43–1,672)
Prednisone	■ 2 mg/kg PO per day with 25% dosage reduction every 4–6 weeks if patient is improving; final goal is 0.25–0.5 mg/kg PO every other day indefinitely or discontinuation	■ Polyphagia, PU/PD, HPA-axis suppression, gastrointestinal tract ulceration, hepatopathy, diabetes mellitus, hyperlipidemia, decreased thyroid hormone, decreased protein synthesis, slowed wound healing, immunosuppression	In combination with methylprednisolone: 602 (45–654)
			In combination with dexamethasone: 570 (2–3,540)

PO, orally; SC, subcutaneously; IV, intravenously; PU/PD, polyuria/polydipsia; HPA, hypothalamic–pituitary–adrenal.

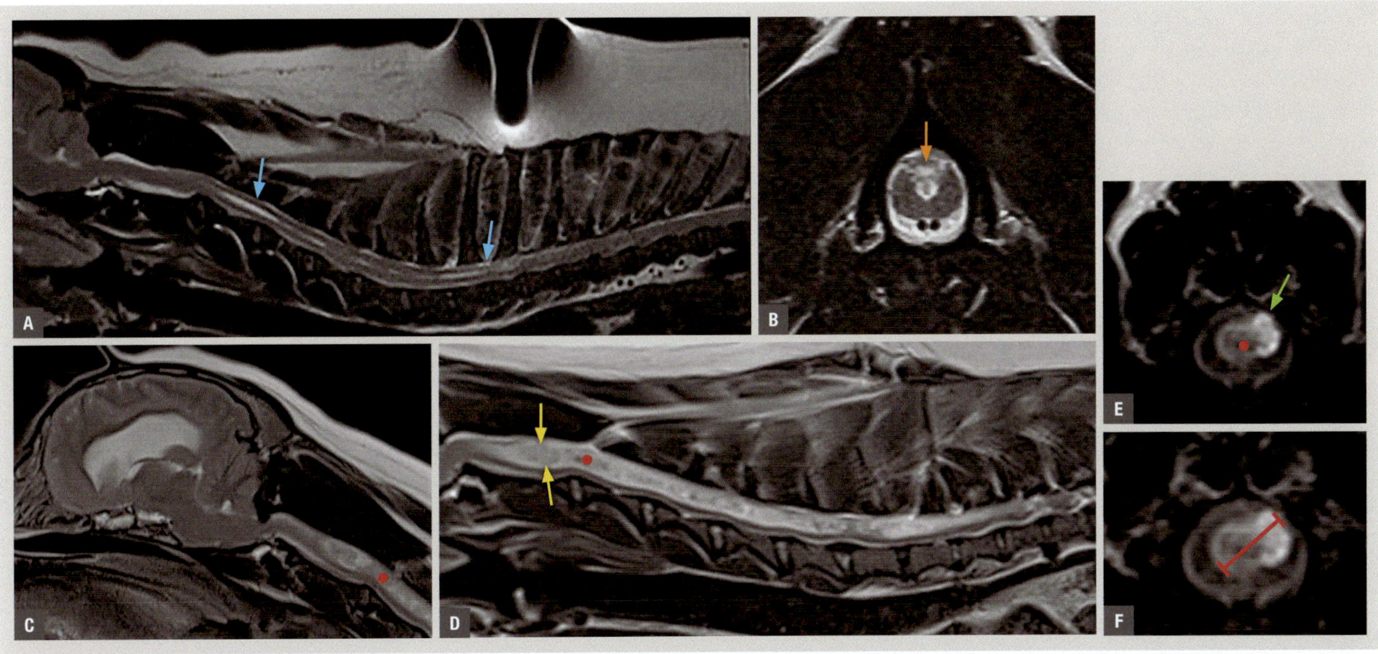

FIG. 27.2 (A, B) Mild (clinically irrelevant) syringomyelia (SM-M). (A) T2-weighted (T2W) image of the midsagittal cervical spine. (B) Transverse T2W image through the spinal cord at C3. The syrinx is small and symmetrical and is developing in the cranial cervical and cranial thoracic regions (blue arrows). There is presyrinx (glymphedema) in the dorsal columns (orange arrow) dorsal to the small symmetrical syrinx. The spinal cord outline is not altered. This 2-year-old male Cavalier King Charles Spaniel was presented with a history of pain and head scratching (signs of Chiari pain). (C–F) Severe (clinically relevant) syringomyelia (SM-S). (C) Parasagittal TW2 image of the brain to the level of C3. (D) Midsagittal TW2 image of the cervical and cranial thoracic spinal cord. (E, F) Transverse T2W images through the spinal cord at the level of C3. There is fluid signal-void sign (FSVS; red dots), the spinal cord outline is expanded (yellow arrows), the maximum diameter of the syrinx (red line) is greater than 4 mm, and there is extension of the syrinx into the superficial dorsal horn (green arrow). FSVS within the syrinx cavity indicates a pulsatile or turbulent flow (slosh[55]), which is a sign of an "active" and filling syrinx, more likely to expand. FSVS refers to signal loss occurring within moving fluids observed on T2W images as "dark" hypointense regions within the "white" hyperintense syrinx. (F) Measurement of width is made on a transverse slice from the widest syrinxes identified on the sagittal images (red line). This 2-year-old male Cavalier King Charles Spaniel was presented at 2 years old with an 18-month history of pain and phantom scratching to the left.

Other diagnostic tests

If there is suspicion of CNS inflammatory disease, CSF analysis should be performed, preferably through lumbar puncture, especially if the cisternal space is small. CSF analysis results may be challenging to interpret because CM and SM are often associated with a marginal elevation in cell counts, including the presence of neutrophils,[28] and elevated CSF protein due to stagnation of flow (Froin's syndrome).

Treatment

Treatment guidelines are formulated based on existing evidence and the author's experience due to a lack of comprehensive studies on the medical and surgical management of CM-P and SM. Current research is limited by small cohorts and short follow-up periods.

Surgical management

Surgical options include: craniocervical decompression surgery (foramen magnum decompression), ventricular to peritoneal shunting, and syrinx shunting to the pleural or subarachnoid space. The types and indications for surgical management of CM-P and SM-S and potential complications are reviewed elsewhere.[29] While the few surgical reports have all noted significant clinical improvement, none provided MRI evidence of sustained postoperative syrinx collapse. If the postoperative MRI shows the syrinx expanding beyond the spinal cord outline, it indicates active syrinx filling. Simply documenting a static syrinx does not confirm surgical efficacy, as many syrinxes reach a dynamic equilibrium. Similarly, the stabilization or improvement of the clinical signs post surgery does not necessarily prove surgical efficacy, as these improvements can also occur with medical management, which many postoperative patients receive.

Medical management

Based on the limited studies available on medical management, it is unlikely that CM-P will improve with the prescription of carprofen (or other nonsteroidal anti-inflammatory drugs) alone. However, a combination of carprofen and gabapentin is more likely to be successful, and there is reasonable evidence supporting improvement with pregabalin alone.[30–32] There is also evidence that pregabalin will reduce SM-associated phantom scratching.[33] If an animal continues to experience pain, other adjuvant analgesics (e.g., topiramate, ketamine, amantadine, and memantine), acupuncture, physical therapy, and physiotherapy may be beneficial. Maropitant, an NK-1 receptor antagonist that blocks the action of substance P in the CNS, can be useful to reduce phantom scratching.[34] However, the positive effect of maropitant is not sustained in most dogs, and the drug accumulates with repeated dosing, so it is recommended that it be used to "top up" the existing therapy on "bad scratching days". For example, many dogs with SM-S can become very distressed attending a groomer because of the stimulation to the affected dermatome. Giving maropitant 2 hours before the event may lessen this distress. Anecdotally, some animals have shown a positive response to antacids such as cimetidine or omeprazole. The hypothesis is that these drugs may reduce CSF production, thereby lessening the driving force behind CM-P and SM. However, there is limited evidence that these drugs achieve a therapeutic concentration in the choroid plexus or affect CSF production.[35,36] Excessive weight gain should be discouraged, and exercise, within the dog's limitations, should be encouraged. Hydrotherapy can be useful for some patients, especially those with weakness or proprioceptive deficits. Treatment algorithms are indicated in **Figures 27.3–27.5** and drugs are discussed in **Table 27.4**.

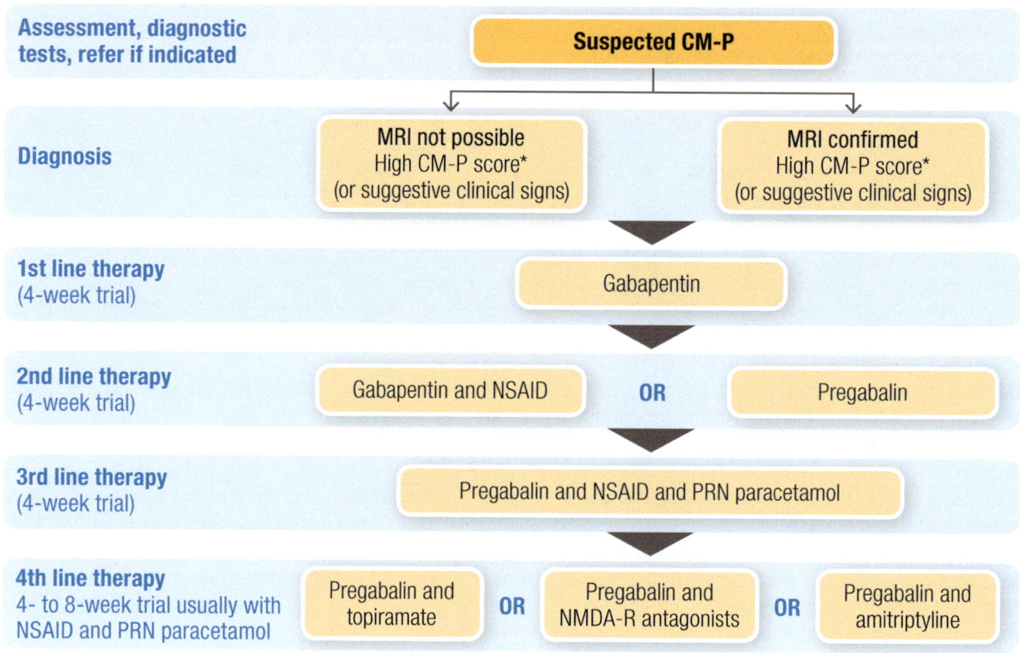

FIG. 27.3 Medical treatment algorithm for Chiari pain (CM-P).

MRI, magnetic resonance imaging; PRN, pro re nata (when required); NSAID, nonsteroidal anti-inflammatory drug; NMDA–R, N-methyl-D-aspartate receptor.
* High CM-P score determined via Chiari Check: caninechiari.com.

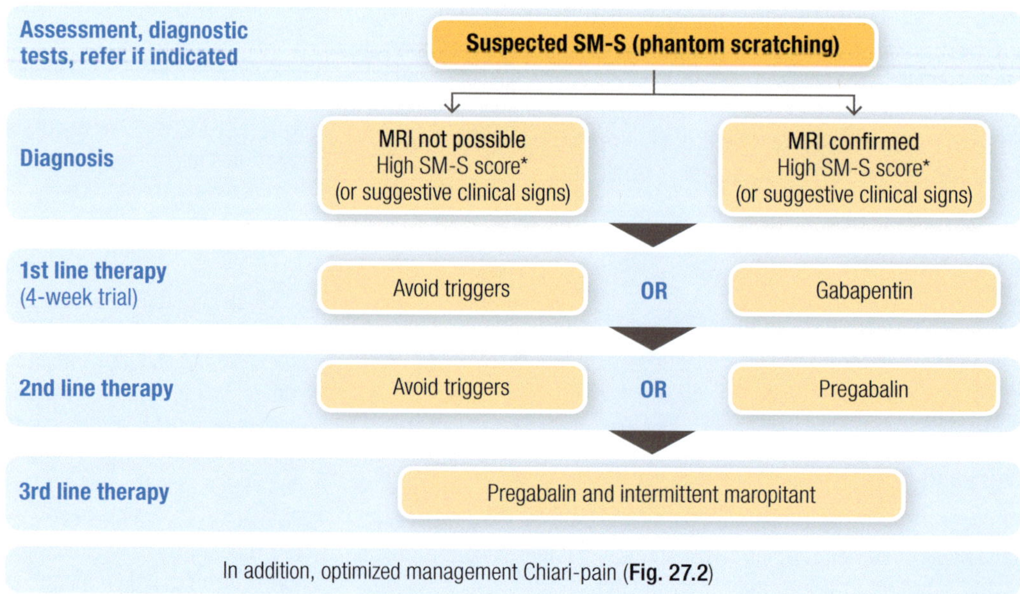

FIG. 27.4 Medical treatment algorithm for severe syringomyelia (SM-S) phantom scratching.

MRI, magnetic resonance imaging; PRN, pro re nata (when required); NSAID, nonsteroidal anti-inflammatory drug; NMDR–R, N-methyl-D-aspartate receptor.
* High SM score determined via Chiari Check: caninechiari.com.

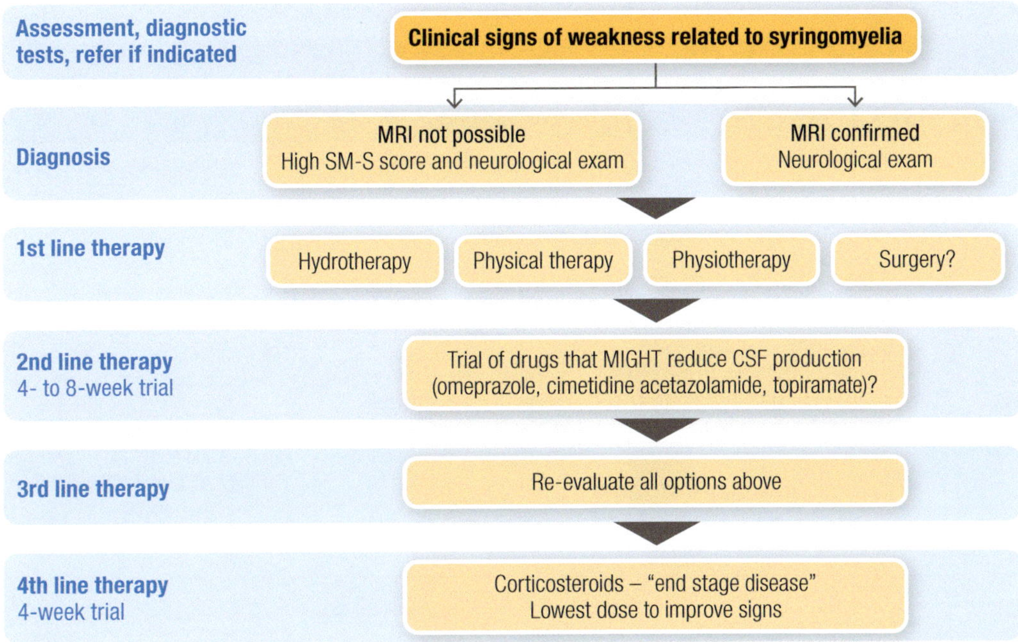

MRI, magnetic resonance imaging; CSF, cerebrospinal fluid.
* High SM score determined via Chiari Check: caninechiari.com.

FIG. 27.5 Medical treatment algorithm for severe syringomyelia (SM-S) weakness.

TABLE 27.4 Adjuvant analgesics and other unlicensed drugs used in the management of Chiari malformation and syringomyelia.

Drug	Dose	Common (dose-related) adverse effects	Less common adverse effects	Monitoring
Adjuvant analgesics				
Gabapentin	■ 10–20 mg/kg PO every 8–12 h (most dogs will require every 8-hour therapy)	■ Sedation, ataxia ■ Gabapentin has minimal hepatic metabolism and is excreted unchanged by the kidney. If chronic kidney disease (IRIS stages 2 and 3), then reduce dose (amount and frequency)[48] ■ Increased appetite and weight gain	■ Gastrointestinal signs (hypersalivation, vomiting, diarrhea) ■ Tremor, myoclonus ■ Respiratory depression (caution if compromised respiratory function)	■ Hematology, serum biochemistry (baseline, then every 6–12 months) ■ Dose is adjusted based on efficacy or adverse effects, but serum concentrations can be measured using human epilepsy therapeutic range as a guide, especially if kidney disease
Pregabalin	■ 4–10 mg/kg PO every 8–12 h or, if switching from gabapentin, halve the current gabapentin mg/kg dose and give at twice daily frequency (e.g., a gabapentin dose of 100 mg every 8 h becomes a pregabalin dose of 50 mg every 12 h)	■ Sedation, ataxia ■ Like gabapentin, pregabalin is excreted unchanged by the kidney. If chronic kidney disease (IRIS stages 2 and 3), then reduce dose (amount and frequency) ■ Increased appetite and weight gain	■ Gastrointestinal signs (hypersalivation, diarrhea) ■ Tremor, myoclonus ■ Respiratory depression (caution if compromised respiratory function)	■ Hematology, serum biochemistry (baseline, then every 6–12 months) ■ Dose is adjusted based on efficacy or adverse effects, but serum concentrations can be measured using human epilepsy therapeutic range as a guide, especially if kidney disease
Topiramate	■ 10 mg/kg PO every 12 h	■ Sedation, ataxia ■ Gastrointestinal signs (inappetence, nausea, diarrhea)	■ In cats, renal tubular acidosis with hypokalemia has been reported with regular formulation[49] and anemia reported with extended-release formulation[50]	■ Hematology, serum biochemistry (baseline, 1 month after initiating, then every 6–12 months) ■ Assay bicarbonate if suspected acidosis ■ Dose is adjusted based on serum concentrations using human epilepsy therapeutic range as guide
Amantadine	■ 3–5 mg/kg PO every 12–24 h ■ At least 3 weeks therapy required to assess effect on neuropathic pain	■ Sedation, ataxia ■ If chronic kidney disease (IRIS stages 2 and 3), then reduce dose (amount and frequency)	■ Gastrointestinal signs (vomiting, diarrhea) ■ Overdose (agitation, tremors, hypersalivation)	■ Hematology, serum biochemistry (baseline, then every 6–12 months). ■ Dose adjusted based on efficacy or adverse effects

Continued.

TABLE 27.4 *Continued.* Adjuvant analgesics and other unlicensed drugs used in the management of Chiari malformation and syringomyelia.

Drug	Dose	Common (dose-related) adverse effects	Less common adverse effects	Monitoring
Adjuvant analgesics				
Memantine	■ 0.3–1 mg/kg every 12 h	■ As for amantadine, there is no reported studies for neuropathic pain in dogs and poor evidence in humans (small effect and adverse effects dizziness). However, compared to amantadine, it is cheaper and easier to dose in larger dogs	■ As for amantadine, there is no reported studies for neuropathic pain in dogs and poor evidence in humans (small effect and adverse effect of dizziness). However, compared to amantadine, it is cheaper and easier to dose in larger dogs	■ Hematology, serum biochemistry (baseline, then every 6–12 months) ■ Dose adjusted based on efficacy or adverse effects
Amitriptyline	■ 0.5–4 mg/kg PO every 12–24 h ■ At least 3 weeks of therapy required to assess effect on neuropathic pain	■ Unpalatable. Consequently, it can be difficult to administer or induce hypersalivation (compounding can help) ■ Sedation, ataxia	■ ECG changes (widened QRS complexes, prolonged PR intervals, flattened T waves) and ventricular arrhythmia ■ Gastrointestinal signs (nausea, vomiting) ■ Hematological (bone marrow suppression, thrombocytopenia, neutropenia) ■ Anticholinergic effects (constipation, urinary retention, hyperexcitability, seizures) ■ Reduced thyroid hormone concentrations	■ Baseline ECG prior to therapy ■ Hematology, serum biochemistry, and thyroid function (baseline, 1 month after initiating, then every 6–12 months) ■ Dose adjusted based on efficacy or adverse effects
Ketamine	■ 0.5 mg/kg SC as "one off" or every 1–4 weeks ■ 24–48 h CRI (0.5 mg/kg IV loading dose then 0.1–0.6 mg/kg/h) for initial management or during acute exacerbation (can be combined with dexmedetomidine or opioid)	■ Vomiting, salivation, vocalization	■ CNS effects (hyperthermia, nystagmus, tremors, myoclonus, hypertonicity, seizures) ■ Respiratory depression ■ Acute congestive heart failure	■ Monitor adverse effects (for at least 30 minutes following SC administration)
Cannabidiol (CBD oil/ hemp extract)	■ 2–9 mg/kg PO every 12 h ■ Absorption is improved in oil or with fatty food. Dose of CBD oil is based on studies that assessed CBD oil for pain associated with osteoarthritis and epilepsy.[51–54] Many commercial preparations do not contain enough compound to be able to achieve this dose easily ■ Not recommended as other agents are more effective with less impact on liver	■ Sedation, ataxia	■ Products with tetrahydrocannabinol (THC) more likely to cause adverse CNS signs ■ Gastrointestinal (hypersalivation, diarrhea, vomiting) ■ Increased serum ALT activity	■ Serum liver enzymes (baseline, 1 month after initiating, then every 6–12 months). In humans with hepatic impairment, a dose reduction of 50% (moderate) to 80% (severe) is recommended[51]
Other				
Prednisone/ prednisolone	■ 0.25–0.5 mg/kg PO every 24 h then decrease to lowest possible. Ideally, alternate day dose that controls signs ■ Chronic therapy (greater than 3 months) not advised	■ Polydipsia, polyuria, and polyphagia, weight gain	■ Adverse effects associated with long-term administration, in particular iatrogenic Cushing's syndrome and potentially predisposition to diabetes mellitus	■ Hematology, serum biochemistry (baseline)
Maropitant	■ 2–8 mg/kg PO PRN up to once daily for 5 days ■ Give 2 hours before known scratching trigger (e.g., grooming) or as soon as possible on "bad scratching day" ■ Administer with food	■ Vomiting and salivation at higher doses (administer with food) ■ Accumulates with repeated dosing	■ Decreased appetite and body weight if given daily ■ Allergic reactions	■ Hepatic metabolism ■ Hematology, serum biochemistry (baseline)
Paracetamol (not cats)	■ Acute 10–20 mg/kg PRN up to every 6 h ■ Chronic 10–15 mg/kg every 12 h	■ Potential for adverse renal, hepatic, gastrointestinal and hematological effects	■ Keratoconjunctivitis sicca	■ Hematology, serum biochemistry (baseline, then every 6–12 months for chronic therapy)
NSAIDs	As per data sheet for individual drugs			

In each case, start at the low end of the dose range/frequency and titrate up. Be sure to fully understand and comply with your country's regulations for controlled or other drugs, especially gabapentinoids, ketamine, and cannabidiol (CBD) oil. PO, per os; IV, intravenous; SC, subcutaneously; CRI, constant rate infusion; ECG, electrocardiogram; CNS, central nervous system; ALT, alanine transaminase; PRN, pro re nata (when required); IRIS, International Renal Interest Society; NSAIDs; nonsteroidal anti-inflammatory drugs. Not recommended for management of Chiari pain or syringomyelia: tramadol, furosemide or long-term acetazolamide, or corticosteroids.

Prognosis

While the width of syrinxes tends to increase over time, the rate of this increase is not consistent. Some syrinxes can rapidly expand within a matter of months or even days, only to remain relatively stable over the course of years, having reached a steady state of hydrodynamic equilibrium. Clinical signs worsen in approximately 75% of dogs, with around 15% being euthanized due to CM-P and SM-S.[32,37,38] However, despite the progression of signs, many dogs experiencing pain and phantom scratching respond well to medical management, and their caregivers often perceive their quality of life as acceptable.[32,37] Anecdotally, despite the persistence of the syrinx, cervicotorticollis can improve gradually.

Genetic factors and breeding advice

CM is a complex trait, and the predisposition to SM involves additional genetic factors.[39–42] Screening for CM-P or risk of future SM through MRI or CT scans may benefit from a machine learning solution to provide an objective measure using a straightforward artificial intelligence tool.[43] SM screening using MRI is available, and many European kennel clubs either enforce or recommend SM screening for predisposed breeds, along with breeding practices aligned with established guidelines.[44] Due to the late onset nature of SM, MRI screening is typically performed at 12 months of age and before breeding. Ideally, breeding dogs should undergo additional MRI screening after reaching 5 years of age. This is because dogs that are free of SM at 12 months of age may not necessarily remain free of SM. Data in the CKCS breed suggests that the prevalence of SM increases from 25% at 12 months to 70% at 72 months.[3] If there were breed-wide screening and contribution to an estimated breeding value scheme, it could be used to predict the risk of SM in descendants. In countries where obligatory screening programs are enforced by law, there is a reduced prevalence of SM in each subsequent generation of offspring.[7,45] However, in some breeds, for example the CKCS, the breed-wide prevalence is so high that vigorous selection against SM and with other prevalent inherited disorders such as mitral valve disease will result in genetic bottlenecking.[46,47] A crossbreeding program to introduce new genetic material is recommended and has been implemented in Scandinavia.

Further resources: The reader is referred to YouTube video resources at https://www.youtube.com/@clare-neurovet for more detailed information on neuropathic pain, drugs used for management of CM-P and SM, up-to-date treatment algorithms, and research updates.

Acknowledgements: The author wishes to thank Ryan Jones and Penny Knowler for their assistance with Fig. 27.2 and Jemima Harrison Passionate Productions for Video 27.1.

KEY POINTS

Canine Chiari malformation (CM) and syringomyelia (SM) are characterized by neuroparenchymal disproportion and CSF pathway obstruction.

Etiology and prevalence

- CM-SM is common in toy brachycephalic breeds such as Cavalier King Charles Spaniels (CKCS), with a CM prevalence of almost 100% and up to 70% SM by 5 years of age. A comparable prevalence is found in other breeds such as the Chihuahua, Pomeranian, and Griffon Bruxellois.

Clinical presentation

- Dogs may show signs of pain, vocalization, or avoidance of physical activity, especially during actions mimicking the Valsalva maneuver. The syndrome of pain is referred to as Chiari-pain (CM-P).
- Clinically relevant SM presents with central spinal cord syndrome, leading to signs such as phantom scratching, scoliosis, and thoracic limb and spinal weakness.

Diagnosis

- MRI is required for detecting CM and SM, though caution is needed to avoid overdiagnosis of clinically silent disease in predisposed breeds.
- Diagnosis of CM-P relies on clinical signs, MRI features, and exclusion of other causes, while clinically relevant SM diagnosis focuses on identifying spinal cord cavities and their impact.

Treatment and prognosis

- Medical management often includes NSAIDs, gabapentin, pregabalin, and adjunct therapies such as acupuncture.
- Surgical options exist, but evidence of long-term efficacy is limited.
- Prognosis varies, with some dogs responding well to medical management despite syrinx progression.

Breeding advice

- CM and SM have genetic components; MRI screening before breeding is recommended to reduce prevalence.
- Crossbreeding programs are suggested to introduce new genetic material and avoid bottlenecks, especially in highly affected breeds such as the CKCS.

References

1. Knowler SP, Gillstedt L, Mitchell TJ, et al. Pilot study of head conformation changes over time in the Cavalier King Charles spaniel breed. *Vet Rec.* 2019 Jan 26;184(4):122.
2. Knowler SP, Dumas E, Spiteri M, et al. Facial changes related to brachycephaly in Cavalier King Charles Spaniels with Chiari-like malformation associated pain and secondary syringomyelia. *J Vet Intern Med.* 2020 Jan;34(1):237–246.
3. Parker JE, Knowler SP, Rusbridge C, et al. Prevalence of asymptomatic syringomyelia in Cavalier King Charles spaniels. *Vet Rec.* 2011 Jun 25;168(25):667.
4. Schulze S, Refai M, Deutschland M, et al. Prevalence of syringomyelia in clinically unaffected Cavalier King Charles Spaniels in Germany (2006-2016). *Tierarztl Prax Ausg K Kleintiere Heimtiere.* 2018 Jun;46(3):157–162.
5. Wijnrocx K, Van Bruggen LWL, Eggelmeijer W, et al. Twelve years of chiari-like malformation and syringomyelia scanning in Cavalier King Charles Spaniels in the Netherlands: Towards a more precise phenotype. *PloS one.* 2017;12(9):e0184893.
6. Cerda-Gonzalez S, Dewey CW, Scrivani PV, Kline KL. Imaging features of atlanto-occipital overlapping in dogs. *Vet Radiol Ultrasound.* 2009 May-Jun;50(3):264–268.
7. Limpens C, Smits VTM, Fieten H, Mandigers PJJ. The effect of MRI-based screening and selection on the prevalence of syringomyelia in the Dutch and Danish Cavalier King Charles Spaniels. *Front Vet Sci.* 2024 Jan 29;11:1326621.
8. British Veterinary Association. *Chiari Malformation/Syringomyelia Scheme (CM/SM Scheme).* Retrieved from: https://www.bva.co.uk/canine-health-schemes/cmsm-scheme/. Last date accessed: June 2024.
9. Kiviranta AM, Rusbridge C, Laitinen-Vapaavuori O, et al. Syringomyelia and Craniocervical Junction Abnormalities in Chihuahuas. *J Vet Intern Med.* 2017 Nov;31(6):1771–1781.
10. Santifort KM, Carrera I, Bossens K, Mandigers PJJ. Phenotypic characterization of Pomeranians with or without Chiari-like malformation and syringomyelia. *Front Vet Sci.* 2023;10:1320942.
11. Freeman AC, Platt SR, Kent M, et al. Chiari-Like Malformation and Syringomyelia in American Brussels Griffon Dogs. *J Vet Intern Med.* 2014 Sep-Oct;28(5):1551–1559.
12. Knowler SP, Kiviranta AM, McFadyen AK, et al. Craniometric Analysis of the Hindbrain and Craniocervical Junction of Chihuahua, Affenpinscher and Cavalier King Charles Spaniel Dogs With and Without Syringomyelia Secondary to Chiari-Like Malformation. *PLoS One.* 2017 Jan 25;12(1):e0169898.
13. Cross HR, Cappello R, Rusbridge C. Comparison of cerebral cranium volumes between cavalier King Charles spaniels with Chiari-like malformation, small breed dogs and Labradors. *J Small Anim Pract.* 2009 Aug;50(8):399–405.
14. Shaw TA, McGonnell IM, Driver CJ, et al. Increase in cerebellar volume in Cavalier King Charles Spaniels with Chiari-like malformation and its role in the development of syringomyelia. *PloS One.* 2012;7(4):e33660.
15. Cerda-Gonzalez S, Olby NJ, Griffith EH. Medullary position at the craniocervical junction in mature cavalier King Charles spaniels: relationship with neurologic signs and syringomyelia. *J Vet Intern Med.* 2015 May-Jun;29(3):882–886.
16. Marino DJ, Loughin CA, Dewey CW, et al. Morphometric features of the craniocervical junction region in dogs with suspected Chiari-like malformation determined by combined use of magnetic resonance imaging and computed tomography. *Am J Vet Res.* 2012 Jan;73(1):105–111.
17. Driver CJ, De Risio L, Hamilton S, et al. Changes over time in craniocerebral morphology and syringomyelia in cavalier King Charles spaniels with Chiari-like malformation. *BMC Vet Res.* 2012;8(1):215.
18. Knowler SP, Cross C, Griffiths S, et al. Use of Morphometric Mapping to Characterise Symptomatic Chiari-Like Malformation, Secondary Syringomyelia and Associated Brachycephaly in the Cavalier King Charles Spaniel. *PLoS One.* 2017 Jan 25;12(1):e0170315.
19. Knowler SP, Galea GL, Rusbridge C. Morphogenesis of Canine Chiari Malformation and Secondary Syringomyelia: Disorders of Cerebrospinal Fluid Circulation. *Front Vet Sci.* 2018 Jul 27;5:171.
20. Cirovic S, Lloyd R, Jovanovik J, et al. Computer simulation of syringomyelia in dogs. *BMC Vet Res.* 2018 Mar 9;14(1):82.
21. Sparks CR, Robertson I, Olby NJ. Morphometric analysis of spinal cord termination in Cavalier King Charles Spaniels. *J Vet Intern Med.* 2019 Mar;33(2):717–725.
22. Rusbridge C, McFadyen AK, Knower SP. Behavioral and clinical signs of Chiari-like malformation-associated pain and syringomyelia in Cavalier King Charles spaniels. *J Vet Intern Med.* 2019 Sep;33(5):2138–2150.
23. Haykowsky MJ, Eves ND, R Warburton DE, Findlay MJ. Resistance exercise, the Valsalva maneuver, and cerebrovascular transmural pressure. *Med Sci Sports Exerc.* 2003 Jan;35(1):65–68.
24. Nalborczyk ZR, McFadyen AK, Jovanovik J, et al. MRI characteristics for "phantom" scratching in canine syringomyelia. *BMC Vet Res.* 2017;13(1):340.
25. Loderstedt S, Benigni L, Chandler K, et al. Distribution of syringomyelia along the entire spinal cord in clinically affected Cavalier King Charles Spaniels. *Vet J.* 2011 Dec;190(3):359–363.
26. Rusbridge C, Stringer F, Knowler SP. Clinical Application of Diagnostic Imaging of Chiari-Like Malformation and Syringomyelia. *Front Vet Sci.* 2018 Nov 28;5:280.
27. Akins PT, Guppy KH. Does Impaired Glymphatic Drainage Cause Glymphedema? A Review Tailored to Neurocritical Care and Neurosurgery. *Neurocrit Care.* 2021 Oct;35(2):545–558.
28. Whittaker DE, English K, McGonnell IM, Volk HA. Evaluation of cerebrospinal fluid in Cavalier King Charles Spaniel dogs diagnosed with Chiari-like malformation with or without concurrent syringomyelia. *J Vet Diagn Invest.* 2011 Mar;23(2):302–307.
29. Rusbridge C, Knower SP. Brain Disorders Associated with Brachycephaly. In: Packer R, O'Neil DC (eds.). *Health and Welfare of Brachycephalic (Flat-faced) Companion Animals. A Complete Guide for Veterinary and Animal Professionals*, 1st ed. Boca Raton: CRC Press; 2021. p. 418.
30. Plessas IN, Volk HA, Rusbridge C, et al. Comparison of gabapentin versus topiramate on clinically affected dogs with Chiari-like malformation and syringomyelia. *Vet Rec.* 2015 Sep 19;177(11):288.
31. Sanchis-Mora S, Chang YM, Abeyesinghe SM, et al. Pregabalin for the treatment of syringomyelia-associated neuropathic pain in dogs: A randomised, placebo-controlled, double-masked clinical trial. *Vet J.* 2019 Aug;250:55–62.
32. Plessas IN, Rusbridge C, Driver CJ, et al. Long-term outcome of Cavalier King Charles spaniel dogs with clinical signs associated with Chiari-like malformation and syringomyelia. *Vet Rec.* 2012 Nov 17;171(20):501.
33. Thoefner MS, Skovgaard LT, McEvoy FJ, et al. Pregabalin alleviates clinical signs of syringomyelia-related central neuropathic pain in Cavalier King Charles Spaniel dogs: a randomized controlled trial. *Vet Anaesth Analg.* 2020 Mar;47(2):238–248.
34. Gilbert E, Mora SS, Pelligand L, et al. Frequency of Phantom Scratching in Cavalier King Charles Spaniels Assessed by Owner Questionnaire Before and During Maropitant Treatment. *BSAVA Congress 2021: Clinical abstract presentations.* British Small Animal Veterinary Association; 2021.
35. Girod M, Allerton F, Gommeren K, et al. Evaluation of the effect of oral omeprazole on canine cerebrospinal fluid production: A pilot study. *Vet J.* 2016;209:119–124.
36. Girod M, Allerton F, Vangrinsven E, et al. CSF omeprazole concentration and albumin quotient following high dose intravenous omeprazole in dogs. *Res Vet Sci.* 2019 Aug;125:266–271.
37. Thøfner MS, Stougaard CL, Westrup U, et al. Prevalence and heritability of symptomatic syringomyelia in Cavalier King Charles Spaniels and long-term outcome in symptomatic and asymptomatic littermates. *J Vet Intern Med.* 2015 Jan;29(1):243–250.
38. Rusbridge C. Chiari-like malformation with syringomyelia in the Cavalier King Charles spaniel: long-term outcome after surgical management. *Vet Surg.* 2007 Jul;36(5):396-405.
39. Kibar Z, Dubé MP, Knowler SP, et al. Preliminary results from syringomyelia (SM) genome wide scans in cavalier King Charles spaniel kindred

and directions for future research. In: Rusbridge C. *Chiari-like Malformation and Syringomyelia*. Dissertation. Utrecht University; 2007. Retrieved from: https://dspace.library.uu.nl/handle/1874/20717. Last date accessed: July 2024.
40. Lemay P, Knowler SP, Bouasker S, et al. Quantitative Trait Loci (QTL) Study Identifies Novel Genomic Regions Associated to Chiari-Like Malformation in Griffon Bruxellois Dogs. *PloS One*. 2014;9(4):e89816.
41. Ancot F, Lemay P, Knowler SP, et al. A genome-wide association study identifies candidate loci associated to syringomyelia secondary to Chiari-like malformation in Cavalier King Charles Spaniels. *BMC Genet*. 2018 Mar 22;19(1):16.
42. Andrino S, Lorenzo V, Dunner S, et al. Syringohydromyelia in Dogs: The Genomic Component Underlying a Complex Neurological Disease. *Animals (Basel)*. 2022 Sep 29;12(19):2622.
43. Spiteri M, Knowler SP, Rusbridge C, Wells K. Using machine learning to understand neuromorphological change and image-based biomarker identification in Cavalier King Charles Spaniels with Chiari-like malformation-associated pain and syringomyelia. *J Vet Intern Med*. 2019 Nov;33(6):2665–2674.
44. British Veterinary Association/Kennel Club. *Chiari malformation/Syringomyelia (CM/SM) Scheme. Appendix 1. Breeding recommendations until relevant EBVs are available*. Retrieved from: https://www.bva.co.uk/media/2803/cm-sm_breeding_recommendations-1-5.pdf. Last date accessed: July 2024.
45. Wijnrocx K, Van Bruggen LWL, Eggelmeijer W, et al. Twelve years of chiari-like malformation and syringomyelia scanning in Cavalier King Charles Spaniels in the Netherlands: Towards a more precise phenotype. *PLoS One*. 2017 Sep 21;12(9):e0184893.
46. Mabunda RS, Makgahlela ML, Nephawe KA, Mtileni B. Evaluation of Genetic Diversity in Dog Breeds Using Pedigree and Molecular Analysis: A Review. *Diversity*. 2022; 14(12):1054
47. Beuchat C. *The Institute of Canine Biology Blog*. Retrieved from: https://www.instituteofcaninebiology.org/. Last date accessed: July 2024.
48. Quimby JM, Lorbach SK, Saffire A, et al. Serum concentrations of gabapentin in cats with chronic kidney disease. *J Feline Med Surg*. 2022 Dec;24(12):1260–1266.
49. Centola SJ, Kaiman G, Rizzo K, et al. Presumptive renal tubular acidosis secondary to topiramate administration in a cat. *J Vet Emerg Crit Care (San Antonio)*. 2022;32(3):420–425.
50. Graham LT, Foss KD, Reinhart JM, et al. The pharmacokinetics of single oral dose extended-release topiramate and adverse effects after multi-dose administration in healthy cats. *J Vet Pharmacol Ther*. 2023;46(4):218–228.
51. Plumb DC. *Cannabidiol (CBD)*. Retrieved from: https://app.plumbs.com/drug/1zvENnoNgv-0V4WuK8v3dGI. Updated June 2022. Last date accessed: July 2024.
52. Verrico CD, Wesson S, Konduri V, et al. A randomized, double-blind, placebo-controlled study of daily cannabidiol for the treatment of canine osteoarthritis pain. *Pain*. 2020 Sep 1;161(9):2191–2202.
53. Deabold KA, Schwark WS, Wolf L, Wakshlag JJ. Single-Dose Pharmacokinetics and Preliminary Safety Assessment with Use of CBD-Rich Hemp Nutraceutical in Healthy Dogs and Cats. *Animals (Basel)*. 2019 Oct 19;9(10):832.
54. Potschka H, Bhatti SFM, Tipold A, McGrath S. Cannabidiol in canine epilepsy. *Vet J*. 2022 Dec;290:105913.
55. Cirovic S, Rusbridge C. Slosh Simulation in a Computer Model of Canine Syringomyelia. *Life (Basel)*. 2021 Oct 14;11(10):1083.

CHAPTER 28

Steroid responsive meningitis-arteritis

Oliver Marsh
BVM BVS, DECVN, MRCVS

Steroid responsive meningitis-arteritis (SRMA) is an immune-mediated disease of dogs.[1] Its ultimate trigger is unknown, though genetic factors may be responsible.[2] It principally affects young dogs (usually less than 18 months of age),[3] with several breeds being predisposed, including Beagles, Boxers, Bernese Mountain Dogs and Whippets, among others.[4]

The most common presentation is acute onset of lethargy, pyrexia, and severe neck pain.[5,6] This is the consequence of aberrant immune activity that culminates in a sterile suppurative leptomeningitis with severe arteritis in the meninges of the spinal cord, typically in the cervical region. A less common chronic, relapsing form of SRMA also exists; this can take a waxing and waning course, and affected dogs may show neurological deficits in addition to neck pain.[1]

There is no single conclusive diagnostic test for SRMA; however, a confident diagnosis can be achieved by collating compatible signalment, clinical signs, clinicopathological data, diagnostic imaging findings, cerebrospinal fluid (CSF) analysis, and ruling out other diseases that could present similarly.

The mainstay of treatment is immunosuppression using corticosteroids, and most acute cases respond well, though relapses can occur.[5–7] Chronic cases are more challenging to treat, conferring a more guarded prognosis.[5,6,8]

Disease definition and etiology

Nomenclature

SRMA has been referred to by numerous terms over the years, including Beagle pain syndrome,[9] necrotizing vasculitis,[10] and canine juvenile polyarteritis syndrome.[11] *SRMA* is now almost universally used; the abbreviation aptly summarizes the pathology and treatment of the condition, and its adoption avoids confusion and facilitates consistency across the scientific literature.

Immune response

SRMA has been established to be an immune-mediated disease.[12] Aberrant Th2-type immune activity occurs, involving a complex interplay between many cell types, cytokines, inflammatory molecules, and autoantibodies. This culminates in arteritis and necrotizing vasculitis in small leptomeningeal vessels, compromise of the blood–central nervous system (CNS) barrier, and influx of nondegenerate neutrophils, typically most severe in the cervical spinal cord. A full description of the immunopathogenesis of SRMA is beyond the scope of this chapter, but it is detailed in a recent review.[1]

Similar arterial lesions may also be seen in the thyroid gland, heart, and mediastinum,[13] and 9–46% of dogs with SRMA have concurrent immune-mediated polyarthritis.[14,15] Myositis is also reported.[9] This suggests that, at least in some dogs, SRMA is one component of a more diffuse systemic inflammatory disease.

Triggers and risk factors

The inciting trigger for the pathological immune activity causing SRMA is not understood. As with meningoencephalomyelitis of unknown origin, many studies have investigated whether various environmental factors or pathogens could be responsible. No risk factors for SRMA associated with infectious agents, neoplasia, vaccination, geographical location, neuter status, or inciting events have been identified.[4,15–17] One case report describes a dog with a sterile neutrophilic meningitis resembling SRMA, presumed to be triggered by *Pasteurella multocida* septic arthritis, though it is not possible to determine how closely the immunopathogenesis underlying the meningitis in that case aligns with spontaneously occurring SRMA.[18]

The only significant risk factor consistently identified for the development of SRMA is breed.[4,19] Strong breed predilections undoubtedly raise the prospect of genetic involvement in disease pathogenesis. Siblings have been reported to be affected by SRMA, including three Petit Bassett Griffon Vendéen littermates[20] and three Bernese Mountain Dog littermates,[21] suggesting heredity in those individuals. A genetic basis has been reported for SRMA in the Nova Scotia Duck Tolling Retriever, specifically mutations in the *PP3CA* and *DAPP1* genes. Both genes regulate T cell activity; the mutations lead to pathologically excessive T cell activation.[2] Testing for these variants is not currently commercially available. Clear evidence of heredity or genetic basis has not yet been established in other breeds of dog, but this is an important area for further investigation.

Clinical features

Prevalence

The data on SRMA prevalence is limited to two reports. A prospective study in a UK referral hospital found that 20 dogs were diagnosed with SRMA over a 2-year period. These comprised 0.6% of all dogs presented to the institution, and 1.6% of dogs seen within the neurology service.[7] A retrospective study at the University of Bern (Switzerland) found that, over an 11-year period, 1.4% (71/5092) of dogs presented to the neurology service had a clinical, presumptive, or histopathological diagnosis of SRMA.[22]

Patient signalment

SRMA is predominantly a disease of young dogs, with 80% of patients being less than 18 months of age.[3] It is occasionally seen in older dogs, with cases in patients of up to 9 years being reported.[6]

Most studies have not demonstrated a sex predilection, though a few have found males to be slightly more frequently affected than females.[3,19,23]

Any breed can be affected, but several are particularly prone. Beagles, Bernese Mountain Dogs, Nova Scotia Duck Tolling Retrievers, Pointers, Boxers, Golden Retrievers, Border Collies, Jack Russell Terriers Whippets, Weimaraners, and Korthal Griffons have all been shown to be overrepresented.[4,5,8,13,24,25]

Clinical signs

Acute form

The acute form of SRMA is by far the most common. The most frequent clinical signs are acute progressive onset of lethargy, inappetence, pyrexia, and neck pain.[3,6,13] The neck pain typically manifests as low head carriage and reluctance to voluntarily move the head and neck in any direction. The patient will often try to follow people and objects by moving the eyes and/or shifting position of the whole body while keeping the neck in a fixed and rigid position. Even gentle palpation and attempts to manipulate the head or neck elicit severe discomfort. More diffuse spinal pain extending into the thoracolumbar region is sometimes found (Fig. 28.1 and Video 28.1). Specific neurological deficits (i.e., abnormal proprioception, deficits of segmental spinal reflexes, and cranial nerve abnormalities) are not usually present. The exception is when the arteritis is so severe that it leads to blood vessel rupture and hemorrhage, with resultant signs of myelopathy.[26]

Chronic form

This is much less common and is less well described than the acute form. It can occur if treatment of acute SRMA is inadequate (for example, corticosteroids given at insufficient doses or of too short duration), if there are repeated relapses that are refractory to standard treatment, or occasionally when the disease waxes and wanes of its own accord

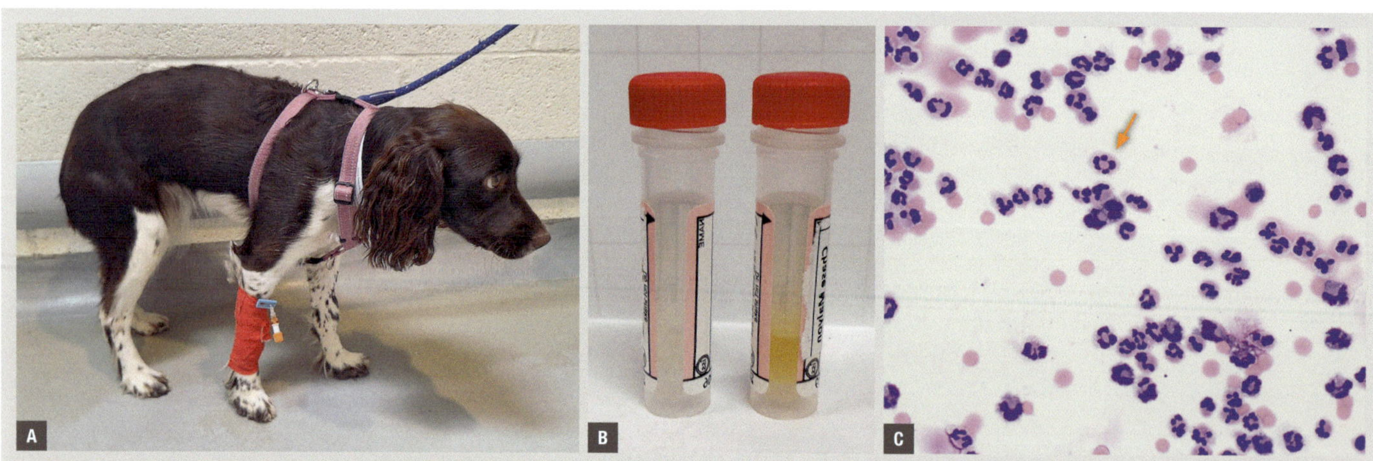

FIG. 28.1 (A) A 13-month-old female entire English Springer Spaniel with steroid-responsive meningitis-arteritis (SRMA). This dog shows a kyphotic posture and low head carriage. The tail is tucked under the body, and the dog is reluctant to move the head or neck in any direction. This posture is overall consistent with pain, particularly affecting the cervical region. (B) Cisternal (left) and lumbar (right) cerebrospinal fluid (CSF) samples. Both samples showed a marked neutrophilic pleocytosis and elevated protein concentration, but these were more severe in the xanthochromic lumbar sample. (C) CSF cytology in a case of SRMA (modified Wright's stain). There is a marked neutrophilic pleocytosis. One of the numerous nondegenerate neutrophils is arrowed. Picture courtesy of Kathleen Tennant, DWR Veterinary Specialists.

Video 28.1

This video shows a young adult Weimaraner diagnosed with steroid-responsive meningitis-arteritis (SRMA). Note the low head carriage, consistent with neck pain. There is no overt ataxia or paresis, but the gait overall appears slightly stiff, reflecting discomfort. Postural reactions, spinal reflexes, and cranial nerve reflexes are not shown but would be expected to be normal. Obvious discomfort is elicited on palpation of the cranial lumbar and thoracic region, and a marked reaction is seen when the neck is extended. Spinal pain, most severe in the neck, is common in SRMA, but, importantly, can be more diffuse, as seen in this case. The authors always recommend that any patient with suspected neck pain is handled using a chest harness rather than neck lead.

over a period of time. Under these circumstances, neurological deficits consistent with myelopathy, radiculopathy, or cranial neuropathy may be seen.[5,6,8]

Neurological deficits occur because chronic disease can lead to fibrosis and mineralization of the meninges, which compresses the spinal cord and/or nerve roots and potentially alters CSF flow dynamics. Chronically inflamed and fibrotic blood vessels also have the potential to compress adjacent nervous tissue, as well as rupture, leading to compression and localized ischemia. The chronic form is more difficult to diagnose than the acute form as its features are less distinct and may mimic other conditions[27] (see Chapter 5 on spinal pain for other important differential diagnoses). Inflammatory infiltrates may extend into the CNS parenchyma, including that of the brain, which rarely can lead to intracranial signs, including epileptic seizures in one case report.[28]

Clinicopathological findings

Hematology

Around 65% of dogs with acute SRMA show hematological abnormalities.[3] Leukocytosis is usually observed together with marked peripheral neutrophilia with a left shift. The presence of hematological abnormalities combined with pyrexia has a 99.5% sensitivity for SRMA but a low specificity of 55%,[3] meaning that almost all dogs with SRMA have hematological abnormalities and are pyrexic, but so do a significant number of dogs that do not have SRMA.

Acute phase proteins and other biomarkers

C-reactive protein (CRP) is usually markedly elevated in SRMA (often over 100 mg/L; reference, 0–10 mg/L) and can be readily and economically tested in practice. Although CRP tends to be higher in dogs with SRMA than in those with other neurological disease, it is not specific for SRMA;[29] rather, it is a marker of systemic inflammation.[27] Any disease of which inflammation is a component (e.g., infection, neoplasia) can result in CRP elevation of a similar magnitude to that seen in SRMA. CRP tends to drop dramatically within a few days of treatment and typically remains within the normal range during remission,[29] though some cases in remission have a CRP concentration slightly above the reference range.[7] Marked elevation in CRP is typically seen in the event of relapse. Serum amyloid A (SAA) shows a similar pattern of elevation at the time of diagnosis, normalization during remission, and increase in the event of relapse,[7] though it is probably less routinely available than CRP measurement. Serum IgA is likely to be elevated in SRMA, though unlike CRP and SAA it can remain increased during remission, making it less valuable for monitoring purposes.[6,7]

Many other biomarkers for SRMA have been investigated in a research setting, including leukocyte subtype populations as well as various acute-phase proteins and cytokines. Very often, the limitation with these, similar to CRP and APP, is their lack of specificity in distinguishing SRMA from other causes of systemic inflammation.[27]

Cerebrospinal fluid analysis

CSF collection and analysis is indicated in suspected SRMA. It should be performed after advanced imaging, preferably magnetic resonance imaging (MRI), to rule out disease or anatomical abnormalities that would make CSF collection difficult or dangerous. The site of collection is a matter of clinician preference, though a higher diagnostic yield has been demonstrated when both cisternal and lumbar samples are obtained (Fig. 28.1b).[30]

CSF may be macroscopically unremarkable or might appear turbid, xanthochromic, or hemorrhagic. Laboratory analysis in acute SRMA cases typically reveals neutrophilic pleocytosis with increased protein concentration (Fig. 28.1c). The pleocytosis is often marked (i.e., over 50 nucleated cells/μL). The neutrophils will be nondegenerate, and bacterial culture, if performed, will be negative. IgA is often detectable in the CSF of SRMA patients. The presence of IgA in both serum and CSF is fairly sensitive for a diagnosis of SRMA (91%), but of limited specificity (78%).[31] This means that detection of IgA in serum and CSF does not rule out other neurological disease, such as meningoencephalomyelitis of unknown origin.

In the chronic form of SRMA, a mixed pleocytosis dominated by mononuclear cells may be seen, but in these cases, CSF may only show albuminocytological dissociation or can be normal.[5,7,32]

Diagnostic imaging

The purpose of advanced imaging in suspected SRMA cases is to gather evidence that supports the putative diagnosis and to rule out other differentials.[25,33] The most comprehensive study on the MRI features of SRMA found that almost all affected dogs (98.6%) had MRI-visible abnormalities. These included enhancement of the meninges, nerve roots, synovium of articular facets, and paravertebral muscles on T1 postcontrast sequences, with saturation techniques increasing the conspicuity of lesions (Fig. 28.2).[33] Other reported MRI abnormalities in SRMA include short tau inversion recovery (STIR) and T2 paraspinal muscle hyperintensities (Fig. 28.3).[25,34]

There is only limited information on the use of other imaging modalities in SRMA. Radiographs of the cervical spine will be normal, and meningeal enhancement may be seen on postcontrast computed tomography (CT) images.[8]

Histopathology

Histological diagnosis is not routinely performed in SRMA cases, as diagnosis can generally be reached by less invasive means than biopsy. Histopathology is generally performed postmortem. Fortunately, the relatively low mortality rate in SRMA means postmortem examination is not commonly required.[22] The key histopathological feature in acute disease is leptomeningeal inflammation, comprising mainly neutrophils with scattered lymphocytes, plasma cells, and macrophages. There is fibrinoid necrotizing arteritis of the meningeal arteries, which may be thrombosed. With chronicity, mononuclear infiltrates are seen, and fibrosis of both the meninges and arterial walls occur; the latter can lead to stenosis of the vessel lumen. Meningeal hemorrhage and hematomyelia might be seen in both acute and chronic cases. Occasionally, the inflammation extends to the cerebral meninges, choroid plexus, and periventricular tissues.[8,13,35]

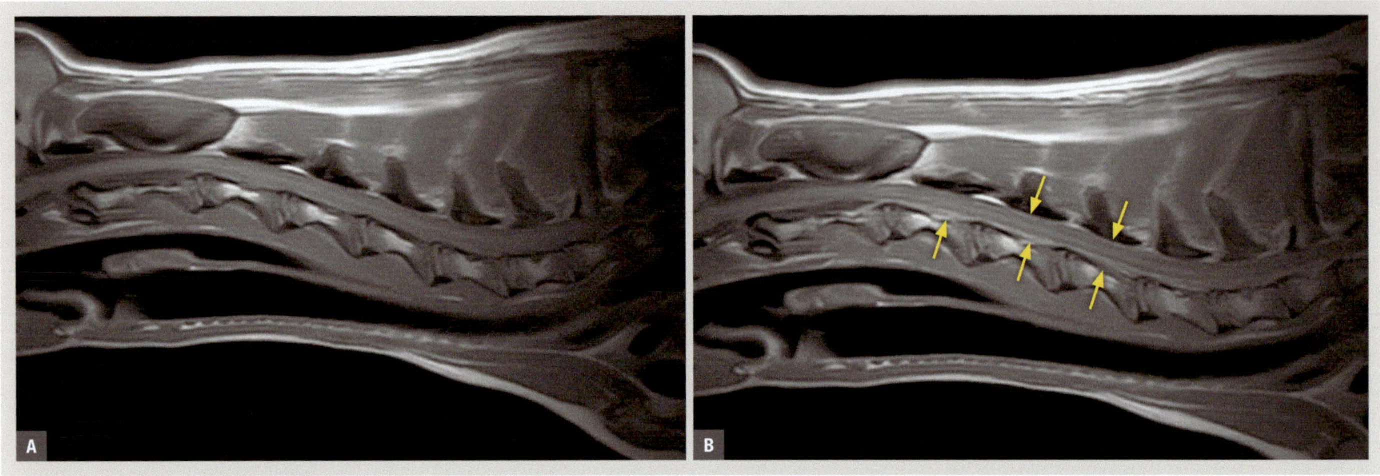

FIG. 28.2 Pre- (**A**) and postcontrast (**B**) T1-weighted midline sagittal magnetic resonance images of the neck of a dog with steroid-responsive meningitis-arteritis. There are no obvious precontrast abnormalities, but meningeal enhancement (arrowed) is present after contrast administration.

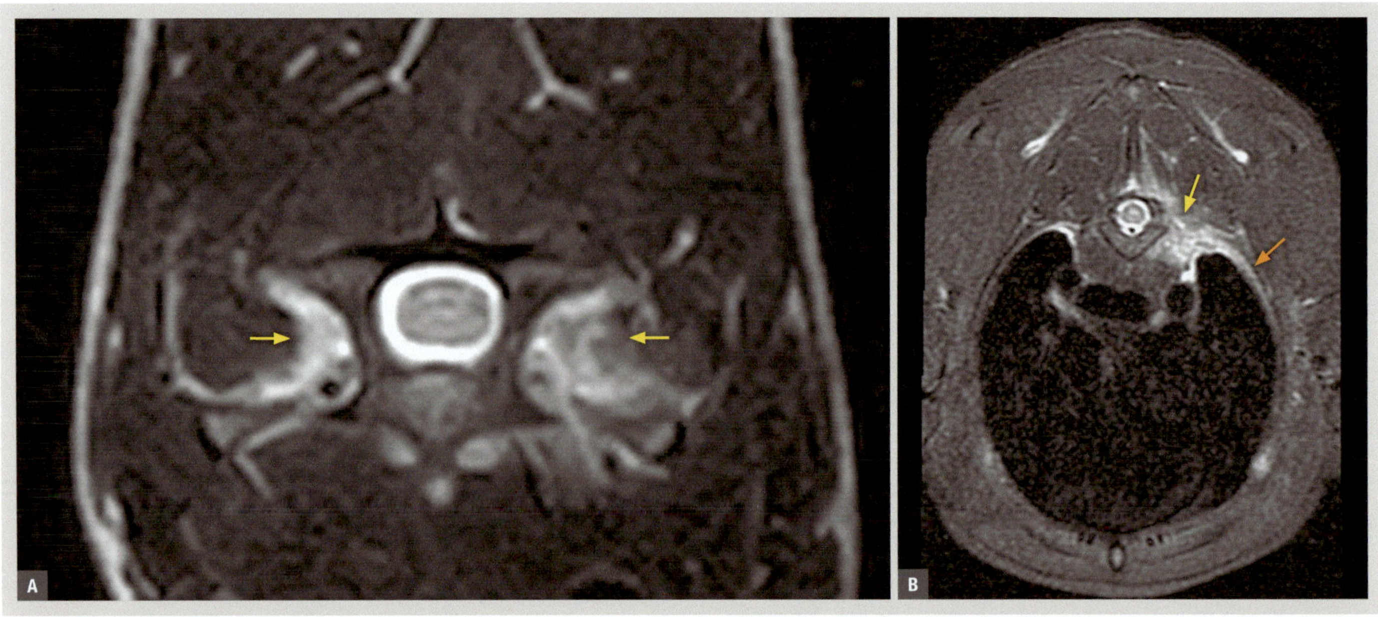

FIG. 28.3 (**A**) T2-weighted transverse magnetic resonance (MR) image of the spine of a dog with steroid-responsive meningitis-arteritis at the level of the C4 vertebra. Bilateral, asymmetrical, irregular, ill-defined hyperintensities within the paraspinal muscles are arrowed. (**B**) Short tau inversion recovery (STIR) transverse MR image at the level of the T4 vertebra. There are left-sided paraspinal muscle hyperintensities (yellow arrow) and pleuritis (orange arrow), showing the potential for inflammation beyond the immediate paraspinal tissues.

Treatment

Immunosuppressive corticosteroids

The mainstay of treatment is immunosuppressive corticosteroids, on a gradually tapering regimen. Until recently, most studies have suggested a treatment protocol lasting around 6 months,[6–8] but a more recent study investigated truncated treatment over 6 weeks.[36]

A "traditional" 6-month protocol is detailed below; this was used in a single-center prospective study including 20 dogs with acute SRMA. Clinical remission was achieved in all dogs, with 4 later experiencing relapse of clinical signs. All 4 of these reentered remission with an increase in the prednisolone dose. All dogs in the study had eventual resolution of disease with a follow-up of 6 months after discontinuation of prednisolone.[7] Other authors have recommended very similar treatment regimes.[6,8]

Six-month prednisolone protocol for SRMA:

- 2 mg/kg per os (PO) every 12 h for 2 days
- 1 mg/kg PO every 12 h for 12 days
- 0.5 mg/kg PO every 12 h for 6 weeks
- 0.5 mg/kg PO every 24 h for 6 weeks
- 0.5 mg/kg PO every 48 h for 6 weeks
- 0.5 mg/kg PO every 72 h for 6 weeks
- Then stop

Prednisolone treatment for SRMA, tapering over 6 weeks, was recently reported by Rose et al.[36] Their prospective, multicenter, blinded study compared a 6-week regime with a 6-month course. Twenty-four dogs were treated for 6 weeks and 20 for 6 months. The 6-month course was the same as that outlined above; the 6-week protocol is detailed below.

Six-week prednisolone protocol:

- 2 mg/kg PO every 12 h for 2 days
- 1 mg/kg PO every 12 h for 12 days
- 0.5 mg/kg PO every 12 h for 7 days
- 0.5 mg/kg PO every 24 h for 7 days
- 0.5 mg/kg PO every 48 h for 7 days
- 0.5 mg/kg PO every 72 h for 7 days
- Then stop

All dogs responded to treatment. Relapse was defined as a recurrence of clinical signs with or without confirmatory investigation. The relapse rates (30% in the 6-month group and 38% in the 6-week group) and incidences of relapse were not significantly different between cohorts, with a 12-month follow-up. This 6-week protocol can be considered as an alternative to 6-month regimes and may be a means to reduce both corticosteroid adverse effects and the burden on owners.

Nonsteroidal anti-inflammatory drugs

Uncommonly, nonsteroidal anti-inflammatory drugs (NSAIDs), rather than steroids, have been used in very mild cases.[8] There is not, however, a detailed description of a treatment regimen or outcome. In all but the least severe cases, NSAIDs may not be sufficient to quell the aberrant immune response. A further potential problem with NSAID use is that, if treatment is unsuccessful, a switch to corticosteroids is indicated. This requires a "wash-out" of varying duration (depending on which NSAID has been used), which will delay institution of more aggressive treatment. Based on the available evidence from the peer-reviewed published literature, the author does not recommend NSAIDs for treatment of SRMA.

Additional immunosuppressive medications

There is limited information on the addition of second immunosuppressive agents to the initial prednisolone treatment regime. In a retrospective study including 26 dogs with acute SRMA, azathioprine was used alongside prednisolone to allow steroid tapering over 3 months and limit side effects. All dogs showed a good clinical response, and relapse, defined as recurrence of clinical signs, was relatively infrequent, occurring in 5/26 dogs (19%).[37] In contrast, a larger retrospective, multicenter study comprising 153 dogs with acute SRMA compared prednisolone treatment with and without azathioprine. The overall relapse rate, again determined by recurrence of clinical signs, was 29.5%, but relapse was significantly more likely in the group receiving azathioprine and prednisolone than in the group on prednisolone monotherapy.[19] The data is currently insufficient to determine whether adding a second immunosuppressive agent to the initial treatment is beneficial.

Supportive treatment

Analgesia is indicated during the first few days of treatment while prednisolone takes its full effect. Acetaminophen (paracetamol) at a dose of 10–15 mg/kg every 8 to 12 hours and gabapentin (10 mg/kg every 8 hours) are both good choices as they can be safely combined with corticosteroids. Supportive treatment such as intravenous fluid therapy may be required until patients are comfortable enough to eat and drink independently. In most uncomplicated cases, hospitalization is only required for a day or two, as a positive response to treatment tends to be seen fairly quickly.

Treatment of a relapse

In the event of a relapse of SRMA, it is generally recommended to return to an earlier stage of treatment at higher prednisolone dosages. In one study, relapsing dogs were returned to the 1 mg/kg PO every 12 hour phase,[7] while in another, relapsers received 2 mg/kg PO every 12 hours.[36] All relapsing dogs in both studies responded to the dosage increases. Second-line immunosuppressive agents including cytarabine[38] and mycophenolate[6] have also been used alongside prednisolone during relapses. The majority of dogs (10/12 on cytarabine and 3/4 on mycophenolate) eventually had resolution of disease and were able to come off treatment. The rationale of a second immunosuppressive agent is that since relapses are considered difficult to treat, more aggressive protocols may be necessary. Also, addition of a second immunosuppressive may allow the prednisolone dose to be tapered more quickly, reducing side effects during what is likely to be a prolonged period of treatment. Currently, the data on the use of second immunosuppressive agents for SRMA relapses is too scant for firm recommendations to be made.

Monitoring during treatment

Regular reexamination is important during treatment of SRMA to ensure that the dog is free of clinical signs (i.e., neurologically normal with no indication of spinal pain, normothermic, showing normal levels of energy, and with a normal appetite), there are no signs of relapse, treatment compliance is optimal, and side effects of medication are manageable for the patient and owner. The author tends to reexamine SRMA patients after the first 2 weeks, then every 4 to 6 weeks depending on the case. Dog owners are instructed to monitor for signs of lethargy, inappetence, and pain and to contact the practice if these occur. The two most commonly used objective measures of response to treatment are CSF analysis[6] and serum CRP measurement.[29] One study showed that dogs that eventually relapsed were more likely to have CSF and serum CRP abnormalities at 3 months post diagnosis than nonrelapsers.[23] Though normal CSF and CRP do not exclude future relapse, those with ongoing abnormalities warrant closer monitoring and probably more conservative tapering of treatment. Compared to CSF, serum CRP measurement is simpler, more widely available, more cost-effective and avoids the (albeit relatively small) risks of a short general anesthetic and CSF collection. There is currently no evidence available to inform frequency of CRP measurement, and this therefore remains a matter of clinician preference, with some clinicians checking it prior to every prednisolone dose reduction and others doing so less regularly. An increase in CRP may be the first sign of SRMA relapse, but it is important to take into account the whole clinical picture, as CRP is such a nonspecific marker, and it will be elevated in many other diseases.

Prognosis

The vast majority of dogs show a marked and rapid improvement in their clinical signs after starting treatment. They are often significantly more comfortable after just one or two administrations of corticosteroids. As many as 98.5% of SRMA patients enter remission.[25] Relapse, however, is not uncommon, and can occur at any stage of treatment, or after discontinuation of medications. The likelihood of relapse probably reduces the older the dog gets and the longer it has been stable without treatment.[23] The rate of relapse has been reported to range from 16% to 60%[5–7,23,25,29] but tends to cluster around 30%. Death due to SRMA is uncommon, with mortality rates of 1.6–8% being reported.[5,23,25] Almost all dogs with SRMA that receive high doses of prednisolone will show adverse effects, impacting owner-perceived quality of life at least for a period of time.[25]

KEY POINTS

- Steroid-responsive meningitis-arteritis (SRMA) is a relatively common immune-mediated disease of young dogs. Any breed can be affected, but certain breeds are predisposed.
- Common clinical signs include acute lethargy, pyrexia, and neck pain; neurological deficits may additionally be seen in the less common chronic form and in the acute form when the arteritis is so severe that it leads to blood vessel rupture and hemorrhage with resultant signs of myelopathy.
- Diagnosis is made on the basis of the compatible clinical signs (listed above), clinicopathological abnormalities (leukocytosis, neutrophilia, and elevated acute phase proteins), MRI abnormalities, and CSF analysis (typically showing neutrophilic pleocytosis).
- Treatment comprises immunosuppression, typically with glucocorticoids, which are tapered over a period of several weeks to months.
- The prognosis is good for the acute form, though relapse can occur. The chronic form is more challenging to treat and carries a less favorable prognosis.

References

1. Wohlsein JC, Tipold A. Steroid-responsive meningitis-arteritis: What have we learned since 2010? A narrative review. *Vet J.* 2023 Oct-Dec;300-302:106030.
2. Wilbe M, Jokinen P, Hermanrud C, et al. MHC class II polymorphism is associated with a canine SLE-related disease complex. *Immunogenetics.* 2009 Aug;61(8):557–564.
3. Grapes NJ, Packer RMA, De Decker S. Clinical reasoning in canine cervical hyperaesthesia: which presenting features are important? *Vet Rec.* 2020 Nov 28;187(11):448.
4. Rose JH, Kwiatkowska M, Henderson ER, et al. The impact of demographic, social, and environmental factors on the development of steroid-responsive meningitis-arteritis (SRMA) in the United Kingdom. *J Vet Intern Med.* 2014 Jul-Aug;28(4):1199–1202.
5. Tipold A, Jaggy A. Steroid responsive meningitis-arteritis in dogs: Long-term study of 32 cases. *J Small Anim Pract.* 1994;35(6):311–316.
6. Cizinauskas S, Jaggy A, Tipold A. Long-term treatment of dogs with steroid-responsive meningitis-arteritis: clinical, laboratory and therapeutic results. *J Small Anim Pract.* 2000 Jul;41(7):295–301.
7. Lowrie M, Penderis J, McLaughlin M, et al. Steroid responsive meningitis-arteritis: a prospective study of potential disease markers, prednisolone treatment, and long-term outcome in 20 dogs (2006-2008). *J Vet Intern Med.* 2009 Jul-Aug;23(4):862–870.
8. Tipold A, Schatzberg SJ. An update on steroid responsive meningitis-arteritis. *J Small Anim Pract.* 2010 Mar;51(3):150–154.
9. Hayes TJ, Roberts GK, Halliwell WH. An idiopathic febrile necrotizing arteritis syndrome in the dog: beagle pain syndrome. *Toxicol Pathol.* 1989;17(1 Pt 2):129–137.
10. Brooks P. Necrotizing vasculitis in a group of Beagles. *Laboratory Animals.* 1984;18:285–290.
11. Felsburg P, HogenEsch H, Somberg R, et al. Immunologic abnormalities in canine juvenile

polyarteritis syndrome: a naturally occurring animal model of Kawasaki disease. *Clin Immunol Immunopathol.* 1992;65(2):110–118.

12. Schwartz M, Moore PF, Tipold A. Disproportionally strong increase of B cells in inflammatory cerebrospinal fluid of dogs with Steroid-responsive Meningitis-Arteritis. *Vet Immunol Immunopathol.* 2008 Oct 15;125(3-4):274–283.
13. De Lahunta A, Glass E, Kent, M (eds.). *De Lahunta's Veterinary Neuroanatomy and Clinical Neurology*, 5th ed. Philadelphia: Elsevier; 2021.
14. Webb AA, Taylor SM, Muir GD. Steroid-responsive meningitis-arteritis in dogs with noninfectious, nonerosive, idiopathic, immune-mediated polyarthritis. *J Vet Intern Med.* 2002 May-Jun;16(3):269–273.
15. Gonçalves R, De Decker S, Walmsley G, et al. Inflammatory Disease Affecting the Central Nervous System in Dogs: A Retrospective Study in England (2010-2019). *Front Vet Sci.* 2022 Jan 27;8:819945.
16. Barber RM, Li Q, Levine JM, et al. Screening for Viral Nucleic Acids in the Cerebrospinal Fluid of Dogs With Central Nervous System Inflammation. *Front Vet Sci.* 2022 Mar 24;9:850510.
17. Rose JH, Harcourt-Brown TR. Screening diagnostics to identify triggers in 21 cases of steroid-responsive meningitis-arteritis. *J Small Anim Pract.* 2013 Nov;54(11):575–578.
18. Albertini G, Marsh O, Raj J, Stabile F. Steroid-responsive meningitis-arteritis secondary to septic arthritis due to *Pasteurella multocida* in a bull terrier puppy. *Vet Rec Case Rep.* 2021;9(4):e184.
19. Hilpert E, Tipold A, Meyerhoff N, et al. Steroid-responsive meningitis-arteritis in dogs in Germany: Are there epidemiological or clinical factors influencing recurrence rate? *Tierarztl Prax Ausg K Kleintiere Heimtiere.* 2020 Feb;48(1):5–12.
20. Voss J, Rentmeister K, Maiolini A, Tipold A. Steroid-responsive meningitis-arteritis in three Petit Basset Griffon Vendeen littermates. *Kleintierpraxis.* 2012;57(4):185–191.
21. Meric S, Child G, Higgins R. Necrotizing vasculitis of the spinal pachyleptomeningeal arteries in three Bernese Mountain dog littermates. *J Am Anim Hosp Assoc.* 1986;22:459–465.
22. Fluehmann G, Doherr MG, Jaggy A. Canine neurological diseases in a referral hospital population between 1989 and 2000 in Switzerland. *J Small Anim Pract.* 2006 Oct;47(10):582–587.
23. Biedermann E, Tipold A, Flegel T. Relapses in dogs with steroid-responsive meningitis-arteritis. *J Small Anim Pract.* 2016 Feb;57(2):91–95.
24. Anfinsen KP, Berendt M, Liste FJ, et al. A retrospective epidemiological study of clinical signs and familial predisposition associated with aseptic meningitis in the Norwegian population of Nova Scotia duck tolling retrievers born 1994-2003. *Can J Vet Res.* 2008 Jul;72(4):350–355.
25. Lau J, Nettifee JA, Early PJ, et al. Clinical characteristics, breed differences, and quality of life in North American dogs with acute steroid-responsive meningitis-arteritis. *J Vet Intern Med.* 2019 Jul;33(4):1719–1727.
26. Zilli J, Olszewska A, Farke D, Schmidt MJ. Successful surgical and medical treatment of a severe, acute epidural bleed in a young dog due to steroid responsive meningitis-arteritis. *Acta Vet Scand.* 2021 Jul 10;63(1):27.
27. Andersen-Ranberg E, Berendt M, Gredal H. Biomarkers of non-infectious inflammatory CNS diseases in dogs: Where are we now? Part 2 - Steroid responsive meningitis-arteritis. *Vet J.* 2021 Jul;273:105692.
28. Wrzosek M, Konar M, Vandevelde M, Oevermann A. Cerebral extension of steroid-responsive meningitis arteritis in a boxer. *J Small Anim Pract.* 2009 Jan;50(1):35–37.
29. Bathen-Noethen A, Carlson R, Menzel D, et al. Concentrations of acute-phase proteins in dogs with steroid responsive meningitis-arteritis. *J Vet Intern Med.* 2008 Sep-Oct;22(5):1149–1156.
30. Carletti BE, De Decker S, Rose J, et al. Evaluation of concurrent analysis of cerebrospinal fluid samples collected from the cerebellomedullary cistern and lumbar subarachnoid space for the diagnosis of steroid-responsive meningitis arteritis in dogs. *J Am Vet Med Assoc.* 2019 Nov 1;255(9):1035–1038.
31. Maiolini A, Carlson R, Schwartz M, et al. Determination of immunoglobulin A concentrations in the serum and cerebrospinal fluid of dogs: an estimation of its diagnostic value in canine steroid-responsive meningitis-arteritis. *Vet J.* 2012 Feb;191(2):219–224.
32. Lowrie M, Penderis J, Eckersall PD, et al. The role of acute phase proteins in diagnosis and management of steroid-responsive meningitis arteritis in dogs. *Vet J.* 2009 Oct;182(1):125–130.
33. Remelli C, Martello A, Valentini A, et al. Magnetic resonance imaging highlights the meningeal involvement in steroid responsive meningitis-arteritis and suggests the inflammation of the surrounding tissues (70 cases). *Front Vet Sci.* 2022 Aug 19;9:957278.
34. Eminaga S, Cherubini GB, Villiers E, et al. STIR muscle hyperintensity in the cervical muscles associated with inflammatory spinal cord disease of unknown origin. *J Small Anim Pract.* 2013 Mar;54(3):137–142.
35. Vandevelde M, Higgins R, Oevermann A. *Veterinary Neuropathology: Essentials of Theory and Practice.* Chichester: Wiley-Blackwell; 2012.
36. Rose JH, Driver CJ, Arrol L, et al. Prospective randomized trial comparing relapse rates in dogs with steroid-responsive meningitis-arteritis treated with a 6-week or 6-month prednisolone protocol. *J Vet Intern Med.* 2024 Jul-Aug;38(4):2221–2227.
37. Giraud L, Girod M, Cauzinille L. Combination of Prednisolone and Azathioprine for Steroid-Responsive Meningitis-Arteritis Treatment in Dogs. *J Am Anim Hosp Assoc.* 2021 Jan 1;57(1):1–7,
38. Günther C, Steffen F, Alder DS, et al. Evaluating the use of cytosine arabinoside for treatment for recurrent canine steroid-responsive meningitis-arteritis. *Vet Rec.* 2020 Jul;187(1):e7.

CHAPTER 29

Intervertebral disc herniation

Natasha Olby
DVM, PhD, MRCVS,
DACVIM (Neurology)

The intervertebral disc (IVD) includes cartilaginous endplates and an external annulus fibrosus (AF) surrounding a gelatinous nucleus pulposus (NP). The whole structure is anchored to the adjacent vertebral endplates via Sharpey's fibers. The AF is composed of concentric collagenous fibers that are well organized in the outer zone and then become progressively more disorganized until the transitional zone blends into the NP. The NP contains physaliferous cells derived from the notochord. These cells lie in a ground substance that has a high glycosaminoglycan content, enabling it to trap water; the NP is 80% water. There is no blood supply to the IVD. Nutrition is provided by diffusion from the microvascular beds in the vertebral endplates; loading of the vertebral column during movement helps this process.[1,2]

The vertebral column has the dual function of protecting the delicate spinal cord while supporting movement. The IVD facilitates movement of the vertebral column; as such, it is subject to loading in different directions and is prone to degeneration and traumatic injury. In addition, in certain dog breeds, there is a strong genetic risk factor that drives premature degeneration of the IVD. Canine IVD disease is an extremely important cause of pain and myelopathy, with a reported lifetime prevalence of 3.5%.[3] More than 20,000 thoracolumbar spinal surgeries are performed in North America per year for acute intervertebral disc extrusions,[4] and intervertebral disc herniations (IVDH) account for 72% of all emergency presentations for nonambulatory paraparesis or paraplegia.[5]

> The term IVDH is an umbrella term relating to displacement of a part of the IVD, either NP or AF or both, into the vertebral canal causing contusion to and compression of the spinal cord. Many different forms of IVDH are now recognized.[6]

The types of IVDH covered in this chapter include:

- Hansen type I acute intervertebral disc extrusion (IVDE)
- Acute noncompressive nucleus pulposus extrusion (ANNPE)
- Hydrated nucleus pulposus extrusion (HNPE)
- Hansen type II chronic intervertebral disc protrusion (IVDP)

Subsets of these conditions, disc-associated extensive epidural hemorrhage (DEEH) and intradural intraparenchymal disc extrusion (IIVDE), are also mentioned.

Hansen type I intervertebral disc extrusion

Etiology and pathophysiology

The most common form of IVDE occurs in chondrodystrophic dog breeds and is associated with expression of an *FGF4* retrogene on chromosome (CFA)12.[7] Indeed, this retrogene is associated with a more than 50-fold increase in risk of IVDH in the Nova Scotia Duck Tolling Retriever.[7] The increase in expression of FGF4 during development of the vertebral column is associated with premature and rapid degeneration of the NP, in which there is transformation of the notochordal cells into chondrocytes (chondroid metaplasia), with subsequent cellular death and calcification. NP degeneration and calcification is present in breeds such as the Dachshund and French Bulldog by 6 months of age, and the number of calcified discs peaks around 2 years of age.[8] The changes to the NP result in an inability to withstand normal forces, there is splitting and damage to the surrounding AF, and calcified nuclear material is extruded into the canal causing spinal cord compression and contusion.[9] The speed of extrusion and volume of extruded material vary greatly between individuals, and the picture can be complicated by laceration of the internal vertebral venous plexus, causing hematoma formation (disc-associated extensive epidural hemorrhage, DEEH), or by such forceful release of disc material that it lacerates the dura mater and comes to rest either within the subarachnoid space or within the spinal cord (intradural intramedullary intervertebral disc extrusion, IIVDE).[6] There are clearly additional factors that precipitate or protect from a disc extrusion, given that the prevalence of the CFA12 *FGF4* retrogene is high in breeds such as the Dachshund and French Bulldog, while the prevalence of IVD disease in Dachshunds is between 15 and 30%. Another factor reported to be associated with the risk of IVDE in chondrodystrophic breeds is the amount and nature of exercise, with more than 30 minutes of exercise a day and certain forms of exercise (e.g., moderate stair climbing) being protective.[10,11] In addition, being neutered is a negative risk factor.[10] IVDE can also occur in nonchondrodystrophic breeds of dogs and in cats that do not have the same genetic risk factor. Nonchondrodystrophic dog breeds and cats are more likely to have a single calcified disc, but the resulting changes in integrity of the IVD have the same outcome, i.e., failure of the AF and extrusion of calcified material into the canal.

Clinical presentation

The onset of signs can be abrupt, but signs typically develop over a few days, with owners first noticing discomfort and reluctance to move. The clinical signs reflect the location of the disc extrusion and range in severity from spinal pain to ataxia and paresis to paralysis with, at the most severe, loss of pain perception. Segmental spinal reflexes are depressed or absent for lesions affecting the brachial or the lumbar intumescence, and in extrusions cranial to L1–L2, the caudal border of the cutaneous trunci reflex shifts cranially to lie just caudal to the level of the lesion. The presence of pain perception should be assessed carefully in both pelvic limbs and in the tail because this is one of the most important prognostic indicators in paralyzed animals (Video 29.1). The clinical picture can be complicated by the presence of spinal shock. This occurs in acutely and severely affected animals, and the most common finding is a reduced withdrawal reflex in the presence of normal patellar and perineal reflexes. In addition, dogs with DEEH tend to have more severe spinal pain.

Cervical disc extrusions are more likely to be associated with severe pain alone, while thoracolumbar disc extrusions are usually associated with pelvic limb, tail, and bladder neurological deficits. Disc extrusions are less common caudal to L5 but if they occur, they can cause pain with less prominent neurological deficits because they are impacting the nerve roots of the cauda equina. Similarly, profoundly lateralized disc extrusions in the thoracolumbar spine cause pain rather than severe neurological deficits because they impact the nerve root or spinal ganglion at the intervertebral foramen. There are numerous schemes for grading clinical signs, but the major categories are provided in Table 29.1.

TABLE 29.1 Categorization of severity of the clinical signs of myelopathy.

Signs grouped according to increasing severity	
Cervical	**Thoracolumbar**
■ Spinal pain ■ Ambulatory tetraparesis and ataxia ■ Nonambulatory tetraparesis ■ Tetraplegia ■ Tetraplegia with hypoventilation	■ Spinal pain ■ Ambulatory paraparesis and ataxia ■ Nonambulatory paraparesis ■ Paraplegia ■ Paraplegia with no pain perception (also known as no deep pain)

Video 29.1

Assessment of deep pain perception in a 2-year-old male castrated mixed-breed dog. The left pelvic limb is tested using hemostatic forceps to apply pressure across a digit, and a withdrawal reflex is readily produced, but the dog remains unaware of the stimulus. When the right pelvic limb is tested in the same way, the dog is very aware of the stimulus and sits up and looks towards the examiner.

Diagnostic imaging

Spinal radiographs are a useful screening tool but not an accurate diagnostic test. The presence of calcified NP confirms the presence of degenerative disc disease. Indicators of acute extrusion include narrowing of the IVD space compared with the spaces immediately cranial and caudal, a change in the shape of the intervertebral foramen, and opacification within the vertebral canal, which is easiest to see in the intervertebral foramen (Fig. 29.1). The presence of a vacuum phenomenon within the narrowed disc space is strongly correlated with the presence of a disc extrusion but is a rare finding.[12]

In order to make a definitive diagnosis, advanced imaging with magnetic resonance imaging (MRI) or computed tomography (CT) is needed. CT is more widely available, is a rapid test that can be performed under sedation in a healthy, young dog, and is less expensive than MRI. CT identifies calcified material and blood as hyperattenuating material in the vertebral canal with a reported sensitivity of 81–100% in dogs with Hansen type 1 IVDE (Fig. 29.2). Accuracy decreases if larger breed and older dogs are included.[12,13] Importantly, if the disc material extruded is not calcified, the CT image will likely be nondiagnostic, and a CT myelogram or MRI scan will be required to identify the site of compression. In addition, CT does not provide additional information on spinal cord parenchyma and does not contribute prognostic information.

MRI is more expensive and less available, but it is extremely accurate. It provides detail on the spinal cord parenchyma and allows identification of both calcified and noncalcified disc extrusions (Fig. 29.3). The longitudinal extent of loss of HASTE signal and T2 parenchymal hyperintensity can be prognostic in deep pain negative dogs, although magnet strength and protocol can influence parameters.[12,13] Myelography can also be used to diagnose IVDE if MRI and CT are not available. The relative invasiveness of introducing contrast into the intrathecal space and the inability to generate cross-sectional views unless combined with CT mean that this diagnostic modality is rarely used at this time.

Prognosis and treatment

Treatment options are conservative management and surgical decompression, and the choice made is based on data on outcomes with both approaches as well as owner preferences and patient comorbidities. A decision-making algorithm is provided, and **Table 29.2** lists the percentage of dogs that recover with different injury severities and management. In this instance, recovery implies pain-free independent ambulation with continence. The rates of incontinence are also provided for surgical management; they are not available for conservative management. There are abundant data available for speed of recovery of thoracolumbar IVDE with surgical management, but little for conservative management. Overall, the majority of nonambulatory paraparetic and paraplegic (with deep pain) dogs recover ambulation within 2 weeks following surgery, while paraplegic deep pain negative dogs that do recover pain perception should be walking by 4 weeks. Further improvement can continue for many weeks. Dogs that do not regain deep pain perception by 4 weeks are unlikely to (although there are exceptions), but close to 40% of these dogs will recover the ability to walk (albeit they will remain fecally and urinary incontinent),[14] and this percentage could be improved to close to 60% with intensive rehabilitation.[15]

When nuclear material is acutely extruded, it typically damages the internal vertebral venous plexus causing hemorrhage. In larger dog breeds as well as in the French Bulldog, it is not unusual for this bleeding to be extensive, causing multilevel hematoma formation (DEEH). In smaller dog

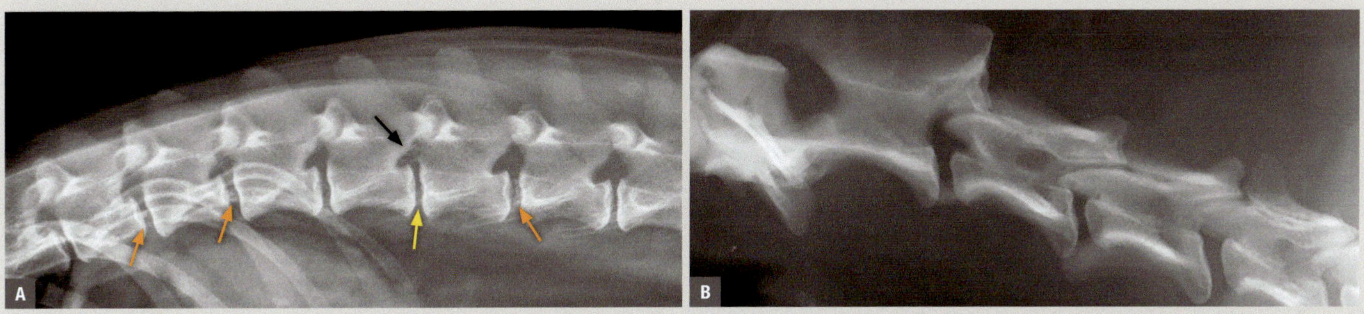

FIG. 29.1 Lateral survey radiographs of the thoracolumbar spine (**A**) and cervical spine (**B**). In (**A**), several of the intervertebral discs have calcification within the nucleus pulposus (orange arrows), the intervertebral foramen at L2–L3 is smaller and contains calcified material (black arrow), and the disc space appears slightly narrowed when compared with the spaces at L1–L2 and L3–L4 (yellow arrow). Cross-sectional imaging confirmed a disc extrusion at L2–L3. In (**B**), the disc space at C3–C4 appears narrowed when compared with the spaces at C2–C3 and C4–C5. There is no obvious calcified nuclear material visible, but cross-sectional imaging revealed a disc extrusion at C3–C4 and calcified material was retrieved at surgery.

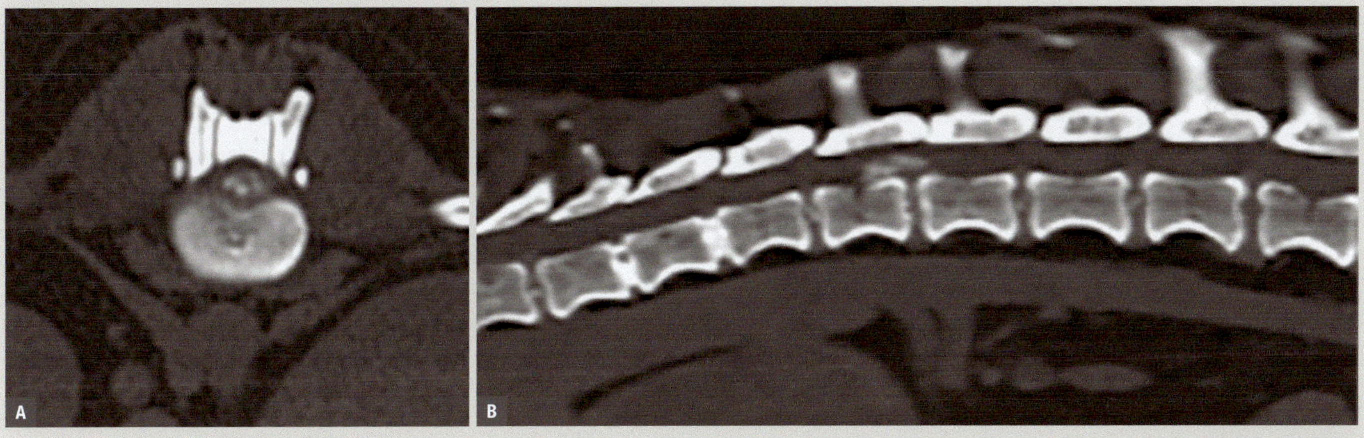

FIG. 29.2 Computed tomography scans of the thoracolumbar spine of a 6-year-old male castrated Dachshund. (**A**) Transverse image at the level of the T13–L1 disc space showing hyperattenuating material in the ventral aspect of the vertebral canal. Calcification of the nucleus pulposus in situ is also visible. (**B**) Sagittal reconstruction of the images clearly showing calcification of the nucleus pulposus in most of the disc spaces and the presence of material within the vertebral canal at T13–L1.

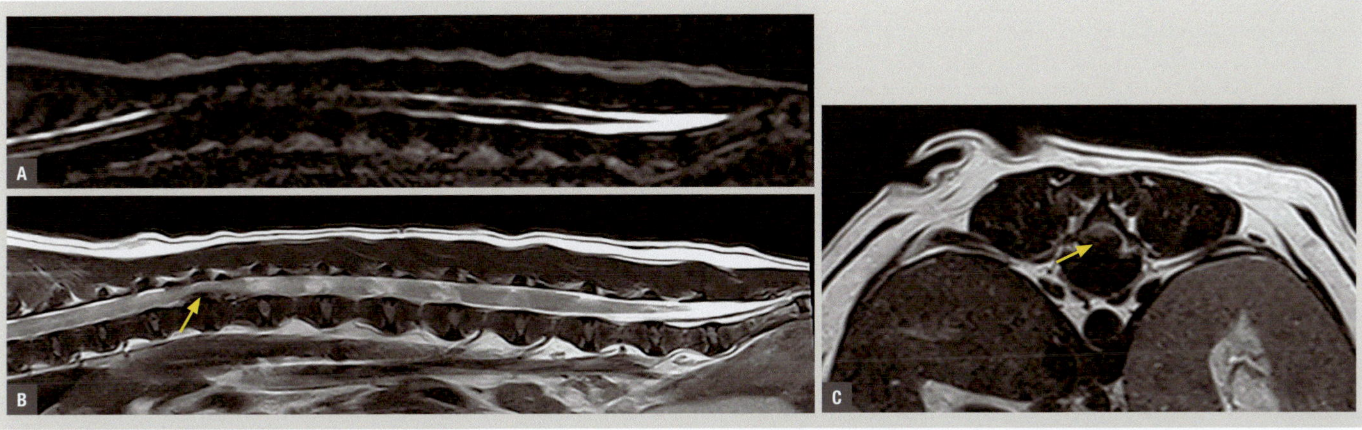

FIG. 29.3 Magnetic resonance (MR) images of the thoracolumbar spine in a 4-year-old male castrated miniature poodle. (**A**) Sagittal HASTE image showing interruption of the subarachnoid space over five vertebrae at the level of the thoracolumbar junction. (**B**) T2-weighted sagittal image. There is a mass of hypointense material centered over the T12–T13 intervertebral disc space. There is some heterogenous signal within the mass. The underlying nucleus pulposus (NP) has lost T2 signal, unlike the rest of the NP visible on the MR image. (**C**) Transverse T2-weighted image at the level of the T12–T13 intervertebral disc space demonstrating compression of the spinal cord by hypointense material on the floor of the canal. Both calcified and fibrous material appear hypointense on MR images and cannot be distinguished from each other.

ALGORITHM 29.1

Suggested decision-making algorithm for considering medical versus surgical management in dogs with acute intervertebral disc extrusions.

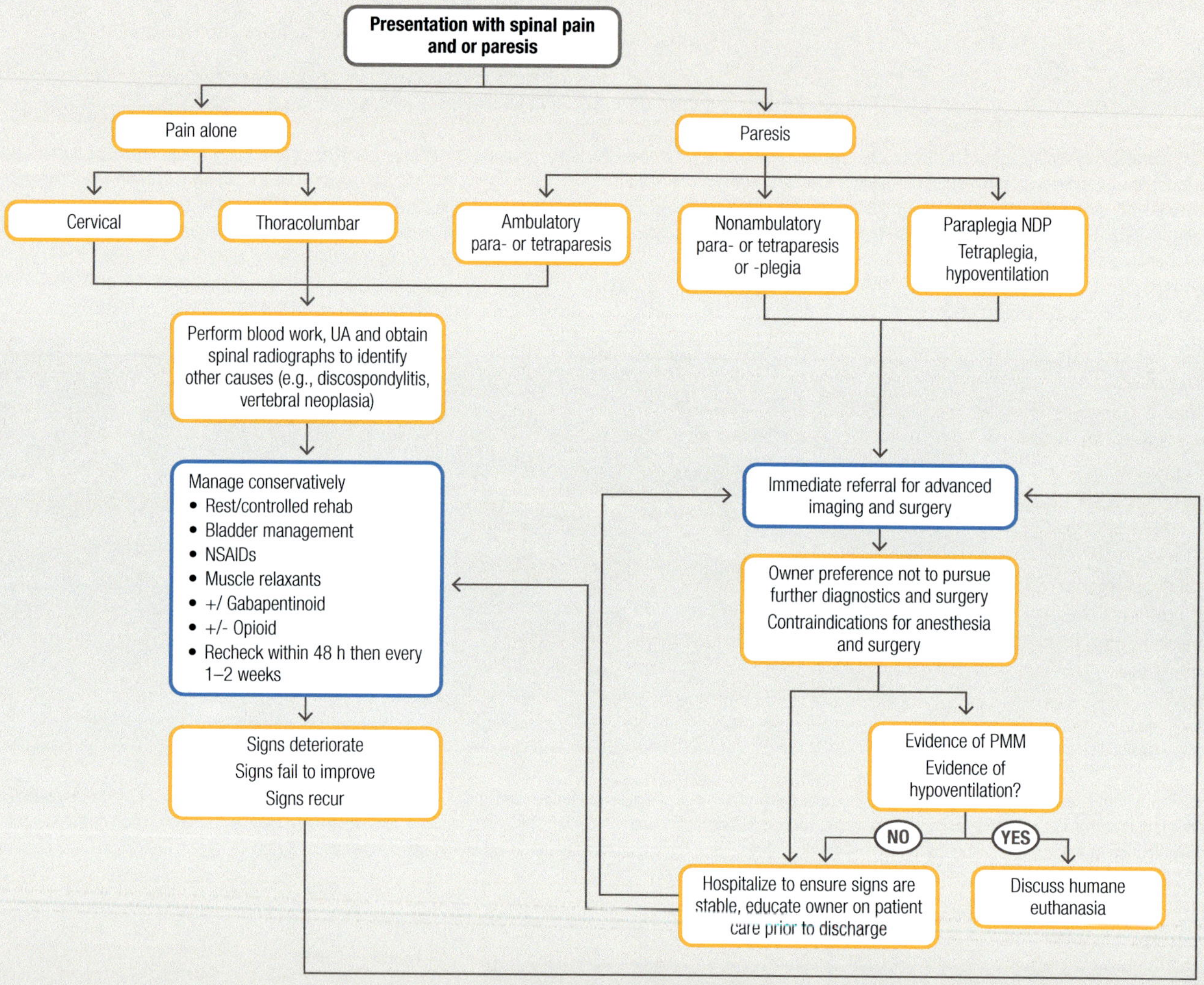

NDP, negative deep pain; UA, urinalysis; NSAIDs, nonsteroidal anti-inflammatory drugs; PMM, progressive myelomalacia.

Diagnostic protocol   Diagnosis   Treatment

TABLE 29.2 Prognoses with conservative versus surgical management. These numbers are derived from numerous publications, many summarized in recent reviews and consensus statements.[13–23] Percentages are rounded to the nearest whole numbers, and ranges reflect conclusions drawn by different studies.

Cervical[16–19]	Conservative	Surgical	Thoracolumbar[14,16,20–23]	Conservative	Surgical		
Pain alone	73%	96%	Pain alone	73–80%	99%		
Ambulatory tetraparesis			Ambulatory paraparesis				
Nonambulatory tetraparesis			Nonambulatory paraparesis	81%	93%	UC: 95%	FC: 97%
Tetraplegia with adequate ventilation			Paraplegia with pain perception	56–60%	93%	UC: 84%	FC: 91%
Tetraplegia with hypoventilation			Paraplegia with no deep pain	21–22%	61%	UC: 61%	FC: 82%
Foraminal	85%	NA	Foraminal	90%	96%*		

* Note these surgically managed cases had failed medical management. NA, not applicable – inadequate data available; UC, urinary continence; FC, fecal continence.

breeds and in less severe grades of injury, this does not appear to influence outcome, but in larger dog breeds or dogs that present paraplegic with or without deep pain, the outcome is negatively affected.[24,25] More detailed reporting of outcomes can be found elsewhere, and it should be noted that there is considerable variation between individuals, and additional recovery will continue over time.[26]

Based on these outcomes, in the case of thoracolumbar IVDE, surgery is usually recommended (but not required) in dogs that are nonambulatory paraparetic or paraplegic. Management of cervical IVDE tends to start with conservative management if the only sign is pain and move to surgical decompression in the face of severe signs (pain or neurological deficits). Most of these dogs present with cervical pain, with or without a nerve root signature or mild gait deficits. Relatively few present as nonambulatory tetraparetic or tetraplegic, and these dogs are usually managed surgically. The severity of signs seems not to affect the outcome, although clearly the need for mechanical ventilation in some dogs poses therapeutic challenges.[16,17]

Conservative management of cervical or thoracolumbar IVDE

The goals of conservative management are to alleviate the clinical signs, to avoid further disc extrusion causing compression of or contusion to the spinal cord while allowing the AF defect to heal, and to support neurological recovery. This is achieved through a combination of pain and bladder management, restricted movement and controlled rehabilitation. Careful nursing to ensure skin health is also vital. Pain control includes a combination of nonsteroidal anti-inflammatory drugs (NSAIDs), muscle relaxants (methocarbamol or diazepam), and neuropathic pain medications (gabapentin or pregabalin). Muscle relaxants are particularly important in the case of cervical IVDE.[13,18] In the instance of severe pain, hospitalization and administration of intravenous opioids might be necessary, and opioids can be administered orally or transdermally (fentanyl patch) when at home.

The use of corticosteroids in disc-associated spinal cord injury is contentious and confusing. Anti-inflammatory doses of corticosteroids do not appear to cause significant side effects as long as they are not used in combination with NSAIDs.[13] Corticosteroids are likely to reduce pain due to nerve root and meningeal inflammation. However, used in this way, they are not neuroprotective and might inhibit healing of the AF. High doses (30 mg/kg) of methylprednisolone sodium succinate have been advocated as a neuroprotectant when used within 8 hours of injury, but a randomized controlled trial did not show a benefit in dogs with IVDE, and this high dose use is not recommended.[13]

Owners need to be educated on the frequency with which dogs should urinate and the warning signs of a urinary tract infection. Dogs that are paraplegic typically cannot urinate voluntarily and will need to be hospitalized until they improve neurologically or their owners have mastered manual expression of their bladder. Most dogs have lesions cranial to the lumbar intumescence and suffer from urine retention due to increased urethral tone ("upper motor neuron bladder"). In this instance, administration of an alpha-adrenergic antagonist (e.g., prazosin, phenoxybenzamine, or tamsulosin) and a skeletal muscle relaxant (diazepam) to decrease tone in the internal and external urethral sphincters can aid manual expression.[13] A smaller proportion of dogs have more caudal disc extrusions and can suffer from loss of tone of the external anal and urethral sphincters and detrusor muscle ("lower motor neuron bladder"). Such animals might leak both urine and feces constantly and can be very challenging to manage. Management revolves around regular expression of the bladder, careful attention to the skin of the perineal and inguinal region to avoid urine scald, and regular changes of absorbent bedding.

It is anticipated that the AF will take several weeks to heal, and so confinement to a crate for 4–6 weeks is recommended to avoid falls, jumps, and other activities that could exacerbate the disc extrusion. However, there is little evidence to support the duration of confinement, and confinement should be combined with controlled, phased rehabilitation. Owners need careful training in patient care, and dogs should be rechecked within a few days and then every 2 weeks. Dogs should show a steady improvement, and a failure to improve over a 2-week period or any deterioration signals a failure in medical management.[13,18]

Surgical management of thoracolumbar IVDE

The goals of surgical management are to decompress the spinal cord and nerve roots and to reduce the risk of a recurrence. The optimal timing of surgery is unclear, with published studies presenting conflicting data.[13,20,21] It likely differs between patients, but we have a poor understanding of the variables that dictate the need for more timely surgery. Overall, timing of surgery does not appear to alter the final outcome in dogs that have incomplete lesions (paraplegic with deep pain and nonambulatory paraparetic). In paraplegic deep pain negative dogs, timing of surgical decompression does not appear to alter the percentage of dogs that recover motor function, but delaying surgery might be a risk factor for the development of progressive myelomalacia (PMM).[20,27] A practical approach to timing involves consideration of the speed of onset and progression of signs, their severity, and the hospital resources in terms of availability of diagnostic equipment and staff to assist in diagnosis and treatment. Typically, neurosurgeons will aim to perform surgery on nonambulatory paraparetic or paraplegic dogs within 24 hours of admission, and dogs that are paraplegic without deep pain or are tetraplegic are addressed within 12 hours of admission. It is important to note that these suggested windows are from the time of admission, not onset, and that this is not intended to imply that the outcome will be altered if surgery is not performed within these windows, or that surgery outside these times should not be considered. Indeed, there is no set threshold beyond which surgery is futile.

The most common surgical technique used to access the vertebral canal is the hemilaminectomy, but variations on this approach include the pediculectomy and partial lateral vertebrectomy, and minimally invasive approaches are now being developed (Fig. 29.4). Currently, the surgical choice is the preference of the surgeon. The value of durotomy to reduce intraparenchymal pressure and reestablish spinal cord perfusion in severe injuries is unclear. There is some evidence that spinal cord blood flow is not improved with a durotomy, and there is conflicting evidence of benefit in deep pain negative dogs looking at two different outcomes, improved functional recovery and the development or progression of PMM (see below).[13,28]

Complications of surgery include neurological deterioration, intraoperative hemorrhage, incisional infections, hematoma formation, recurrence of disc extrusion, discospondylitis, aspiration pneumonia, and vascular events. Subluxation at the surgical site is unlikely but can occur if the dog suffers from articular process hypoplasia or bilateral decompression is needed (e.g., if addressing a same site but contralateral recurrence). In the latter instance, either a pediculectomy is needed on the contralateral side to avoid bilateral removal of the articular processes, or surgical stabilization is needed.

There is evidence that fenestration of degenerate or calcified discs reduces the risk of recurrence, and fenestration of the affected site at minimum is strongly recommended.[14,18] The approach to fenestration differs between neurologists and surgeons, with approximately 70% of neurologists routinely performing fenestrations of at-risk disc spaces compared with 36% of surgeons.[4] Historically, fenestration alone was used to treat IVDE, and laser-induced destruction of the NP is used by some groups as a therapy and prophylactic for IVDE in dogs with a less severe grade of injury.[29]

Postoperative care largely mirrors conservative management with the addition of care of the surgical incision. Perioperative pain management strategies can be employed to reduce the severity of intraoperative and early postoperative pain. These include preoperative erector spinae plane (ESP) blocks, incisional intramuscular bupivacaine (2 mg/kg), or preservative free morphine (0.1 mg/kg) injected into sterile absorbable hemocollagen sponges and placed in the laminectomy defect. Standard postoperative management of pain includes a combination of 24–48 hours of an opioid, a nonsteroidal drug (or continuation of an anti-inflammatory dose of a corticosteroid if the patient is already receiving one at presentation), gabapentin or pregabalin, and a muscle relaxant. Diazepam can serve both as a muscle relaxant and as an aid to bladder expression. Trazodone can be used as an anxiolytic. Ice packing of the incision every 6–8 hours for 24–48 hours followed by hot packing can help control pain and improve wound healing. Other interventions such as pulsed electromagnetic fields and cold laser can also help with wound healing and pain control. These protocols are summarized elsewhere.[13]

Bladder management follows the guidelines provided under conservative management; however, while hospitalized, intermittent or indwelling catheters can be used to facilitate bladder emptying and recovery in paraplegic patients or in animals that are difficult to manually express. Early intervention with phased rehabilitation can be undertaken safely.[30] This can be performed in house, or rehabilitation plans can be designed for owners to perform at home. While dogs with incomplete injuries have an excellent prognosis for recovery with or without customized rehabilitation, dogs with more severe injuries (paraplegic with loss of deep pain) or concurrent orthopedic disease and larger dogs are likely to benefit from more specific expert rehabilitation.

PMM is a fatal complication of thoracolumbar disc extrusions that owners should be made aware of. This complication occurs at a rate of around 10% in dogs presenting paraplegic with no deep pain, with higher rates in French Bulldogs (as high as 33%). Caudal lumbar disc herniations and injury severity are important risk factors. PMM manifests as extension of neurological deficits both caudally and cranially, with progressive loss of pelvic limb and perineal reflexes, loss of abdominal tone, cranial migration of the cutaneous trunci reflex caudal border, difficulty righting from lateral recumbency, and ultimately, development of tetraparesis, hypoventilation, and Horner's syndrome.[31] Signs of PMM at time of presentation should be taken very seriously. Suspicion should be raised when the neurological examination suggests a more extensive lesion than a focal myelopathy, for example, a cutaneous trunci reflex cut-off cranial to T10 (most commonly, IVDE occurs caudal to T10) or loss of the patellar reflex combined with a cutaneous trunci cut-off suggestive of a caudal thoracic myelopathy. Such signs are reflected on MRI by extensive loss of the HASTE signal and longitudinally extensive T2 hyperintensity. There is conflicting evidence

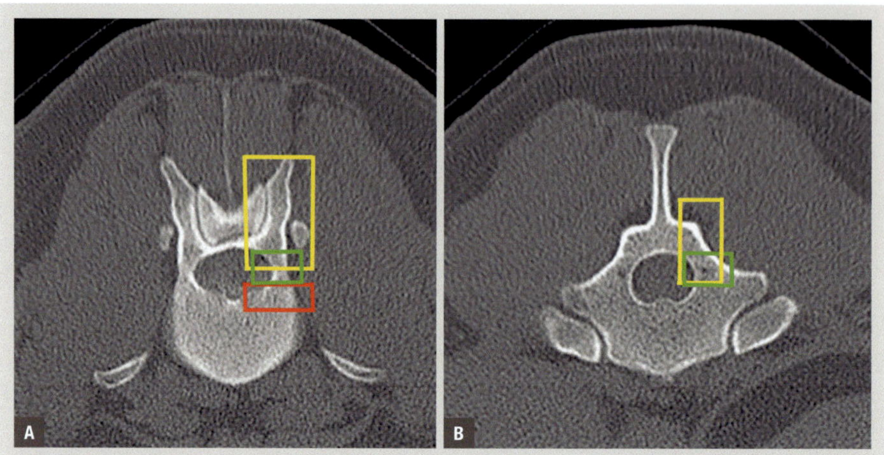

FIG. 29.4 Transverse computed tomography images of the lumbar spine midvertebral body (A) and at the level of the intervertebral disc (B) showing outlines of the bone removed for a hemilaminectomy (yellow), a pediculectomy and mini-hemilaminectomy (green), and a partial lateral vertebrectomy (red).

that performing durotomies at the time of decompressive surgery will reduce the prevalence of PMM, and that progression of clinically evident PMM can be halted by performing extensive durotomies to include the full extent of HASTE interruption.[13,32,33] Most commonly, PMM results in hypoventilation and is fatal.

Surgical management of cervical IVDE

The decision-making process for surgical versus conservative management of cervical disc extrusions differs slightly from thoracolumbar IVDE. Cervical disc extrusions are less likely to be associated with significant paresis but are associated with much more severe and persistent pain that might respond to pain medications but can recur the minute they are discontinued. As such, surgery in the form of a ventral slot is frequently performed for pain alone. While it is never wrong to attempt to manage cervical pain with muscle relaxants, anti-inflammatory drugs, and neuropathic pain medications, persistence of the signs in the face of this approach or recurrence as they are tapered is a strong indication for surgery. Risks of surgery include intraoperative hemorrhage, which can be significant due to the position of the internal vertebral venous plexus, neurological deterioration, intraoperative arrythmias, or Horner's syndrome.[34] The ventral slot is effective at removing disc material from ventral to the spinal cord, but extremely lateralized material has to be retrieved via a dorsal or lateral approach, both of which can be more challenging surgical approaches.[35] Fenestration of at-risk discs at the time of decompression is relatively straightforward when compared with this procedure in the thoracolumbar spine, but there is little information available on recurrence rates with or without fenestration.

Acute noncompressive nucleus pulposus extrusion (ANNPE)

Etiology and pathophysiology

This condition is typically associated with strenuous exercise that involves some form of leaping and twisting in medium to large breed dogs. A small volume of nuclear material is abruptly ejected through the AF and contuses the spinal cord. The presence of the dorsal longitudinal ligament on the floor of the canal deflects the extruded material laterally, producing a very asymmetrical injury. The association with exercise suggests changes in intradiscal pressure underly this condition. It occurs more commonly in the thoracolumbar spine but can be cervical. The disc material is usually hydrated NP, but it can be somewhat degenerate, consistent with aging.[6]

Clinical signs

The onset of paresis is peracute, usually during exercise. Dogs frequently cry out at the time and appear extremely anxious, even agitated. Deficits are clearly lateralized and reflect the location of the disc extrusion, with spinal shock complicating the assessment of segmental spinal reflexes, because of the speed of onset of signs and presentation to the veterinarian. Mild spinal pain might be present.[36] Dogs with thoracolumbar injuries might be monoparetic if the lesion is extremely lateralized, although typically, the other pelvic limb is not normal. When testing the segmental reflexes, it is important to assess the cutaneous trunci reflex to identify the level of the focal myelopathy (Video 29.2).

Extremely lateralized cervical lesions present as hemiplegia with minimal hemiparesis on the contralateral side. Such cases will exhibit differential hyperthermia due to damage to the sympathetic tracts in the lateral funiculus. These dogs also demonstrate positional dystonia, likely due to unilateral loss of the vestibulospinal tract. This manifests as a strong preference to lie on the more affected side. When turned, these dogs appear distressed, their limbs on the less affected side extend, and they turn their head to the less affected side and attempt to turn back over.[37] These cervical disc explosions are more likely to be precipitated by trauma.

Diagnostic imaging

The clinical suspicion for ANNPE is usually high based on the history and neurological findings. Spinal radiographs and CT are unrewarding, but in some instances, mild narrowing of the affected IVD space is apparent. The diagnosis is made from MRI. Classic findings include lateralized T2 hyperintensity within the spinal cord directly overlying a disc space. The NP of that disc is typically hydrated but has a slightly reduced volume when compared to adjacent discs. Careful inspection of the vertebral canal reveals small amounts of material in the epidural space at the level of the T2 hyperintensity (Fig. 29.5). The main differential for this clinical history and the presence of lateralized intraparenchymal T2 hyperintensity is fibrocartilaginous embolism (FCE). However, the T2 hyperintensity is more likely to be focused on the grey matter in FCE, can be more diffuse or even multifocal, and will not overlie the IVD directly with no disruption of the epidural fat. In spite of these differences, in some cases it is difficult to distinguish these differentials, particularly on images acquired with low-field (i.e., <1.5 Tesla) MRI. CT is not useful for the diagnosis of ANNPE or FCE.

Treatment and prognosis

This is not a surgical disease. Treatment rests on supportive care as described for IVDE, confinement to an area where the patients cannot fall and hurt themselves, and rehabilitation. Improvement is initially rapid but slows and plateaus over 4–6 weeks. Animals with severe myelopathies will show improvement over a longer period of time. Prognosis for recovery is excellent in animals that have some residual motor function. For dogs with cervical disease, the asymmetry of the injury can pose real problems during recovery, and rehabilitation is especially important. Paraplegic dogs with intact deep pain perception do typically recover ambulation with time and assistance from rehabilitation, but approximately 85% of dogs recover full urinary continence, and more notably, approximately 50% recover fecal continence.[26] Information on recovery of paraplegic deep pain negative dogs is lacking.

Video 29.2

Neurological examination in a 4-year-old male castrated mixed-breed dog with acute onset of monoparesis affecting the right pelvic limb due to a right lateralized acute noncompressive nucleus pulposus extrusion at the level of L1–L2. The dog has proprioceptive placing and hopping deficits of the right pelvic limb, with intact patellar and withdrawal reflexes but a cutaneous trunci reflex cut-off on the right around L2.

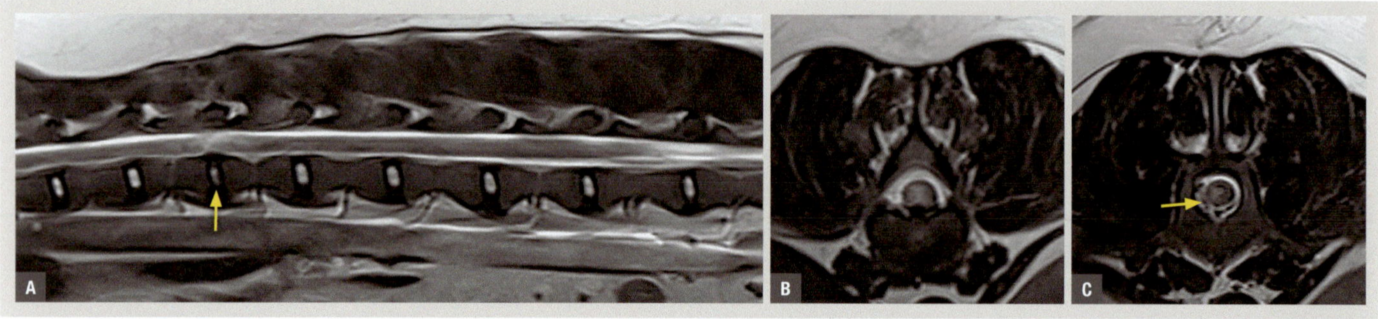

FIG. 29.5 Magnetic resonance images of the thoracolumbar spine in a 7-year-old female spayed Labrador Retriever. (**A**) Sagittal T2-weighted image showing focal T2 hyperintensity within the spinal cord parenchyma at T13–L1. The T13–L1 intervertebral disc has a reduced volume of T2 hyperintense nucleus pulposus and a narrowed disc space (arrow). (**B**) T2-weighted transverse image directly over T13–L1 demonstrating a slightly lateralized T2 hyperintensity within the spinal cord. (**C**) Another T2-weighted transverse image taken just caudal to image B showing persistence of the T2 hyperintensity within the spinal cord and presence of disc material within the epidural space (arrow).

Hydrated nucleus pulposus extrusion (HNPE)

Etiology and pathophysiology

The causes of this type of IVDH are poorly understood. It happens most commonly in the cervical spine in middle-aged to older small- to medium-sized dogs. A moderate amount of hydrated although often partially degenerate NP is extruded into the vertebral canal causing compression of the overlying spinal cord. The hydration status of the material ranges from extremely fluid to more proteinaceous and may contain solid fibrocartilage. It does not appear to be caused by exertion or trauma.[6]

Clinical presentation

Owners report an acute onset of rapidly progressive tetraparesis (or less commonly, paraparesis) that is usually symmetrical. It is not unusual for severely affected dogs to have respiratory compromise and present with a gulping breathing pattern (Video 29.3). Dogs do not typically present signs of spinal pain.

Diagnostic imaging

The lack of calcification of the material means it cannot be detected on radiographs or CT images, and a spinal MRI is needed to establish the diagnosis. The extruded material is T2 hyperintense, and because it does not disrupt the midline meningovertebral ligament, it produces a classic seagull shape on transverse images (Fig. 29.6). The appearance of the hydrated material varies on HASTE imaging according to the protein content and fluidity (Fig. 29.6). Compression of the spinal cord can be severe.

Video 29.3

Nine-year-old male castrated mixed-breed dog presented for acute onset of tetraplegia due to a hydrated nucleus pulposus extrusion. At presentation, the dog had an open-mouth, gasping breathing pattern.

Treatment and prognosis

Given the fluid nature of the compressive disc material, it is reasonable to expect regression of the compression over time, and this type of disc extrusion can be managed medically or surgically (ventral slot or hemilaminectomy depending on the location) with similar outcomes. Typically, surgery is reserved for those with more severe clinical signs and severe compression. Medical management follows the same protocols outlined for IVDE. More than 95% of dogs are reported to recover with either surgical or medical management.[6]

Hansen type II intervertebral disc protrusion (IVDP)

Etiology and pathophysiology

This type of disc degeneration and protrusion is associated with aging and occurs particularly at sites with more mobility such as the caudal cervical spine (disc-associated Wobbler syndrome, see Chapter 32), the lumbosacral junction (a component of degenerative lumbosacral stenosis, see Chapter 33), and the thoracolumbar junction and lumbar spine (covered here). Classically, this condition affects older medium to large breed dogs such as the German Shepherd, but smaller dog breeds can be affected as well. The IVD undergoes age-associated changes in the composition of the NP with decreased hydration, gradual transformation to fibrocartilage, increased fibrous content, and progressive splitting and bulging of the AF into the canal, often with fragments of the fibrous NP within the protruding annular material.[9,38] It is not unusual for multiple IVDs to be affected.

Clinical signs

The onset of signs of proprioceptive ataxia and paraparesis is usually insidious but can be acute. Indeed, it is not unusual to encounter the syndrome of "acute on chronic", in which there is acute onset of severe signs, often triggered by activity, with an imaging finding of a chronic IVDP. Signs might lateralize or be symmetrical, and while overt signs of pain might not be present, the dog usually has spinal pain on palpation.

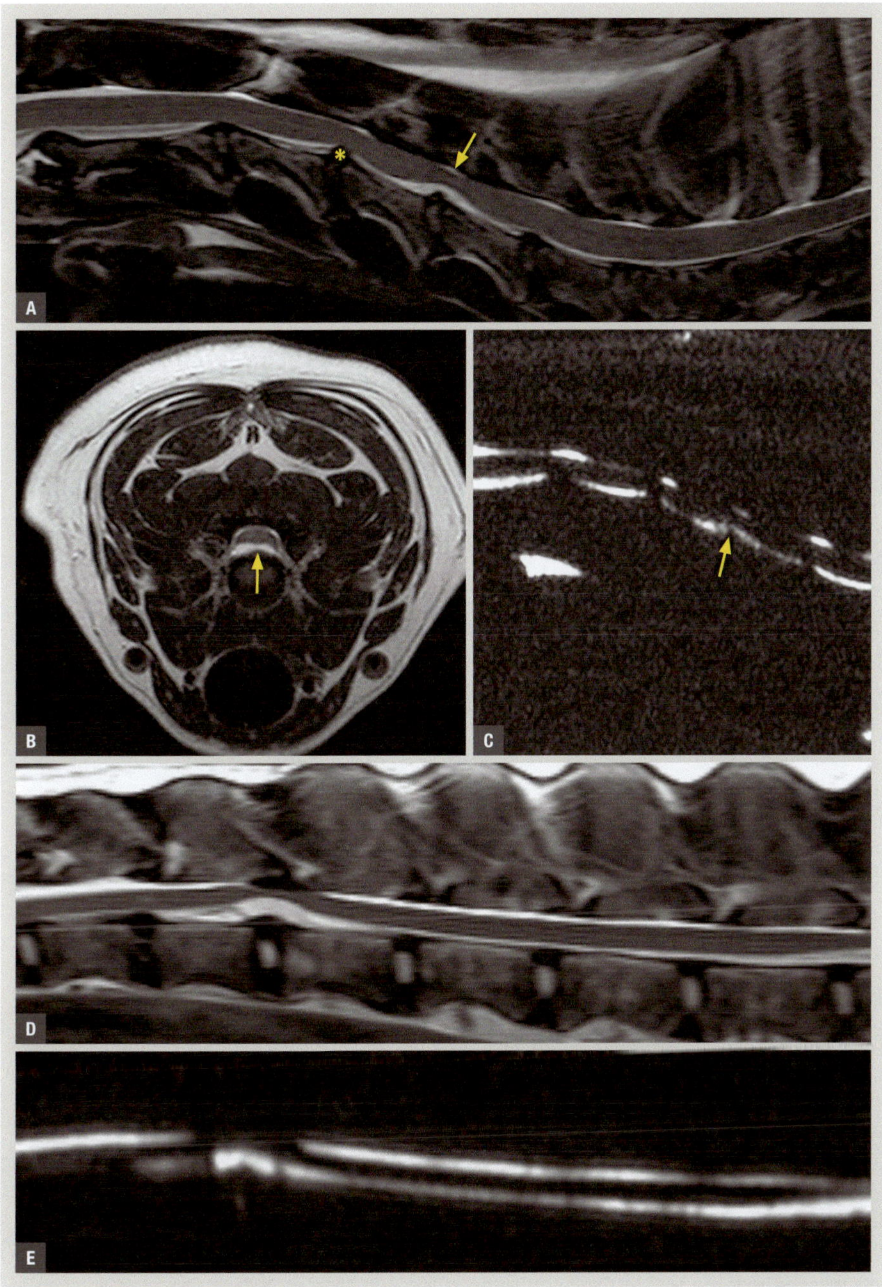

FIG. 29.6 (**A–C**) Magnetic resonance images of the cervical spine of a 7-year-old male castrated mixed-breed dog with acute onset tetraplegia. (**A**) T2-weighted sagittal image of the cervical spine demonstrating a hyperintense ventrally extradural compressive lesion at C4–C5 causing severe spinal cord compression with slight T2 hyperintensity within the overlying spinal cord (arrow). Note the T2 hypointense extradural lesion with smooth margins (asterisk): mild type II intervertebral disc protrusion. (**B**) Transverse T2 image at the level of the C4–C5 showing the hyperintense material located ventrally with a classic seagull-like appearance due to the intact meningovertebral ligament (arrow). (**C**) Sagittal HASTE image showing the material ventral to the spinal cord at C4–C5 is hyperintense but not as hyperintense as the fluid within the subarachnoid space (arrow). At surgery, extremely soft, hydrated nucleus pulposus was removed. (**D, E**) Magnetic resonance image of the thoracolumbar spine of an 8-year-old female spayed Saluki with acute onset paraplegia. (**D**) Sagittal T2-weighted image showing the marked compression of the spinal cord at L1–L2 by extradural T2 hyperintense material. (**E**) HASTE image of the same region; the compressive lesion is isointense to the subarachnoid space, and at surgery, a large amount of clear fluid was released.

Signs are typically progressive, although they can wax and wane, and the true clinical course of thoracolumbar IVDP is not well described in the literature. Given these are often older dogs, the clinical picture can be complicated and magnified by orthopedic disease, and a very careful orthopedic examination should be performed.

Diagnostic imaging

While one would suspect that IVDP is associated with chronic degenerative changes on spinal radiographs, there is actually a poor correlation between radiographic findings and the presence of disc protrusions. Given the fibrous nature of the protruded material, it is not visible on CT, and MRI is needed. Myelography and CT myelograms can also be used but, as noted earlier, are not recommended. MRI findings include spinal cord atrophy and compression by T2 hypointense material with smooth borders centered over the disc space. The protruding annular material can be midline or lateralized, and multiple protrusions can be present. The NP in the underlying disc has lost its T2 hyperintensity reflecting dehydration (Fig. 29.7). The spinal cord can have centrally located T2 hyperintensity reflecting chronic loss of grey matter and associated gliosis.

Treatment and prognosis

Treatment options focus on medical management versus surgical decompression. Compared with acute IVDE, there is relatively little information published on outcomes in this group of dogs, but those case series available suggest medical management may initially be effective (associated with an

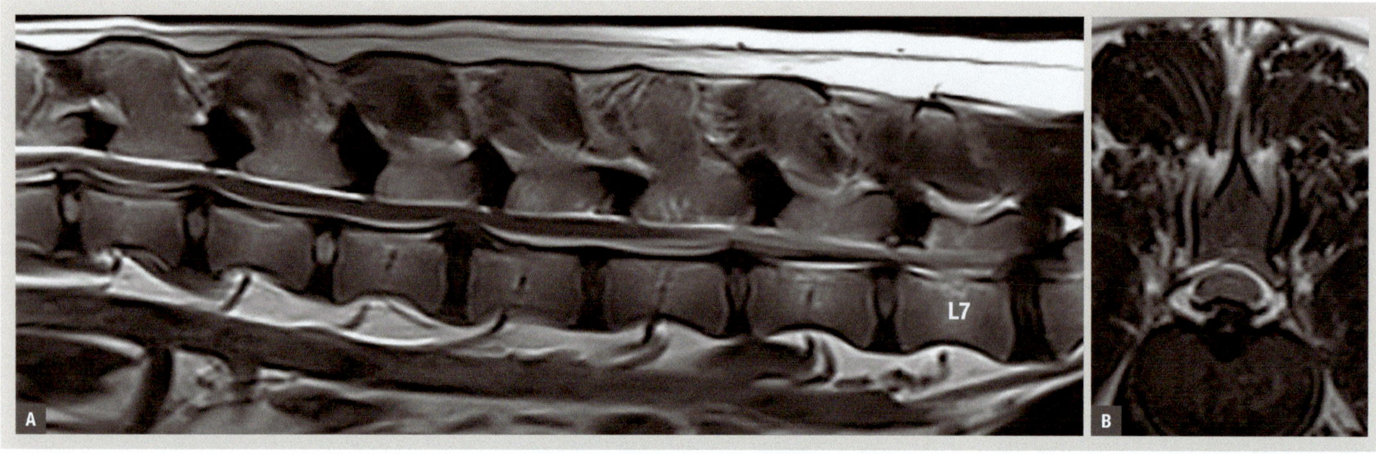

FIG. 29.7 Magnetic resonance images of the thoracolumbar spine of a 5-year-old male castrated German Shepherd dog. (**A**) Sagittal T2-weighted image showing bulging of the hypointense annulus fibrosus at L1–L2 (mild), L3–L4, and L7–S1. The smooth outline of this material centered directly over the disc space is consistent with an intervertebral disc protrusion. The nucleus pulposus has lost T2 signal at L3–L4 through L7–S1. (**B**) Transverse T2-weighted image at the center of L3–L4 showing hypointense material ventral to the spinal cord. This centrally located material lies under the dorsal longitudinal ligament.

improvement) in approximately 40% of dogs, although a large proportion subsequently deteriorate within 12 months with a 12-month success rate of around 30%.[39] This is compared to surgical decompression, in which success rates of as high as 82% have been reported 2 months after surgery, dropping to around 70% when followed for approximately a year.[39–41] These success rates can be difficult to compare because they are derived from retrospective data, and the populations are therefore different. In general, the dogs managed medically have less severe signs but are more likely to have multilevel disease with numerous disc protrusions.[39,42]

Suggested medical management

Medical management has traditionally involved strict confinement without rehabilitation. Typically, dogs are confined for 4 to 6 weeks with anti-inflammatory and gabapentinoid drugs for pain as needed. Given the compressive nature of the disc material, avoiding further injury through managing the environment so that slips and jumping and twisting activities are eliminated is important. However, in a chronic condition, it is vital to address core strength and build both proprioceptive and motor aspects of gait. Given the growth of veterinary rehabilitation as a specialty, it is likely that case series reporting outcomes with rehabilitation will emerge, and outcomes might improve with this approach.

Surgical management

A variety of different surgical approaches have been reported, and it is important to understand that, unlike disc extrusions, the disc material is annular and firmly attached to the vertebral floor with the spinal cord draped over, making it challenging to remove disc material without impacting the spinal cord. In addition, the internal vertebral venous plexus can be extremely distended and lie directly adjacent to the protruding material. The spinal cord has already suffered long-term compressive injury, and there might be less safety factor for the surgeon. As such, owners should be warned that neurological deterioration immediately postoperatively is anticipated, and while these signs should be reversible over a period of 1–2 weeks, in rare cases, deterioration can be severe and permanent. Typical approaches include hemilaminectomy alone or combined with annulectomy, discectomy, and stabilization. Approaching the site more laterally to do a partial lateral corpectomy is challenging to learn but is successful and can be performed via a minimally invasive approach.[41,43]

Conclusions

Veterinary neurology and neurosurgery have entered a new era of understanding of IVD disease. Knowledge of genetic risk factors provides a new avenue to prevent IVDEs, improved understanding of the different types of disc herniation that occur allows more specific treatment, and the combination of improved imaging via MRI, advancement of surgical techniques, and the development of veterinary rehabilitation should improve the overall outcomes.

KEY POINTS

- Intervertebral disc disease disease is the most common cause of myelopathy and pain in dogs.
- Intervertebral disc extrusions can be treated surgically or medically depending on the severity of signs.
- Acute noncompressive nucleus pulposus extrusions cause abrupt onset of lateralized signs and surgical management is not indicated.
- Hydrated nucleus pulposus extrusions are more commonly cervical and can be managed surgically or medically.
- Overall acute disc extrusions have a good prognosis with appropriate treatment in all but the most severely affected animals.
- Chronic disc protrusions cause more insidious signs and pose greater therapeutic challenges, both medically or surgically.

References

1. Bray JP, Burbidge HM. The canine intervertebral disk: part one: structure and function. *J Am Anim Hosp Assoc.* 1998 Jan-Feb;34(1):55–63.
2. Bergknut N, Meij BP, Hagman R, et al. Intervertebral disc disease in dogs - part 1: a new histological grading scheme for classification of intervertebral disc degeneration in dogs. *Vet J.* 2013 Feb;195(2):156–163.
3. Bergknut N, Egenvall A, Hagman R, et al. Incidence of intervertebral disk degeneration-related diseases and associated mortality rates in dogs. *J Am Vet Med Assoc.* 2012 Jun 1;240(11):1300–1309.
4. Moore SA, Early PJ, Hettlich BF. Practice patterns in the management of acute intervertebral disc herniation in dogs. *J Small Anim Pract.* 2016 Aug;57(8):409–415.
5. Rossi G, Stachel A, Lynch AM, Olby NJ. Intervertebral disc disease and aortic thromboembolism are the most common causes of acute paralysis in dogs and cats presenting to an emergency clinic. *Vet Rec.* 2020 Nov 14;187(10):e81.
6. Fenn J, Olby NJ; Canine Spinal Cord Injury Consortium (CANSORT-SCI). Classification of Intervertebral Disc Disease. *Front Vet Sci.* 2020 Oct 6;7:579025.
7. Brown EA, Dickinson PJ, Mansour T, et al. *FGF4* retrogene on CFA12 is responsible for chondrodystrophy and intervertebral disc disease in dogs. *Proc Natl Acad Sci U S A.* 2017 Oct 24;114(43):11476–11481.
8. Jensen VF, Arnbjerg J. Development of intervertebral disk calcification in the dachshund: a prospective longitudinal radiographic study. *J Am Anim Hosp Assoc.* 2001 May-Jun;37(3):274–282.
9. Smolders LA, Bergknut N, Grinwis GC, et al. Intervertebral disc degeneration in the dog. Part 2: chondrodystrophic and non-chondrodystrophic breeds. *Vet J.* 2013 Mar;195(3):292–299.
10. Packer RM, Seath IJ, O'Neill DG, et al. DachsLife 2015: an investigation of lifestyle associations with the risk of intervertebral disc disease in Dachshunds. *Canine Genet Epidemiol.* 2016 Nov 5;3:8.
11. Jensen VF, Ersbøll AK. Mechanical factors affecting the occurrence of intervertebral disc calcification in the dachshund--a population study. *J Vet Med A Physiol Pathol Clin Med.* 2000 Jun;47(5):283–296.
12. da Costa RC, De Decker S, Lewis MJ, Volk H. Canine Spinal Cord Injury Consortium (CANSORT-SCI). Diagnostic Imaging in Intervertebral Disc Disease. *Front Vet Sci.* 2020 Oct 22;7:588338.
13. Olby NJ, Moore SA, Brisson B, et al. ACVIM consensus statement on diagnosis and management of acute canine thoracolumbar intervertebral disc extrusion. *J Vet Intern Med.* 2022 Sep;36(5):1570–1596.
14. Olby N, Levine J, Harris T, et al. Long-term functional outcome of dogs with severe injuries of the thoracolumbar spinal cord: 87 cases (1996-2001). *J Am Vet Med Assoc.* 2003 Mar 15;222(6):762–769.
15. Gallucci A, Dragone L, Menchetti M, et al. Acquisition of Involuntary Spinal Locomotion (Spinal Walking) in Dogs with Irreversible Thoracolumbar Spinal Cord Lesion: 81 Dogs. *J Vet Intern Med.* 2017 Mar;31(2):492–497.
16. Bach FS, Mai W, Weber LFS, et al. Association between spinal cord compression ratio in magnetic resonance imaging, initial neurological status, and recovery after ventral slot in 57 dogs with cervical disc extrusion. *Front Vet Sci.* 2023 Jan 6;9:1029127.
17. Hillman RB, Kengeri SS, Waters DJ. Reevaluation of predictive factors for complete recovery in dogs with nonambulatory tetraparesis secondary to cervical disk herniation. *J Am Anim Hosp Assoc.* 2009 Jul-Aug;45(4):155–163.
18. Moore SA, Tipold A, Olby NJ, et al. Current Approaches to the Management of Acute Thoracolumbar Disc Extrusion in Dogs. *Front Vet Sci.* 2020 Sep 3;7:610.
19. Bersan E, McConnell F, Trevail R, et al. Cervical intervertebral foraminal disc extrusion in dogs: clinical presentation, MRI characteristics and outcome after medical management. *Vet Rec.* 2015;176:597–597.
20. Jeffery ND, Barker AK, Hu HZ, et al. Factors associated with recovery from paraplegia in dogs with loss of pain perception in the pelvic limbs following intervertebral disk herniation. *J Am Vet Med Assoc.* 2016 Feb 15;248(4):386–394.
21. Martin S, Liebel FX, Fadda A, et al. Same-day surgery may reduce the risk of losing pain perception in dogs with thoracolumbar disc extrusion. *J Small Anim Pract.* 2020 Jul;61(7):442–448.
22. Langerhuus L, Miles J. Proportion recovery and times to ambulation for non-ambulatory dogs with thoracolumbar disc extrusions treated with hemilaminectomy or conservative treatment: A systematic review and meta-analysis of case-series studies. *Vet J.* 2017 Feb;220:7–16.
23. Silva S, Guevar J, José-López R, et al. Clinical signs, MRI findings and long-term outcomes of foraminal and far lateral thoracolumbar intervertebral disc herniations in dogs. *Vet Rec.* 2022 Jun;190(12):e1529.
24. Bridges J, Windsor R, Stewart SD, et al. Prevalence and clinical features of thoracolumbar intervertebral disc-associated epidural hemorrhage in dogs. *J Vet Intern Med.* 2022 Jul;36(4):1365–1372.
25. Woelfel CW, Robertson JB, Mariani CL, et al. Outcomes and prognostic indicators in 59 paraplegic medium to large breed dogs with extensive epidural hemorrhage secondary to thoracolumbar disc extrusion. *Vet Surg.* 2021 Apr;50(3):527–536.
26. Olby NJ, da Costa RC, Levine JM, et al. Prognostic Factors in Canine Acute Intervertebral Disc Disease. *Front Vet Sci.* 2020 Nov 26;7:596059.
27. Castel A, Olby NJ, Ru H, et al. Risk factors associated with progressive myelomalacia in dogs with complete sensorimotor loss following intervertebral disc extrusion: a retrospective case-control study. *BMC Vet Res.* 2019 Dec 3;15(1):433.
28. Jeffery ND, Rossmeisl JH, Harcourt-Brown TR, et al. Randomized Controlled Trial of Durotomy

as an Adjunct to Routine Decompressive Surgery for Dogs With Severe Acute Spinal Cord Injury. *Neurotrauma Rep.* 2024 Feb 20;5(1):128–138.

29. Bartels KE, Higbee RG, Bahr RJ, et al. Outcome of and complications associated with prophylactic percutaneous laser disk ablation in dogs with thoracolumbar disk disease: 277 cases (1992-2001). *J Am Vet Med Assoc.* 2003 Jun 15;222(12):1733–1739.
30. Zidan N, Sims C, Fenn J, et al. A randomized, blinded, prospective clinical trial of postoperative rehabilitation in dogs after surgical decompression of acute thoracolumbar intervertebral disc herniation. *J Vet Intern Med.* 2018 May;32(3):1133–1144.
31. Castel A, Olby NJ, Mariani CL, et al. Clinical Characteristics of Dogs with Progressive Myelomalacia Following Acute Intervertebral Disc Extrusion. *Vet Intern Med.* 2017 Nov;31(6):1782–1789.
32. Hirano R, Asahina R, Hirano T, et al. Outcomes of extensive hemilaminectomy with durotomy on dogs with presumptive progressive myelomalacia: a retrospective study on 34 cases. *BMC Vet Res.* 2020 Dec 7;16(1):476.
33. Nakamoto Y, Uemura T, Hasegawa H, et al. Outcomes of dogs with progressive myelomalacia treated with hemilaminectomy or with extensive hemilaminectomy and durotomy. *Vet Surg.* 2021 Jan;50(1):81–88.
34. Rossmeisl JH, White C, Pancotto TE, et al. Acute adverse events associated with ventral slot decompression in 546 dogs with cervical intervertebral disc disease. *Vet Surg.* 2013 Oct;42(7):795–806.
35. Rossmeisl JH, Lanz OI, Inzana KD, et al. A modified lateral approach to the canine cervical spine: procedural description and clinical application in 16 dogs with lateralized compressive myelopathy or radiculopathy. *Vet Surg.* 2005 Sep-Oct;34(5):436–444.
36. Fenn J, Drees R, Volk HA, et al. Comparison of clinical signs and outcomes between dogs with presumptive ischemic myelopathy and dogs with acute noncompressive nucleus pulposus extrusion. *J Am Vet Med Assoc.* 2016 Oct 1;249(7):767–775.
37. Griffiths IR. A syndrome produced by dorso-lateral "explosions" of the cervical intervertebral discs. *Vet Rec.* 1970;87:737–741.
38. Kranenburg H-JC, Grinwis GCM, Bergknut N, et al. Intervertebral disc disease in dogs - part 2: comparison of clinical, magnetic resonance imaging, and histological findings in 74 surgically treated dogs. *Vet J.* 2013 Feb;195(2):164–171.
39. Crawford AH, Decker SD. Clinical presentation and outcome of dogs treated medically or surgically for thoracolumbar intervertebral disc protrusion. *Vet Rec.* 2017 Jun 10;180(23):569.
40. Downes CJ, Gemmill TJ, Gibbons SE, et al. Hemilaminectomy and vertebral stabilisation for the treatment of thoracolumbar disc protrusion in 28 dogs. *J Small Anim Pract.* 2009 Oct;50(10):525–535.
41. Ferrand F-X, Moissonnier P, Filleur A, et al. Thoracolumbar partial lateral corpectomy for the treatment of chronic intervertebral disc disease in 107 dogs. *Ir Vet J.* 2015 Dec 1;68:27.
42. Macias C, McKee WM, May C, et al. Thoracolumbar disc disease in large dogs: a study of 99 cases. *J Small Anim Pract.* 2002 Oct;43(10):439–446.
43. Guevar J, Olby N. Minimally invasive microsurgical decompression of an intervertebral disc protrusion in a dog. *Vet Surg.* 2020 Jun;49 Suppl 1:086-092.

CHAPTER 30

Fibrocartilaginous embolic myelopathy

Sarah A. Moore
DVM, DACVIM
(Neurology)

Disease definition/etiology

Fibrocartilaginous embolic myelopathy (FCEM) is a common neurological disorder due to the sudden obstruction of blood vessels within the spinal cord by fragments of fibrocartilaginous material. The condition typically arises when a portion of the intervertebral disc, which is composed of fibrocartilage, herniates and ruptures, leading to the release of these fragments into the bloodstream. Once these fragments enter the spinal cord's circulation, they can obstruct small blood vessels, ultimately resulting in decreased blood flow and oxygen supply to the affected area.[1]

As the fibrocartilaginous emboli impede blood flow, the neurons and supporting cells within the spinal cord undergo ischemia and infarction, leading to tissue damage and dysfunction. The injury occurs suddenly and may manifest as acute onset paralysis, typically in the pelvic limbs. Secondary mechanisms of tissue injury, such as those seen with other mechanisms of spinal cord injury (e.g., oxidative stress, ionic imbalances, lipid peroxidation, and inflammatory responses), can be triggered, causing further cell death and perpetuating damage to the spinal cord tissue.[2] These secondary injury mechanisms can also lead to swelling and increased pressure within the spinal cord, further exacerbating neurological deficits. As the fibrocartilaginous material breaks down and is absorbed by the body over time, dogs usually experience a partial or near complete recovery of neurological function in all but the most severe of cases.[3]

Video 30.1

Seven-year-old spayed female German Shepherd dog presented for a sudden onset of severe paresis of her left pelvic limb of less than 12 hours' duration. The dog was playing out in the yard with a housemate when she was heard crying out by the owner and was immediately noted to have difficulty moving her left pelvic limb. The neurological examination revealed a severely left lateralized T3–L3 myelopathy with an absence of paraspinal hyperesthesia. Fibrocartilaginous embolic myelopathy was considered the most likely diagnosis.

Clinical presentation/features

Predisposing factors

FCEM occurs in dogs of any breed or age, but it is most commonly seen in large and giant breeds. An increased disposition to the condition has also been observed in several small breeds, including the Miniature Schnauzer and the Shetland Sheepdog.[3,4] There appears to be a male sex predilection for the condition, and about 30% of owners report a history of trauma or vigorous exercise immediately prior to the onset of signs. The condition is much more common in nonchondrodystrophic breeds, in which the nucleus pulposus maintains its normal physiological, hydrated status well into adulthood.[5]

Onset and progression

FCEM typically presents as an acute (<24 hours) onset of nonprogressive neurological deficits. Affected dogs may experience a sudden loss of pelvic limb coordination, paresis, or paralysis. The presentation is often unilateral or severely lateralized, particularly in less severely affected animals, so dogs can appear to have neurological signs impacting only one side of the body (Video 30.1). While it was more classically described as a condition of the cervical or lumbar intumescences, recent reports suggest that the most common location for FCEM is the thoracolumbar region (T3–L3).[3] Occasionally, dogs with FCEM may appear to have a multifocal myelopathy due either to showering of embolic material to multiple foci through the neuraxis[6] or to the presence of a T3–L3 myelopathy with concurrent spinal shock in the acute phase of the condition.[7] Clinical signs will vary with the severity of the embolism and can range from mild ataxia and paresis to paraplegia with or without preserved nociception in the affected limbs.

A hallmark of FCEM is that the clinical signs do not progress substantially after their initial onset, as occurs with other vascular lesions of the central nervous system but as opposed to what is seen with other differentials such as intervertebral disc disease, neoplasia, or inflammatory conditions. A brief progressive period can be observed in up to 30% of patients; however, for animals in which the clinical signs continue to progress for more than 36 hours, differentials beyond FCEM should be strongly considered.[3]

Presence of spinal pain

FCEM is classically considered a nonpainful condition, although approximately 10% of owners report their pet appearing to be in pain at the onset of clinical signs.[3] Clinicians may also observe the presence of paraspinal hyperesthesia on neurological examination in about 25% of cases in the period immediately after the onset of signs; it usually resolves within the first 12 hours. In a small number of cases, paraspinal hyperesthesia has been noted to persist longer than 12 hours after the onset of signs. This finding might correlate with hyperintensity noted on magnetic resonance imaging (MRI) in the longissimus, iliocostalis thoracis, and transversospinal muscles putatively associated with muscle spasm or infarction.[8]

Other findings

In animals with severe lateralized lesions of the cervical or high thoracic spinal cord, a unique complement of clinical signs can be observed, related to a loss of sympathetic innervation to the affected side of the head and neck due to damage to the lateral tectotegmental spinal tract as it traverses centrally within the cervical and high thoracic spinal cord. These animals may present with ipsilateral Horner's syndrome (miosis, ptosis, enophthalmos, elevation of the third eyelid) due to a loss of sympathetic innervation to the eye. They might also display transient ipsilateral vasodilation of the cutaneous vasculature due to a loss of sympathetic tone to the blood vessels in the area. This can be observed clinically as skin on the affected side of the body appearing red or flushed and feeling palpably warm to the touch (Fig. 30.1). This phenomenon is most easily observed on the unhaired skin on the inside of the ear pinna. It generally resolves within a few days of the injury.

Clinicopathological findings

Routine clinicopathological testing in animals with FCEM is typically normal. Occasionally, mild to moderate elevations in serum creatine kinase (CK) can be observed secondary to recumbency. Anecdotally, this author has observed marked liver enzyme elevations in a dog with FCEM that was observed at necropsy to have emboli in various other organs throughout the body, including the liver.

Diagnostic imaging findings

Radiographs of the vertebral column will not reveal specific findings associated with FCEM but may be useful in ruling out other causes of acute myelopathy, such as a vertebral lytic neoplasm or fracture. Computed tomography images are also typically unremarkable (they have been reported to be normal in more than half of cases) but, when coupled with a myelogram, may reveal segmental swelling of the spinal cord at the site of infarction.[3,9,10] MRI is the diagnostic modality of choice for FCEM and typically shows intraparenchymal changes within the affected portion of the spinal cord, which may appear as hypointense (dark) areas on T1-weighted images and as hyperintense (bright) areas on T2-weighted images. These areas represent the site of the fibrocartilaginous emboli that have caused a blockage in the blood vessels within the spinal cord and subsequent decreased perfusion to the area. These lesions can contain foci of hemorrhage evidenced as signal voids on a gradient echo sequence and might display contrast enhancement within or adjacent to the parenchymal lesion. MRI can rarely be normal in cases of FCEM, particularly if imaging is performed using a low field magnet or if it is performed in the first 24–48 hours after the onset of signs.[1]

There is substantial overlap between the MRI findings of FCEM and those of acute noncompressive nucleus pulposus extrusion (ANNPE), although certain imaging characteristics may be more consistent with ANNPE, including disruption of epidural fat overlying the intervertebral disc space, narrowing of the intervertebral disc space, presence of minimally compressive extruded disc material within the vertebral canal at the site of the intraparenchymal lesion, and decreased volume of the nucleus pulposus of the intervertebral disc space. In reality, some cases of FCEM and ANNPE may be indistinguishable from each other on imaging. Although some studies report slight differences in outcome, particularly related to the return of fecal and urinary continence,[11] both are managed similarly and the distinction might therefore be of little consequence for most patients.

Other diagnostic procedures

Cerebrospinal fluid (CSF) analysis may be performed to rule out other conditions that might cause similar MRI changes in the spinal cord, such as myelitis. CSF findings in FCEM are relatively nonspecific and may be normal, reveal albuminocytological dissociation (increased protein concentration with a normal total nucleated cell count) secondary to vascular disruption, or show marked inflammation, particularly in cases in which severe necrosis of the spinal cord is present.[1,3]

Treatment

Treatment of FCEM primarily involves supportive care, which includes physical therapy to improve mobility, and bladder care for animals who are severely affected and cannot void their bladder voluntarily. Steroids are not indicated in the treatment of FCEM, and analgesia is not required as the condition is typically nonpainful. Surgical decompression is not indicated for dogs with FCEM because there is no compressive lesion associated with the condition.

Nursing care

For dogs that are initially nonambulatory secondary to FCEM, proper nursing care is important for preventing and reducing the incidence of complications of recumbency such as aspiration pneumonia, decubital ulcers, and urine or fecal scalding. Patients should be kept on a thickly padded surface and, for those that are unable to do so on their own, should be flipped 4–5 times daily to prevent pressure sores. Animals should be kept clean and dry and should be kept in sternal recumbency as much as possible to lessen the chance of aspiration.

Bladder and bowel management

For dogs with mild to moderate neurological signs that maintain the ability to move their limbs after injury, specific approaches to bladder and bowel management are less commonly needed. However, in the initial phase after the injury, for dogs with FCEM causing paralysis and involving the cervical or T3–L3 spinal cord segments, management of an upper motor neuron bladder will be required. Clinical signs associated with upper motor neuron bladder dysfunction are generally related to increased

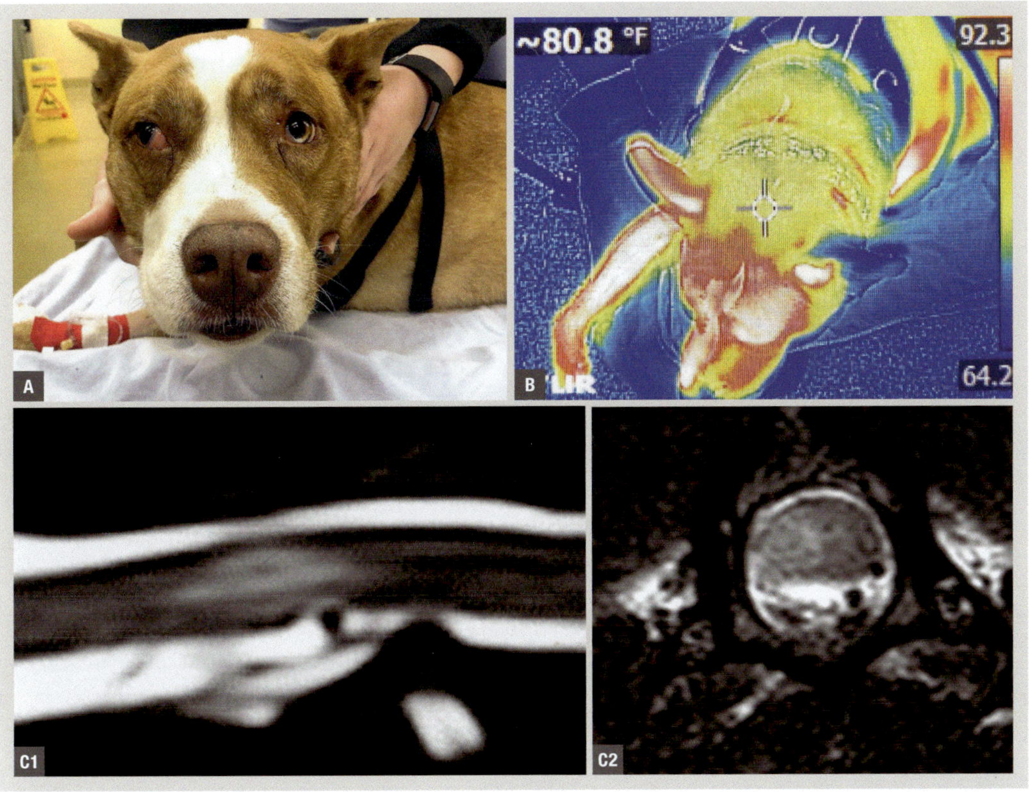

FIG 30.1 Eight-year-old neutered male, large mixed breed dog presented for a sudden onset of nonambulatory tetraparesis and severely right lateralized cervical myelopathy. Horner's syndrome was apparent in the right eye (**A**) and the skin of the right ear and face were warm to the touch. Thermography (**B**) confirmed differential hyperthermia of the right side of the face and head compared to the left. Magnetic resonance images (**C**) confirmed a T2-weighted hyperintensity of the cervical spinal cord at the level of C2–C3, mostly on the right. The appearance was consistent with either fibrocartilaginous embolic myelopathy or acute noncompressive nucleus pulposus extrusion.

muscle tone in the bladder and the urinary sphincters. This heightened tone can result in increased resistance to urine flow, making it difficult for the bladder to relax properly during the storage phase and for the sphincters to open effectively during voiding. Treatments aimed at managing this aspect of FCEM should focus on preventing overfilling of the bladder by ensuring proper emptying to limit urinary retention and on reducing the risk of urinary tract infection. Dogs with urinary incontinence related to an upper motor neuron bladder typically benefit from drugs that relax the urethral sphincter to assist with voiding.

Dogs with FCEM of the L4–S3 spinal cord segments will require management of a lower motor neuron bladder. In contrast to an upper motor neuron bladder, a lower motor neuron bladder typically lacks the spontaneous, coordinated contractions needed for efficient bladder emptying. The bladder may not contract on its own during the voiding phase. There is also reduced muscle tone in the bladder and urinary sphincters, leading to sphincter incontinence and thus persistent urine dribbling. Dogs with urinary incontinence related to lower motor neuron bladder dysfunction will benefit from medications that tighten the urethral sphincter to prevent

TABLE 30.1 Medications commonly used for the pharmacological management of urinary incontinence in the acute phase of recovery after spinal cord injury.[14–16]

Drug		Mechanism of action	Dose	Side effects/notes
Upper motor neuron bladder management	Diazepam	Relaxes skeletal muscle and reduces anxiety	■ 0.2–2.0 mg/kg PO 30 minutes prior to voiding/expressing bladder	■ Sedation ■ Caution in patients with liver dysfunction
	Phenoxybenzamine	Relaxes smooth muscle, nonspecific α-antagonism	■ 0.25–1 mg/kg PO every 8–24 h	■ Tachycardia, miosis, hypotension (most pronounced with first dose) ■ Might take up to 5 days to see effect
	Prazosin	Relaxes smooth muscle, α_1-antagonism	■ 1 mg/dog <15 kg PO every 8–12 h ■ 2 mg/dog >15 kg PO every 8–12 h	■ Hypotension, nausea, sedation ■ Caution in patients with kidney or heart disease
	Tamsulosin	α_{1A}-antagonism, smooth muscle relaxation	■ 0.01–0.2 mg/kg PO every 12–24 h	■ Hypotension
Lower motor neuron bladder management	Bethanechol	Parasympathomimetic, increases contractility of detrusor muscle	■ 2.5–25 mg per dog every 8 h	■ Diarrhea, vomiting, hypersalivation, bradycardia ■ Titrate dose upwards to lessen side effects
	Phenylpropanolamine	Sympathomimetic, increases urethral tone	■ 1.5 mg/kg PO every 8–12 h	■ Urine retention, hypertension

urine dribbling and that enhance bladder wall contraction. Medications typically employed to assist with the management of both upper and lower motor neuron bladder dysfunction in cases of FCEM are detailed in Table 30.1.

While constipation or the inability to void feces are not typically observed in dogs with FCEM causing cervical or thoracolumbar lesions, fecal incontinence may occur. Two types of fecal incontinence are typically reported: urge incontinence, where the dog becomes acutely aware of the need to defecate but is unable to prevent the defecation reflex, or unconsciously dropping stool. For most owners, this is not a major complaint, as it is often manageable with timed feeding, and most owners learn to anticipate the toileting needs of their dog.

Dogs with a lower motor neuron lesion of the anal sphincter have a weak or absent sphincter tone, which can manifest as constant leakage of feces. This is much harder for owners to manage and can be a reason for euthanasia if the dog's fecal incontinence does not improve with time.

Activity restriction

While commonly recommended as a pillar of management for compressive causes of myelopathy such as intervertebral disc herniation (IVDH), strict activity restriction is not typically required for dogs with FCEM. Due to reduced mobility, dogs will likely limit themselves with respect to activity in the acute period after injury, and they should be kept away from stairs until they are stable enough to navigate them without assistance. However, unlike with acute IVDH, there is no tear in the annulus fibrosus that needs to heal. For this reason, animals with FCEM are typically advised to participate in controlled, low impact activity as soon as possible to encourage mobility and limit muscle atrophy and other comorbidities associated with being unable to walk. For animals in which ANNPE remains a possible diagnosis based on the imaging findings, a stricter course of activity restriction is warranted.

Physiotherapy

While no prospective study has demonstrated the benefits of physiotherapy on the outcome of dogs with FCEM, it stands to reason that patients with this condition could benefit from targeted rehabilitation approaches.[12] One retrospective study has evaluated the association between physiotherapy and locomotor outcome in FCEM and suggested that institution of early physiotherapy might speed recovery.[13]

Prognosis

Locomotor recovery

The prognosis for recovery from FCEM is good to excellent in most cases, with 85% of dogs regaining the ability to walk without assistance a median time of 14 days after diagnosis, although persistent neurological deficits are common.[3,12] Dogs presenting with loss of nociception because of the condition appear to have a worse outcome than those that retain nociception.[3,13] While no prospective studies have specifically evaluated recovery in these more severely affected dogs, one systematic review[3] noted recovery rates between 10% and 43% for dogs reported in the veterinary literature, depending on the inclusion criteria used.

Recovery of bladder and bowel continence

The prognosis for recovery of urinary continence in dogs with FCEM has been reported to be similar to that in dogs with a compressive injury to the spinal cord such as an intervertebral disc extrusion, in which >90% of dogs with intact nociception are expected to regain urinary continence. Fecal incontinence appears to be much more common in the chronic phase of recovery in dogs with noncompressive causes of myelopathy such as FCEM and ANNPE, in which vascular lesions induce a more centrally located damage within the cord and are more likely to affect descending inhibitory control of the defecation reflex.[11] As such, clinicians should discuss the potential of persistent fecal incontinence with owners of dogs presented for FCEM.

KEY POINTS

- Dogs with fibrocartilaginous embolic myelopathy present with acute (<24 hours), relatively nonprogressive, nonpainful neurological signs.
- Neurological signs may be unilateral or heavily lateralized and may include sympathetic dysfunction if the cervical cord is involved.
- Magnetic resonance imaging is the diagnostic modality of choice.
- Treatment is supportive in nature.
- Prognosis for recovery of ambulation is good, as long as nociception is preserved.

References

1. De Risio L, Platt SR. Fibrocartilaginous embolic myelopathy in small animals. *Vet Clin North Am Small Anim Pract.* 2010;40:859–869.
2. Park EH, White GA, Tieber LM. Mechanisms of injury and emergency care of acute spinal cord injury in dogs and cats. *J Vet Emerg Crit Care (San Antonio).* 2012;22:160–178.
3. Bartholomew KA, Stover KE, Olby NJ, Moore SA. Clinical characteristics of canine fibrocartilaginous embolic myelopathy (FCE): a systematic review of 393 cases (1973-2013). *Vet Rec.* 2016;179:650.
4. Hawthorne JC, Wallace LJ, Fenner WR, Waters DJ. Fibrocartilaginous embolic myelopathy in miniature schnauzers. *J Am Anim Hosp Assoc.* 2001;37:374–383.
5. De Risio L. A Review of Fibrocartilaginous Embolic Myelopathy and Different Types of Peracute Non-Compressive Intervertebral Disk Extrusions in Dogs and Cats. *Front Vet Sci.* 2015;2:24.
6. Axlund TW, Isaacs AM, Holland M, O'Brien DP. Fibrocartilaginous embolic encephalomyelopathy of the brainstem and midcervical spinal cord in a dog. *J Vet Intern Med.* 2004;18:765–767.
7. Full AM, Heller HLB, Mercier M. Prevalence, clinical presentation, prognosis, and outcome of 17 dogs with spinal shock and acute thoracolumbar spinal cord disease. *J Vet Emerg Crit Care (San Antonio).* 2016;26:412–418.
8. Martens SM, Nykamp SG, James FMK. Magnetic resonance imaging muscle lesions in presumptive canine fibrocartilaginous embolic myelopathy. *Can Vet J.* 2018;59:1287–1292.
9. Grunenfelder FI, Weishaupt D, Green R, Steffen F. Magnetic resonance imaging findings in spinal cord infarction in three small breed dogs. *Vet Radiol Ultrasound.* 2005;46:91–96.
10. Fenn J, Drees R, Volk HA, Decker SD. Inter- and Intraobserver Agreement for Diagnosing Presumptive Ischemic Myelopathy and Acute Noncompressive Nucleus Pulposus Extrusion in Dogs using Magnetic Resonance Imaging. *Vet Radiol Ultrasound.* 2016;57:33–40.
11. Mari L, Behr S, Shea A, et al. Outcome comparison in dogs with a presumptive diagnosis of thoracolumbar fibrocartilaginous embolic myelopathy and acute non-compressive nucleus pulposus extrusion. *Vet Rec.* 2017;181:293.
12. Spinella G, Bettella P, Riccio B, Okonji S. Overview of the Current Literature on the Most Common Neurological Diseases in Dogs with a Particular Focus on Rehabilitation. *Vet Sci.* 2022;9:429.
13. Gandini G, Cizinauskas S, Lang J, et al. Fibrocartilaginous embolism in 75 dogs: clinical findings and factors influencing the recovery rate. *J Small Anim Pract.* 2003;44:76–80.
14. Lane IF. Diagnosis and management of urinary retention. *Vet Clin North Am Small Anim Pract.* 2000;30:25–57, v.
15. Granger N, Olby NJ, Nout-Lomas YS, Canine Spinal Cord Injury Consortium. Bladder and Bowel Management in Dogs With Spinal Cord Injury. *Front Vet Sci.* 2020;7:583342.
16. Plumb DC. *Plumb's Veterinary Drugs.* https://app.plumbs.com. Accessed December 15, 2023.

CHAPTER 31

Spinal malformations

Steven De Decker
DVM, PhD, MvetMed, DECVN, FHEA, PGCert VetEd, MRCVS

A variety of vertebral and spinal malformations have been reported in dogs (Tables 31.1 and 31.2). The most common vertebral malformations are hemivertebrae, caudal articular process dysplasia, and atlantoaxial instability, while the most common spinal malformations are spinal arachnoid diverticulum and meningeal fibrosis.

Vertebral malformations

There is a high prevalence of vertebral malformations in neurologically normal small brachycephalic breeds. They can therefore often be considered incidental findings, and the correlation between diagnostic imaging abnormalities and clinical signs is important. The most common vertebral malformations are hemivertebrae, caudal articular process dysplasia, and transitional vertebrae. Atlantoaxial instability is a specific vertebral malformation, which occurs commonly in toy breeds. Atlantoaxial instability is typically associated with neurological signs and should not be considered an incidental finding on diagnostic imaging studies.

Hemivertebra

Disease definition

Hemivertebrae or vertebral body malformations result from an uneven growth between the two halves of a vertebral body during embryologic development, resulting in an incompletely formed or even absent vertebral body. Up to 10 subtypes of hemivertebrae have been described, including ventral aplasia or "dorsal hemivertebra", ventral hypoplasia or "wedged vertebra", and ventral and median aplasia or "butterfly vertebra".[1–4] A hemivertebra can result in kyphosis or an abnormal dorsoventral curvature of the vertebral column.[1,2] These vertebral body malformations occur most often in the mid-thoracic region. Hemivertebrae are also commonly seen in the lumbosacral area of neurologically normal screw-tailed brachycephalic breeds, such as French and English Bulldogs.[5] Thoracic hemivertebrae are almost omnipresent in neurologically normal French Bulldogs. Depending on the study population, 78% to 100% of neurologically normal French Bulldogs are affected by one or multiple hemivertebrae.[3,6,7] Thoracic hemivertebrae are also commonly seen in neurologically normal English Bulldogs and to a lesser extent in Pugs.[7] This indicates that most hemivertebrae observed on diagnostic imaging studies should be considered incidental findings (Fig. 31.1). Kyphosis occurs in up to 30% of neurologically normal French Bulldogs.[8] Despite their common occurrence on diagnostic imaging studies, hemivertebrae with kyphosis are a relatively uncommon clinical diagnosis.

Clinical presentation

Hemivertebrae occur most often in small brachycephalic dogs, such as the French Bulldog, Pug, and English Bulldog. The Pug seems especially prone to the development of neurological signs. Severe kyphosis and the Pug breed have both been associated with an increased likelihood of clinical signs when a hemivertebra is observed on diagnostic imaging studies (Fig. 31.2).[9,10] Most dogs will demonstrate clinical signs in their first year of life, with slowly progressive ataxia and paresis of the pelvic limbs being the most common clinical presentation. Spinal hyperesthesia is often absent. Although hemivertebra with kyphosis is an uncommon cause of neurological signs in French Bulldogs, this abnormality can contribute to the development of other spinal conditions, such as acute thoracolumbar intervertebral disc extrusion.[8]

Diagnostic imaging findings

Hemivertebrae can be readily observed on spinal radiographs and computed tomography (CT) images. The very high prevalence of hemivertebrae in neurologically normal small brachycephalic dogs is however associated with a realistic risk of making a false positive diagnosis. Although survey radiographs or CT images therefore cannot be used to confirm a diagnosis of hemivertebra, kyphosis exceeding 35 degrees is associated with a high likelihood of clinical signs.[9] MRI is the diagnostic modality of choice and has the additional benefit of allowing for screening of concurrent spinal disorders. CT can be used to assist in surgical planning.

Treatment

Dogs with a hemivertebra can be treated medically or surgically. It has been suggested that young dogs with mild clinical signs could experience clinical stabilization when they become skeletally mature. However, all dogs in one study experienced progressive deterioration of their clinical signs.[11] Surgery should thus likely be the treatment modality of choice. Although the pathophysiology of hemivertebrae is considered multifactorial, vertebral instability or the presence of dynamic spinal cord compression is considered an important factor. Vertebral stabilization has therefore been considered a key aim of surgical treatment. Multiple surgical techniques have been described and include intrathoracic vertebral stabilization and dorsal stabilization techniques.[12–15] Decompressive surgery by dorsal laminectomy without additional stabilization is currently not recommended. It has been postulated that this could aggravate preexisting vertebral instability. It is currently unclear if (partial) realignment of the kyphotic vertebral segment is necessary to improve the surgical outcome.

Prognosis

Although it is possible that medical management will result in acceptable outcomes for dogs with mild clinical signs, all dogs in one study showed continued progression of clinical signs, with most dogs becoming nonambulatory.[11] Several studies have reported favorable outcomes after surgical stabilization with or without additional decompression.[12–15]

TABLE 31.1 Types of vertebral malformations and their characteristics.

	Definition	Breed predisposition	Diagnostic imaging findings	Clinical relevance	Comments
Hemivertebra	Incomplete formation of the vertebral body	Small brachycephalic breeds	Abnormally short and shaped vertebral bodies with or without kyphosis	Common finding in neurologically normal dogs	Occurrence in Pugs and severe kyphosis is associated with clinical signs
Block vertebra	Incomplete separation of the vertebral bodies	Small brachycephalic breeds	Fused vertebral bodies without disc space	Unlikely to be associated with neurological signs	Unclear if associated with altered vertebral biomechanics
Caudal articular process dysplasia	Absence (aplasia) or incomplete formation (hypoplasia) of the caudal articular processes	Pugs, other small brachycephalic breeds, toy breeds, small breeds, medium-sized breeds	Caudal articular processes absent or smaller than normal	Common finding in neurologically normal dogs. Potential contribution to development other spinal disorders	Clinical relevance is unclear. Has been associated with meningeal fibrosis and intervertebral disc protrusion
Transitional vertebra	Vertebrae possessing anatomical characteristics of different vertebra types	Pugs, German Shepherds	Variable: presence of ribs on first lumbar vertebra, absence of ribs on last thoracic vertebra with rudimentary transverse processes, transverse processes on first sacral vertebra, etc.	Unlikely to result in clinical signs. Predisposing factor for degenerative lumbosacral stenosis	Wide variety of possible anatomical characteristics
Thoracic vertebral canal stenosis	Absolute or relative stenosis of the thoracic vertebral canal	Molosser dog breeds, screw-tail brachycephalic breeds	Hypertrophy of the dorsal lamina, hypertrophy and abnormal orientation of the articular processes. Normal anatomy possible in relative stenosis	Can occur in dogs with no neurological signs	Can be a component of cervical spondylomyelopathy
Spina bifida	Incomplete closure of the vertebral arch	Pugs, screw-tailed brachycephalic breeds	Bony defect in the dorsal arch with incompletely fused spinous process.	Commonly seen at T1 in neurologically normal Pugs	Clinical signs occur only when there is protrusion of the meninges or neural tissue
Vertebral vascular aplasia	Defect in ossification of the vertebral body, centered around the vascular canal	French and English Bulldogs	Bony defect in vascular canal region	Commonly seen in neurologically normal French and English Bulldogs	Clinical relevance uncertain
Atlantoaxial instability	Cranial and dorsal displacement of C2 relative to C1	Toy breeds	Increased distance between the spinous processes of C1 and C2. Craniodorsal displacement of C2. Abnormal or absent dens	Likely to result in neurological signs	Can be associated with an abnormal dens or ligamentous support

TABLE 31.2 Types of spinal malformations and their characteristics.

	Definition	Breed predisposition	Diagnostic imaging findings	Clinical relevance	Comments
Spinal arachnoid diverticulum	Focal dilation of the subarachnoid space filled with CSF	Rottweilers, French Bulldogs, Pugs	Teardrop- or scalpel-shaped expansion of the subarachnoid space	Typically associated with neurological signs	Can be congenital or acquired
Meningeal fibrosis	Dense intradural fibrotic bands	Pugs	Irregular subarachnoid space, linear intradural hypointense bands, spinal cord distortion, pockets of CSF, bilateral V-shaped ventrolateral extradural lesions	Typically associated with neurological signs	Possible genetic and mechanical factors involved
Meningocele and meningomyelocele	Protrusion of meninges or neural tissue through bony defect (spina bifida)	Screw-tailed brachycephalic breeds	Dorsal extension meninges with or without neural tissue through spina bifida defect	Typically associated with neurological signs	Often localized at the lumbosacral junction
Dermoid sinus	Failure of separation between the skin and neural tube	Rhodesian Ridgebacks	Fluid-filled tract extending from skin ventrally to varying depth	Typically associated with clinical signs. Absence of signs possible in noncommunicating tracts	Type of clinical signs dependent on depth of sinus tract

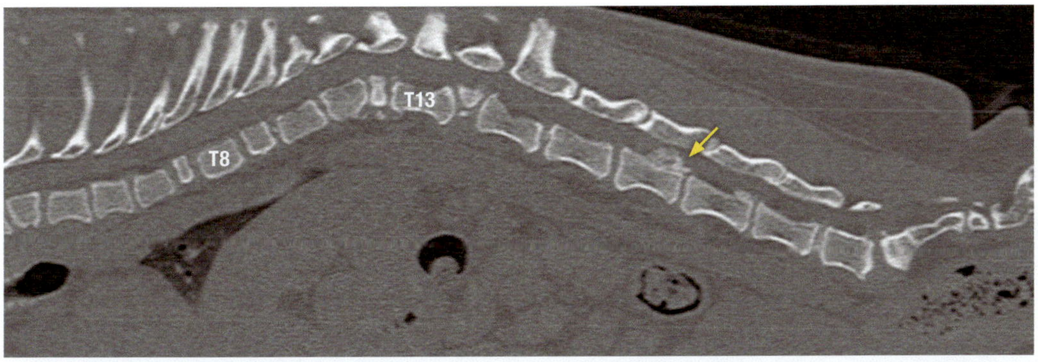

FIG. 31.1 Sagittal reconstructed computed tomography (CT) scan (bone window) of a 4-year-old French Bulldog with acute onset nonambulatory paraparesis. Vertebrae T7, T9, T12, and L1 are hemivertebrae, and the T12 hemivertebra is associated with kyphosis. The dog's clinical signs are however caused by an L4–L5 intervertebral disc extrusion (arrow). This CT scan illustrates that hemivertebrae should be considered an incidental imaging abnormality in most cases.

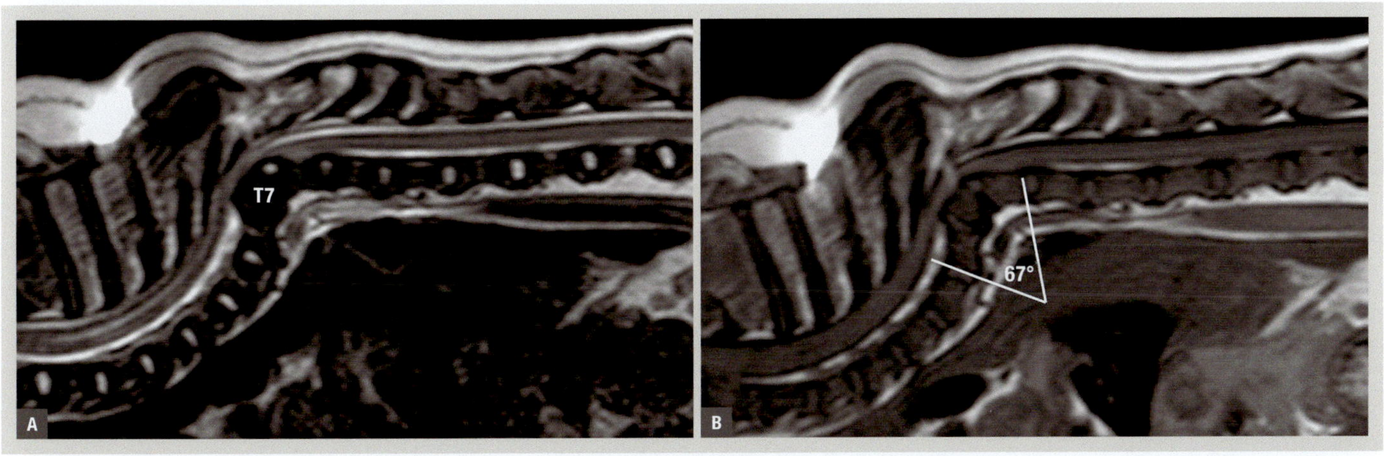

FIG. 31.2 Sagittal T2-weighted (**A**) and T1-weighted (**B**) magnetic resonance imaging sequences of an 11-month-old Pug with chronic progressive ataxia and paresis of the pelvic limbs. A T7 hemivertebra with severe kyphosis is evident. The severity of the kyphosis can be quantified by the Cobb angle, which is 67 degrees in this dog. Hemivertebrae in Pugs and kyphosis exceeding 35 degrees are associated with an increased likelihood of clinical signs.

Caudal articular process dysplasia

Disease definition

Caudal articular process dysplasia is characterized by a complete (aplasia) or partial (hypoplasia) absence of one or more caudal articular processes (Fig. 31.3).[16] Although this vertebral malformation has been heavily associated with the Pug breed, it is also common in other small brachycephalic breeds, toy breeds, other small breeds, and medium breeds.[17,18] One study identified one or more vertebrae with caudal articular process dysplasia in 97% of neurologically normal Pugs, 70.4% of French Bulldogs and 84.1% of neurologically normal English Bulldogs.[17]

Pathophysiology

The clinical relevance of caudal articular process dysplasia is currently unclear. It has been suggested that this vertebral malformation could result in low-grade and repetitive vertebral instability. This could then potentially lead to the formation of intradural fibrotic bands, which could result in progressive constriction of the spinal cord.[16] This condition has been referred to as "meningeal fibrosis" or "constrictive myelopathy" (see below). Other spinal conditions that have been associated with caudal articular process dysplasia are intervertebral disc protrusion and spinal arachnoid diverticula (see below).[19] It is therefore not surprising that the caudal articular processes of the caudal thoracic region are most often affected in dogs with neurological signs. However, studies have been unable to demonstrate a direct causative relationship between caudal articular process dysplasia and other spinal conditions;[18,20] caudal articular process dysplasia is almost omnipresent in neurologically normal small brachycephalic breeds,[17] and all the conditions mentioned above can also occur without concurrent vertebral anomalies.[20,21]

Clinical presentation

Most dogs with caudal articular process dysplasia will not show or develop neurological signs. If this anomaly is associated with a concurrent spinal disorder such as meningeal fibrosis, affected animals will often demonstrate slowly progressive pelvic limb ataxia and paresis. Spinal hyperesthesia is typically not present, and dogs with advanced disease can display urinary and fecal incontinence.[21]

Diagnostic imaging findings

Caudal articular process dysplasia can be readily observed on spinal radiographs and CT images.[16] Since this vertebral malformation is common in neurologically normal animals and cannot be considered a primary cause of neurological signs, the mere observation of hypoplastic or aplastic caudal articular processes does not confirm a clinical diagnosis. MRI is the diagnostic modality of choice as it allows visualization of concurrent spinal disorders, such as meningeal fibrosis, intervertebral disc protrusion, and spinal arachnoid diverticulum.

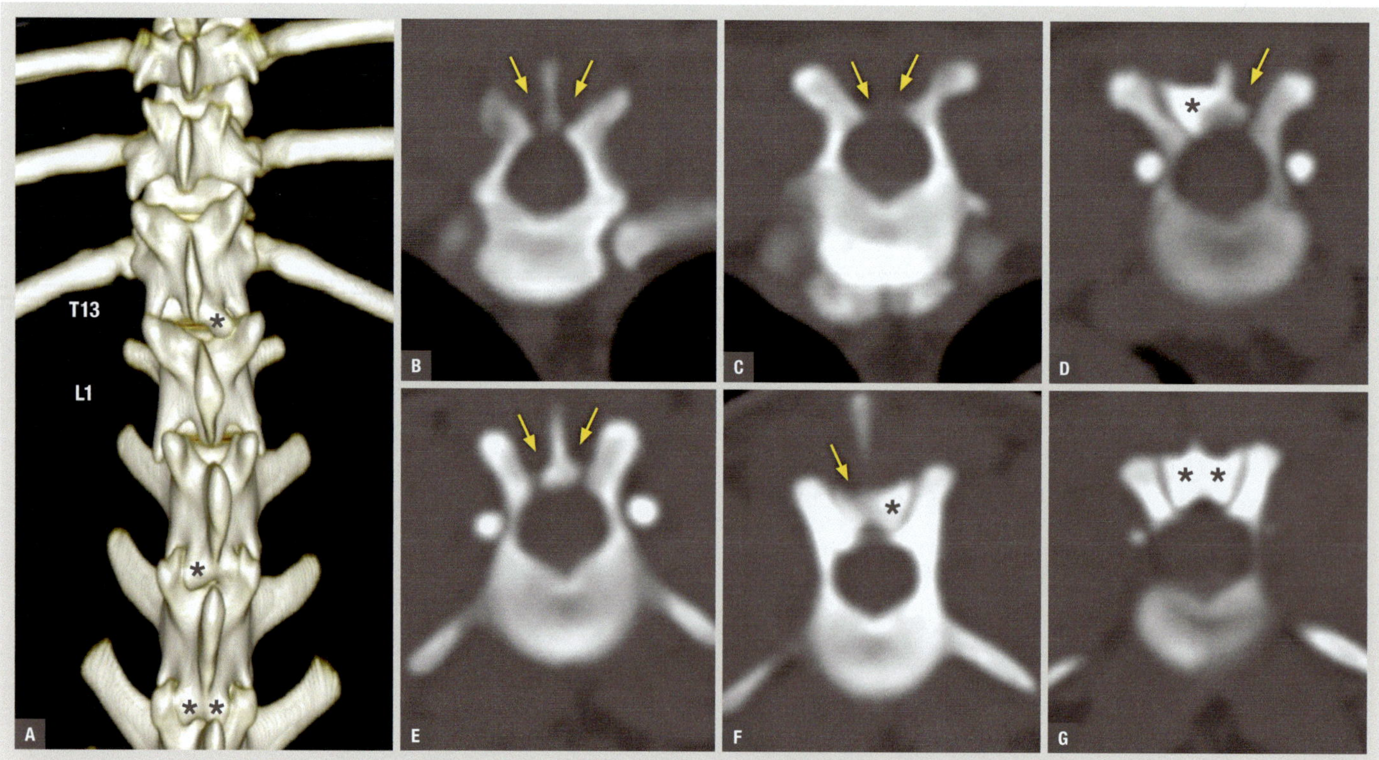

FIG. 31.3 Three-dimensional reconstructed (A) and transverse computed tomography (CT) images (B–G) of a 9-year-old neurologically normal Pug with multiple sites of caudal articular process dysplasia. (A) Bilateral caudal articular process aplasia at the levels of T11–T12, T12–T13, and L1–L2. Left-sided caudal articular process aplasia at the level of T13–L1 and right-sided caudal articular process hypoplasia at the level of L2–L3. The normal caudal articular processes are indicated by an asterisk (*). (B, C) Bilateral caudal articular process aplasia (arrows) at the level of T11–T12 (B) and T12–T13 (C). (D) Normally developed right-sided caudal articular process (asterisk) and severely hypoplastic left-sided caudal articular process (arrow) at the level of T13–L1. (E) Bilateral caudal articular process aplasia (arrows) at the level of L1–L2. (F) Normally developed left-sided caudal articular process (asterisk) and hypoplastic right-sided caudal articular process (arrow) at the level of L2–L3. (G) Bilaterally normal caudal articular processes (asterisks) at the level of L2–L3.

Treatment

The type of treatment in dogs with neurological signs is primarily dictated by the presence and nature of concurrent spinal disorders. Vertebral instability has been demonstrated intraoperatively in Pugs with caudal articular process dysplasia.[22] It has therefore been suggested to consider vertebral stabilization in dogs with caudal articular process dysplasia that undergo surgery for spinal disease.

Prognosis

The prognosis is dictated by the presence and nature of concurrent spinal disorders. It is currently unclear how the presence of caudal articular process dysplasia influences the outcome of surgery for spinal disorders.

Transitional vertebrae

Transitional vertebrae are vertebrae that possess symmetrical or asymmetrical anatomical characteristics of two different types of vertebrae. They are therefore seen at the junction between two divisions of the vertebral column, such as the thoracolumbar and lumbosacral junction. Examples include the presence of one or two ribs on the first lumbar vertebra, the absence of one or two ribs on the last thoracic vertebra in association with rudimentary transverse processes, and rudimentary transverse processes on the first sacral vertebra. Transitional vertebrae are unlikely to directly result in clinical signs. They can, however, complicate diagnostic procedures or surgical planning. Transitional vertebrae have also been considered to alter the biomechanical characteristics of the vertebral column and are considered a risk factor for the development of degenerative lumbosacral stenosis in dogs and cats.[23,24] A specific type of transitional vertebra occurs commonly in Pugs (46% in one study) and is characterized by the presence of cervical ribs on C7.[25] This is referred to as homeotic transformation of C7 and is rare in other breeds.

Thoracic vertebral canal stenosis

Disease definition

Cranial thoracic vertebral canal stenosis has been described in both dogs and cats. Absolute stenosis is characterized by a vertebral canal that is narrow enough for the osseous structures to cause direct spinal cord compression.[26] Affected animals typically develop clinical signs early in life. Relative stenosis is characterized by a narrowed vertebral canal that does not cause direct spinal cord compression.[26] However, the spinal cord can become compressed when relatively mild (clinically irrelevant under normal circumstances) compressive lesions occur, such as age-related intervertebral disc herniation or ligamentum flavum hypertrophy. Affected animals typically develop clinical signs later in life.

Pathophysiology

Absolute vertebral canal stenosis is often caused by malformation and hypertrophy of the dorsal lamina and articular processes, resulting in dorsal or dorsolateral spinal cord compression (Fig. 31.4). It most commonly affects the vertebral canal between T2 and T4.[27] Affected dogs often present with clinical signs within the first year of life. Cranial thoracic vertebral canal stenosis can be a component of osseous-associated cervical spondylomyelopathy.[28] Relative vertebral canal stenosis can be associated with relatively modest or no appreciable vertebral column abnormalities.[29]

Clinical presentation

Young dogs of molosser breeds (e.g., Bullmastiffs) and screw-tailed brachycephalic breeds, (e.g., French and English Bulldogs) are most often affected.[27,30] Chronic progressive ataxia with ambulatory paraparesis is the most common clinical presentation. Spinal hyperesthesia can be present, especially in the early stages of disease.[29]

Diagnostic imaging findings

The nature of anatomical abnormalities is best appreciated on imaging studies that allow transverse imaging, such as CT and MRI (Fig. 31.4). Imaging findings compatible with thoracic vertebral canal stenosis are not always associated with spinal cord compression and are commonly encountered in neurologically normal French and English Bulldogs.[30] Care should thus be taken to correlate imaging findings with neurological signs. In animals with neurological signs, MRI can reveal a focal intraparenchymal spinal hyperintensity.

Treatment and prognosis

Surgical decompression by dorsal laminectomy or hemilaminectomy can result in clinical improvement, although residual gait abnormalities can remain. Response to medical management is variable.[27,29–31]

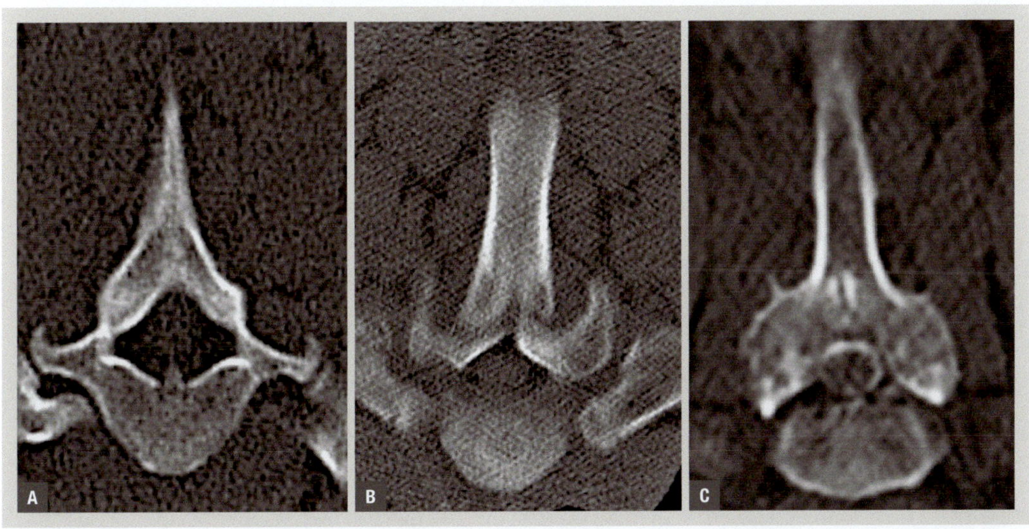

FIG. 31.4 Transverse computed tomography (CT) images at the level of T2 of a neurologically normal 18-month-old Bullmastiff (A) and a neurologically normal 4-year-old Dogue de Bordeaux (B), and CT-myelogram (C) of an 11-month-old Bullmastiff with progressive ataxia and paresis of the pelvic limbs. (A) Normal vertebral anatomy. (B) Hypertrophic dorsal lamina and abnormal oblique orientation of the articular processes. (C) Hypertrophy of the articular processes. The intrathecal contrast medium has resulted in only partial and faint delineation of the spinal cord contour, which was considered compatible with mild spinal cord compression. Imaging abnormalities compatible with cranial thoracic stenosis can also be seen in neurologically normal dogs.

Atlantoaxial instability

Disease definition

This condition is characterized by a dorsal and cranial displacement of the axis relative to the atlas.[32]

Pathophysiology

Atlantoaxial subluxation is often associated with congenital abnormalities of the dens, such as aplasia or dorsal angulation, and failure of ligamentous support.[32]

Clinical presentation

Atlantoaxial instability most often affects toy breed dogs, such as Chihuahuas, Yorkshire Terriers and Pomeranians, and most animals will present with clinical signs within the first year of life.[33,34] Clinical signs can vary from intermittent cervical hyperesthesia to tetraparesis and tetraplegia. Clinical signs can have an acute or more protracted onset. Clinical signs can also occur acutely after minor trauma.

Diagnostic imaging findings

A diagnosis can be confirmed by radiography, CT, or MRI. Gentle flexion might be necessary to achieve a radiographic diagnosis (Fig. 31.5). However, excessive cervical flexion in a dog with atlantoaxial instability can have devastating and even fatal consequences. Inducing gentle flexion is typically not necessary when using CT or MRI to obtain a diagnosis of atlantoaxial subluxation (Fig. 31.4). The lack of (protective) muscle tone when inducing general anesthesia for diagnostic procedures is associated with risk of iatrogenic neurological injury. Gentle manipulation is therefore necessary.

Treatment

Selected cases can be treated medically with analgesia, strict rest, and external splinting. Several surgical techniques have been reported, with no clear evidence of superiority for any specific surgical technique.[32–34] Medical management is occasionally considered a temporary treatment strategy to delay surgery until the patient is more skeletally mature.

Outcome

Although surgery is technically demanding, this type of treatment can result in excellent outcomes with rapid recovery.

Spinal malformations

Spinal arachnoid diverticula

Disease definition

Spinal arachnoid diverticula (SAD) are likely the most common spinal malformation and are characterized by a cerebrospinal fluid (CSF)–filled, focal, teardrop-shaped dilation of the subarachnoid space. This can cause progressive spinal cord compression.[35]

Pathophysiology

SAD can be congenital in nature or acquired, secondary to another spinal disorder. Acquired SAD have been associated with vertebral malformations, spinal fracture and luxation, intervertebral disc disease, and inflammatory spinal disease.[35] Although SAD can occur over the entire length of the vertebral column, they are most commonly found in the cranial cervical or thoracolumbar region. Large breed dogs are most

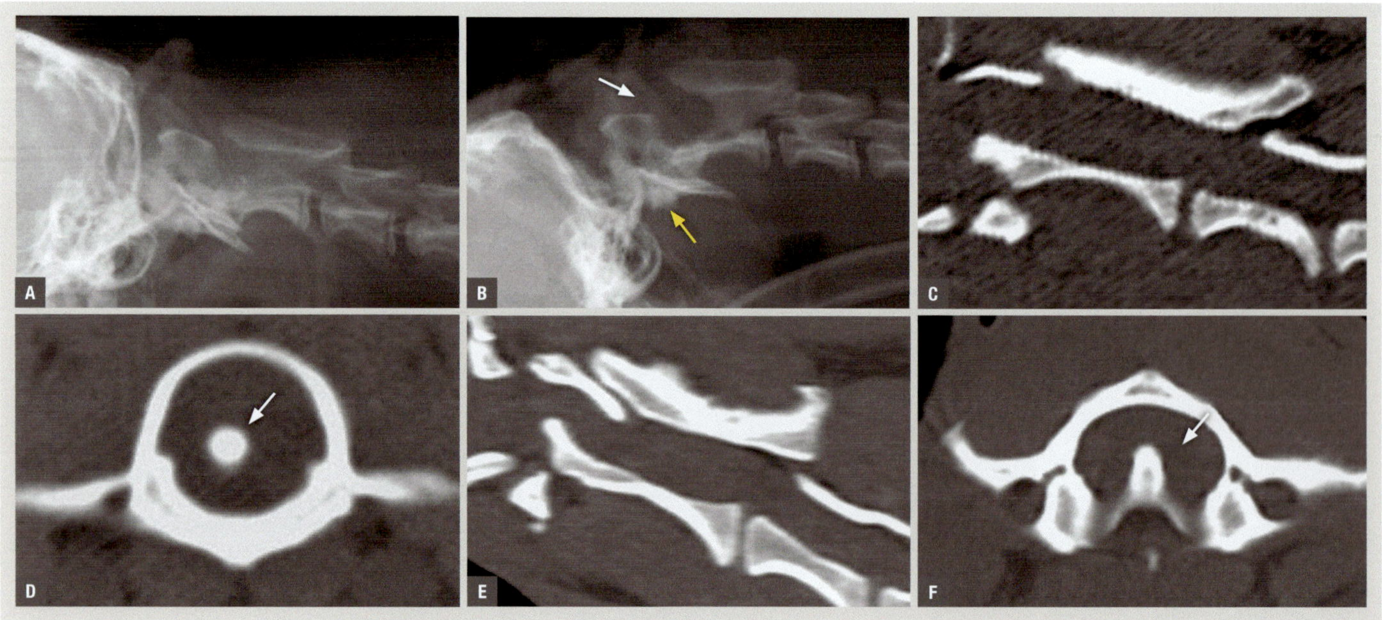

FIG. 31.5 (A, B) Survey radiographs of a 4-month-old Shih-Tzu with intermittent cervical hyperesthesia. (A) No obvious instability or subluxation can be appreciated in a neutral position. (B) Gentle flexion reveals an increased distance between the dorsal spinous processes of C1 and C2 (white arrow) and a dorsal and cranial displacement of C2 relative to C1 (yellow arrow). (C) Sagittal reconstructed computed tomography (CT) image (bone window) of a 7-month-old Pomeranian with atlantoaxial instability. Cranial and dorsal displacement of C2 relative to C1 can be seen in a neutral position. (D) Transverse CT image (bone window) of the same dog as (C) illustrating the abnormal dorsal position of the dens (arrow). (E) Sagittal reconstructed and (F) transverse CT images (bone window) of a 6-month-old Chihuahua with atlantoaxial instability. Atlantoaxial instability can be associated with abnormalities of the dens, such as dorsal angulation into the vertebral canal (arrow).

often affected by cervical SAD and small breed dogs by thoracolumbar SAD.[35] In young Pugs, SAD are however also regularly seen in the cervical region.[36] Although multiple lesions and alternative directions are possible, SAD is most typically a single lesion with a midline dorsal localization. Rottweilers, Pugs, and French Bulldogs are considered to be predisposed.[35]

Video 31.1

Clinical presentation, diagnostic imaging findings, surgical treatment, and early postoperative outcome in a 1.5-year-old Pug with a thoracolumbar spinal arachnoid diverticulum.

Clinical presentation

The nature of the clinical signs is influenced by the location of the SAD along the vertebral column. Affected animals typically demonstrate a slowly progressive proprioceptive ataxia (Video 31.1). Although this is unusual for lesions located in the thoracolumbar region, approximately 20% of dogs with a thoracolumbar SAD have urinary or fecal incontinence.[35] Incontinence in animals with SAD is possibly related to the midline dorsal location of these malformations. Spinal hyperesthesia is uncommonly observed. Because of the multifactorial etiology of SAD and the heterogenous character of the potential underlying spinal conditions, there is a wide variation in the age of onset of the clinical signs.

Diagnostic imaging findings

SAD can be diagnosed by myelography, CT myelography, or MRI.[37] Spinal radiographs or conventional CT images are expected to be normal in animals with SAD. If, during myelography, the subarachnoid contrast medium can fill the SAD, it will appear as a typical teardrop-shaped dilation of the subarachnoid space. MRI can demonstrate a focal teardrop, or scalpel blade–shaped widening of the subarachnoid space (Fig. 31.6). This widening of the subarachnoid space has the intensity characteristics of CSF on all sequences. MRI also allows visualization of the adjacent spinal cord parenchyma and the eventual presence of syringomyelia, presumed to be secondary to SAD. Nonetheless, it can be difficult to reliably detect a SAD on conventional MRI sequences and to differentiate the lesion from the surrounding epidural fat. Addition of a single-shot turbo spin-echo sequence or use of three-dimensional constructive interference in steady state (CISS) MRI have been suggested to increase confidence in making a diagnosis of SAD.[38,39]

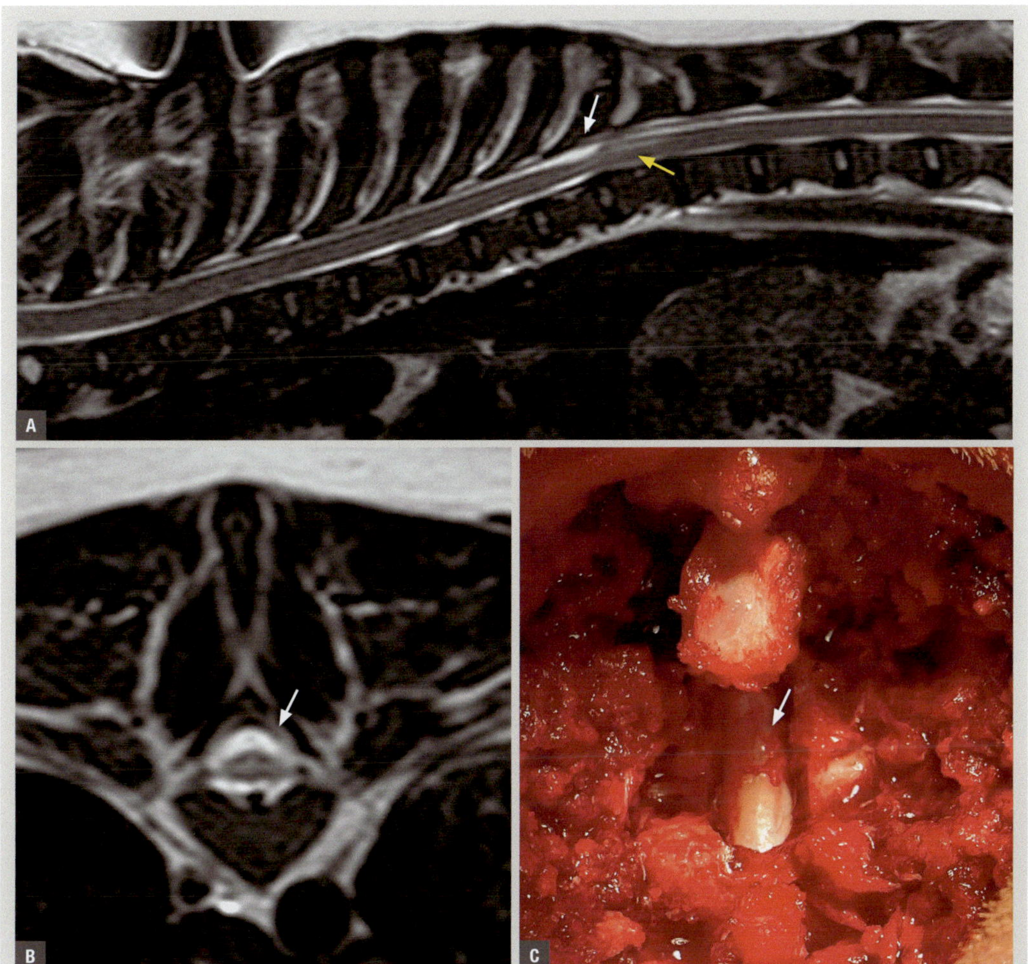

FIG. 31.6 (A) Sagittal and (B) transverse T2-weighted magnetic resonance images of a 2-year-old Staffordshire Bull Terrier with chronic, progressive ataxia and paresis of the pelvic limbs. The spinal arachnoid diverticulum appears as a focal teardrop or scalpel-shaped expansion of the subarachnoid space filled with cerebrospinal fluid (white arrows). (A) Mild syringomyelia can also be observed (yellow arrow). (C) Intraoperative image of the same dog showing the spinal arachnoid diverticulum (arrow).

Treatment

Medical and surgical treatment options can be considered. Medical treatment typically consists of administration of anti-inflammatory doses of prednisolone. The rationale for administering prednisolone is to decrease the rate of CSF production. Several surgical techniques have been described, which include durotomy, durectomy, or marsupialization (see **Video 31.1**).[40] There is no clear evidence of superiority of one surgical technique over the others.

Prognosis

Although transient early postoperative neurological deterioration is common, most dogs will experience long-term improvement. In one study, 82% of dogs treated surgically experienced long-term neurological improvement, while 3% remained stable and 16% deteriorated. After medical management, 30% of dogs experienced long-term improvement, while 30% remained stable and 40% deteriorated.[41] Late-onset recurrence of clinical signs is possible but rare. Although surgery has been associated with good outcomes in most dogs, it has been suggested that Pugs with thoracolumbar SAD have a worse long-term prognosis after surgery with a high rate of recurrence of signs.[42] It is currently unclear why Pugs could have a more unfavorable prognosis.

Meningeal fibrosis

Disease definition

Meningeal fibrosis or constrictive myelopathy is characterized by the formation of dense intradural bands of fibrotic tissue.[16,21] This condition is associated with the Pug breed and concurrent caudal articular process dysplasia.[16]

Pathophysiology

Meningeal fibrosis is associated with intradural adhesions between the arachnoid and pia mater, which causes progressive constriction of the spinal cord and vasculature.[21] It has been suggested that meningeal fibrosis occurs secondary to low-grade vertebral instability associated with caudal articular process dysplasia.[16] However, meningeal fibrosis has also been reported in Pugs without caudal articular process dysplasia or any other vertebral malformation.[21] The causative relationship between meningeal fibrosis and caudal articular process dysplasia is therefore unclear. Although mechanical factors are possibly involved in the development of meningeal fibrosis, a genetic predisposition has been suggested. Multiple candidate genes have been identified in Pugs with chronic and progressive thoracolumbar myelopathy.[43] Pathological and histopathological findings in Pugs with meningeal fibrosis include circumferential fibrosis with focal malacia, syringomyelia, lymphohistiocytic inflammation, and arachnoid diverticulum formation.[21]

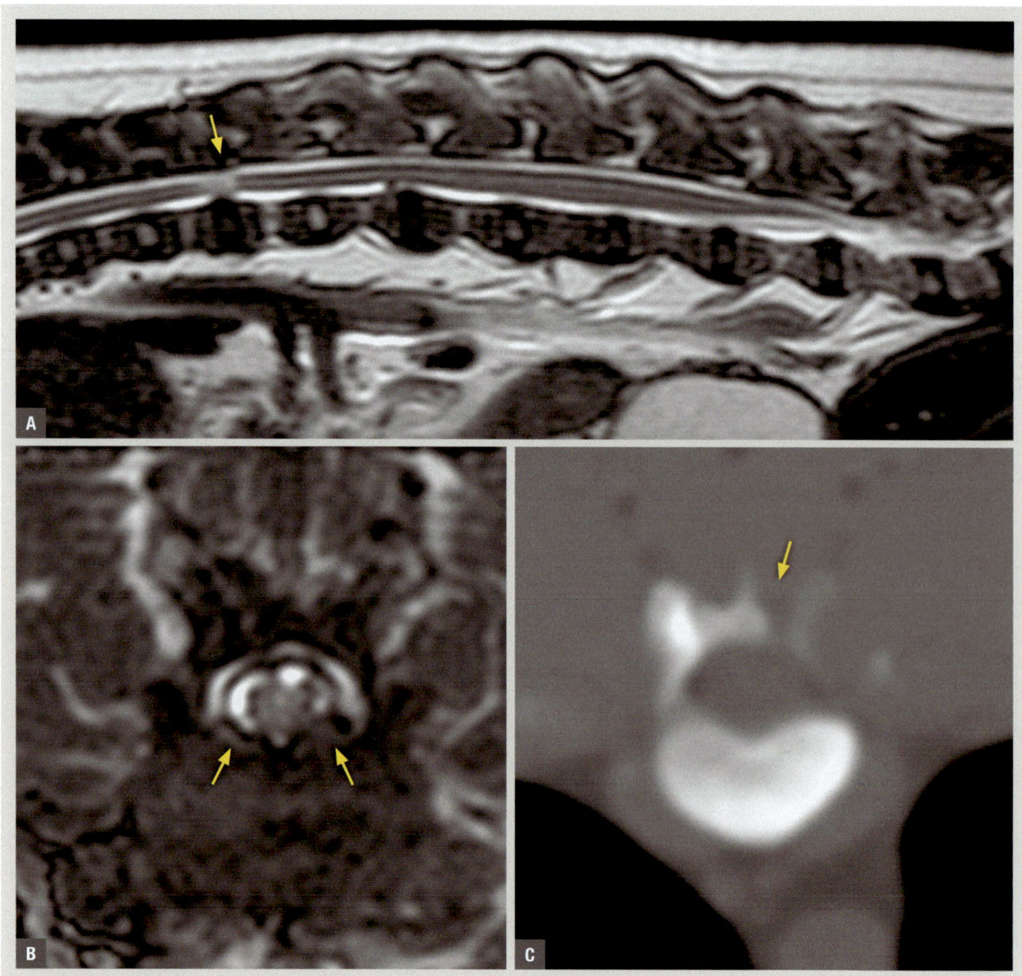

FIG. 31.7 (**A**) Sagittal T2-weighted magnetic resonance image in an 8-year-old Pug with meningeal fibrosis or constrictive myelopathy at the level of T12–T13. A dorsoventral narrowing of the spinal cord and a focal T2-weighted intraparenchymal hyperintensity can be observed (arrow). (**B**) BALT-GRAD sequence (thin-slice T2-weighted) at the level of T12–T13 revealing distortion and compression of the spinal cord, an irregular subarachnoid space, multiple linear hypointense bands extending from the arachnoid to the pia mater, cerebrospinal fluid accumulation in pockets, and bilateral V-shaped ventrolateral extradural lesions (arrows). (**C**) Transverse computed tomography image (bone window) at the same level showing unilateral caudal articular process dysplasia (arrow). The causative relationship between meningeal fibrosis and caudal articular process dysplasia is currently unclear.

Clinical presentation

Pugs are overrepresented for this disorder, and affected animals develop clinical signs later in life (around 7.5 years). A chronic onset of slowly progressive paraparesis and ataxia of the pelvic limbs is the most common presentation. Urinary and fecal incontinence can be seen, especially in advanced disease. Spinal hyperesthesia is typically not present.[16,21] The characteristic clinical presentation of an adult to older Pug with chronic and slowly progressive spinal disease localized to the T3–L3 spinal cord segments has been referred to as "Pug dog thoracolumbar myelopathy".[20,43]

Diagnostic imaging findings

Spinal radiographs or CT images do not reveal any abnormalities suggestive for meningeal fibrosis. MRI is necessary to confirm this diagnosis. The MRI abnormalities associated with meningeal fibrosis include an irregular subarachnoid space with mixed intensity, multiple linear, hypointense bands that extend from the arachnoid to the pia mater, spinal cord distortion and compression, cerebrospinal fluid accumulation in multiple pockets, and bilateral V-shaped ventrolateral extradural lesions (Fig. 31.7). An intraparenchymal hyperintense signal is often present at the site of spinal cord compression.[19,44] It is common for multiple conditions to be present and contribute to clinical signs of progressive ataxia and paraparesis.[20] An advantage of MRI is the possibility to detect concurrent spinal conditions, such as intervertebral disc disease and spinal arachnoid diverticulum.

Treatment

Medical or surgical treatment can be considered for dogs with meningeal fibrosis. A short course of an anti-inflammatory dose of corticosteroids can be considered in order to decrease inflammation, CSF production, and vasogenic edema. Suggested surgical techniques include vertebral stabilization with or without additional decompression or placement of a subarachnoid shunt to bridge the site of CSF obstruction.[45,46]

Prognosis

Although little is known about the natural progression or results of medical management in dogs with meningeal fibrosis, clinical signs are expected to slowly progress over time. Surgical treatment, as described above, can result in clinical improvement or stabilization of mild clinical signs.[45,46] Incontinence can however be irreversible.[45] Decompressive surgery followed by dissection of the intradural fibrotic band has been associated with a poor outcome.[16] It is currently unclear how the presence of multiple concurrent spinal disorders affects the outcome or progression of clinical signs.

KEY POINTS

- Vertebral malformations are commonly seen in small brachycephalic dog breeds, such as the French Bulldog and the Pug.
- Vertebral malformations, such as hemivertebrae and caudal articular process dysplasia, can often be considered incidental findings on diagnostic imaging studies.
- Hemivertebra is more likely to cause clinical signs in Pugs and when the associated kyphosis exceeds 35 degrees.
- In dogs with neurological signs and vertebral malformations (e.g., hemivertebra, caudal articular process dysplasia), MRI is the diagnostic modality of choice as it can detect concurrent spinal disorders.
- Spinal arachnoid diverticula and meningeal fibrosis are the most common spinal malformations.
- The etiology of meningeal fibrosis is still unknown, and its relationship with caudal articular process dysplasia is unclear.

References

1. Gutierrez-Quintana R, Guevar J, Stalin C, et al. A proposed radiographic classification scheme for congenital thoracic vertebral malformations in brachycephalic "screw-tailed" dog breeds. *Vet Radiol Ultrasound* 2014 Nov-Dec;55(6):585–591.
2. Ryan R, Gutierrez-Quintana R, Ter Haar G, De Decker S. Relationship between breed, hemivertebra subtype, and kyphosis in apparently neurologically normal French Bulldogs, English Bulldogs, and Pugs. *Am J Vet Res.* 2019 Feb;80(2):189–194.
3. Brown JD, Podadera J, Ward M, et al. The presence, morphology and clinical significance of vertebral body malformations in an Australian population of French Bulldogs and Pugs. *Aust Vet J.* 2021 Sep;99(9):378–387.
4. Lackmann F, Forterre F, Brunnberg L, Loderstedt, S. Epidemiological study of congenital malformations of the vertebral column in French bulldogs, English bulldogs and pugs. *Vet Rec.* 2022 Jan;190(1):e509.
5. Bertram S, Ter Haar G, De Decker S. Congenital malformations of the lumbosacral vertebral column are common in neurologically normal French Bulldogs, English Bulldogs, and Pugs, with breed-specific differences. *Vet Radiol Ultrasound.* 2019 Jul;60(4):400–408.
6. Moissonnier P, Gossot P, Scotti S. Thoracic kyphosis associated with hemivertebra. *Vet Surg.* 2011 Dec;40(8):1029–1032.
7. Ryan R, Gutierrez-Quintana R, Ter Haar G, De Decker S. Prevalence of thoracic vertebral malformations in French bulldogs, Pugs and English bulldogs with and without associated neurological deficits. *Vet J.* 2017 Mar;221:25–29.
8. Inglez de Souza MCCM, Ryan R, Ter Haar G, et al. Evaluation of the influence of kyphosis and scoliosis on intervertebral disc extrusion in French bulldogs. *BMC Vet Res.* 2018 Jan 5;14(1):5.

9. Guevar J, Penderis J, Faller K, et al. Computer-assisted radiographic calculation of spinal curvature in brachycephalic "screw-tailed" dog breeds with congenital thoracic vertebral malformations: reliability and clinical evaluation. *PloS One.* 2014 Sep 8;9(9):e106957.
10. De Decker S, Packer RMA, Capello R, et al. Comparison of signalment and computed tomography findings in French bulldogs, pugs, and English bulldogs with and without clinical signs associated with thoracic hemivertebra. *J Vet Intern Med.* 2019 Sep;33(5):2151–2159.
11. Wyatt S, Gonçalves R, Gutierrez-Quintana R, De Decker S. Results of non-surgical treatment for congenital vertebral body malformations: 13 dogs (2009-2016). *J Am Vet Med Assoc.* 2018 Sep 15;253(6):768–773.
12. Aikawa T, Kanazono S, Yoshigae Y, et al. Vertebral stabilization using positively threaded profile pins and polymethylmethacrylate, with or without laminectomy, for spinal canal stenosis and vertebral instability caused by congenital thoracic vertebral anomalies. *Vet Surg.* 2007 Jul;36(5):432–441.
13. Charalambous M, Jeffery ND, Smith PM, et al. Surgical treatment of dorsal hemivertebrae associated with kyphosis by spinal stabilisation with or without decompression. *Vet J.* 2014 Nov;202(2):267–273.
14. Mathiesen CB, de la Puerta B, Groth AM, et al. Ventral stabilization of thoracic kyphosis through bilateral intercostal thoracotomies using SOP (String of Pearls) plates contoured after a 3-dimensional print of the spine. *Vet Surg.* 2018 Aug;47(6):843–851.
15. Mariné, AF, De Risio L, Mascort J, et al. Transthoracic vertebral distraction and stabilization in 10 dogs with congenital thoracic vertebral malformations. *Vet Comp Orthop Traumatol.* 2021 Sep;34(5):367–374.
16. Fisher SC, Shores A, Simpson ST. Constrictive myelopathy secondary to hypoplasia or aplasia of the thoracolumbar caudal articular processes in Pugs: 11 cases (1993-2009). *J Am Vet Med Assoc.* 2013 Jan 15;242(2):223–229.
17. Bertram S, Ter Haar G, De Decker S. Caudal articular process dysplasia of thoracicvertebrae in neurologically normal French bulldogs, English bulldogs, and Pugs: prevalence and characteristics. *Vet Radiol Ultrasound.* 2018 Jul;59(4):396–404.
18. Ban J, Park J, Kim H, et al. Investigation of canine caudal articular process dysplasia of thoracic vertebrae using computed tomography: prevalence and characteristics. *Front Vet Sci.* 2023 Feb 15;10:1066420.
19. Driver CJ, Rose J, Tauro A, et al. Magnetic resonance imaging in pug dogs with thoracolumbar myelopathy and concurrent caudal articular process dysplasia. *BMC Vet Res.* 2019 May 31;15(1):182.
20. Wachowiak IJ, Patterson JS, Winger KM, et al. Thoracolumbar myelopathies in pug dogs. *J Vet Intern Med.* 2023 Mar;37(2):618–625.
21. Rohdin C, Ljungvall I, Häggström J, et al. Thoracolumbar meningeal fibrosis in pugs. *J Vet Intern Med.* 2020 Mar;34(2):797–807.
22. Aikawa T, Miyazaki, Y, Kihara, et al. Vertebral stabilisation for thoracolumbar vertebral instability associated with cranial and caudal articular process anomalies in pugs: Seven cases (2010–2019). *J Small Anim Pract.* 2022 Sep;63(9):699–706.
23. Flückiger MA, Damur-Djuric N, Hässig M, et al. A lumbosacral transitional vertebra in the dog predisposes to cauda equina syndrome. *Vet Radiol Ultrasound.* 2006 Jan-Feb;47(1):39–44.
24. Harris G, Ball J, De Decker S. Lumbosacral transitional vertebrae in cats and its relationship to lumbosacral vertebral canal stenosis. *J Feline Med Surg.* 2019 Apr;21(4):286–292.
25. Brocal J, De Decker S, José-López R, et al. C7 vertebra homeotic transformation in domestic dogs – are Pug dogs breaking mammalian evolutionary constraints? *J Anat.* 2018;233:255–265.
26. Bailey CS, Morgan JP. Congenital spinal malformations. *Vet Clin North Am Small Anim Pract.* 1992 Jul;22(4):985–1015.
27. Johnson P, De Risio L, Sparkes A, et al. Clinical, morphologic, and morphometric features of cranial thoracic spinal stenosis in large and giant breed dogs. *Vet Radiol Ultrasound.* 2012 Sep-Oct;53(5):524–534.
28. Da Costa RC, Echandi RL, Beauchamp D. Computed tomography myelographic findings in dogs with cervical spondylomyelopathy. *Vet Radiol Ultrasound.* Vet Radiol Ultrasound. 2012 Jan-Feb;53(1):64–70.
29. Gillespie S, De Decker S. Thoracic vertebral canal stenosis in cats: clinical features, diagnostic imaging findings, treatment and outcome. *J Feline Med Surg.* 2020 Dec;22(12):1191–1199.
30. Conte A, Bernardini M, De Decker S, et al. Thoracic vertebral canal stenosis associated with vertebral arch anomalies in small brachycephalic screw tail dog breeds. *Vet Comp Orthop Traumatol.* 2021 May;34(3):191–199.
31. Carletti BE, Espadas I, Sanchez-Masian D. Thoracic vertebral canal stenosis due to articular process hypertrophy in two cats treated by hemilaminectomy with partial osteotomy of the spinous process. *J Feline Med Surg Open Rep.* 2019 Aug 13;5(2):2055116919863176.
32. Stalin C, Gutierrez-Quintana R, Faller K, et al. A review of canine atlantoaxial joint subluxation. *Vet Comp Orthop Traumatol.* 2015;28(1):1–8.
33. Platt SR, Chambers JN, Cross A. A modified ventral fixation for surgical management of atlantoaxial subluxation in 19 dogs. *Vet Surg.* 2004 Jul-Aug;33(4):349–354.
34. Tabanez J, Gutierrez-Quintana R, Kaczmarska A, et al. Evaluation of a novel dorsal-cemented technique for atlantoaxial stabilisation in 12 dogs. *Life (Basel)* 2021 Oct 2;11(10):1039.
35. Mauler DA, De Decker S, De Risio L, et al. Signalment, clinical presentation, and diagnostic findings in 122 dogs with spinal arachnoid diverticula. *J Vet Intern Med.* 2014 Jan-Feb;28(1):175–181.
36. Rohdin C, Nyman HT, Wohlsein P, Hultin Jäderlund K. Cervical spinal intradural arachnoid cysts in related, young pugs. *J Small Anim Pract.* 2014 Apr;55(4):229–234.
37. Galloway AM, Curtis NC, Sommerlad SF, Watt PR. Correlative imaging findings in seven dogs and one cat with spinal arachnoid cysts. *Vet Radiol Ultrasound.* 1999 Sep-Oct;40(5):445–452.
38. Seiler GS, Robertson ID, Mai W, et al. Usefulness of a half-fourier acquisition single-shot turbo spin-echo pulse sequence in identifying arachnoid diverticula in dogs. *Vet Radiol Ultrasound.* 2012 Mar-Apr;53(2):157–161.
39. Tauro A, Jovanovik J, Driver CJ, Rusbridge C. Clinical application of 3D-CISS MRI sequences for diagnosis and surgical planning of spinal arachnoid diverticula and adhesions in dogs. *Vet Comp Orthop Traumatol.* 2018 Feb;31(2):83–94.
40. Jones B, Behr S, Shaw T, et al. Surgical techniques used in the management of intra-arachnoid diverticula in dogs across four referral centres and their immediate outcome. *J Small Anim Pract.* 2022 Jul;63(7):520–525.
41. Mauler DA, De Decker S, De Risio L, et al. Spinal arachnoid diverticula: outcome in 96 medically or surgically treated dogs. *J Vet Intern Med.* 2017 May;31(3):849–853.
42. Alisauskaite N, Cizinauskas S, Jeserevics J, et al. Short- and long-term outcome and magnetic resonance imaging findings after surgical treatment of thoracolumbar spinal arachnoid diverticula in 25 Pugs. *J Vet Intern Med.* 2019 May;33(3):1376–1383.
43. Brandel G, Rohdin C, Bianchi M, et al. Multiple genetic loci associated with pug dog thoracolumbar myelopathy. *Genes.* 2023 Feb 1;14(2):385.
44. Lourinho F, Holdsworth A, McConnell JF, et al. Clinical features and MRI characteristics of presumptive constrictive myelopathy in 27 pugs. *Vet Radiol Ultrasound.* 2020 Sep;61(5):545–554.
45. Tauro A, Rose J, Rusbridge C, Driver CJ. Surgical management of thoracolumbar myelopathies in Pug dogs with concurrent articular facet dysplasia. *Vet Comp Orthop Traumatol Open.* 2019;2:e60-e72.
46. Meren IL, Chavera JA, Alcott CJ, Barker AK, Jeffery ND. Shunt tube placement for amelioration of cerebrospinal fluid flow obstruction caused by spinal cord subarachnoid fibrosis in dogs. *Vet Surg.* 2017 Feb;46(2):289–296.

CHAPTER 32

Cervical spondylomyelopathy

Ronaldo Casimiro da Costa
DVM, MSc, PhD,
DACVIM (Neurology)

Cervical spondylomyelopathy (CSM) is a challenging disease common in the cervical vertebral column of large and giant breed dogs. In spite of significant research over the past 20 years, it is the only spinal disease of dogs that is still associated with a relatively short survival time despite medical or surgical treatment. Controversial in nature, it has been referred to by no fewer than 14 different names, *wobbler syndrome* being the most popular, but also *common cervical stenotic myelopathy*, *cervical vertebral instability*, *cervical malformation/malarticulation syndrome*, or *disc-associated wobbler syndrome*. Its challenging nature is also illustrated by the fact that, to this day, no fewer than 35 surgical techniques have been reported as treatment options for CSM.

Etiology

Several etiologies have been proposed, including genetic and congenital factors, body conformation, and nutritional causes. The latter two appear to not be significant in the development of CSM. There is enough evidence to support a congenital etiology that is likely linked to a genetic basis, though this has only been documented in Doberman Pinschers.

Despite some degree of overlap, the pathophysiology of spinal cord compressions can generally be divided into osseous- or disc-associated compressions.[1,2]

Disc-associated compressions are caused by a combination of intervertebral disc protrusion with or without ligament hypertrophy (either the dorsal longitudinal ligament or ligamentum flavum) (Fig. 32.1). Three factors explain together the pathophysiology of disc-associated CSM (DA-CSM):

- Relative vertebral canal stenosis
- Greater torsion in the caudal cervical spine leading to intervertebral disc degeneration
- Protrusion of larger-volume discs in the caudal cervical vertebral column

Affected dogs are apparently born with congenital stenosis of the vertebral canal. Stenosis of the vertebral canal by itself does not lead to clinical signs but predisposes to their development.[3] Most disc-associated spinal cord compressions are located in the caudal cervical vertebral column, affecting discs C5–C6 and C6–C7.[3]

The pathophysiology of osseous-associated CSM (OA-CSM) is quite different. Firstly, it is seen in much younger dogs, typically of giant breeds, such as Great Danes. These dogs usually have severe absolute vertebral canal stenosis secondary to proliferation of the vertebral arch (dorsally), articular facets (dorsolaterally), or articular facets and pedicles (laterally) (Fig. 32.2). The cause of the compression appears to be a combination of vertebral malformation and/or osteoarthritic/osteoarthrotic changes at the level of the articular facets.

Recently, 25% of dogs with CSM have been shown to present with a combination of DA-CSM and OA-CSM (Fig. 32.3).[4] Another important recent development is the fact that dorsal ligamentous compressions are increasing in prevalence.[5]

Clinical features

Signalment and historical findings

CSM is primarily a disease of large and giant breed dogs. It is also occasionally seen in older small and medium breed dogs. Most large breed dogs (e.g., Weimaraners, Dalmatians, Dobermans) are older than 3 years at presentation, whereas giant breeds (Great Danes and Mastiffs) are usually seen at a younger age. Recently, the juvenile form of CSM (i.e., affecting dogs younger than 1 year of age) seems to be increasing in prevalence in both Dobermans and Great Danes.[6] Similarly, German Shepherds have become one of the most commonly affected breeds in the USA.[5] It is very easy to miss signs of CSM in German Shepherds as they tend to be affected at an older age and frequently have other concurrent neurological and orthopedic diseases. A chronic progressive history (several weeks to months) is typical. Acute presentations are usually associated with cervical pain and more commonly seen with disc-associated CSM.

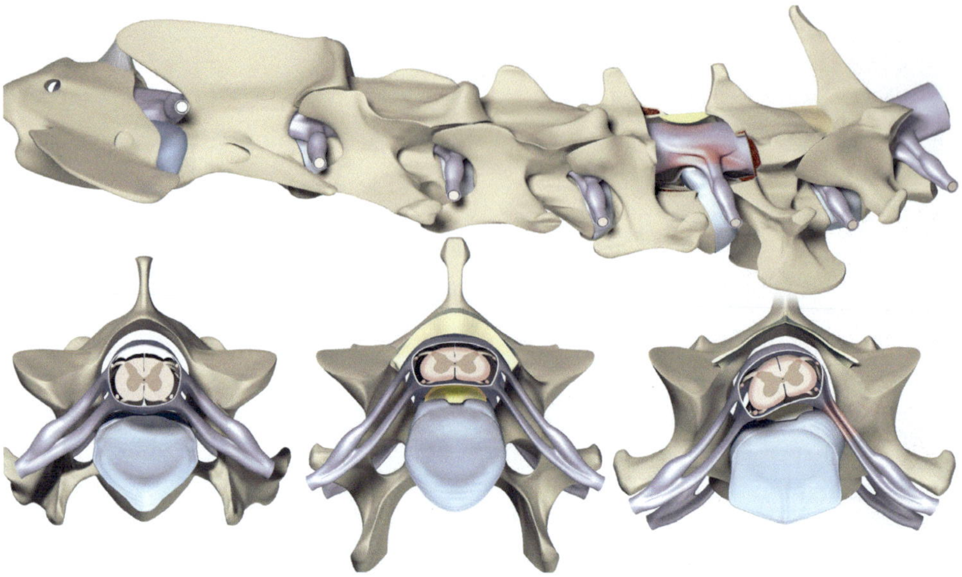

FIG. 32.1 Disc-associated cervical spondylomyelopathy. (**A**) The image shows ventral spinal cord compression and nerve root compression at C5–C6 caused by intervertebral disc protrusion. Dorsally, hypertrophy of the ligamentum flavum causes mild spinal cord compression. (**B**) Transverse section at the level of the C4–C5 disc region, showing a normal spinal cord and vertebral canal. (**C**) Ventral compression at the C5–C6 region caused by intervertebral disc protrusion and hypertrophy of the dorsal longitudinal ligament and ligamentum flavum (causing mild dorsal compression). (**D**) Asymmetric intervertebral disc protrusion at C6–C7 causing spinal cord and nerve root compressions.

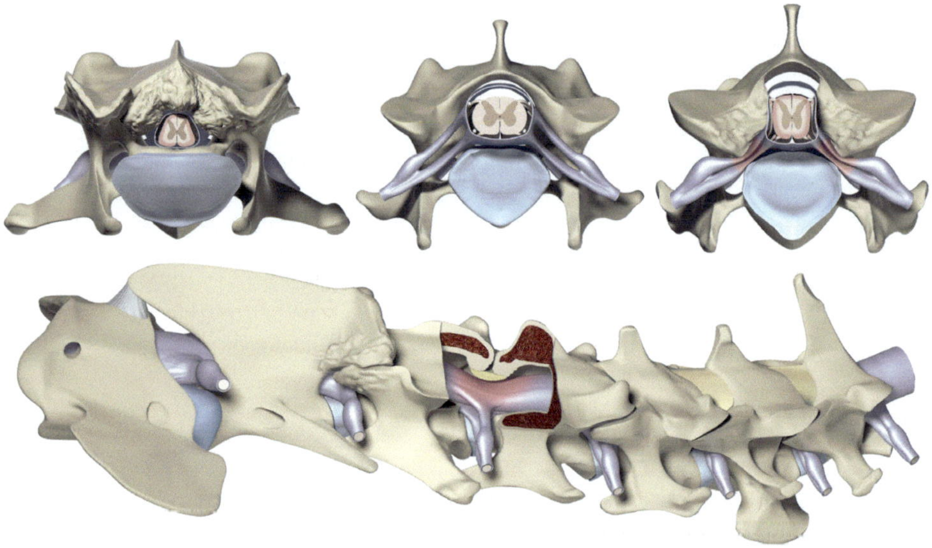

FIG. 32.2 Osseous-associated cervical spondylomyelopathy. (**A**) Severe dorsolateral spinal cord compression at C2–C3 caused by osseous malformation and osteoarthritic changes. (**B**) Normal C3–C4 disc region. (**C**) Bilateral compression at C4–C5 caused by osteoarthritic changes and medial proliferation of the facets causing absolute vertebral canal stenosis and foraminal stenosis leading to spinal cord and nerve root compressions, respectively. (**D**) Dorsal spinal cord compression at C3–C4 caused by lamina malformation and hypertrophy of the ligamentum flavum. Osteoarthritic changes are also shown at C2–C3.

Clinical signs

Cervical pain is part of the clinical findings in approximately 65–70% of Dobermans and in 40–50% of other breeds, but it is rarely the primary complaint (only in 5–10% of dogs with CSM).[7] Forceful manipulations of the cervical spine are unnecessary to document the presence of pain and can lead to neurological decompensation. Careful assessment of posture, palpation of the intervertebral spaces, and evaluation of the voluntary range of motion (side-to-side, ventrally, and dorsally) using food treats are recommended to assess and document cervical pain.

Gait evaluation is the most important component of the examination in dogs suspected of suffering from CSM because it reliably identifies proprioceptive ataxia, even in the absence of conscious proprioceptive deficits (Videos 32.1 and 32.2). Proprioceptive ataxia is seen in most dogs with CSM. Dogs with lesions in the cranial or midcervical spine tend to present with ataxia affecting all four limbs equally. Typically, however, affected dogs have obvious pelvic limb ataxia with milder abnormalities in the thoracic limbs. In some cases, the thoracic limb ataxia or weakness may be very mild in comparison with the pelvic limb signs, making thoracic limb abnormalities go unnoticed. The thoracic limb gait can appear short-strided or, on the contrary, spastic with a pseudohypermetric ("floating") appearance. Occasionally, thoracic limb lameness can be seen, suggesting nerve root entrapment. The pelvic limb gait is often wide based (abducted) and markedly uncoordinated. The stride length of the pelvic limbs is prolonged, causing the swaying movements of the hind end, typical of the disease. Scuffing of the pelvic or thoracic limb toes/nails can also be seen. Postural reaction deficits (proprioceptive positioning deficits) are seen in most dogs with CSM but may not be evident in those with a chronic history despite the presence of proprioceptive ataxia. Assessment of proprioceptive positioning in the thoracic limbs is technically difficult due to the size and weight of typical patients with CSM; hopping is therefore a valid alternative to assess conscious proprioceptive pathways, primarily in the thoracic limbs. In a number of cases, postural reactions are normal in the thoracic limbs. Approximately 10% of dogs with CSM present initially with nonambulatory tetraparesis.[1,2]

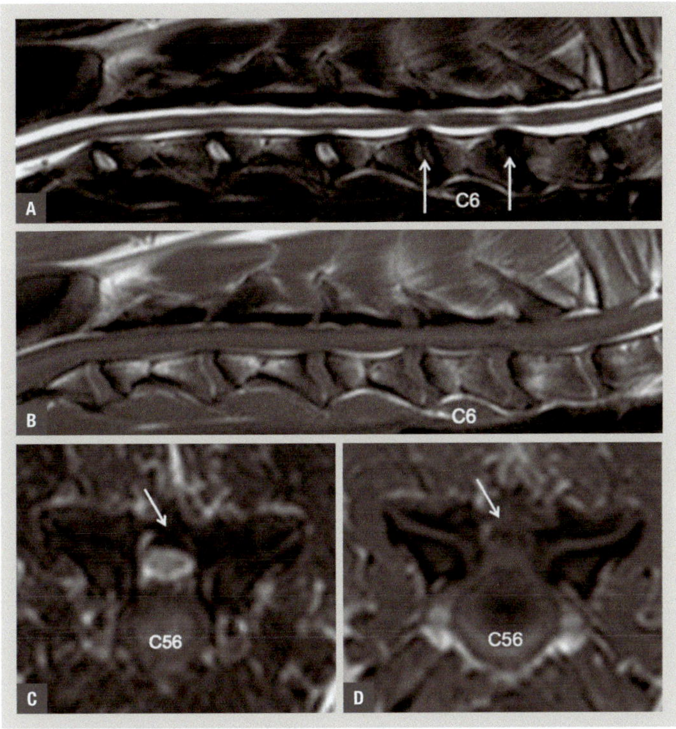

FIG. 32.3 Sagittal and transverse T1- and T2-weighted magnetic resonance images from a 6-year-old Bernese Mountain Dog with combined disc- and osseous-associated cervical spondylomyelopathy with concurrent ligamentous hypertrophy. Note a C5–C6 ventrodorsal and C6–C7 ventral compression of the spinal cord, with hyperintensity at both sites. The dorsolateral compression at C5–C6 (arrows) is caused by a combination of articular facet and soft tissue/ligamentous proliferation (note the isointense signal on the T1-weighted image).

Video 32.1

Three-year-old female spayed Great Dane with osseous-associated cervical spondylomyelopathy.

Video 32.2

Nine-year-old female spayed Doberman Pinscher with disc-associated cervical spondylomyelopathy.

Clinicopathological findings

Diagnostic imaging

Radiographs

Survey radiographs can only be used as a screening test to rule out other differential diagnoses for cervical myelopathies, such as osseous neoplasia, trauma, vertebral osteomyelitis, or discospondylitis. The radiographic findings seen in DA-CSM are primarily changes in the shape of the vertebral body (which assumes a triangular shape in severe cases), narrowing of the intervertebral disc space, and vertebral canal stenosis. Osteoarthritic, sclerotic changes of the articular facets are the radiographic hallmarks in giant breed dogs with osseous compressions and can be seen on lateral and ventrodorsal views. Some of the radiographic findings seen in dogs with CSM (e.g., vertebral tipping) are also seen in normal dogs.[1]

Myelography

Myelography is no longer the method of choice to diagnose CSM. It can be used when computed tomography (CT) and magnetic resonance imaging (MRI) are not available, but these other tests, primarily MRI, offer significant advantages over plain myelography. If myelography is to be performed, lateral and ventrodorsal views should be obtained. Postmyelographic seizures occur in 25% of dogs with CSM. The risk of seizures can be minimized by restricting the total volume of contrast medium and injecting the contrast in the lumbar region.[1,8]

Computed tomography

CT is a rapid test that allows visualization of transverse sections of the cervical vertebral column. Noncontrast CT can be diagnostic depending on the nature of the compressive lesions, but ideally, it should be combined with myelography (CT-myelography) to identify the exact location of the compressive lesion(s). It provides superior visualization of the direction and severity of the spinal cord compression compared with myelography and allows identification of spinal cord atrophy. Plain CT can be performed without general anesthesia with sedation only, which may be useful when general anesthesia is contraindicated or for long-term assessment of osseous compressive lesions.[9]

Magnetic resonance imaging

MRI is the gold standard test for evaluation of dogs suspected of having CSM, due to its superior ability to detail soft tissues. The main advantage of MRI is that it detects spinal cord signal changes and thus allows assessment of the spinal cord parenchyma. These parenchymal signal changes are seen in approximately 50% of dogs with CSM and allow precise identification of the site that is most severely affected. The presence of spinal cord signal changes, namely hyperintensity on T2-weighted images (T2WIs), is associated with severity and chronicity of the clinical signs and severity of spinal cord compression. Hyperintensity on T2WIs does not appear to correlate with prognosis in dogs, but preliminary evidence suggests that the combination of hyperintensity on T2WIs and hypointensity on T1WIs may be associated with a worse prognosis.[10]

In some cases, the degree of spinal cord compression is minimal relative to the severity of the clinical signs. Dynamic spinal cord compressions are assumed to be present in such cases. It has recently been shown that kinematic MRI is a very important tool in the diagnostic evaluation of dogs with DA-CSM and OA-CSM. MRI in extension revealed new compressive sites and documented worsening of dorsal and ventral compressions.[11] It is easy to understand why MRI in extension is so valuable. Normally, dogs tend to keep their head and neck elevated in relation to their thoracic spine. MRI in dorsal recumbency with the cervical and thoracic spine at the same level removes this normal extended position and can limit visualization of all compressive lesions.

Additional diagnostic tests

Many large breed dogs may suffer from concurrent medical conditions that can potentially increase the anesthetic or surgical risk or affect long-term prognosis. In the case of affected Doberman Pinschers, testing for hypothyroidism, von Willebrand disease, and dilated cardiomyopathy should be part of the routine assessment of dogs suspected of having CSM, primarily if surgical treatment is being considered.

Treatment

Ideally, the natural history of a disease should be known to properly decide on treatment recommendations. Unfortunately, the natural history of CSM has not yet been clearly defined. We now know that it is quite complex, and the disease can progress, regress, or remain static with medical management. It also appears that the disease progresses slowly in many dogs with DA-CSM and OA-CSM, with two recent studies indicating that OA-CSM progresses more slowly than DA-CSM.[9,12]

Conservative (medical) treatment

The most important component of medical management is exercise restriction to minimize high impact activities that would exacerbate the dynamic component of spinal cord compression. Dogs can be leash walked, but free, unsupervised activity is strongly discouraged. A body harness should be worn instead of a neck collar. Cage confinement is not necessary and is contraindicated since it can hasten muscle atrophy.[1]

Corticosteroids appear to benefit dogs with CSM, and anti-inflammatory dosages of prednisone are often used (0.5 to 1.0 mg/kg every 12–24 hours), progressively tapering the dosage over the course of 2–3 weeks.[1] Corticosteroids, particularly dexamethasone, improve neurological function in chronic spinal cord compression predominantly by decreasing vasogenic edema. Other proposed mechanisms include protection from glutamate toxicity and reduction of neuronal and oligodendroglial apoptosis. Despite the potential benefits associated with corticosteroid therapy, the use of corticosteroids, particularly for long periods, can be associated with important adverse effects.[11] Nonsteroidal anti-inflammatory drugs (NSAIDs) can be used in place of corticosteroids if neck pain appears to be a main component of the syndrome or if the adverse effects of the corticosteroids cannot be tolerated. Independent of the NSAID used, corticosteroids and NSAIDs should never be used in combination. Physical therapy can also be considered as an adjunct treatment for dogs with CSM.

The author typically starts all ambulatory dogs on medical management to evaluate the dog's response and give owners an opportunity to plan and decide about surgery. The response to medical management (usually with corticosteroids and exercise restriction) can be used to indirectly assess the degree of reversible spinal cord lesions.[1,7,13]

Surgical treatment

Surgical treatment is generally assumed as the treatment of choice for CSM. As most affected dogs have spinal cord compression, decompressing the spinal cord would, in theory, lead to definitive treatment. The decision to recommend surgical treatment should, however, be based on several factors such as severity of the neurological signs, pain, type and severity of compressive lesion(s), response (or lack of response) to medical management, short- and long-term expectations of the owner, and presence of other concurrent neurological or orthopedic problems or extraneurological diseases (e.g., dilated cardiomyopathy) that would affect the long-term outcome.[14] It is very important to stress the importance of screening for dilated cardiomyopathy, because almost 50% of Dobermans older than 6 years are affected. It is quite unfortunate when dogs have surgery and decline 3 months later due to cardiac failure.

The decision on the specific surgical technique can be complicated. More than 35 surgical techniques have been proposed to treat CSM. It is important to consider that a significant proportion of dogs worsen approximately 2–3 years after surgery. Therefore, whenever possible, the surgical technique should allow long-term postoperative imaging using MRI.[12] All metallic implants, except those made of titanium, will cause significant artifacts, precluding the use of MRI. Polymethyl methacrylate (PMMA) or titanium implants (screws, plate, or artificial disc) cause minimal artifacts, allowing postoperative MRI.

Treatment recommendations can generally be made based on the source and direction of compression, which are broadly classified as disc-associated or osseous-associated.

DA-CSM

DA-CSM is the most common form of CSM and the one with the largest number of surgical techniques proposed to treat it. Many, if not most, of the surgical techniques have been based on the concept of static or dynamic lesions, following stress or traction myelography, which is highly subjective and probably incorrect. Nevertheless, the outcome for most surgical techniques is quite similar and generally positive.[15] Ventral static compressions are usually treated with the traditional ventral slot or the inverted cone slot. Dynamic compressions can be treated with distraction–stabilization techniques, such as a cage with locking plate or pins/screws with PMMA. Multiple compressive sites can be treated with distraction–stabilization techniques.[14] Dorsal laminectomy is also an alternative for multiple ventral compressions. A relatively new technique, artificial disc arthroplasty, is an option for single or multiple lesions.[16] More recently, combined dorsal and ventral fixation has been proposed with the theoretical advantage of better outcomes, though the 1-year outcome was similar to that achieved with previous techniques.[17]

Osseous compressions

Typically, these compressions are thought to be primarily static and, as such, direct decompression of the affected sites is recommended.[14] This is typically achieved by dorsal laminectomy, but it can also be achieved by cervical hemilaminectomy. Another way to treat osseous lesions is by distraction–stabilization of the affected segments ventrally.[18] Stabilization and fusion of the affected segments does not directly decompress the affected sites but eliminates the dynamic component of the spinal cord compression. This technique was associated with a high rate of recurrence in multiple compressive lesions and, although it was claimed to allow regression of the osseous and ligamentous lesions over time, this could not be proven with postoperative long-term CT studies.

Pure ligamentous compressions

Ligamentous hypertrophy is usually combined with either disc- or osseous-associated compressions. Pure ligamentous compression typically causes dorsal compression, and it is best treated with direct decompression via dorsal laminectomy.[14]

Surgical complications

Surgical treatment can lead to several complications, including death. Postoperative deterioration has been reported in up to 78% of dogs with OA-CSM treated with dorsal laminectomy,[19] possibly related to the technique chosen, although the author's experience indicates a much lower prevalence. Hypotension and hemorrhage may be responsible for a large proportion of the cases with intraoperative and perioperative complications. Aggressive monitoring and maintenance of appropriate arterial blood pressure transoperatively is essential to minimize complications. When instrumentation is used, penetration of the vertebral canal or transverse foramina with implants and implant failure can also be observed, with an incidence ranging from 7.5 to 30%.[15]

Prognosis

The outcome of surgical treatment for DA-CSM is usually successful, with approximately 80% (70–90%) of dogs improving after surgery. No surgical technique stands out as being clearly superior, even for dogs with DA-CSM (not even the most complex and time-consuming techniques). Considering the success rates of surgical and medical treatments for CSM, surgery more consistently leads to clinical improvement and should always be considered in the treatment of dogs with CSM. Surgery, however, does not appear to alter the long-term survival of dogs with CSM. The survival time of 76 dogs with CSM (33 dogs treated surgically and 43 dogs treated medically) was reported, and the median survival time of dogs with CSM was identical (36 months), regardless of whether the dog was treated medically or surgically.[7] This finding indicates that CSM continues to progress regardless of the method of treatment and that the clinical deterioration seen months to years after treatment may not be due solely to failure of the surgery or development of adjacent segment disease, but it may also occur secondary to other mechanisms, such as ischemia, apoptosis, or other molecular changes within the spinal cord.

KEY POINTS

- Cervical spondylomyelopathy (CSM) is primarily a disease of large and giant breed dogs and the only spinal disease of dogs that is still associated with a relatively short survival time despite medical or surgical treatment.
- The disease may be disc-associated (DA-CSM) and osseous-associated (OA-CSM).
- The clinical signs of CSM include cervical pain and proprioceptive ataxia, which is typically more obvious in the pelvic limbs.
- MRI is the gold standard test for evaluation of dogs suspected of having CSM and allows assessment of the spinal cord parenchyma.
- Medical management mainly involves exercise restriction and administration of corticosteroids, which may replaced by nonsteroid anti-inflammatory drugs if neck pain appears to be a main component of the syndrome or if the adverse effects of the corticosteroids cannot be tolerated.
- More than 35 surgical techniques have been proposed to treat CSM, and the decision on the specific surgical technique can be complicated. Use of metallic implants should be avoided to allow long-term postoperative imaging using MRI.
- Surgical treatment most consistently leads to clinical improvement than medical treatment, although it does not appear to alter the long-term survival of dogs with CSM.

References

1. da Costa RC. Cervical spondylomyelopathy (Wobbler syndrome). *Vet Clin North Am Small Anim Pract.* 2010;40(5):881–913.
2. De Decker S, da Costa RC, Volk HA, et al. Current insights and controversies in the pathogenesis and diagnosis of disc-associated cervical spondylomyelopathy in dogs. *Vet Rec.* 2012;171(21):531–537.
3. da Costa RC, Parent J, Partlow G, et al. Morphologic and morphometric magnetic resonance imaging features of Doberman pinscher dogs with and without clinical signs of cervical spondylomyelopathy. *Am J Vet Res.* 2006;67(9):1601–1612.
4. Bonelli MA, da Costa RC. Magnetic resonance imaging and neurologic characterization of combined osseous- and disc-associated cervical spondylomyelopathy in dogs. *J Vet Intern Med.* 2023;37(4):1418–1427.
5. Bonelli MA, da Costa RC. Clinical and magnetic resonance imaging features of cervical spondylomyelopathy in German shepherd dogs: 10 cases (2006-2018). *J Am Vet Med Assoc.* 2019;255(11): 1263–1269.
6. Bonelli MA, da Costa RC. Clinical and magnetic resonance imaging characterization of cervical spondylomyelopathy in Juvenile Dogs. J Vet Intern Med 2019;33(5): 2160–2166.
7. da Costa RC, Parent JM, Holmberg DL, Sinclair D, Monteith G. Outcome of medical and surgical treatment in dogs with cervical spondylomyelopathy: 104 cases (1988-2004). *J Am Vet Med Assoc.* 2008 Oct 15;233(8):1284–1290.
8. De Decker S, Gielen IM, Duchateau L, et al. Intraobserver, interobserver, and intermethod agreement for results of myelography, computed tomography-myelography, and low-field magnetic resonance imaging in dogs with disk-associated wobbler syndrome. *J Am Vet Med Assoc.* 2011;238(12):1601–1608.
9. Vansteenkiste DP, Martin-Vaquero P, Bonelli M, et al. Long-term clinical and computed tomography follow-up study in Great Danes with signs of cervical spondylomyelopathy. *BMC Vet Res.* 2019;15(1):1–8.
10. Martin-Vaquero P, da Costa RC. Magnetic resonance imaging features of Great Danes with and without clinical signs of cervical spondylomyelopathy. *J Am Vet Med Assoc.* 2014;245(4):393–400.
11. Provencher M, Habing A, Moore SA, et al. Kinematic Magnetic Resonance Imaging for Evaluation of Disc-Associated Cervical Spondylomyelopathy in Doberman Pinschers. *J Vet Intern Med.* 2016;30(4): 1121–1128.
12. Nye C, Hostnik E, Parker E, et al. Long-term clinical and magnetic resonance imaging follow-up of dogs with osseous-associated cervical spondylomyelopathy. *J Vet Intern Med.* 2020;34(5):2012–2020.
13. De Decker S, Bhatti SF, Duchateau L, et al. Clinical evaluation of 51 dogs treated conservatively for disc-associated wobbler syndrome. *J Small Anim Pract.* 2009;50(3):136–142.
14. Platt SR, da Costa RC. Cervical spine. In: Tobias KM, Johnston SA (eds.). *Veterinary Surgery: Small Animal.* Philadelphia, PA: Elsevier; 2011. pp. 410–448.
15. Jeffery ND, McKee WM. Surgery for disc-associated wobbler syndrome in the dog - an examination of the controversy. *J Small Anim Pract.* 2001;42(12):574–581.
16. Adamo PF. Cervical arthroplasty in two dogs with disk-associated cervical spondylomyelopathy. *J Am Vet Med Assoc.* 2011;239(6):808–817.
17. Falzone C, Tranquillo V, Gasparinetti N. Comparison of Two Surgical Techniques for the Treatment of Canine Disc Associated-Cervical Spondylomyelopathy. *Front Vet Sci.* 2022 Jun 20;9:880018.
18. Lewis M, Olby NJ, Sharp NJ, Early P. Long-term effect of cervical distraction and stabilization on neurological status and imaging findings in giant breed dogs with cervical stenotic myelopathy. *Vet Surg.* 2013;42(6):701–709.
19. Taylor-Brown FE, Cardy TJ, Liebel FX, et al. Risk factors for early post-operative neurological deterioration in dogs undergoing a cervical dorsal laminectomy or hemilaminectomy: 100 cases (2002-2014). *Vet J.* 2015;206(3):327–331.

CHAPTER 33

Lumbosacral stenosis

Frank Steffen
DVM, DECVN

Lumbosacral stenosis can result from congenital narrowing of the L7–S1 canal and/or intervertebral foramina but is more frequently caused by degenerative changes at the lumbosacral spine. Degenerative lumbosacral stenosis (DLSS) is an acquired, multifactorial condition in which compression of the cauda equina occurs as a result of progressive proliferation of bony and soft tissue structures. DLSS is most common in medium to large breeds of middle and older age, especially in working dogs. The condition can be debilitating and, in a retrospective study of 976 military working dogs, DLSS was the cause of euthanasia or death in 15% of the population.[1]

Etiology and pathophysiology

Degenerative changes, which most commonly start in the intervertebral disc (IVD), are mandatory for development of clinical signs. Loss of the normal structure of the IVD gives rise to further degenerative changes within the lumbosacral junction, including narrowing of the disc space due to bulging of the annular fibers into the central canal, formation of bony osteophytes near the ventral and lateral endplates, and thickening of the ligaments and joint capsule (Fig. 33.1). Remodeling of the facet joints also occurs with advanced ageing and is observed as an enlargement of the facet join angle in the dorsal plane.[2] Complete rupture of the disc with free disc material in the vertebral canal (Hansen type 1 disc extrusion) is uncommon. Bulging of the IVD and proliferation of bony and soft tissue structures may result in mechanical compression of the nerve roots of the cauda equina. Nerve root dysfunction occurs as a consequence of compression and/or tethering and impairment of radicular blood flow. Similarly, traction on the nerve roots caused by abnormal lumbosacral motion or tethering causes pain and dysfunction. A variety of structural and functional changes occur in the nerve root and dorsal root ganglion due to compression; these changes include venous stasis, edema and subsequent intra- and perineural fibrosis. Subsequent demyelination and axon loss may result in functional deficits. In unmyelinated fibers, mechanical stress may cause ectopic discharges, which are experienced as neuropathic pain.[2]

A second mechanism not associated with nerve root compression but with low back pain is the production of inflammatory mediators and upregulation of various inflammatory genes associated with degeneration of bony and soft tissue structures at L7–S1. These proinflammatory and pain-related products promote ingrowth and stimulation of sensory nerve fibers in various structures. In addition, these molecular mechanisms are responsible for the progressive natural course of DLSS by continuous apoptosis and degradation of the disc tissue.[3]

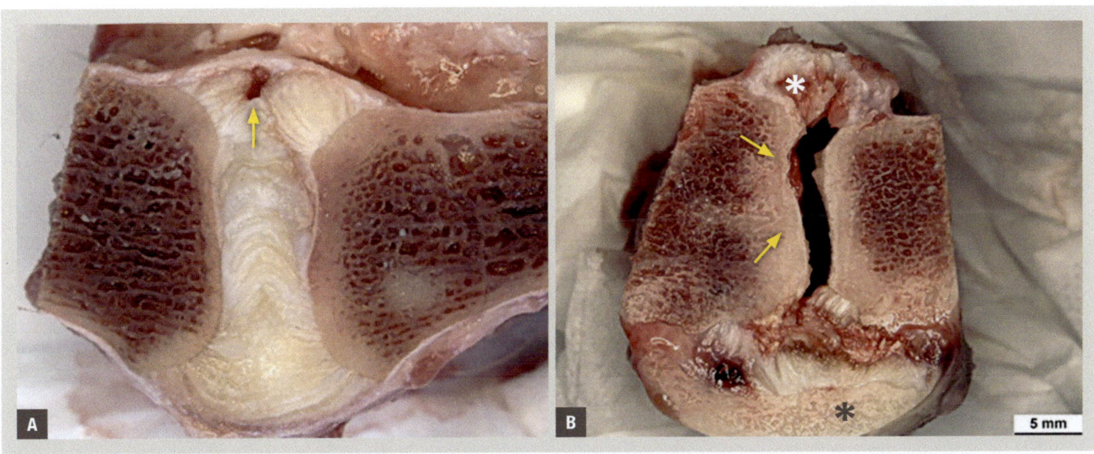

FIG. 33.1 Midsagittal sections of the lumbosacral discs of dogs with degenerative lumbosacral stenosis with different grades of degeneration. **(A)** Mild bulging of the dorsal annulus into the vertebral canal along with ruptured lamellae (arrow) and loss of the gelatinous structure of the nucleus pulposus. **(B)** Almost complete loss of disc tissue with collapse of the intervertebral disc space, protrusion of the remnants of the dorsal annulus (white asterisk), sclerosis of the endplates (arrows), and new bone formation (black asterisk) at the ventral aspect of the segment all represent end-stage degeneration.

Clinical presentation

In general, dogs with lumbosacral disease can be divided into two broad categories based on the clinical signs. The first and by far the largest group consists of dogs with low back pain and lameness only. The second group includes dogs with neurological deficits in addition to the previously cited signs (cauda equina syndrome).

Lower back pain manifests as a characteristic posture (arched back); difficulties jumping and rising into a standing position on all fours or the hindlimbs and a stilted pelvic limb gait are the first and most consistent clinical signs in dogs with DLSS (Video 33.1).[3] In some dogs, pain occurs only with heavy exercise and disappears with return to normal physical activity.

In most cases, localized pain can be reproduced by applying digital pressure on the lumbosacral junction and by using the lordosis test (extension of the pelvic limbs while applying downward pressure on the lumbosacral junction). This test does not differentiate hip pain from lumbosacral pain. To avoid stress on the hip joints during lordosis, the pelvic limbs may be supported in a flexed position while applying downward pressure. Traction or extension of the tail and palpation of the ventral aspect of the lumbosacral joint through the rectum can also aid in detecting lumbosacral pain. Neurological deficits are usually not observed in this category.

Neurological dysfunction in dogs with DLSS may be motor, sensory, and/or autonomous in nature and depends on which nerves of the cauda equina are compromised. More than one nerve root is usually affected, but dysfunction of a single root may also result in clinical signs. In addition, the same nerve root may be compressed or stretched at different levels, rendering identification of the specific site of compression within the cauda equina difficult.[4] The gait is often stiff and stilted, although proprioceptive ataxia as seen with thoracolumbar myelopathies is not a feature of DLSS. Accordingly, proprioceptive tests are often normal. Severely affected dogs exhibit lower motor neuron signs. If the lesion involves the sciatic nerve roots (L6–S2), clinical signs include muscle atrophy of the gluteal and hamstring muscle groups, paraparesis manifested as dragging of the toes, reduced flexor reflex and exaggerated patellar reflex (pseudohyperreflexia), and altered skin sensation over the associated dermatomes. A reduced flexor reflex is often evident with decreased flexion of the hock, while adduction in the hip is normal.

Video 33.1

Eight-year-old male castrated Beauceron with long-standing, severe lumbosacral stenosis due to disc protrusion and proliferation of adjacent bony and soft tissue structures (including thickened sacral and pudendal nerve roots) diagnosed with magnetic resonance imaging. The gait examination shows only mild paraparesis with mild hypometria of the hindlimbs.

Video 33.2

Clinical signs include severe paresis of the tail with retained sensory function, reduced perineal reflexes, and reduced urethral resistance when the bladder is expressed manually (fecal and urinary incontinence). Paw repositioning in the hindlimbs is mildly delayed. Spinal reflexes are intact, but hock flexion is reduced when withdrawal is tested (not shown).

Lesions restricted to the seventh lumbar or first sacral nerve root often present as neurogenic lameness only and thus strongly mimic the presence of an orthopedic condition. Dysfunction of the pudendal nerve roots (S1–S3) results in a decreased perineal reflex and perineal skin sensation and reduced anal and urethral sphincter tone. Involvement of the parasympathetic fibers of the pelvic nerve results in atony of the urinary bladder and reduced sphincter tone. Caudal nerve root lesions (Cd1–5) frequently cause weak tail tone, tail paresis or plegia, reduced tail sensation, or paresthesia of the tail (Video 33.2).[2,4,5]

Regarding the natural history of DLSS, the disease progresses over variable periods of time, with some clinical signs and radiographic parameters changing significantly with time.[6]

Diagnostic imaging

Imaging is crucial for diagnosis of DLSS. The purpose of imaging tests is to provide accurate morphological information and influence therapeutic decision-making. Both computed tomography (CT) and magnetic resonance imaging (MRI) are superior to conventional radiography, myelography, and epidurography because they provide precise morphological information due to their sensitivity and ability to generate views in different planes.

However, plain radiography remains a first and low-cost imaging modality to rule out other diseases associated with lumbosacral signs, such as fractures/luxations, discospondylitis, and bone neoplasia.

Disorders predisposing for DLSS such as translational vertebrae, osteochondrosis-dissecans of the sacral endplate, and diffuse idiopathic spinal hyperostosis (DISH) can be identified on radiographs and provide a basis for subsequent diagnostic and therapeutic measures.

Computed tomography

CT imaging allows excellent evaluation of vertebral body and facet joint degeneration and of stenosis of the vertebral canal and intervertebral foramina. Abnormalities found on CT include loss of epidural fat, increased soft tissue opacity, bulging of the intervertebral disc, new bone proliferations, narrowed intervertebral foramen and vertebral canal, thickened articular facets, and articular facet subluxation.[7] Using volumetric analysis and dynamic imaging moving the lumbosacral junction from a flexed to an extended position, CT provides reliable diagnostic information about foraminal stenosis. However, stenosis originating from soft tissue proliferations is underestimated on CT studies. A foraminal volume <90 mm^3 had a 75% positive predictive value for clinically relevant foraminal stenosis, while a volume >90 mm^3 was associated with an 86% negative predictive value in German Shepherd dogs. A median reduction in the foraminal volume of 79% during dynamic positioning was found in German Shepherds unaffected by DLSS, while an 85% reduction was observed in affected German Shepherds.[8]

Magnetic resonance imaging

MRI is the most sensitive modality for detection of various degrees of disc degeneration and abnormalities of soft tissues, including the lumbosacral spine nerve roots and surrounding tissues.[9] Stenosis in the vertebral canal and intervertebral foramen is readily identified in the presence of a reduced epidural fat signal on T2-weighted images (Fig. 33.2). Because almost all DLSS cases have dynamic lesions with a maximal narrowing of the vertebral and foraminal canal during extension, it is

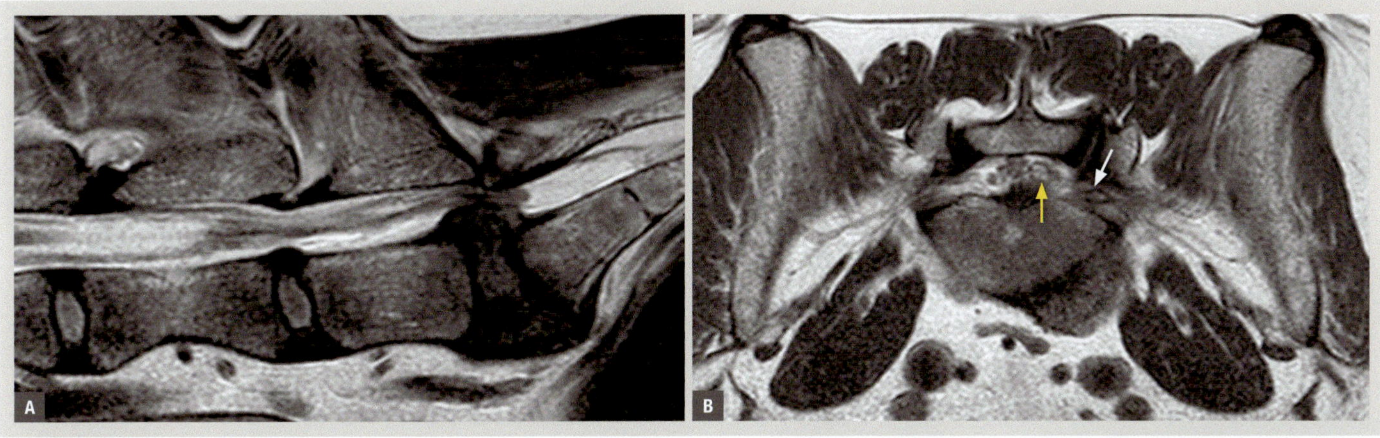

FIG. 33.2 Midsagittal (A) and transverse (B) T2-weighted magnetic resonance images of the lumbosacral junction of a 10-year-old Rhodesian Ridgeback with low back pain and neurogenic lameness on the left pelvic limb. There is protrusion of the degenerated intervertebral disc into the vertebral canal, with severe stenosis and compression of the cauda equina nerve roots and dural sac (A). Note the enlargement and hyperintensity of the left S1 root (yellow arrow) and complete loss of the fat signal in the left neurovascular foramen (white arrow).

recommended to obtain images with the dog in dorsal recumbency and the lumbosacral junction in extension for diagnosis. However, the degree of stenosis must be interpreted with caution as stenosis in the vertebral canal and loss of intraforaminal fat signal have been found in up to 85% and 54% of healthy dogs, respectively.[10] Nerve root abnormalities such as enlargement and T2-hyperintensity are likely to be more strongly associated with clinical signs of DLSS than narrowing of the vertebral canal and intervertebral foramina. In a study using low-field MRI in a large population of clinically affected dogs, radiculopathy of the L7 root was identified in 87.9% of a total of 364 foramina with a reduced fat signal.[10] A significant association of a history of low back pain and neurogenic lameness was found in dogs with MRI abnormalities of the L7 and S1 nerve roots.

Electrodiagnostic examinations

Electromyography of the pelvic limbs, tail, and pelvic diaphragm myotomes is a tool for mapping the distribution of denervation in dogs with DLSS and may help in excluding dogs with orthopedic diseases that may mimic DLSS. In one study, electromyography was not able to discriminate between dogs with painful foraminal stenosis and those without.[11] Similarly, analysis of the compound muscle action potentials (CMAP) recorded during motor stimulation of the tibial nerve did not reveal a difference between affected and unaffected dogs. Cord dorsum potential onset latency, F-wave onset latency and F-ratio were increased in dogs with lumbosacral foraminal stenosis versus those without this condition, although there was an overlap of values between groups. Delayed cord dorsum potential latency, was found to be more sensitive than F-wave abnormalities; the former is therefore probably the most useful parameter to diagnose dysfunction of the nerve roots contributing axons to the tibial nerve.[11] Based on this information, cord dorsum potential analysis can complement clinical and MRI examination findings and further support the diagnosis of DLSS. As many dogs affected with DLSS present with pain and neurogenic lameness only, confirmation of nerve root dysfunction with electrodiagnostic testing can provide a more objective diagnosis.

Treatment

Once the diagnosis of DLSS has been established, a decision on the most appropriate treatment option is warranted. Medical and surgical procedures are usually available. The effectiveness of each treatment modality has been examined in a review of two studies investigating the outcome of dogs treated either medically or surgically for DLSS.[12] Based on this limited information, it was concluded that both treatment options can improve the outcome, but statements about the effectiveness of each modality in the long term are not possible.

Medical treatment

The results of medical treatment using a combination of NSAIDs, gabapentin, and exercise restriction have been reported in a large population of dogs affected with DLSS. A successful outcome was observed in 55% of dogs, while the failure rate was 32%.[13] To address the inflammatory component of DLSS, which occurs in the epidural space as a consequence of mechanical compression and degeneration of various anatomical structures, local infiltration of the epidural space with corticosteroids can provide temporary relief of pain. In a clinical investigation, most of the 32 affected dogs (84%) improved after a single-dose injection of methylprednisolone acetate (1 mg/kg) at L7/S1. While 74% of dogs had a relapse within 6 months of the injection, 15% had a sustained improvement with a mean follow-up of more than 9 months.[14] Alternatively, corticosteroid injection can be performed at the exit zone of the L7 nerve root to address foraminal stenosis.

Surgical treatment

There is consensus that a surgical strategy is indicated after recurrent episodes of pain with medical treatment and in dogs unresponsive to conservative measures. Two contrasting strategies are available for the management of DLSS: decompression of the cauda equina with and without instrumented stabilization of the lumbosacral spine. Dorsal laminectomy is the decompressive procedure most frequently performed; it is often combined with annulectomy of the protruding disc, disc fenestration, or partial discectomy of L7/S1. Good to excellent results have been reported in most dogs having undergone dorsal laminectomy.[4] However, a 2017 investigation by Rapp et al. using postoperative CT and MRI in dogs treated with widespread laminectomy (including the entire laminae of L7 to S1, the dorsal spinous processes, and the associated ligaments) yielded severe imaging abnormalities. Advanced spondylosis, osteoarthritis of the facet joints, and contrast accumulation in the paraspinal tissues and L7 roots were observed in most dogs. A severe and clinically relevant finding was bilateral fracture of the facet joints in 4/13 dogs.[15] It should be noted that in humans, this "classical" variant of dorsal laminectomy is no longer used because it involves removing supporting structures and resecting large amounts of soft tissue. Another study using a more limited, partial laminectomy—whereby only the most caudal part of the L7 lamina was removed, and the dorsal ligaments and spinous processes were spared—avoided most of the imaging abnormalities described by Rapp et al. at 10 months MRI follow-up.[16]

Lesions affecting the neurovascular foramen at L7/S1 are frequently encountered in dogs with DLSS. Lateral formation of osteophytes and bony and soft tissue proliferations of the facet joints are the most frequent pathologies compressing the L7 root.[10] As foraminal stenosis cannot be adequately addressed with dorsal laminectomy, a lateral foraminotomy technique with no need to remove the facet joint can be performed.[5] Long-term complete resolution of the preoperative signs was reported in 97% of cases. Lateral foraminotomy can be performed bilaterally and combined with dorsal laminectomy if multilevel stenosis is present at the lumbosacral junction.

Several procedures for surgical stabilization have been reported. The main goal of all of them is to prevent motion of the lumbosacral junction in order to control pain during exercise and dynamic compression of the nerve roots.

Transarticular fixation of the facet joints using pins or screws is frequently used by specialists. The technique is easy to perform and can be combined with a partial laminectomy. Dorsal fusion can be encouraged by debriding articular cartilage and applying a bone graft procured from the wing of the ilium. The clinical outcome is reportedly similar to dorsal laminectomy but bending, fracture, and pullout of screws have been observed in up to 30% of cases in a follow-up study using CT.[2] This suggests that this procedure should be restricted to dogs under 15 kg of body weight because it does not provide enough rigidity in larger dogs.

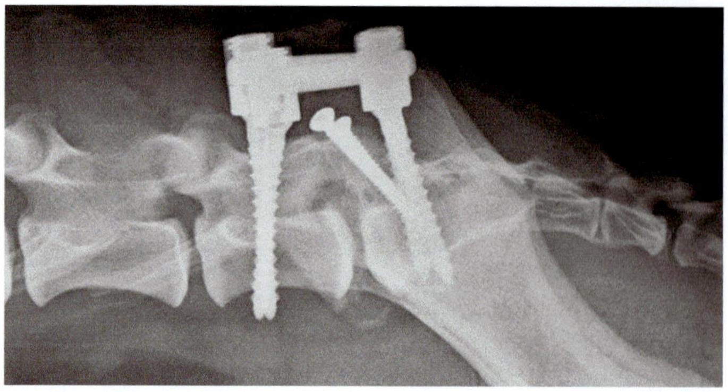

FIG. 33.3 Postoperative radiograph of a dog after implantation of a pedicle screw rod-system and transarticular screw fixation. This construct provides rigid stabilization of the lumbosacral junction and can be used in combination with dorsal laminectomy and/or lateral foraminotomy.

Stabilization with screw placement dorsally in L7 and S1 plus transarticular fixation followed by use of bone cement for bondage results in a biomechanically rigid construct. The clinical outcome was excellent in a clinical study and implant failure was observed in only 2% of patients.[17] Alternatively, pedicle-screw rod fixation (PSRF) systems can be used with identical success rates (Fig. 33.3). A PSRF system requires less muscle resection and can be adapted to the specific anatomy of each patient thanks to polyaxial screw heads. Improvement was noted in all dogs without implant failure in a 2019 study.[2] Distraction and stabilization of the lumbosacral joint to address foraminal stenosis has also been reported. However, because the intervertebral foramen is located cranial to the intervertebral disc space at L7/S1, ongoing compression of the L7 root at the exit zone may persist. In a cadaveric study, foraminal volume was shown to increase more after foraminotomy than after distraction-stabilization.[18]

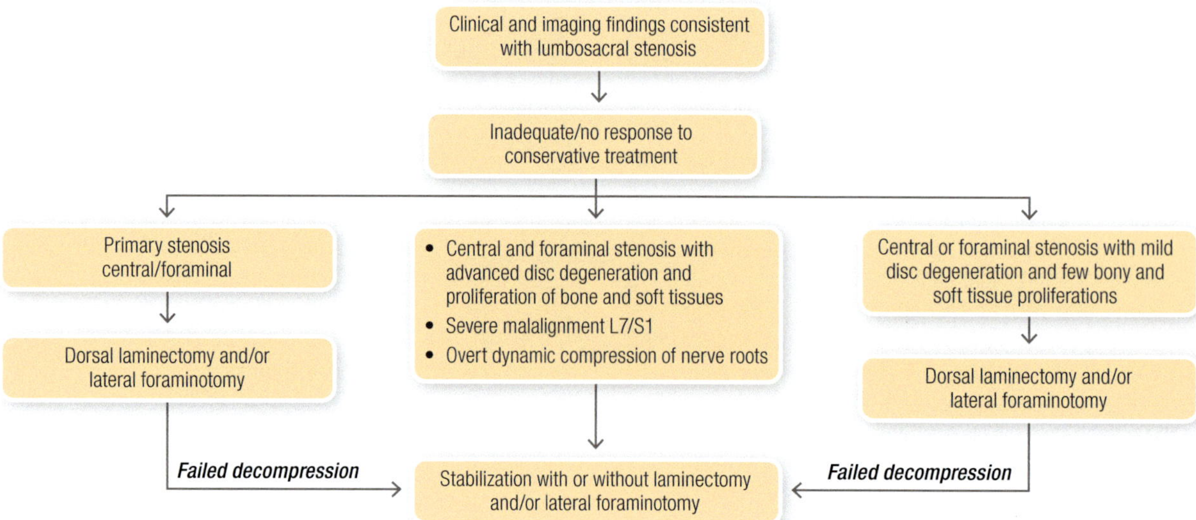

FIG. 33.4 Suggested decision-making algorithm for treatment of lumbosacral stenosis. Note that reliable preoperative indicators for treatment procedures are not available.

Currently, there is no definitive cure for DLSS, and all measures are aimed at pain relief only. Recent investigations have focused on control of the inflammatory microenvironment within the lumbosacral disc by intradiscal injection of anti-inflammatory drugs or mesenchymal stem cells.[2,16] Despite good clinical results, robust evidence on the long-term effectiveness of these new treatment modalities is not available yet. A suggested decision-making algorithm for treatment of lumbosacral stenosis is shown in **Figure 33.4**.

KEY POINTS

- Degenerative lumbosacral stenosis is the most common disorder of the canine lumbar spine.
- The most frequent and early clinical sign is low back pain, which may progress to cauda equina syndrome after a variable period of time in some dogs.
- Diagnosis is based on the correlation of history, clinical signs, and advanced imaging findings.
- Epidural corticosteroid infiltration is more effective than systemically administered medication.
- Surgical options include decompression of the nerve roots with or without stabilization, with both being effective in most cases.
- There is no definitive cure for DLSS.

References

1. Moore GE, Burkman KD, Carter MN, et al. Causes of death or reasons for euthanasia in military working dogs: 927 cases (1993-1996). *J Am Vet Med Assoc.* 2001;219:209–214.
2. Worth A, Meij B, Jeffery N. Canine Degenerative Lumbosacral Stenosis: Prevalence, Impact And Management Strategies. *Vet Med (Auckl).* 2019 Nov 19;10:169–183.
3. Bitterli T, Schmid D, Ettinger L, et al. Targeted screening of inflammatory mediators in spontaneous degenerative disc disease in dogs reveals an upregulation of the tumor necrosis superfamily. *JOR Spine.* 2023 Nov 23;7(1):e1292.
4. Suwangkong N, Meij BP, Voorhout G, et al. Review and retrospective analysis of degenerative lumbosacral stenosis in 156 dogs treated by dorsal laminectomy. *Vet Comp Orthop Traumatol.* 2008;21:285–293.
5. Gödde T, Steffen F. Surgical treatment of lumbosacral foraminal stenosis using a lateral approach in twenty dogs with degenerative lumbosacral stenosis. *Vet Surg.* 2007;36:705–713.
6. Steffen F, Hunold K, Scharf G, et al. A follow-up study of neurologic and radiographic findings in German Shepherd Dogs with and without degenerative lumbosacral stenosis. *J Am Vet Med Assoc.* 2007:231(10);1529–1533.
7. Da Costa RC, Samii VF. Advanced imaging of the spine in small animals. *Vet Clin North Am.* 2010;40:765–790.
8. Worth AJ, Hartman A, Bridges JP, et al. Effect of dorsal laminectomy and dorsal annulectomy with partial lumbosacral discectomy on the volume of the lateral intervertebral neuroforamina in dogs when the lumbosacral junction is extended. *Vet Surg.* 201;46(2):265–270.
9. Lampe R, Foss KD, Hague DW, et al. Dynamic MRI is reliable for evaluation of the lumbosacral spine in healthy dogs. *Vet Radiol Ultrasound.* 2020;61:555–565.
10. Lichtenhahn V, Richter, Gödde T, et al. Evaluation of L7-S1 nerve root pathology with low-field MRI in dogs with lumbosacral foraminal stenosis. *Vet Surg.* 2020;49:247–257.
11. Harcourt-Brown TR, Granger NP, Fitzpatrick N et al. Electrodiagnostic findings in dogs with apparently painful lumbosacral foraminal stenosis. *J Vet Int Med.* 2019; Sep-Oct; 33(5): 2167–2174.
12. Goh K. Comparing clinical outcomes of dogs suffering from degenerative lumbosacral stenosis upon surgical or nonsurgical treatment. *Veterinary Evidence.* 2023;8(2).
13. De Decker S, Wawrzenski LA, Volk HA. Clinical signs and outcome of dogs treated medically for degenerative lumbosacral stenosis: 98 cases (2004-2012). *J Am Vet Med Assoc.* 2014 Aug 15;245(15):408–413.
14. Gomes SA, Lowrie M, Targett M. Single dose epidural methylprednisolone as a treatment and predictor of outcome following subsequent decompressive surgery in degenerative lumbosacral stenosis with foraminal stenosis. *Vet J.* 2020 Mar;257:105451.
15. Rapp M, Loy CL, Hansson K, et al. Postoperative computed tomography and low-field magnetic resonance imaging findings in dogs with degenerative lumbosacral stenosis treated by dorsal laminectomy. *Vet Comp Orthop Traumatol.* 2017 Mar 20;30(2):143–152.
16. Steffen F, Bertolo A, Affentranger R, et al. Treatment of Naturally Degenerated Canine Lumbosacral Intervertebral Discs with Autologous Mesenchymal Stromal Cells and Collagen Microcarriers: A Prospective Clinical Study. *Cell Transplant.* 2019 Feb;28(2):201–211.
17. Tanoue H, Shimada M, Ichinohe T, et al. Postoperative outcomes of combined surgery comprising dorsal laminectomy, transarticular screws, pedicle screws and polymethylmethacrylate for dorsal fixation in 21 dogs with degenerative lumbosacral stenosis. *J Am Vet Med Assoc.* 2022 Jun 28;260(14):1813–1819.
18. Smolders LA, Knell SC, Park B, et al. The effects of foraminotomy and intervertebral distraction on the volume of the lumbosacral intervertebral neurovascular foramen: An ex vivo study. *Vet J.* 2020 Feb;256:105435.

CHAPTER 34

Degenerative myelopathy

Joan R. Coates
DVM, MS, DACVIM (Neurology)

Canine degenerative myelopathy (DM) is an inherited, adult-onset neurodegenerative disease, which begins in the central nervous system (CNS), most severely affecting the thoracolumbar spinal cord and later progressing to involve the peripheral nervous system (PNS). Clinical signs consist in progressive paresis and paralysis of the pelvic limbs and eventually all limbs. Canine DM was first described in German Shepherd Dogs by Averill in 1973.[1] The disease was also recognized to affect the nerve roots and cause signs of patellar hyporeflexia.[2] Hence, DM is synonymous with the terms German Shepherd Dog myelopathy and canine degenerative radiculomyelopathy. Canine DM is recognized as a common neurological disorder in a number of pure and mixed breeds, with an overall prevalence of 0.19%.[3] There is no sex predisposition and the mean age of onset of neurological signs is 9 years old in large dog breeds.[1,2] A study in Pembroke Welsh Corgis, a smaller dog breed, reported a mean age of onset of 11 years.[3]

Etiology

Genetics

In 2009, Awano et al. identified a *c.118G>A* transition of glutamate to lysine in exon 2 of the superoxide dismutase 1 gene (*SOD1*), which predicted an E40K amino acid substitution in the SOD1 protein and underlies most cases of canine DM.[4] Homozygosity for the A variant was associated with DM. SOD1 is a ubiquitous intracellular protein functioning as a free radical scavenger. Mutations in *SOD1* have been linked to some forms of familial amyotrophic lateral sclerosis (ALS) in people. *Amyotrophy* means "muscles without nourishment", while lateral is the location within the spinal cord of axonal disease, and *sclerosis* refers to replacement of diseased axons by sclerotic or "scar" tissue. ALS, the most common adult motor neuron disease, is characterized by a loss of motor neurons causing stiffness and slowing of muscle movements, difficulty speaking and swallowing, muscle atrophy, and severe weakness.

Not all *SOD1:c.*118A homozygotes (A/A) develop neurological signs. DM appears to be an age-related, incompletely penetrant autosomal recessive disease, whereas most human *SOD1* mutations are autosomal dominant.[4] Thus, homozygosity for the E40K mutation is a major risk factor for canine DM. Less commonly, some dogs of certain breeds heterozygous (A/G) for the E40K mutation have also developed DM.[5] Since its discovery, the mutant *SOD1*:c.118A allele has been identified in 188 different dog breeds.[5] Based on genotypes from over 100,000 dogs, the frequency of the *SOD1*:c.118A allele is approximately 7.8% in mixed breed dogs and 5.4% in purebred dogs, which makes this allele by far the most common known molecular genetic cause for a canine Mendelian disease.[6] Ivansson et al.[7] reported a modifier locus with the SP110 nuclear body protein that affects risk and age of onset of DM in Pembroke Welsh Corgis *SOD1*:c.118A homozygotes and is associated with altered expression that may be relevant in disease progression. In 2011, a second nonsynonymous *SOD1* variant (*SOD1*:c.52A>T) that predicted a T18S amino acid substitution was identified in Bernese Mountain Dogs to cause DM in the homozygous state[8] or as a compound heterozygote in combination with the *SOD1*:c.118A allele.[5] Laboratories around the world offer DNA tests that genotype individual dogs with respect to the c.118G/A variant. These tests are intended to help breeders avoid matings likely to produce puppies at risk for developing DM and to help veterinarians with the diagnosis of dogs showing signs of presumptive DM.[9]

Histopathology

The pathological features of DM include axonal degeneration with secondary demyelination and astroglial proliferation in all funiculi, although it is most severe in the dorsal portion of the lateral and dorsal funiculi of the middle to lower thoracic spinal cord (Fig. 34.1).[1,2,10,11] Regional axonal loss is severe in the spinal cord of DM-affected dogs, with complete loss of axonal and myelin profiles and replacement by large areas of astrogliosis.[1,2,10,12] Lesions in the ascending and descending pathways within the dorsal portion of the lateral funiculus and the ascending pathways within the dorsal funiculus would explain the loss of general proprioception and paraparesis. More severely affected dogs show significantly greater axonal degeneration and loss in the thoracic spinal cord segments and progression to the cervical and lumbar spinal cord.[10] Neuronal cell body degeneration or loss in the ventral horn of the spinal cord becomes apparent in terminal disease.[13] Neurons in affected dogs contain cytoplasmic aggregates that stain with anti-SOD1 antibodies (Fig. 34.2). Histopathological studies in dogs with neuromuscular signs have revealed denervation atrophy in muscle, nerve fiber loss with axonal degeneration and loss, and secondary myelin loss in the myelinated fibers of peripheral nerves.[4,14] Studies on thoracic motor and sensory neurons have found that sensory neuron (dorsal root ganglion) degeneration did precede motor neuron pathology.[15] Involvement of both the upper motor neuron (UMN) and lower motor neuron (LMN) systems and the central and peripheral motor and sensory neurons classifies DM as a multisystem disease.[16]

Multifactorial pathogenesis

The pathogenesis of DM is multifactorial in onset and progression and may involve diverse forms of cellular abnormalities including protein aggregation, disturbances of protein degradation, mitochondrial dysfunction, oxidative stress, altered neuronal excitability, and altered axonal transport. These events activate and recruit nonneuronal cells (astrocytes, microglia, and oligodendroglia), which exert both neuroprotective and neurotoxic effects on the neurons.[17] Unlike many other mutations, *SOD1* mutations do not lead to disease by loss of normal enzyme function. Instead, these mutations lead to misfolded protein, which accumulates in the neurons and glia.[18] The mutant misfolded SOD1 may induce neurodegeneration by forming insoluble aggregates that alter intracellular function or alter the enzyme substrate specificity and generate toxic by-products. Mutant canine SOD1 remains enzymatically active

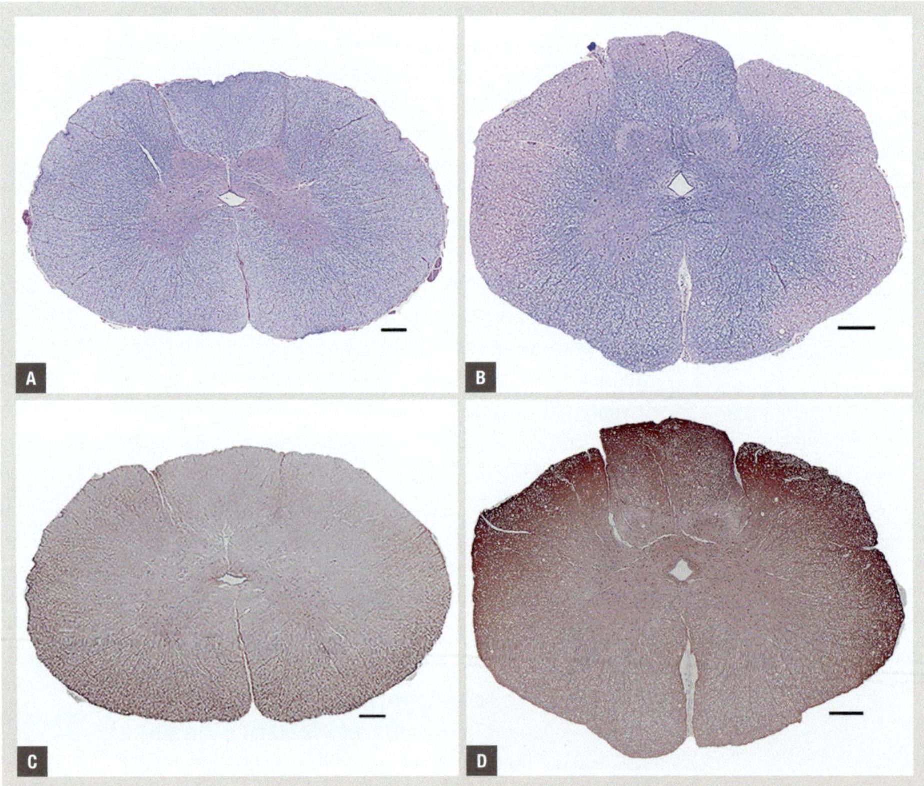

FIG. 34.1 Histopathology of the thoracic spinal cord. Comparison of Luxol fast blue with a periodic acid–Schiff counterstain (LFB/PAS) staining (**A** and **B**) and immunohistochemistry detecting glial fibrillary acidic protein (GFAP) (C and D) from a normal unaffected 15.1-year-old female neutered Pembroke Welsh Corgi (**A** and **C**), and a 11.5-year-old, male neutered Pembroke Welsh Corgi with signs of stage 4 degenerative myelopathy and flaccid tetraplegia (**B** and **D**). The loss of myelinated axons in the dorsal and lateral white matter is depicted by a loss of blue color and increased pallor (**B**) and increased areas of astrogliosis (**D**). The bars represent 400 micrometers.

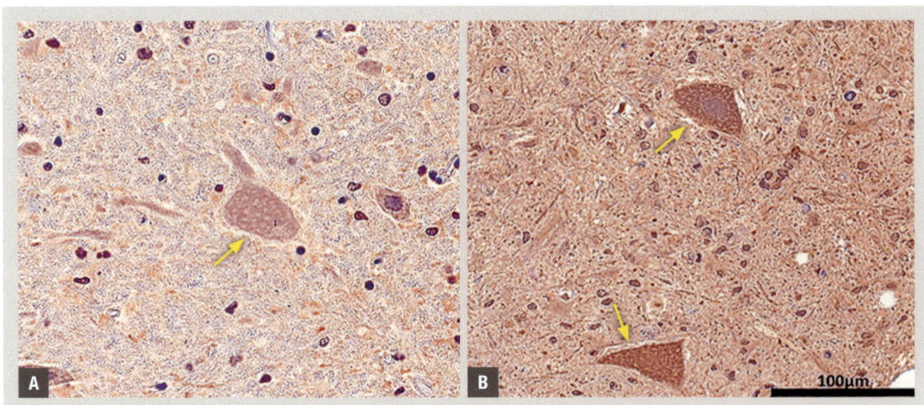

FIG. 34.2 Immunohistochemical staining with anti-SOD1 antibody of the spinal cords from a G/G homozygous normal 13-year-old female neutered mixed-breed (**A**) and an A/A homozygous 11.5-year-old male neutered Pembroke Welsh Corgi with degenerative myelopathy (**B**). The neurons (see arrows) containing cytoplasmic aggregates stained with anti-SOD1 antibodies appear as dark clumps (**B**).

with a tendency for intracellular aggregation, supporting the hypothesis of a toxic gain-of-function mutation.[19] Furthermore, *SOD1* mutations promote protein aggregation, possibly involving structural destabilization, reduction of net negative charge, or production of disulfide-linked oligomers.[20,21] However, whether this mechanism of toxicity is sufficient for the multisystem degeneration observed in DM remains to be elucidated. Ogawa et al.[13] showed that expression of a glutamate transporter (GLT-1) was significantly decreased in the ventral horns of late-stage DM-affected Pembroke Welsh Corgis when compared to that in normal dogs. These results indicate that excitotoxicity related to the reduced expression of the excitatory amino acid transporter 1 (GLT-1) may be involved in neuron loss in DM. The absence of significant differences between unaffected dogs with the *SOD1* mutation and dogs without the mutation also indicates that decreased GLT-1 expression is a secondary event to disease onset and may be involved in the disease progression rather than in its onset.[13]

Clinical features

The clinical course of DM is uniform after the presumptive diagnosis, and progression is divided into four stages (Table 34.1 and Video 34.1).[16] The duration of the clinical course varies depending on when the pet owner elects euthanasia.

Early disease (upper motor neuron signs)

The earliest clinical signs noted by pet owners include asymmetric scuffing of the claws, wearing of nails, and pelvic limb weakness. An asymmetric general proprioceptive ataxia and mild spastic paresis in the pelvic limbs are characteristic early in the disease course (stage 1).[1] Postural reaction testing shows asymmetric paw replacement (proprioceptive positioning) and hopping deficits. At disease onset, spinal reflexes localize the lesion between T3 and L3. Patellar reflexes may be normal or exaggerated to clonus; however, hyporeflexia early in the course of the disease has also been reported.[22] Involvement of the dorsal roots of the femoral nerve may inhibit sensory impulses from stretch receptors located in the quadriceps muscle.[15] Flexor (withdrawal) reflexes may also be normal or show crossed extension (suggestive of chronic upper motor neuron dysfunction). Progress from ambulatory to nonambulatory paraparesis (stage 2) occurs within a median time of 10 months (95% confidence interval; range, 9–12) from the onset of signs.[23] The onset of urinary and fecal incontinence is variable but frequently spared until paraplegia.

Late disease (lower motor neuron signs)

If the DM-affected dog is not euthanized early, clinical signs will progress to lower motor neuron paraplegia and ascend to affect the thoracic limbs within 18 to 24 months (stage 3). Lower motor neuron signs emerge as hyporeflexia of the patellar and withdrawal reflexes, flaccid paralysis,

TABLE 34.1 Pattern of clinical progression of canine degenerative myelopathy.

Disease stage	Clinical signs	Duration of signs from onset (months)
1	**GP ataxia and UMN paraparesis** ■ Progressive GP ataxia ■ Asymmetric spastic paresis ■ Intact spinal reflexes (patellar reflex may be decreased) ■ Lack of paraspinal hyperesthesia	9–12
2	**LMN paraparesis to paraplegia** ■ Nonambulatory paraparesis ■ Decreased or absent PL spinal reflexes ■ Loss of muscle mass in PL ■ +/- Urinary and fecal incontinence	12–18
3	**LMN paraplegia to TL weakness** ■ Signs of TL weakness ■ Flaccid paraplegia ■ Severe loss of PL muscle mass ■ Urinary and fecal incontinence	14–24
4	**LMN tetraplegia and brainstem signs** ■ Flaccid tetraplegia ■ Absent spinal reflexes all limbs ■ Decreased or absent cutaneous trunci reflex ■ Generalized muscle wasting ■ Urinary and fecal incontinence	>36

GP, general proprioceptive; UMN, upper motor neuron; LMN, lower motor neuron; PL, pelvic limbs; TL, thoracic limbs.

and widespread muscle atrophy beginning in the pelvic limbs as the patients become nonambulatory. The paresis becomes symmetric and progresses to flaccid tetraplegia (stage 4).[4,13,24,25] Widespread and severe loss of muscle mass occurs in the axial and appendicular musculature. Previous reports attributed the loss of muscle mass to disuse, but flaccidity in patients with protracted disease suggests denervation and sarcopenia.[14] Eventually, the disease progresses to the brainstem, with cranial nerve signs that include tongue paresis, dysphagia, and an inability to bark. In terminal disease, hypoventilation occurs due to dysfunction of the intercostal muscles reflected by a change of respiration to an abdominal breathing pattern.[25]

Diagnosis

Currently, DM is only definitively diagnosed postmortem by histopathology of the spinal cord. A presumptive diagnosis of DM is based on ruling out other diseases that can cause progressive myelopathy. Diagnosis

Video 34.1

The first part of the video shows a 7-year-old female spayed Rhodesian Ridgeback with early signs of degenerative myelopathy. Note the mild asymmetric general proprioceptive ataxia. Mild spasticity in the pelvic limbs is also observed in the long stride length. Both pelvic limbs show postural reaction deficits, which are slightly more severe on the left side. The spinal reflexes are intact in all limbs. Palpation of the spine did not reveal evidence of spinal hyperesthesia. The neuroanatomical localization is T3 to L3. The second part of the video shows an 8.5-year-old German Shepherd with more severe signs of degenerative myelopathy. The dog is considered nonambulatory paraparetic and needs support in the pelvic limbs, in which postural reactions are absent. The muscle mass in these limbs is atrophied. Pelvic limb tone is somewhat reduced and patellar reflexes are reduced.

can be challenging because many acquired spinal cord diseases and polyneuropathy mimic the initial clinical presentation of DM. It is not uncommon for older dogs with DM to have coexisting orthopedic (e.g., hip dysplasia, cruciate ligament disease) and neurological diseases (e.g., degenerative lumbosacral stenosis, polyneuropathy), which confound the interpretation of the neurological examination. Paw replacement is a useful test that distinguishes between orthopedic and neurological diseases because it does not require weight bearing. It is important to perform a careful neurological examination to differentiate between a T3–L3 and a L4–S2 (e.g., degenerative lumbosacral stenosis) myelopathy. Pelvic limb dysfunction often precedes thoracic limb deficits in generalized neuromuscular disease and caudal cervical spinal cord disease. A key feature when establishing a differential diagnosis early in the course of DM is the absence of paraspinal hyperesthesia, which rules out the involvement of pain-sensitive tissues (e.g., nerve root, disc, periosteum, joint, meninges, muscle). Common differentials causing a T3–L3 nonpainful myelopathy in older dogs include intervertebral disc herniation, spinal cord neoplasia, subarachnoid diverticulum, and other miscellaneous compressive myelopathies.

Diagnostic testing is typically performed in the early stage of disease. Algorithm 34.1 reflects the decision-making process when a dog presents with general proprioceptive ataxia and paresis in the pelvic limbs. A presumptive diagnosis of DM is made by eliminating other neurological diagnoses based on a lack of abnormal findings on thoracic and lumbar magnetic resonance imaging (MRI), electrodiagnostic testing, cerebrospinal fluid (CSF) analysis and DNA testing, along with a stereotypic pattern of disease progression. DNA testing for homozygosity of the risk allele will complement the described diagnostic testing procedures but does not definitively diagnose DM (see Chapter 12).

Typically, the MRI scan is performed between the T3 and S3 spinal cord segments and reviewed for compressive lesions and signal intensity changes in the spinal cord parenchyma indicative of other diseases. Spinal imaging not uncommonly reveals intervertebral disc protrusions, which may confound a diagnosis of DM. Ultimately, the clinician must be guided by the amount of compression, presence or absence of paraspinal hyperesthesia, and clinical experience to assess the severity of myelopathy and speed of disease progression. The reduction in size of the dorsal root ganglion on MRI was shown to provide a noninvasive and quantitative assessment of neurodegeneration in this structure, which may be of diagnostic utility.[26] Additionally, diffusion tensor imaging has shown decreases in fractional anisotropy in regions of spinal cord with severe DM, which correlated with disease grade.[27]

Electrodiagnostic testing is useful for diagnosing neuromuscular diseases and ruling out an underlying polyneuropathy. In DM, electromyography and nerve conduction studies should be within normal limits when upper motor neuron signs predominate. When lower motor signs emerge later in the disease course, electromyography shows spontaneous activity consisting of positive sharp waves and fibrillation potentials in the appendicular musculature.[4,14] Recording of the compound muscle action potentials from stimulation of mixed sensory and motor nerves has shown decreases in amplitude consistent with axonopathy and slowing of conduction velocity and temporal dispersion that indicate demyelination.[4]

Analysis of a CSF sample from a DM-affected dog may show mild increases in protein concentration, which is a nonspecific finding of an active neurological disease. Given the progressive central and peripheral axonal degeneration and loss, phosphorylated neurofilament heavy and neurofilament light in blood and CSF have been shown as potential biomarkers for DM.[28,29]

Treatment and management

To date, no therapy has been shown to slow the clinical progression of DM. Therapies including drugs and nutritional supplements for canine DM have been empiric, with lack of evidence-based medicine approaches for determining efficacy. Physiotherapy improves quality of life and may extend time of ambulation.[30] Kathmann et al.[31] reported survival data from 22 DM-affected dogs that received varying degrees of physiotherapy. Dogs that received intensive physiotherapy had significantly longer survival times compared to dogs that received moderate or no physiotherapy. The main limitations to this study were a lack of randomization and definitive diagnosis, a small group size, and bias from owner perception; however, results warrant further investigation into the efficacy of rehabilitation in dogs affected by DM.

Physiotherapy typically consists of paw protection and active and passive exercises (see Chapter 15).[30,32] Two major goals should be considered in cases of DM: slowing of disuse muscle atrophy and minimization of overuse injury.[33] In dogs with general proprioceptive ataxia, paw protection will prevent injury to the dorsum of the paws and prevent wearing of nails. Paw protection can be achieved using a variety of products tailored to individual dogs based on fit, resistance, and support. The product should be fitted properly and have properties that promote hygiene, water resistance, and durability. Passive range-of-motion (PROM) exercises are performed before active exercises and in affected dogs lacking voluntary movement or strength. Regularly performing PROM exercises maintains joint health, slows contracture, enhances mobility of soft tissues and circulation, and reduces pain and spasticity. Before PROM exercises, the limbs should be warmed and massaged using stroking and pressure techniques. The therapist should gently grasp and slowly and steadily move the limb. PROM exercises are recommended at all stages of progression of DM. Extreme stretching exercises should be performed with caution in denervated muscle to prevent further muscle damage.

Active exercises are recommended for DM-affected dogs when spinal reflexes and at least some voluntary movements remain intact. Active exercises improve muscle mass and strength, neuromuscular balance, and coordination. Such therapies include sit-to-stand and standing exercises, weight shifting, and ambulation exercises. Hydrotherapy, such as walking on an underwater treadmill, allows support of the dog's body weight through buoyancy effects, while the water provides resistance to movement for muscle strengthening and increases limb vascular circulation. Dynamic balance exercises for proprioception include balance balls, rolls, or a balance board. Other proprioceptive exercises include standing or walking on an uneven surface or weaving through obstacles. Balance exercises and coordination activities also strengthen core muscles of the trunk and reduce the exaggerated tone in antigravity muscles of the limbs. Caution must be taken during therapeutic exercises, as these dogs can be easily fatigued, and without care, can accelerate muscle injury.

When a DM-affected dog becomes nonambulatory paraparetic, supportive care is necessary to minimize the secondary consequences of DM, such as contracture, decubitus ulcers, and pneumonia. Assistive devices include an array of equipment to help pet owners with ambulation of their pets and to improve quality of life for the pets. Slings are available commercially and should have a soft lining and be fitted properly. Two- and four-wheel carts are available to provide mobility independence when the dogs are unable to ambulate. Bedding must be supportive enough to distribute the dog's weight evenly over bony prominences to prevent decubitus ulceration. The skin over bony prominences should be assessed twice daily for redness and other evidence of ulceration. Body rotation should be performed every

ALGORITHM 34.1

Diagnostic approach for a dog presenting with a progressive asymmetric pelvic limb general proprioceptive ataxia and spastic paresis. Importantly, genetic testing (dotted line) complements the overall diagnostic approach but does not definitively diagnose degenerative myelopathy. A presumptive diagnosis of degenerative myelopathy is made by ruling out other myelopathies.

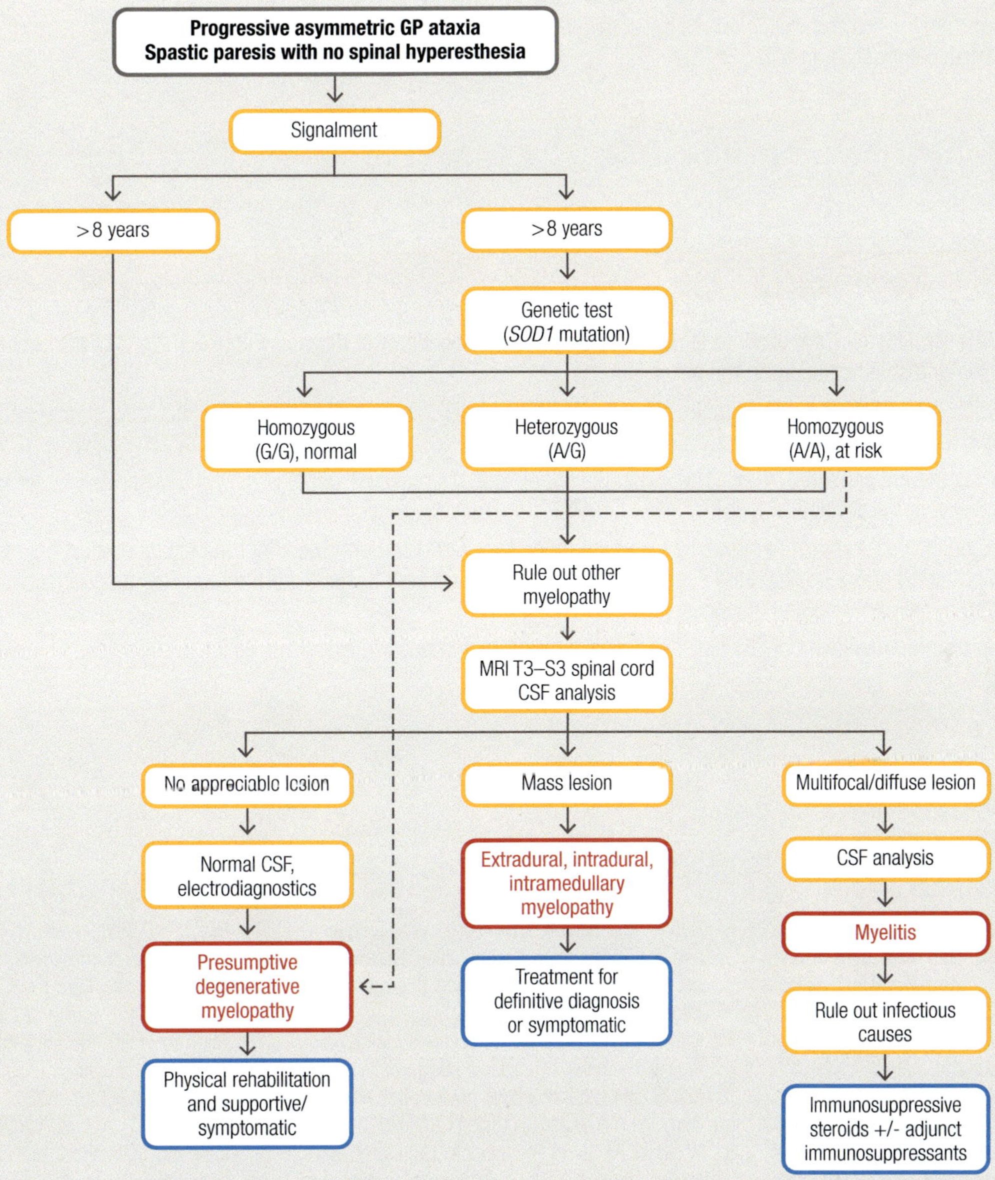

GP, general proprioceptive; MRI, magnetic resonance imaging; CSF, cerebrospinal fluid, T3, third thoracic spinal cord segment; S3, third sacral spinal cord segment.

Diagnostic protocol | Diagnosis | Treatment

4 to 6 hours if the dog is unable to rotate itself. When the dog becomes incontinent, cleanliness is important to prevent fecal and urine scalding. Absorbent materials (diaper pads) should be placed between the dog and the bedding and changed frequently. In late-stage disease, when the dog becomes tetraplegic, dysphagia will predispose to aspiration pneumonia. After discovery of the *SOD1* mutations, DM may serve as a naturally occurring disease model for therapy development in ALS. Many diseases in companion dogs offer a ready clinical population on which therapies can be evaluated using methods similar to those of human clinical trials. As an intermediate-sized model of ALS, dogs with DM could be valuable for temporal studies of disease progression and evaluation of targeted therapies and disease measures used in both ALS and DM.

Prognosis

The long-term prognosis of DM is poor. As a DM-affected dog progresses through the disease stages, the owner encounters the challenges of at-home management and providing appropriate daily care for their dog. Ultimately, the owner will need to make the decision for humane euthanasia, which is often guided with assistance from their primary care veterinarian.

KEY POINTS

- Canine degenerative myelopathy (DM) is an adult-onset, inherited neurodegenerative disease with initial signs of asymmetric general proprioceptive ataxia and spastic paresis in the pelvic limbs.
- During disease progression, the initial upper motor neuron signs in the pelvic limbs progress to lower motor signs and paraplegia, and eventually tetraplegia and brainstem signs.
- Homozygosity for the mutant variant (*SOD1*:c.118G>A) in the superoxide dismutase 1 gene (*SOD1*) is a major risk factor for DM; however, not all homozygotes develop DM.
- A presumptive diagnosis of DM should be made by ruling out other acquired disorders that affect the spinal cord. A neurological examination, MRI of the T3 and S3 spinal cord segments, CSF analysis, and genetic testing are the current standards of care for obtaining an appropriate antemortem diagnosis of DM.
- Physical rehabilitation in management of DM typically consists of active and passive exercises, which are modified in intensity during disease progression.

References

1. Averill DR, Jr. Degenerative myelopathy in the aging German Shepherd dog: clinical and pathologic findings. *J Am Vet Med Assoc.* 1973;162(12):1045–1051.
2. Griffiths IR, Duncan ID. Chronic degenerative radiculomyelopathy in the dog. *J Small Anim Pract.* 1975;16(8):461–471.
3. Coates JR, March PA, Oglesbee M, et al. Clinical characterization of a familial degenerative myelopathy in Pembroke Welsh Corgi dogs. *J Vet Intern Med.* 2007;21(6):1323–1331.
4. Awano T, Johnson GS, Wade CM, et al. Genome-wide association analysis reveals a SOD1 mutation in canine degenerative myelopathy that resembles amyotrophic lateral sclerosis. *Proc Natl Acad Sci U S A.* 2009;106(8):2794–2799.
5. Zeng R, Coates JR, Johnson GC, et al. Breed distribution of SOD1 alleles previously associated with canine degenerative myelopathy. *J Vet Intern Med.* 2014;28(2):515–521.
6. Donner J, Anderson H, Davison S, et al. Frequency and distribution of 152 genetic disease variants in over 100,000 mixed breed and purebred dogs. *PLoS Genet.* 2018;14(4):e1007361.
7. Ivansson EL, Megquier K, Kozyrev SV, et al. Variants within the SP110 nuclear body protein modify risk of canine degenerative myelopathy. *Proc Natl Acad Sci U S A.* 2016;113(22):E3091-3100.
8. Wininger FA, Zeng R, Johnson GS, et al. Degenerative myelopathy in a Bernese Mountain Dog with a novel SOD1 missense mutation. *J Vet Intern Med.* 2011;25(5):1166–1170.
9. Bouché TV, Coates JR, Moore SA, et al. Diagnosis and management of dogs with degenerative myelopathy: A survey of neurologists and rehabilitation professionals. *J Vet Intern Med.* 2023;37(5):1815–1820.
10. March PA, Coates JR, Abyad RJ, et al. Degenerative myelopathy in 18 Pembroke Welsh Corgi dogs. *Vet Pathol.* 2009;46(2):241–250.
11. Braund KG, Vandevelde M. German Shepherd dog myelopathy--a morphologic and morphometric study. *Am J Vet Res.* 1978;39(8):1309–1315.
12. Johnston PEJ, Barrie JA, McCulloch MC, et al. Central nervous system pathology in 25 dogs with chronic degenerative radiculomyelopathy. *Vet Rec.* 2000;146(22):629–633.
13. Ogawa M, Uchida K, Yamato O, et al. Neuronal loss and decreased GLT-1 expression observed in the spinal cord of Pembroke Welsh Corgi dogs with canine degenerative myelopathy. *Vet Pathol.* 2014;51(3):591–602.
14. Shelton GD, Johnson GC, O'Brien DP, et al. Degenerative myelopathy associated with a missense mutation in the superoxide dismutase 1 (SOD1) gene progresses to peripheral neuropathy in Pembroke Welsh corgis and boxers. *J Neurol Sci.* 2012;318(1-2):55–64.
15. Morgan BR, Coates JR, Johnson GC, et al. Characterization of thoracic motor and sensory

neurons and spinal nerve roots in canine degenerative myelopathy, a potential disease model of amyotrophic lateral sclerosis. *J Neurosci Res.* 2014;92(4):531–541.

16. Coates JR, Wininger FA. Canine degenerative myelopathy. *Vet Clin North Am Small Anim Pract.* 2010;40(5):929–950.
17. Toedebusch CM, Snyder JC, Jones MR, et al. Arginase-1 expressing microglia in close proximity to motor neurons were increased early in disease progression in canine degenerative myelopathy, a model of amyotrophic lateral sclerosis. *Mol Cell Neurosci.* 2018;88:148–157.
18. Kobatake Y, Sakai H, Tsukui T, et al. Localization of a mutant SOD1 protein in E40K-heterozygous dogs: Implications for non-cell-autonomous pathogenesis of degenerative myelopathy. *J Neurol Sci.* 2017;372:369–378.
19. Crisp MJ, Beckett J, Coates JR, Miller TM. Canine degenerative myelopathy: biochemical characterization of superoxide dismutase 1 in the first naturally occurring non-human amyotrophic lateral sclerosis model. *Exp Neurol.* 2013;248:1–9.
20. Kimura S, Kamatari YO, Kuwahara Y, et al. Canine SOD1 harboring E40K or T18S mutations promotes protein aggregation without reducing the global structural stability. *PeerJ.* 2020;8:e9512.
21. Wakayama K, Kimura S, Kobatake Y, et al. Molecular mechanisms of aggregation of canine SOD1 E40K amyloidogenic mutant protein. *Molecules.* 2022;28(1):156.
22. Griffiths IR, Duncan ID. Age changes in the dorsal and ventral lumbar nerve roots of dogs. *Acta Neuropathol(Berl).* 1975;32(1):75–85.
23. Kanazono S, Pithua P, Johnson GC, et al. Clinical progression of canine degenerative myelopathy. ACVIM Forum Research Abstracts Program. *J Vet Int Med.* 2013;27(3):673–674.
24. Matthews NS, de Lahunta A. Degenerative myelopathy in an adult miniature poodle. *J Am Vet Med Assoc.* 1985;186(11):1213–1215.
25. Oyake K, Kobatake Y, Shibata S, et al. Changes in respiratory function in Pembroke Welsh Corgi dogs with degenerative myelopathy. *J Vet Med Sci.* 2016;78(8):1323–1327.
26. Naito E, Nakata K, Sakai H, et al. Diffusion tensor imaging-based quantitative analysis of the spinal cord in Pembroke Welsh Corgis with degenerative myelopathy. *J Vet Med Sci.* 2022;84(2):199–207.
27. Johnson PJ, Miller AD, Cheetham J, et al. In vivo detection of microstructural spinal cord lesions in dogs with degenerative myelopathy using diffusion tensor imaging. *J Vet Intern Med.* 2021;35(1):352–362.
28. Toedebusch CM, Bachrach MD, Garcia VB, et al. Cerebrospinal fluid levels of phosphorylated neurofilament heavy as a diagnostic marker of canine degenerative myelopathy. *J Vet Intern Med.* 2017;31(2):513–520.
29. Panek WK, Gruen ME, Murdoch DM, et al. Plasma neurofilament light chain as a translational biomarker of aging and neurodegeneration in dogs. *Molecular Neurobiology.* 2020;57(7):3143–3149.
30. Pancotto TE. Rehabilitation therapy for the degenerative myelopathy patient. *Vet Clin North Am Small Anim Pract.* 2023;53(4):845–856.
31. Kathmann I, Cizinauskas S, Doherr MG, et al. Daily controlled physiotherapy increases survival time in dogs with suspected degenerative myelopathy. *J Vet Intern Med.* 2006;20:927–932.
32. Steinberg HS, Coates JR. Diagnosis of and treatment options for disorders of the spine. In: Zink C, Van Dyke JB (eds.). *Canine Sports Medicine and Rehabilitation*, 2nd ed. Hoboken, NJ: John Wiley & Sons, Inc; 2018. pp. 425–453.
33. Coates JR, Kanazono S. Canine degenerative myelopathy. In: Bonagura JD, Twedt DC (eds.). *Kirk's Current Veterinary Therapy XV.* St. Louis, MO: Elsevier; 2014. pp. 1075–1081.

CHAPTER 35

Myopathies and junctionopathies (myasthenia gravis)

Lara A. Matiasek
Dr. med. vet., DECVN

Myopathies

Muscle pathology can be primary, due to muscle disease, or secondary, resulting from neurogenic damage. Muscle atrophy can occur as a consequence of the myopathy itself, be due to disuse (disuse atrophy), or happen secondary to denervation in nerve disease (neurogenic atrophy). Primary muscle disease may be inherited/breed-specific or acquired. Inflammatory/infectious, endocrine, metabolic, and degenerative etiologies are most prevalent in dogs.

A detailed description of all myopathies is beyond the scope of this book; therefore, only the most common myopathies are discussed below in this chapter.

Clinical presentation

Myopathies are usually generalized, but they can be focal, affecting particular muscle types or regions. In the neurological examination of a patient with polymyopathy, assessment of gait, spinal reflexes, and muscle tone and trophism are of paramount importance. Generalized weakness is often the predominant sign; however, muscle stiffness may occur. Postural reactions are usually normal, although they may be difficult to evaluate in weak patients. Hence, the animal should be adequately supported during the examination. Flexor withdrawal reflexes are usually intact in acute stages but may become weak upon repeated examination, and they are often reduced in chronic phases. In these phases, muscle atrophy and fibrosis are common. In early stages as well as in some specific myopathies, muscle hypertrophy may occur. Myalgia can be a presenting or accompanying complaint.

General diagnostic approach

Signalment, history, and a clinical and neurological examination help to list the differential diagnoses and are the base for investigating myopathies.

Clinicopathological findings

Comprehensive hematology and serum biochemistry (including creatine kinase [CK], electrolytes, lactate, and C-reactive protein) should always be performed. Testing for infectious diseases is recommended (in all cases for *Toxoplasma gondii* and *Neospora caninum*, and also for others such as *Hepatozoon*, *Leishmania*, and *Sarcocystis* species depending on the geographical area). When indicated, thyroid assessment and adrenocorticotropic hormone stimulation/low-dose dexamethasone suppression testing should be added. Genetic testing is available for some inherited myopathies. In the case of suspicion of masticatory muscle myositis (MMM), the presence of serum type IIM antibodies should be investigated. Specific blood tests are listed in the appropriate disease section below.

Serum CK is a very labile enzyme—with a half-life of just over 24 hours in dogs—that indicates muscle fiber damage. It is primarily increased in inflammatory muscle conditions and particularly high in necrotizing or dystrophic myopathies, but CK levels within the reference range do not exclude myopathy. It can also be elevated after surgery, intramuscular injections, prolonged recumbency, and extensive exercise.

Some muscle diseases might also affect the myocardium, in which case cardiac isoforms of troponin may be elevated.

Electrodiagnostic findings

Electromyography (EMG) is of primary importance for the diagnosis of myopathies, but nerve conduction studies and repetitive nerve stimulation should always be performed to differentiate axonal neuropathies and to evaluate for the possibility of simultaneous disease affecting two neuromuscular compartments. The most common EMG findings in myopathies are nonspecific spontaneous activity in the form of fibrillation potentials and positive sharp waves. Complex repetitive discharges may be associated in particular with Cushing's myopathy. Myotonic potentials are characteristic of myotonia congenita. The insertion potential can be prolonged in myopathies or absent in fibrotic muscles. However, a normal EMG does not exclude myopathy.

Diagnostic imaging findings

Chest radiographs are indicated in cases of dysphagia or regurgitation to evaluate for megaesophagus (Fig. 35.1) and aspiration pneumonia. Fluoroscopy provides clearer evidence of dysphagia.

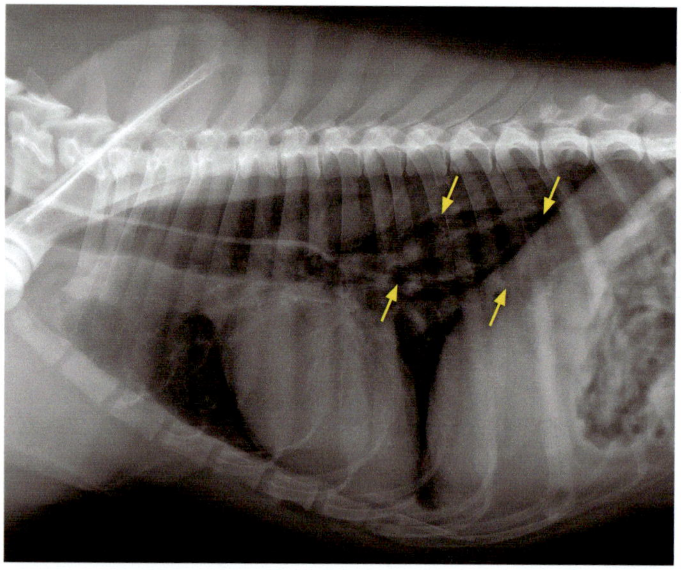

FIG. 35.1 Laterolateral thoracic radiograph of a 10-year-old castrated male crossbreed dog with megaesophagus (arrows). This can be seen in some forms of myopathies and, especially, in dogs affected by acquired myasthenia gravis.

Computed tomography (CT) and magnetic resonance imaging (MRI) can help to select appropriate areas for biopsy but are not classically part of the muscle diagnostic workup.

Muscle biopsy

In most muscle diseases, a biopsy is necessary to provide an etiological diagnosis. In addition, biopsy allows staging of the disease in terms of chronicity, presence of fibrosis, and therefore prognosis. The muscles that are most representative of the ongoing disease should be selected.

Treatment

Etiological treatment should be pursued whenever possible. In case of myalgia or recumbency, appropriate pain management and supportive care are indicated. Physiotherapy is important to prevent permanent dysfunction and chronicity. L-carnitine, coenzyme Q10, and riboflavin can support muscle metabolism and are usually prescribed as generic treatment for many myopathies.

Inflammatory myopathies

Inflammatory myopathies can be immune-mediated (e.g., idiopathic polymyositis, MMM, extraocular myositis) or infectious.

Idiopathic polymyositis

Idiopathic polymyositis may occur at any age and in any breed. Genetic/breed predisposition exists in the Hungarian Vizsla, Dutch Shepherd Dog, Boxer, Newfoundland, Pembroke Welsh Corgi, and Nederlandse Kooikerhondje (Kooiker).[1–5] Polymyositis should also be considered pre- or paraneoplastic, with Boxers being overrepresented.[3]

Weakness and exercise intolerance are usually progressive and may worsen acutely. A stiff, stilted gait is present, and kyphosis and ventroflexion of the neck may occur. Muscle atrophy is common. The myopathy is usually generalized, but it may be focal—for example, affecting the laryngeal, pharyngeal, esophageal, or tongue muscles and resulting in dysphagia, regurgitation, dysphonia, and inspiratory stridor. Patients may also show myalgia. Pyrexia occasionally occurs, possibly due to aspiration pneumonia. Vizsla polymyositis is characterized by pharyngeal dysphagia, salivation, megaesophagus, and atrophy of masticatory muscles.[1] Laryngeal, pharyngeal, and esophageal dysfunction commonly occurs in Newfoundlands.[3] In Corgis, severe tongue and facial muscle atrophy is often seen.[4] Kooikerhondje dogs usually present with locomotor signs and dysphagia.[5]

CK will typically be elevated at least 5- to 10-fold. Tests for infectious diseases should exclude an active infection. EMG shows nonspecific spontaneous activity. Muscle biopsy findings are characterized by inflammation with mononuclear cell infiltration.[6] Chronicity in terms of fiber loss and fibrosis influences the prognosis.

Early diagnosis and aggressive immunosuppressive therapy are prerequisites for a good outcome. Initial treatment usually consists of oral prednisolone (1–2 mg/kg every 12 hours). Other immunosuppressive agents such as azathioprine may be considered. CK normalization and resolution of clinical signs is the time point until which immunosuppression is required. The prognosis is less favorable with megaesophagus, dysphagia, or late treatment. Long-term treatment is usually required, and relapses may occur.[7]

Masticatory muscle myositis

MMM is characterized by the production of antibodies against unique type IIM myofibers, affecting the digastricus, temporalis, and masseter muscles.[8]

Any breed or age can be affected, with a predisposition in large-breed young adults (especially German Shepherds). This condition has been described in Cavalier King Charles Spaniels as young as 3 months of age.[9] Patients with the acute form show bilateral swelling of the masticatory muscles, occasional exophthalmos, and inability to open the mouth (trismus), mainly due to pain. Signs may initially be unilateral, without trismus. The chronic form is characterized by marked bilateral masticatory muscles atrophy, and nonpainful trismus can occur with fibrosis (Video 35.1).[8]

The etiological diagnosis is based on the presence of serum type IIM antibodies (specificity 100%, sensitivity 85–100%[8]). Previous corticosteroid therapy may lead to false-negative results. CK can be elevated in the acute phase. EMG can confirm selective masticatory muscles involvement. In late stages, type IIM antibodies may be absent and EMG normal. MRI and CT are helpful in ruling out other causes of trismus, but they are not routinely performed. Muscle biopsy can confirm the diagnosis (especially in chronic cases with low antibody levels) and provide prognostic information. In the acute phase, there are multifocal, mixed inflammatory infiltrates accompanied by necrosis and phagocytosis; with chronicity, fibrosis may predominate.[8]

In acute MMM, immunosuppression with prednisolone at 1–2 mg/kg per os (PO) every 12 hours is recommended until CK levels and jaw opening are normal. The dose is gradually tapered to the lowest every-other-day

Video 35.1

Labrador Retriever with chronic masticatory muscle myositis. Note the severe muscle atrophy of the masseter and temporalis muscles. The inability to open the mouth is a consequence of the muscle fibrosis that developed after the acute inflammatory phase. Video courtesy of Dr. Gualtiero Gandini.

dose, which should then be maintained for 4–5 months. Serum antibody titers can guide treatment. Other immunosuppressive agents such as azathioprine (1–2 mg/kg PO every 24 hours) can be used if dogs fail to respond or relapse.[8] In chronic phases, anti-inflammatory prednisolone for 1 month and physical jaw therapy are recommended. Adequate water and food intake must be assured. Corticosteroid therapy itself may cause masticatory muscles atrophy, which is not necessarily indicative of disease progression. If early recognized and aggressively treated in the acute phase, the prognosis is good to excellent. Dogs treated in the chronic phase have a guarded prognosis.[8]

Extraocular myositis

Inflammation of the extraocular muscles is presumably immune-mediated. Initially, exophthalmos, strabismus, and decreased ocular motility occurs, with marked strabismus in chronic cases. Golden Retrievers seem to be overrepresented. Diagnosis is made by MRI and ultrasonography. This condition often responds to corticosteroid therapy.[10]

Infectious myopathies

Infectious myopathies are primarily due to protozoa such as *Neospora caninum* or, more rarely, *Toxoplasma gondii*, mostly affecting young or immunocompromised animals. Old cases referred in the literature as toxoplasmosis are most likely neosporosis cases. More sporadically, *Hepatozoon* species, *Leishmania infantum*, bacterial (e.g., leptospiras), or rickettsial infections may be encountered.[10,11]

Clinical signs are typically multisystemic, with diffuse muscle disease and myalgia, and fever may be present. Particularly in patients with neosporosis or toxoplasmosis, radiculoneuritis and central nervous system involvement may occur. A congenital form caused of neosporosis may occur in puppies, where polyradiculoneuritis and myositis lead to ascending paralysis with rigid pelvic limb hyperextension (Video 35.2).[10] Serology can support suspicion, and rising antibody titers are considered confirmative. Polymerase chain reaction (PCR) testing provides evidence of active infection. Elevated serum CK levels and abnormal EMG are nonspecific. Muscle biopsy is often required for definitive diagnosis.[10,11]

The prognosis is good only with adequate early treatment in nonrecumbent patients. However, especially in animals with muscle fibrosis, dysfunction may remain. For protozoal myositis, trimethoprim–sulfonamide (15 mg/kg PO every 12 hours based on sulfonamide) is recommended for at least 4 weeks, possibly combined with pyrimethamine (0.25 mg/kg PO every 24 hours) for 2 weeks. Alternatively, or in addition, clindamycin (10 mg/kg every 8 hours) is an option.[11] Prolonged treatment may be required.

Necrotizing myopathies, rhabdomyolysis, and myoglobinuria

The main histopathological feature of necrotizing myopathies is muscle fiber necrosis in the absence of primary inflammatory infiltrates. It may result from a variety of causes, including muscular dystrophies (MDs), inherited metabolic disorders, exposure to toxins/drugs, infections, or occur after hyperthermic episodes (e.g., heat stroke or malignant hyperthermia; the latter being an inherited disorder of calcium homeostasis in the skeletal muscle).[11–13] CK levels are markedly elevated (up to 100-fold). In severe cases, rhabdomyolysis and myoglobinuria (possibly leading to renal failure) occur and cardiomyopathy may be present.[12] Rhabdomyolysis is the clinical syndrome of muscle necrosis with severely swollen and painful muscles, leading to weakness and collapse. Associated myoglobinuria must be treated with aggressive intravenous fluid therapy. Depending on the etiology, some dogs may recover in 2–3 weeks with supportive care. In other instances, such as in case of MD, the outcome is usually fatal.[12]

Video 35.2

Three-month-old male American Staffordshire Terrier with congenital neosporosis. Note the severe muscle contracture due to muscle fibrosis, particularly pronounced in the quadriceps muscles. There is movement limitation of the limbs and reduced range of motion of the affected joints. Note the inability to flex the stifle joint. Video courtesy of Dr. Gualtiero Gandini.

Endocrine myopathies

Hypothyroid myopathy

In hypothyroidism, muscle catabolism increases, and weakness, stiffness, and muscle wasting can occur, sometimes in association with the typical generalized clinical signs (lethargy, weight gain, and seborrhea). Often, hypothyroid myopathy is subclinical. CK levels are variably elevated, and nonspecific EMG changes may be present. A complete thyroid panel must be performed to exclude nonthyroid illness. Treatment consists of adequate thyroxin supplementation. The prognosis is good, and recovery can be expected within a few weeks.[14]

Cushing's myopathy and corticosteroid myopathy

Both hypercortisolism (Cushing's disease) and chronic corticosteroid administration can result in muscle weakness and atrophy due to increased muscle catabolism.[14] General clinical signs (skin and hair changes, pendulous abdomen) usually occur (Fig. 35.2). Rarely, the gait can be severely stiff due to increased muscle tone, especially in the pelvic limbs (Video 35.3). Hypertrophy of the proximal limb muscles may infrequently occur in case of hypercortisolism. In dogs receiving corticosteroids, atrophy of the masticatory muscles can be prominent.

Diagnosis of hyperadrenocorticism is made by low-dose dexamethasone suppression testing and adrenal gland imaging. Serum CK levels may be

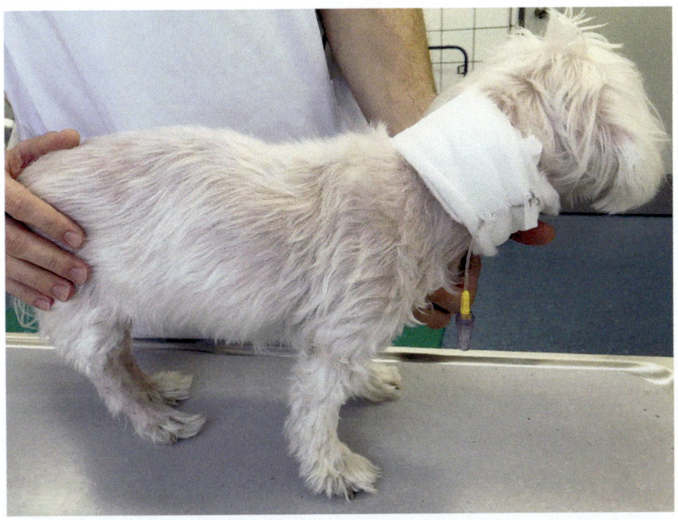

FIG. 35.2 Eleven-year-old spayed female Maltese dog with general clinical signs of Cushing's disease (typical hair coat and skin, pendulous abdomen), muscle atrophy, and weakness.

mildly elevated. EMG in patients with hypercortisolism sometimes reveals complex repetitive discharges, particularly in the proximal limb muscles. In iatrogenic corticosteroid myopathy, muscle signs are reversible, and reducing steroids and possibly switching to other immunomodulatory drugs is the treatment of choice. Improvement may take weeks. In Cushing's disease, adequate treatment of hypercortisolism must be maintained; even if general clinical signs resolve, muscular signs may persist or take months to resolve.

Addison's disease

Adrenal insufficiency results in impaired muscle carbohydrate metabolism and water and electrolyte imbalance (hyperkalemia with depletion of intracellular muscle potassium), leading to muscular weakness and possibly cramping. Signs may occur episodically, including reversible megaesophagus and dysphagia.[11] Diagnosis is made by adrenocorticotropic hormone stimulation testing and adrenal gland imaging. The prognosis is good with appropriate treatment.

Metabolic myopathies

The underlying pathophysiology of this group of rare myopathies is a biochemical defect of myocyte metabolism, which is considered inborn or possibly inherited. For some breeds, specific genetic tests are available.

Mitochondrial myopathies

Mitochondriopathy should be considered in the presence of concurrent central nervous system and muscular disease. Pyruvate dehydrogenase deficiency has been observed in Clumber and Sussex Spaniels, and altered cytochrome c oxidase activity has been confirmed in Old English Sheepdog littermates.[15] A mutation in the acyl-coenzyme A dehydrogenase gene in German Hunting Terriers has also been reported.[16] Changes in resting and postexercise lactate/pyruvate levels and blood gas analysis may aid in the diagnosis, which is confirmed by the detection of red-ragged fibers on muscle biopsy. Electron microscopy allows evaluation of mitochondria. Supportive treatment with L-carnitine (50 mg/kg PO every 12 hours), coenzyme Q10 (100 mg PO every 24 hours), and riboflavin (100 mg PO every 24 hours) is recommended and may result in temporary stabilization.[11]

Lipid storage myopathy

Fatty acid oxidation is an essential source of energy, and carnitine transport into the mitochondria is a prerequisite. Lipid storage myopathy is rare, and affected dogs show myalgia, weakness, and muscle atrophy. Excessive lipid droplets can be detected on oil red O staining of muscle biopsies, while plasma, urine, and muscle carnitine levels can determine a specific metabolic abnormality.[15] Treatment is the same as for mitochondrial myopathies. Prognosis is fair to guarded.

Glycogen storage disease

Various rare defects of glycogen metabolism have been reported in dogs.[7] Fasting hypoglycemia can occur, as can neuromuscular signs and seizures. Even though experimental studies exist, no effective treatment is currently available.

Degenerative myopathies

Degenerative myopathies include MDs and nondystrophic inherited myopathies (e.g., centronuclear myopathy in Labrador Retrievers and Great Danes, X-linked myotubular myopathy).

Muscular dystrophies

MDs are a heterogeneous group of rare degenerative, inherited disorders, and dogs are a spontaneous model for human disease. Gene defects include those associated with the sarcolemma (dystrophin-deficient MD and sarcoglycan-deficient limb-girdle MD) and with the extracellular matrix (congenital MDs associated with defects in collagen 6, laminin α2, and α-dystroglycan).[17] Dystrophin-deficient MD is X-linked, with male dogs clinically affected, while other MDs affect both sexes and are mainly inherited in an autosomal recessive manner. CK level elevations up to 100,000 IU/L and high-grade spontaneous electrical activity in EMG occur with sarcolemmal defects. Absence of structural proteins detected by immunohistology or genetic testing confirms the diagnosis. Clinical signs are usually evident within the first months after birth and, in most cases, progress rapidly, being incompatible with life; however, some MD dogs may live into adulthood. No specific treatment exists, and the prognosis is overall poor.

Dystrophin deficiency has been best studied in humans (Duchenne muscular dystrophy) and in dogs; it was first described in the Golden Retriever and has now been identified in several other breeds.[17] Diffuse muscle atrophy with hypertrophy of certain muscles occurs. Exercise intolerance, bunny hopping, dysphagia, and regurgitation are reported, and cardiomyopathy may result in heart failure. Gene therapy is currently under investigation.[18]

Centronuclear myopathy in Labrador Retrievers and Great Danes

Centronuclear myopathy is an autosomal recessive myopathy primarily described in young Labrador Retrievers and Great Danes.[7] Affected dogs show an insidious onset of slowly progressive weakness, exercise intolerance, and stiff/bunny hopping gait (Video 35.4). In Labradors, ventroflexion of the neck, absent patellar reflex, and decreased flexor reflexes are reported. Signs are exacerbated by cold environments, exercise, and excitement. Great Danes have fawn or brindle coats, present with a stance of legs tucked under the abdomen and extended tail carriage, and show tremors at rest.

CK levels can be normal, and EMG changes are nonspecific. Diagnosis is confirmed by genetic testing. Treatment is supportive (L-carnitine, coenzyme Q, and riboflavin). The prognosis for Labradors is fair, as signs stabilize at around 1 year of age. In Great Danes, the course is

Video 35.3

Gait evaluation in a dog with hypercortisolism showing severe muscle stiffness (Cushing's myotonia). Note the hopping stiff gait, the severe persistent extensor rigidity even when lying down, and the difficulty flexing the pelvic limb joints due to the sustained muscle contraction. Video courtesy of Dr. Gualtiero Gandini.

Video 35.4

Gait examination in a 7-month-old female Labrador Retriever with centronuclear myopathy. Note the progressive exercise intolerance characterized by a low head carriage, a short-strided gait, and the increasing necessity to rest. Note also the absence of ataxia. Diagnosis was confirmed by muscle biopsy and genetic testing. Video courtesy of Dr. Gualtiero Gandini.

progressive, although, in milder forms, survival for up to 55 months has been reported.[19]

X-linked myotubular myopathy

A more severe X-linked myotubular myopathy clinically indistinguishable from centronuclear myopathy has been described in male Labradors, but also in Manchester Terriers and Rottweilers. Diagnosis is made via muscle biopsy, and a gene defect has been found in the Labrador Retriever. The prognosis is generally poor.

Miscellaneous myopathies

Other sporadic congenital/presumed inherited myopathies with protein accumulation in canine muscles have been described (e.g., nemaline rod myopathy, myofibrillary myopathy). Gross muscle hypertrophy with myostatin deficiency has been reported in Whippets.

Myotonia congenita

Myotonia is the prolonged contraction or delayed relaxation of muscles after stimulation or exercise. Clinical signs include stiffness and muscle dimpling. Congenital forms are commonly due to reduced chloride conductance across muscle membranes. CK levels are normal, but electrophysiological tests show classical waxing and waning myotonic discharges. In some breeds (e.g., Miniature Schnauzer) genetic testing is available. Treatment with procainamide (40–50 mg/kg PO every 8–12 hours) or mexiletine (8.3 mg/kg PO every 8 hours) can be attempted,[11] with variable prognosis.

Fibrotic myopathies

Fibrotic myopathy is characterized by a unilateral or bilateral, acquired, sporadically occurring, palpable fibrous band within a specific muscle.[11] It is mostly seen in male German Shepherds and may be related to excessive physical activity. Dogs affected by gracilis and semitendinosus/semimembranosus myopathy show a classic gait characterized by a shortened pelvic limb stride and rapid medial rotation of the paw, due to the inability to extend the fibrotic muscles (mechanical lameness) (Video 35.5). Typically, this myopathy is not painful, and affected dogs can live a normal life. Both infraspinatus and iliopsoas myopathies result in lameness and can be painful in the early stages. Neurological examination is normal, and EMG of the respective muscles shows lack of insertion potential. Tenectomies may be performed, but the prognosis for recovery of normal gait is poor.

Vascular myopathies

In contrast to cats, dogs very rarely suffer from ischemic (neuro-)myopathy due to thrombosis/thromboembolism of the terminal aorta/iliac arteries. Dogs with ischemic (neuro-)myopathy show various degrees of lameness and/or gait anomaly of the affected limbs and may not have pain. The diagnostic approach includes ultrasound or cross-sectional imaging of the region of the affected vessels and investigation of hypercoagulability. Treatment and prognosis depend on the underlying cause.

Video 35.5

Five-year-old female German Shepherd with bilateral gracilis and semitendinosus fibrotic myopathy. Note the medial rotation of the stifle joint and the external rotation of the hock joint due to the inability to extend the fibrotic muscles. The dog is not painful.

Junctionopathies (myasthenia gravis)

Diseases affecting neuromuscular transmission may act presynaptically, synaptically, or postsynaptically. The most common junctionopathy is acquired immune-mediated myasthenia gravis (MG). More rarely, congenital myasthenic syndromes (CMSs),[20] toxins such as organophosphates or carbamate, botulism, and tick paralysis have been reported as causes of junctionopathy.[21]

Acquired immune-mediated myasthenia gravis

MG is an autoimmune disease in which neuromuscular transmission is impaired by autoantibodies against the neuromuscular junction. The acetylcholine receptor (AChR) is the most common target, but autoantibodies may also be directed against other components of the neuromuscular junction, such as the muscle-specific kinase; however, these other autoantibodies are not routinely measured. Therefore, subclassification as seronegative MG is suggested. In addition, MG may be associated with thymoma or, less frequently, other neoplasia (paraneoplastic syndrome), leading to further subclassification (Table 35.1).[20]

Acquired MG typically occurs in dogs older than 6 months. Three clinical forms have been described: focal, generalized, and acute fulminant.[20,21]

- Focal MG selectively involves one or more nonappendicular skeletal muscle groups (facial, esophageal, pharyngeal, or laryngeal), resulting in facial weakness, cranial nerve deficits, dysphagia, dysphonia, and regurgitation/megacsophagus (see Fig. 35.1).
- In generalized MG, (mild to severe) appendicular skeletal muscle weakness occurs with or without additional focal signs. Classically, exercise-induced weakness up to collapse is present (see Chapter 7). The stride becomes progressively shorter, and the gait appears stiff and stilted before the animal needs to rest or collapses. After resting for a while, the dog is usually able to stand up again and walk a few steps before the next episode of exercise-induced weakness occurs (Video 35.6). On neurological examination, spinal reflexes may decrease after repeated elicitation.

TABLE 35.1 Classification of myasthenia gravis (MG) in dogs.

Focal MG	Non–thymoma associated
	Thymoma associated
Generalized MG	Non–thymoma associated
	Thymoma associated
	Seronegative*
Acute fulminant MG	Non–thymoma associated
	Seronegative*

* Seronegative: clinical, neurological, pharmacological, and electrophysiological findings consistent with MG, normalization of clinical signs with acetylcholinesterase inhibitor treatment, and at least twice negative testing for acetylcholine receptor autoantibodies via radioimmunoassay.[20]

- The acute fulminant form is generalized and rapidly progressive, with possible focal components, resulting in recumbency, and may be associated with respiratory failure and death.[20]

The gold standard for the diagnosis of acquired immune-mediated MG is the detection of serum autoantibodies against AChRs (>0.6 nmol/L) by radioimmunoassay,[21] which is highly sensitive and specific. Immunosuppressive treatment can cause false-negative results. Clinical suspicion may be supported by a positive neostigmine test (40 µg/kg intramuscularly [IM] or 20 µg/kg intravenously) (Video 35.7), but this test is neither sensitive nor specific. Repetitive nerve stimulation supports the diagnosis of MG by showing a compound muscle action potential decrement greater than 10%.[20,21]

Dogs suspected of having MG should have a chest radiograph performed to assess for megaesophagus and aspiration pneumonia. Treatment consists of supportive care, symptomatic treatment with acetylcholinesterase inhibitors, and possibly immunosuppression. In acute fulminant MG patients, therapeutic plasma exchange, human intravenous immunoglobulins, and immunoadsorption have been reported.[22–24] If a thymoma is present, thymectomy should be performed. Supportive care includes elevated food/water bowls (specially designed feeding supports can be used), keeping the patient upright for 10–20 minutes after feeding, or gastrostomy tube placement. In severe cases, particularly those with acute fulminant MG, mechanical ventilation might be required. The acetylcholinesterase inhibitor pyridostigmine should be administered at 0.5 mg/kg PO every 8–12 hours. To avoid side effects (gastrointestinal, salivation, weakness at high doses) and cholinergic crisis, a low starting dose is recommended.[21] If necessary, neostigmine can be injected (0.04 mg/kg IM every 6 hours).[11] In dogs, anticholinesterase treatment is generally successful, producing the clinical remission of exercise intolerance. However, many dogs tend to have persistent megaesophagus despite treatment. Immunosuppressive drugs should be carefully considered in those cases that do not respond to symptomatic treatment. Anti-inflammatory doses of corticosteroids (prednisolone 0.5 mg/kg PO every 24 hours) may initially be used in the absence of aspiration pneumonia. If necessary, corticosteroids can be gradually increased every 2 weeks up to an immunosuppressive dose (2 mg/kg PO every 24 hours) under careful observation. Once clinical remission is achieved, slow well-controlled tapering over weeks can be considered.[11] If corticosteroids have an inadequate response, the addition of azathioprine has been suggested (2 mg/kg PO every 24 hours). Use of cyclosporine as well as mycophenolate mofetil has also been described.[11,23] Overall, there is limited data describing effective immunosuppression in dogs with MG.

Video 35.6

Dog with acquired myasthenia gravis before a neostigmin test. Note the short-strided gait and the need to rest after a few steps (exercise-induced weakness). Video courtesy of Dr. Velia Hülsmeyer.

Video 35.7

Same dog as in Video 35.6 after intramuscular administration of neostigmin. Weakness and exercise intolerance have completely disappeared. Video courtesy of Dr. Velia Hülsmeyer.

Serial AChR antibody measurements guide treatment in nonimmunosuppressed animals. Relapses may occur. Although spontaneous clinical and immunological remission has been reported in up to 89% cases within an average of 6.4 months,[21] aspiration pneumonia and respiratory failure remain common causes of death, with 1-year mortality rates ranging from 40% to 60%.[20] The long-term outcome in dogs with thymoma-associated MG appears to be less favorable.[20]

Congenital myasthenic syndromes

CMSs have been reported in a variety of breeds, with an identified or suspected genetic cause (inherited autosomal recessive). They can be subcategorized in presynaptic, synaptic, and postsynaptic disorders. Presynaptic CMSs are associated with a defect in acetylcholine synthesis (gene identified in the Old Danish Pointer). Synaptic CMSs are due to acetylcholinesterase deficiency (gene identified in the Labrador and Golden Retriever). Postsynaptic CMSs are caused by AChR deficiency (gene identified in the Jack Russel Terrier and Heideterrier).[20] The onset of clinical signs occurs in the first few weeks to months of life. Affected dogs show skeletal muscle weakness and fatigability, and testing for AChR autoantibodies is negative. Acetylcholinesterase inhibitors may be effective in postsynaptic CMSs, ineffective in presynaptic CMSs, and may even worsen signs in synaptic CMSs. Repetitive nerve stimulation testing is expected to show decremental changes. The prognosis for most CMSs is unfavorable/fatal; however, postsynaptic forms may respond to treatment.[19] A reversible CMS has been reported in young Smooth-Haired Miniature Dachshunds.[21]

KEY POINTS

- Polymyopathies can be primary or secondary to neuropathic disorders.
- Primary polymyopathies can be further divided into inflammatory/infectious and noninflammatory (endocrine, metabolic, degenerative inherited myopathies).
- Clinical signs are mostly generalized and consist mainly of weakness, exercise intolerance, and possibly myalgia.
- The most important focal myopathy is immune-mediated masticatory muscle myositis (MMM).
- Elevation of serum creatine kinase (CK) levels is dependent upon integrity of the sarcolemma and is particularly pronounced in necrotizing myopathies. CK levels within the reference range do not exclude myopathies.
- Electromyography (EMG) may show nonspecific spontaneous activity in the presence of normal nerve conduction velocity. Normal EMG findings do not exclude myopathies.
- With some exceptions (e.g., acute form of MMM, endocrine myopathies), diagnosis is made via muscle biopsy or genetic testing.
- Etiologic treatment should be pursued when possible.
- Supportive treatment is recommended and primarily consists of L-carnitine, coenzyme Q10, and riboflavin.
- The prognosis depends on the etiology, but early diagnosis of the disease often plays a critical role.
- Acquired myasthenia gravis (MG) is the most common junctionopathy in the dog.
- Acquired MG has three clinical forms: focal, generalized, and acute fulminant.
- Diagnosis of MG is made by measuring autoantibodies against acetylcholine receptors. Neostigmine testing may support the suspicion of MG but is not specific nor sensitive.
- Treatment of acquired MG is symptomatic. Most affected dogs achieve clinical remission, but megaesophagus often persists.
- Immunosuppressive treatment of acquired MG should be carefully considered if there is no response to symptomatic treatment.

References

1. Tauro A, Addicott D, Foale RD, et al. Clinical features of idiopathic inflammatory polymyopathy in the Hungarian Vizsla. *BMC Vet Res.* 2015 Apr 21;11:97.
2. Shelton GD, Minor KM, Li K, et al. A mutation in the mitochondrial aspartate/glutamate carrier leads to a more oxidizing intramitochondrial environment and an inflammatory myopathy in Dutch Shepherd dogs. *J Neuromuscul Dis.* 2019;6(4):485–501.
3. Evans J, Levesque D, Shelton GD. Canine inflammatory myopathies: a clinicopathologic review of 200 cases. *J Vet Intern Med.* 2004 Sep–Oct;18(5):679–691.
4. Toyoda K, Uchida K, Matsuki N, et al. Inflammatory myopathy with severe tongue atrophy in Pembroke Welsh Corgi dogs. *J Vet Diagn Invest.* 2010 Nov;22(6):876–885.
5. Opmeer Y, Grinwis GCM, Shelton GD, et al. An inflammatory myopathy in the Dutch Kooiker dog. *Animals (Basel).* 2023 Apr 29;13(9):1508.
6. Pumarola M, Moore PF, Shelton GD. Canine inflammatory myopathy: analysis of cellular infiltrates. *Muscle Nerve.* 2004 Jun;29(6):782–789.
7. Dewey CW, Talarico LR. Myopathies: disorders of skeletal muscle. In: Dewey CW, Da Costa RC (eds). *Practical Guide to Canine and Feline Neurology*, 3rd ed. Iowa, USA: Wiley-Blackwell; 2016. pp. 481–520.
8. Melmed C, Shelton GD, Bergman R, Barton C. Masticatory muscle myositis: pathogenesis, diagnosis, and treatment. *Compend Contin Educ Vet.* 2004;26(8):590–605.
9. Pitcher GD, Hahn CN. Atypical masticatory muscle myositis in three cavalier King Charles spaniel littermates. *J Small Anim Pract.* 2007 Apr;48(4):226–228.
10. Podell M. Inflammatory myopathies. *Vet Clin North Am Small Anim Pract.* 2002 Jan;32(1):147–167.
11. Platt S, Shelton GD. Exercise intolerance and collapse. In: Platt S, Olby N (eds). *BSAVA Manual of Canine and Feline Neurology*, 4th ed. Gloucester, UK: BSAVA; 2013. pp. 342–367.
12. Shelton GD. Rhabdomyolysis, myoglobinuria, and necrotizing myopathies. *Vet Clin North Am Small Anim Pract.* 2004 Nov;34(6):1469–1482.
13. Brunson DB, Hogan KJ. Malignant hyperthermia: a syndrome not a disease. *Vet Clin North Am Small Anim Pract.* 2004 Nov;34(6):1419–1433.
14. Platt SR. Neuromuscular complications in endocrine and metabolic disorders. *Vet Clin North Am Small Anim Pract.* 2002 Jan;32(1):125–146.
15. Platt SR, Garosi LS. Neuromuscular weakness and collapse. *Vet Clin North Am Small Anim Pract.* 2004 Nov;34(6):1281–1305.
16. Lepori V, Mühlhause F, Sewell AC, et al. A nonsense variant in the *ACADVL* gene in German Hunting Terriers with exercise induced metabolic myopathy. *G3 (Bethesda).* 2018 May 4;8(5):1545–1554.
17. Shelton GD, Minor KM, Friedenberg SG, et al. Current classification of canine muscular dystrophies and identification of new variants. *Genes (Basel).* 2023 Jul 29;14(8):1557.
18. Nghiem PP, Kornegay JN. Gene therapies in canine models for Duchenne muscular dystrophy. *Hum Genet.* 2019 May;138(5):483–489.
19. Lujan Feliu-Pascual A, Shelton GD, Targett MP, et al. Inherited myopathy of great Danes. *J Small Anim Pract.* 2006 May;47(5):249–254.

20. Mignan T, Targett M, Lowrie M. Classification of myasthenia gravis and congenital myasthenic syndromes in dogs and cats. *J Vet Intern Med.* 2020 Sep;34(5):1707–1717.
21. Shelton GD. Myasthenia gravis and disorders of neuromuscular transmission. *Vet Clin North Am Small Anim Pract.* 2002 Jan;32(1):189–206.
22. Vitalo A, Buckley G, Londoño L. Therapeutic plasma exchange as adjunct therapy in 3 dogs with myasthenia gravis and myasthenia-like syndrome. *J Vet Emerg Crit Care (San Antonio).* 2021 Jan;31(1):106–111.
23. Penderis J, Martin-Vaquero P. Junctionopathies: disorders of the neuromuscular junction. In: Dewey CW, Da Costa RC (eds). *Practical Guide to Canine and Feline Neurology*, 3rd ed. Iowa, USA: Wiley-Blackwell; 2016. pp. 521–557.
24. Sänger F, Dörfelt S, Giani B, et al. Successful emergency management of a dog with ventilator-dependent acquired myasthenia gravis with immunoadsorption. *Animals (Basel).* 2023 Dec 21;14(1):33.

CHAPTER 36

Neuropathies

Lluís Sánchez
DVM, MRCVS, DECVN

This chapter focuses on the most common neuropathies in dogs and divides them into generalized, cranial, and single-limb neuropathies. Table 36.1 provides a list of generalized neuropathies. Although optic neuritis is strictly speaking not a neuropathy, it will be included in this chapter.

Generalized neuropathies

Acute canine polyradiculoneuritis

Acute canine polyradiculoneuritis (ACP), also known as Coonhound paralysis or acute idiopathic polyradiculoneuritis, is the most common acute polyneuropathy in dogs and shares a lot of similarities with Guillain–Barré syndrome in humans. In this disease, an immune-mediated reaction to the axons and/or myelin of the spinal roots and nerves is suspected, with the ventral roots being the most severely affected of these structures, especially in the lumbosacral region.[1] The immune-mediated reaction may be induced either by molecular mimicry or the production of autoantibodies against certain components of the membrane of axons or Schwann cells, especially the GM2 gangliosides.[2]

The trigger for ACP is usually unknown, but reported precipitating causes and risk factors include raccoon bites, respiratory or gastrointestinal infections, consumption of raw chicken (potentially associated with *Campylobacter* spp. infection), and vaccination, although the etiological role of the latter has been questioned.[1,2] ACP is found worldwide, and seasonality has been reported. Dogs of different breeds and ages (puppies and adults) have been reported to be affected by ACP.[2]

Clinical signs usually start in the pelvic limbs and progress to the thoracic limbs. A stilted, stiff, short-strided gait may initially be seen, and within 2–10 days, a lower-motor-neuron (LMN) tetraparesis of varying degrees (or even tetraplegia), with intact sensation, develops (Video 36.1).[1] Affected dogs may be unable to lift their heads but typically remain able to wag their tails.[1] On rare occasions, a life-threatening respiratory paresis or paralysis may develop.[1,2]

Facial nerve involvement may be observed, and dysphonia is common. In the acute phase, some animals demonstrate hyperesthesia on palpation or manipulation of their lumbar vertebral column or limbs, and conscious urination and defecation are spared.[1]

The main differential diagnoses for ACP include fulminant myasthenia gravis, botulism, and, depending on the geographical area, tick paralysis.[1] The measurement of serum anti-GM2 ganglioside antibodies may have diagnostic value, but this is not commercially available yet.[2] Electromyography (EMG) reveals denervation potentials (fibrillation potentials and positive sharp waves) in the affected muscles (especially after day 4 of disease), and electroneurography shows abnormalities on motor nerve conduction studies and F-wave evaluation that are indicative of proximal demyelination and a motor axonopathy, with the proximal portions of the nerves, ventral roots or both being more severely affected than the distal portions.[1] Lumbar cerebrospinal fluid (CSF) analysis may reveal albuminocytological dissociation. Nerve biopsies

TABLE 36.1 Common differential diagnoses for generalized neuropathies.

Neuropathies	Common differential diagnoses
Inflammatory, idiopathic	■ Acute canine polyradiculoneuritis ■ Chronic inflammatory demyelinating polyneuropathy ■ Sensory polyganglioradiculoneuritis ■ Others
Infectious	■ Protozoal polyradiculoneuritis (mainly secondary to neosporosis)
Metabolic	■ Diabetic neuropathy[a] ■ Hypothyroidism ■ Hypoglycemia[b]
Toxic	■ Heavy metals (e.g., mercury, thallium, lead) ■ Antibiotics (e.g., lasalocid, nitrofurantoin, salinomycin) ■ Pesticides (e.g., organophosphates) ■ Organic solvents ■ Chemicals (e.g., acrylamide, hexacarbons) ■ Vitamins (e.g., pyridoxine) ■ Antineoplastic drugs (e.g., vincristine, vinblastine, cisplatin)
Neoplastic	■ Paraneoplastic neuropathy (mainly insulinoma) ■ Lymphoma and other round cell neoplasms
Degenerative	■ Various types

[a] Usually subclinical in dogs. [b] Associated with insulinoma.

Video 36.1

Six-month-old entire male Cocker-Poodle with acute canine polyradiculoneuritis exhibiting generalized weakness. Note the intact sensation.

usually reveal no abnormalities or nonspecific findings, but nerve root biopsies (albeit rarely necessary) may be performed.[1]

Treatment is mainly supportive and includes physiotherapy, nursing care, and appropriate nutrition.[1] Owners should pay special attention to body-weight management and the development of contractures and decubitus ulcers. While corticosteroids have not been shown to be beneficial in ACP,[1] the administration of intravenous immunoglobulin, especially at a higher dose, may shorten the recovery time in dogs with this disease, with rare side effects.[3] The prognosis for full recovery is usually favorable and typically occurs within 3–6 weeks but may be prolonged to months.[1] Relapses have been reported.[1,3]

Chronic inflammatory demyelinating polyneuropathy

Chronic inflammatory demyelinating polyneuropathy is a polyneuropathy of likely immune-mediated origin that affects adult dogs of any gender or breed.[4] Clinical signs are typically characterized by a chronic, slowly progressive, and sometimes relapsing-remitting LMN tetraparesis, with the pelvic limbs being commonly affected first.[4,5] Some animals may present with cranial nerve deficits such as dysphonia, laryngeal paralysis, megaesophagus, or facial paralysis. The diagnosis is based on the clinical history, electrophysiological changes, muscle/nerve biopsies, and exclusion of other causes of polyneuropathy. The main pathological finding in nerve biopsies is the presence of demyelination.[5] Many dogs respond to corticosteroid treatment at immunosuppressive dosages, but response may be incomplete.[5]

Hypothyroid neuropathy

Albeit rarely, neuromuscular signs may be associated with hypothyroidism.[5,6] Possible underlying pathophysiological mechanisms include axonal damage and demyelination secondary to thyroid hormone deficiency, and compression of cranial nerves by mucinous deposits in the soft tissues.[5]

Clinical signs of hypothyroid neuropathy include paresis or rarely lameness of one or various limbs and dysfunction of one or multiple cranial nerves (e.g., facial paresis, vestibular signs, and trigeminal nerve dysfunction), often unilaterally.[5] Although hypothyroidism has been associated with megaesophagus and laryngeal paralysis, a cause-and-effect relationship for these has not been demonstrated. Extraneural signs of hypothyroidism (e.g., weight gain and alopecia) may or may not be present. The diagnosis is based on the confirmation of the hypothyroidism, electrophysiological changes, muscle/nerve biopsies, exclusion of other causes of polyneuropathy, and response to treatment.[5]

Electrophysiological testing reveals abnormal spontaneous activity on EMG, reduced motor and sensory nerve conduction velocities on electroneurography, and possibly abnormal brainstem auditory evoked responses. Muscle biopsies may reveal type I and II fiber atrophy (i.e., denervation atrophy) or a selective type II fiber atrophy. Nerve biopsies may show axonal degeneration and demyelination.[5] For a detailed discussion on the diagnosis of hypothyroidism, the reader is referred to comprehensive reviews of this topic. Treatment consists of levothyroxine administration. Prognosis is favorable, and most dogs improve neurologically within several days and in up to 3–8 weeks. The cranial nerve deficits, megaesophagus, and laryngeal paralysis may not improve.[5]

Diabetic neuropathy

Diabetes mellitus may lead to a clinical or subclinical neuropathy, especially in poorly regulated patients.[5] Diabetic neuropathy is less frequently symptomatic in dogs than in cats.[5] The pathophysiology of diabetic neuropathy includes multiple theories.[5] The most common clinical sign is tibial nerve paresis, which leads to tarsal overflexion and a plantigrade posture.[6] Other clinical signs in dogs include, among others, paraparesis (with this possibly progressing to tetraparesis), pelvic limb ataxia, a palmigrade posture, decreased postural reactions and segmental spinal reflexes, distal muscle atrophy, and Horner's syndrome.[5,6] Albeit poorly recognized, paresthesias and hyperesthesia secondary to sensory nerve dysfunction may also be a feature of diabetic neuropathy in animals.[5]

The diagnosis is based on the confirmation of a polyneuropathy in a dog with diabetes mellitus (electrodiagnostics and muscle/nerve biopsies). While electroneurography consistently reveals abnormalities in motor and sensory nerve conduction studies, as well as in F-wave and cord dorsum assessment, EMG may only show, if any, subtle or patchy spontaneous activity in the affected muscles.[5] These findings mainly reflect demyelination, which is confirmed on histopathological analysis of nerve biopsies.[5] Clinical signs often resolve when diabetes mellitus is well controlled.[6]

Paraneoplastic neuropathy

Paraneoplastic neuropathies are cancer-associated alterations in nerve structure and/or function that are not directly related to the physical effects of the primary or metastatic tumor.[7] Paraneoplastic neuropathies are presumptively caused by immune-mediated host responses to the tumor and nerves.[5] Paraneoplastic neuropathies are often subclinical,[7] but clinical forms have been described, mainly with insulinoma; however, other tumors have also been reported to lead to symptomatic paraneoplastic neuropathies.[5] In dogs with insulinoma, hypoglycemia may also play a role in the pathophysiology of the neuropathy.[5] A paraneoplastic syndrome may be the first clinical sign of malignancy and clinical paraneoplastic neuropathies are characterized by diffuse LMN signs.[7] The diagnosis of a paraneoplastic neuropathy is based on the clinical history, electrophysiological changes, muscle/nerve biopsies, identification of the underlying neoplasia and exclusion of other causes of polyneuropathy. Nerve biopsies may reveal excessive paranodal/segmental demyelination and remyelination, or excessive axonal degeneration with myelin ovoids and globules.[7] Paraneoplastic neuropathies may or may not resolve when the tumors are successfully treated.[7] Immunomodulatory therapies such as corticosteroids or intravenous immunoglobulin may also be considered to treat the underlying immune-mediated etiology.[5] Relapses of previously resolved paraneoplastic syndromes may indicate tumor recurrence, even before this is clinically detectable.[7]

Degenerative polyneuropathies

A number of rare inherited and sporadic degenerative polyneuropathies have been recognized in young and old dogs.[5,8] Some of these inherited degenerative polyneuropathies are limited to specific breeds, and most are suspected to have an autosomal recessive mode of inheritance.[8]

Over the last few years, the genetic basis for some of these diseases has been elucidated. Some degenerative polyneuropathies are a consequence of primary peripheral nervous system pathology, and others are a consequence of degeneration of central nervous system nuclei.[6] Degenerative polyneuropathies may present clinically as part of a more generalized degenerative process of the nervous system, including both the central and peripheral nervous systems (e.g., globoid cell leukodystrophy) and are known as syndromic degenerative polyneuropathies. Others present exclusively with signs of polyneuropathy and are known as nonsyndromic degenerative polyneuropathies.[8] Degenerative polyneuropathies may be motor, sensory, or both, and some may be associated with autonomic dysfunction.[8] Some degenerative polyneuropathies may manifest initially with focal clinical signs such as laryngeal paralysis and megaesophagus.[8]

In general, the diagnosis is based on the signalment, clinical history, electrophysiological testing, muscle/nerve biopsies, exclusion of other types of polyneuropathies and, depending on the case, genetic testing. Treatment is usually symptomatic (e.g., surgery for laryngeal paralysis or physical therapy), and prognosis is in general grave, but in some animals the disease may progress very slowly or become static.

Cranial neuropathies

Optic neuritis

Optic neuritis (i.e., inflammation of the optic nerves, chiasm, and/or tracts) is typically caused by meningoencephalitis of unknown origin (MUO), especially granulomatous meningoencephalitis (the ocular or disseminated form). In this chapter, optic neuritis secondary to MUO will be referred to as noninfectious, idiopathic optic neuritis (NION). Other causes include, among others, infections (e.g., with *Toxoplasma gondii*), neoplasia, orbital inflammation, trauma, nutritional etiologies (e.g., hypovitaminosis A) and toxins (e.g., ivermectin).[9,10] Middle-aged dogs are overrepresented.[9,10] Bilateral or unilateral blindness is observed and usually associated with an acute presentation and abnormal pupillary light reflexes (PLR).[9] Other neurological abnormalities may be present; however, abnormal findings during physical examination are rare unless the cause is a microbial infection.[9] Fundoscopy most commonly reveals optic disc swelling and elevation (Fig. 36.1), usually representing papillitis, but the optic disc may be normal if the optic nerves are proximally affected.[9,10] Other changes include optic disc hemorrhage or atrophy, abnormalities in the contiguous retina and chorioretinal lesions.[9]

Hematology and biochemistry are usually normal, except in microbial infections.[9] Magnetic resonance imaging (MRI) or, less preferably, computed tomography of the head should be performed in cases of optic neuritis, and findings depend on the etiology. Potential MRI findings of NION include optic disc swelling, optic nerve or chiasm enlargement, retrobulbar changes, absent CSF signal within the optic nerve sheath complex, optic nerve or chiasm hyperintensities, contrast enhancement of the optic nerves or chiasm, and, in multifocal cases, central nervous system changes suggestive of meningoencephalomyelitis.[10,11] However, studies may be normal.[10,11] CSF analysis may be normal or reveal pleocytosis and/or an increased protein concentration (reportedly up to 3,340 nucleated cells/µL and 564 mg/dL, respectively, for NION).[9,10] Other diagnostic procedures include electroretinography (ERG) or colorimetric PLR testing, ideally performed prior to advanced diagnostic imaging in cases without additional neurological abnormalities, and no fundic lesions.

Treatment depends on the underlying disorder and usually includes a tapering course of corticosteroids with or without additional immunosuppressive agents (e.g., cytosine arabinoside) for NION.[9,10] Vision may partially or completely return in 23–64% of cases of NION, but recurrences are possible.[9,10,12] A younger age, a nonabsent (normal or incomplete) PLR, a normal fundoscopy, and a lower pleocytosis have been associated with complete vision recovery.[12]

Idiopathic trigeminal neuropathy/trigeminal neuritis

Idiopathic trigeminal neuropathy/trigeminal neuritis (ITN) describes dogs with self-limiting signs of trigeminal nerve dysfunction. An immune-mediated neuritis is the suspected cause.[13,14] The diagnosis of ITN is less likely in any dog over 10 years.[14] Motor and, less frequently, sensory signs of unilateral or bilateral trigeminal nerve dysfunction are observed. Cases of bilateral motor trigeminal nerve dysfunction typically present with acute onset dropped jaw and inability to close the mouth (Fig. 36.2), and many of them also exhibit depression, vomiting, diarrhea, dehydration, dyspnea, and scleral injection, among other systemic signs.[13]

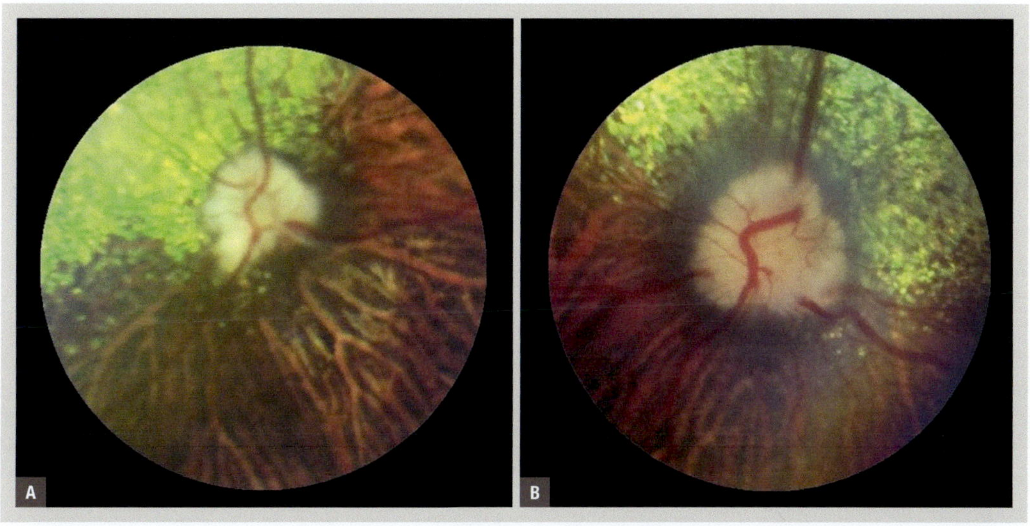

FIG 36.1 Normal fundus (left) and abnormal fundus (right), with marked optic disc swelling and elevation, retinal vascular engorgement and peripapillary edema in an 8-year-old neutered male Bichon Frisé. Images courtesy of Alberto Palella and Marisa Pérez.

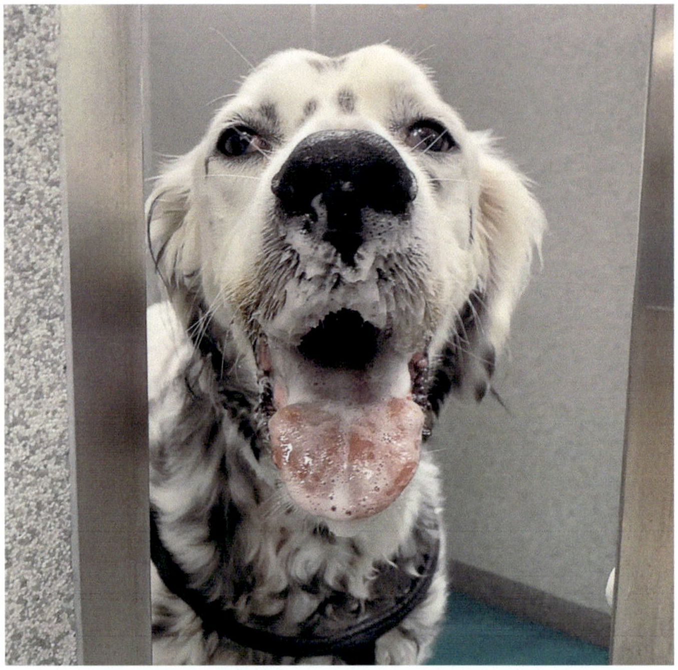

FIG 36.2 Eight-year-old neutered male mixed-breed dog with idiopathic trigeminal neuropathy/neuritis and inability to close the jaw. Picture courtesy of Cristina Toni.

Horner's syndrome, facial nerve deficits, and signs of vestibular dysfunction may also be encountered.[13,14]

MRI of the trigeminal nerves is usually normal in bilateral cases (with these demonstrating possible mild to moderate contrast enhancement), but unilateral cases commonly display diffuse enlargement of the affected nerve.[14] However, some unilateral cases present with normal nerve signal characteristics and morphology. Cisternal CSF analysis in most dropped jaw cases reveals a mildly to moderately increased protein concentration and mild, predominantly lymphocytic, pleocytosis.[13] Unilateral cases may display no abnormalities on CSF analysis.[14]

Treatment mainly involves supportive care, especially if the animal is unable to close its mouth, which may affect eating or drinking.[13] In the most severe cases, placement of a feeding tube could be considered. Feeding should be assisted with balls of wet food in dogs with dropped jaw. Information on how to perform oral and ophthalmic care and recognize signs of aspiration and corneal ulceration should be provided. The prognosis is favorable as the dropped jaw has been reported to resolve within 4 days to 9 weeks, and although relapses are possible, these are rare.[13]

Idiopathic facial neuropathy

Idiopathic facial neuropathy (IFN) is the most common cause of facial nerve dysfunction in dogs, with this accounting for up to 75% of cases.[15] Nerve fiber loss is identified[16] but is thought to represent the consequence of a more proximal neuritis[6] or damage remaining following previous pathology.[17] IFN shares a lot of similarities with Bell's palsy in humans. Middle-aged to older dogs are mostly affected, and Cocker Spaniels are overrepresented.[15] Clinical signs include acute onset unilateral or bilateral paresis or plegia of the muscles affecting the facial expression and, depending on the region of the affected facial nerve, concurrent signs of parasympathetic dysfunction may be observed.[15–17] Affected dogs typically present with an acute inability to blink (Video 36.2), a drooping of the ear and lip, and drooling on the affected side.[18] Ipsilateral peripheral vestibular syndrome is also observed in up to 89% of dogs.[15]

MRI of the head may reveal contrast enhancement of the affected facial nerve and atrophy and increased enhancement of the caudal portion of the ipsilateral digastric muscle, which may appear hyperintense on T2-weighted (T2W) and precontrast T1-weighted (T1W) sequences.[15,16] Cisternal CSF analysis reveals albuminocytological dissociation in 69% of dogs with both IFN and peripheral vestibular syndrome.[16]

Corticosteroids may or may not help improve prognosis. The prognosis for functional recovery is guarded, with <50% of dogs making a full recovery, often within weeks to months.[15] Quality of life is not significantly impaired, but some dogs require long-term eye lubrication to prevent corneal ulceration, and some may develop hemifacial contracture.[15] Relapses involving the contralateral side are possible.[16] The T2W and precontrast T1W hyperintensity of the caudal portion of the ipsilateral digastric muscle has been correlated with a poorer prognosis for return to normal facial nerve function.[15] It is important to remind owners that dogs unable to blink are more susceptible to trauma in their affected eyes.

Acquired idiopathic laryngeal paralysis

Acquired idiopathic laryngeal paralysis (AILP) (also known as geriatric onset laryngeal paralysis polyneuropathy) represents an early, prominent sign of a generalized neuropathy.[6,19] A dying-back axonopathy, predominantly affecting long neurons, is suspected.[6] The cause is unknown and the pathogenesis may differ between individuals.[6] Many dogs have chronic hypothyroidism, but the relationship between this and AILP is not well understood.[6] Recurrent laryngeal neuropathy leads to denervation of the cricoarytenoideus dorsalis muscle, which is essential in opening the glottis during inspiration.[6,19] AILP occurs in middle-aged to older large-breed dogs[6,19] and is more frequent in males than females.[19] Clinical signs of laryngeal paralysis include:[18,19]

- Inspiratory stridor (Videos 36.3 and 36.4).
- Dysphonia (weak, hoarse bark).
- Exercise intolerance.
- Respiratory distress and cyanosis, especially during excitement, exercise, and periods of hot weather.
- Coughing and gagging, especially while drinking, which may lead to aspiration pneumonia, particularly if pharyngeal weakness is also present.

The degree of laryngeal paralysis may be variable, and clinical signs may be worsened by secondary laryngeal edema and inflammation. Unilateral laryngeal paralysis (mostly left-sided) is only symptomatic during strenuous activity.[19] Signs of laryngeal paralysis may be accompanied by other neuromuscular signs (e.g., sciatic neuropathy), but these are mild and do not typically prevent ambulation.[6] In addition, decreased esophageal

Video 36.2

Three-year-old neutered male Chihuahua with idiopathic facial neuropathy on the right side. Note the lack of blinking upon palpebral reflex testing, but the presence of eyeball retraction and prolapse of the third eyelid, which indicates the trigeminal nerve (afferent arm of the palpebral reflex) is intact.

motility is present but may be subclinical,[19] and some dogs present with concurrent megaesophagus.[6]

Diagnostic investigations should rule out hypothyroidism and focal myasthenia gravis,[6,19] but the latter is rarely associated with laryngeal paralysis.[19] Thoracic radiographs may be performed if aspiration pneumonia or megaesophagus are suspected. Laryngeal paralysis is best confirmed by directly observing the laryngeal function (e.g., with a laryngoscope) under a light plane of anesthesia (Videos 36.5 and 36.6).[19]

AILP may be life-threatening if untreated.[6] The treatment of choice consists in unilateral cricoarytenoid cartilage lateralization (Video 36.7).[6,19] However, this may lead to severe postoperative complications, especially aspiration pneumonia in approximately 8–24% of dogs.[6,19] Emergency treatment for dogs with acute respiratory distress includes oxygen supplementation, sedation, cooling, temporary tracheostomy or intubation, and corticosteroids. Conservative treatment may be applied in older dogs with minimal to moderate clinical signs and involves anti-inflammatories, a weight loss program, and lifestyle and environmental changes.[19] "Little and often" walks are preferred to long walks, and walks during the hottest time of the day should be avoided, as well as the use of neck leads. Eventually, the dog's ability to perform normally may be impaired by the progression of the generalized neuropathy.[6] However, obvious signs of general neuropathy and dysphagia may take months to years to develop.[19]

Video 36.3

Ten-year-old neutered male Labrador with severe bilateral laryngeal dysfunction. Note the stridor present on inspiration and the concerned appearance as the dog is suffering with dyspnea. Video courtesy of Dr. William Robinson.

Video 36.4

Three-year-old male Leonberger with severe bilateral laryngeal dysfunction. Note the severe inspiratory stridor. Video courtesy of Dr. Gualtiero Gandini.

Video 36.5

12-year-old neutered male Cocker Spaniel with severe bilateral laryngeal dysfunction upon inspection. Note how the arytenoid cartilages move inward during inspiration due to negative intraglottic pressure (paradoxical movement). Video courtesy of Dr. William Robinson.

Video 36.6

For comparison with the dog in Video 36.5, this is a dog with normal laryngeal function. Note how the arytenoid cartilages abduct actively during inspiration and adduct passively during expiration. Video courtesy of Dr. William Robinson.

Video 36.7

The same dog as in Video 36.3, following unilateral cricoarytenoid cartilage lateralization. Note the improvement in the clinical signs but that some degree of laryngeal noise is considered normal. Video courtesy of Dr. William Robinson.

Single-limb neuropathies

Brachial plexus injury

Brachial plexus injury follows traumatic events such as road traffic accidents and falls from heights.[20,21] Traumatic nerve injury may be divided into neurapraxia, axonotmesis, and neurotmesis:[22]

- Neurapraxia represents transient functional loss (conduction block) without loss of nerve continuity and is associated with an excellent prognosis in days to weeks.
- Axonotmesis represents the interruption of axons and loss of myelin, but the perineurium and epineurium remain intact. Wallerian degeneration occurs distally, but the perineurium, epineurium, and endoneurium guide reinnervation. Prognosis depends on the degree of axonal loss and possibly the distance between the lesion and the muscle to reinnervate.
- Neurotmesis is the complete rupture of a nerve, and recovery is not possible without surgery.

Nerve root avulsion represents a form of neurotmesis and is irreversible.[22] In traumatic events, nerve roots are more frequently affected than nerves due to the relative lack of connective tissue.

The animal's posture, gait, and muscle mass and tone may indicate what nerves of the brachial plexus may be specifically affected. However, the only nerve that leads to significant gait abnormalities is the radial nerve. Monoparesis secondary to radial nerve injury is characterized by knuckling of the paw, decreased or absent carpal extension, carpal hypotonia or atonia, and loss of weight bearing (decreased or absent elbow extension) (Video 36.8). The degree of paresis depends on the severity of the injury. Atrophy of the triceps brachii and cranial antebrachial muscles will also be observed.

The presence or absence of nociception in the affected limb should also be evaluated. This is best accomplished by applying a noxious stimulus to the 2nd and 5th digits of the paw, which are innervated by the radial and median nerves (2nd digit) and ulnar nerve (5th digit). The withdrawal reflex may be evaluated at the same time as nociception testing. The cutaneus trunci reflex may be decreased or absent when ipsilaterally stimulated. Cranial nerve examination may reveal ipsilateral partial or total Horner's syndrome if the postganglionic sympathetic fibers to the eye are affected.

Electrodiagnostics may allow more precise identification of the affected nerves and assessment of the severity of their damage.[22]

Treatment mainly includes physiotherapy, but cases with permanent loss of function may require limb amputation.[21] If sufficient extension of the elbow for weight bearing is achieved but lack of carpal extension is observed, carpal panarthrodesis or the use of external devices such as casts, with external protection of the toes, may also be considered. The development of trophic or traumatic injuries to the paw (e.g., abrasions and infections) will have to be treated accordingly, and analgesia against neuropathic pain will have to be considered in the acute and chronic stages. Along these lines, owners should be asked to keep an eye on the development of signs consistent with paresthesia or dysesthesia.

It is difficult to establish a prognosis and determine whether spontaneous recovery will occur, or whether reconstructive surgery or amputation is required. Spontaneous improvement may only occur in animals with neurapraxia or axonotmesis.[22] Clinically, it is extremely challenging to distinguish between neurapraxia, axonotmesis, and neurotmesis/nerve root avulsion unless spontaneous recovery occurs, but recovery may

Video 36.8

This video (in slow motion for the first 68 seconds) shows a dog following a left brachial plexus injury. Note how the dog has a left thoracic limb monoparesis. The dog is carrying the limb flexed at the elbow and is able to advance it by extending the shoulder; however, the carpus is bouncing on the floor, most of the time on its dorsal surface, because the dog is unable to extend it. Gait analysis in this dog is compatible with left radial nerve dysfunction. Video courtesy of Dr. María Ortega.

take months, if at all.[22] It is important to stress that the radial nerve is the only nerve vital for weight bearing and gait, and so prognosis will be determined by the degree of its injury.

Lack of nociception has been reported as a negative prognostic indicator,[20] and the absence of cutaneus trunci reflex and presence of spontaneous activity in the paraspinal muscles on EMG are associated with severe axonotmesis, neurotmesis, or nerve root avulsion in the radial nerve.[22]

Video 36.9

Eight-year-old female Labrador with a presumptive right-sided nerve sheath tumor. Note the severe atrophy in the muscles of mastication (masseter and temporal) on the right side, as well as the right facial hypo-/anesthesia. Video courtesy of Dr. Gualtiero Gandini.

Nerve sheath tumors

Nerve sheath tumors (NSTs) may arise from Schwann cells, perineurial cells, or intraneural fibroblasts. Schwannomas, neurofibromas, and neurofibrosarcomas have been described.[23] NSTs may be benign or malignant, and in dogs they are usually histologically and biologically aggressive. Despite this, metastases are rare.[23] NST may affect any nerve (usually unilaterally), but the trigeminal nerve and nerve roots or nerves of the brachial and lumbar plexi are frequently affected (Video 36.9). Secondary tumors (e.g., lymphoma [especially T-cell], malignant sarcomas, histiocytic sarcoma, and hamartomas) have occasionally been reported.[23] Middle-aged to older medium breed and large breed dogs are predisposed.[23] The clinical signs depend on the nerve affected and are chronic and progressive. For brachial or lumbosacral plexus NSTs, lameness may be observed initially. Signs of myelopathy (often asymmetric) are possible if the tumor invades the vertebral canal, and signs of pain on palpation or paresthesia are frequent.[23] For NSTs affecting the brachial plexus, a mass may sometimes be palpated. For cranial nerve tumors, the brainstem may also be involved.[23]

MRI is the most useful imaging technique; however, the use of ultrasound, computed tomography (CT) and CT-myelography has also been described. MRI may reveal thickening of one or various nerves (forming tubular lesions) or a discrete mass, and postcontrast sequences may identify subtle tumors.[23] On some occasions, signs of vertebral canal invasion and spinal cord compression or invasion may be observed (Fig. 36.3).

Histopathological examination is required to obtain a definitive diagnosis. For paraspinal or plexus NSTs, surgery may be performed depending on their location. They may be completely resected by amputation, compartmental resection with limb sparing, laminectomy, or combinations of techniques.[23] Volumetric modulated arc radiotherapy has also been described. Nerve lymphomas may respond to radiation or chemotherapy.[23]

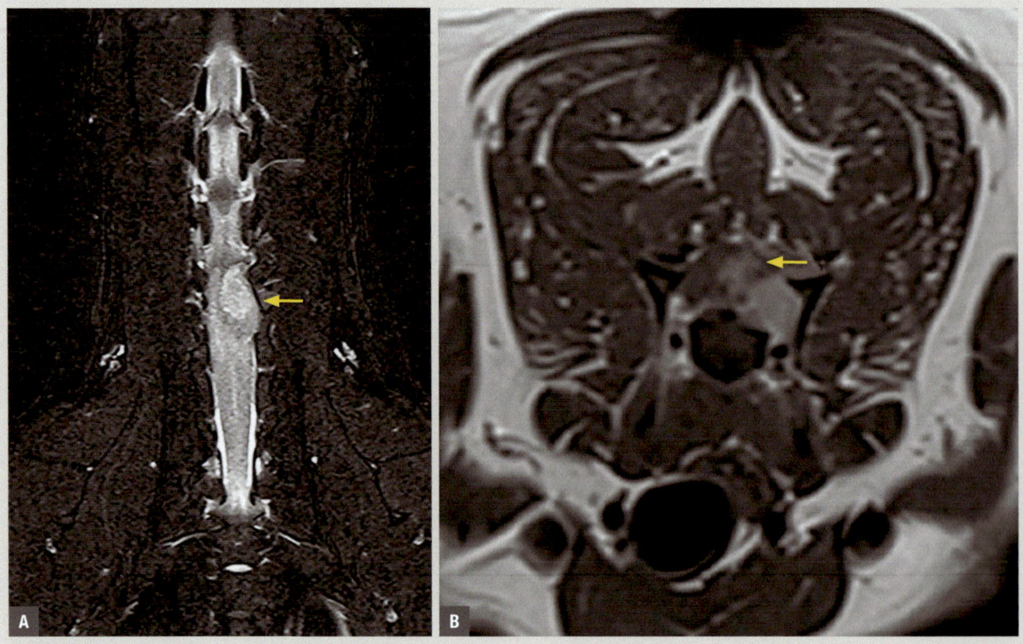

FIG. 36.3 (A) Dorsal dixon and (B) T1-weighted images after contrast administration of an 8-year-old spayed, female mixed-breed dog with a suspected nerve sheath tumor (arrows) at the level of the left C6 foramen. Note the severe compression/invasion of the spinal cord.

Negative prognostic indicators include proximity to and invasion of the vertebral canal and the presence of tumor infiltrated margins following compartmental resection. The median survival time is usually 6 months, but long-term survival is possible following complete resection.[23] Volumetric modulated arc radiotherapy may lead to a mean progression-free survival time of 8 months.[23]

For trigeminal NSTs, if no treatment is applied, the survival time may be up to 18 months without significant clinical progression. Surgery or, ideally, radiotherapy may be performed. Stereotactic radiotherapy may lead to median survival times of 745 and 441 days, depending on the study.[23]

KEY POINTS

- The most common neuropathies in dogs are somatic motor and may affect cranial and/or spinal nerves.
- The most common canine generalized neuropathy is acute canine polyradiculoneuritis, characterized by the acute onset of severe nonambulatory tetraparesis or tetraplegia. Treatment consists of physiotherapy and nursing care, and prognosis is favorable.
- Other chronic polyneuropathies include chronic inflammatory demyelinating polyneuropathy, metabolic neuropathies secondary to hypothyroidism and diabetes mellitus, paraneoplastic neuropathies, and degenerative neuropathies.
- The most common cranial neuropathies involve cranial nerves II, V, VII, and X in the form of optic neuritis, idiopathic trigeminal neuropathy, idiopathic facial neuropathy, and acquired idiopathic laryngeal paralysis, respectively, but other cranial neuropathies are possible.
- The most frequently encountered single-limb neuropathies include brachial plexus injury following traumatic events and nerve sheath tumors.

References

1. Añor S. Acute lower motor neuron tetraparesis. *Vet Clin North Am Small Anim Pract.* 2014;44(6):1201–1222.
2. Halstead SK, Gourlay DS, Penderis J, et al. Serum anti-GM2 and anti-GalNAc-GD1a IgG antibodies are biomarkers for acute canine polyradiculoneuritis. *J Small Anim Pract.* 2022;63(2):104–112.
3. Hirschvogel K, Jurina K, Steinberg TA, et al. Clinical course of acute canine polyradiculoneuritis following treatment with human IV immunoglobulin. *J Am Anim Hosp Assoc.* 2012;48(5):299–309.
4. Olby N. Tetraparesis. In: Platt S, Olby N (eds.) *BSAVA Manual of Canine and Feline Neurology*, 4th ed. Gloucester, UK: BSAVA; 2013.
5. Mariani CL. Peripheral Neuropathies. In: Côte E, Ettinger SJ, Feldman EC (eds.) *Ettinger's Textbook of Veterinary Internal Medicine*, 9th ed. Philadelphia: Elsevier; 2024.
6. de Lahunta A, Glass E, Kent M. (eds.) *de Lahunta's Veterinary Neuroanatomy and Clinical Neurology*, 5th ed. Philadelphia: Elsevier; 2021.
7. Bailey DB. Paraneoplastic Syndromes. In: Vail DM, Thamm DH, Liptak JM (eds.) *Withrow & MacEwen's Small Animal Clinical Oncology*, 6th ed. St. Louis, Missouri: Elsevier; 2020.
8. Granger N. Canine inherited motor and sensory neuropathies: an updated classification in 22 breeds and comparison to Charcot-Marie-Tooth disease. *Vet J.* 2011;188(3):274–285.
9. Smith SM, Westermeyer HD, Mariani CL, et al. Optic neuritis in dogs: 96 cases (1983-2016). *Vet Ophthalmol.* 2018;21(5):442–451.
10. Bedos L, Tetas R, Crespo V, et al. Presumed optic neuritis of non-infectious origin in dogs treated with immunosuppressive medication: 28 dogs (2000-2015). *J Small Anim Pract.* 2020;61(11):676–683.
11. Muñiz Moris L, Cherubini GB, Caine A. Low-Field Magnetic Resonance Imaging Findings in 18 Dogs With Presumed Optic Neuritis. *Front Vet Sci.* 2021;7:585828.
12. Posporis C, Beltran E, Dunning M, et al. Prognostic Factors for Recovery of Vision in Canine Optic Neuritis of Unknown Etiology: 26 Dogs (2003-2018). *Front Vet Sci.* 2019;6:415.
13. Mayhew PD, Bush WW, Glass EN. Trigeminal neuropathy in dogs: a retrospective study of 29 cases (1991-2000). *J Am Anim Hosp Assoc.* 2002;38(3):262–270.
14. Musso C, Le Boedec K, Gomes E, et al. Diagnostic Values of Clinical and Magnetic Resonance Findings in Presumptive Trigeminal Neuropathy: 49 Dogs. *J Am Anim Hosp Assoc.* 2020;56(2):106–113.
15. McGregor O, Plested MJ, Beltran E. Magnetic resonance imaging of the caudal portion of the digastric muscle in canine idiopathic facial neuropathy. *Vet Radiol Ultrasound.* 2021;62(4):455–462.
16. Jeandel A, Thibaud JL, Blot S. Facial and vestibular neuropathy of unknown origin in 16 dogs. *J Small Anim Pract.* 2016;57(2):74–78.
17. Smith PM, Gonçalves R, McConnell JF. Sensitivity and specificity of MRI for detecting facial nerve abnormalities in dogs with facial neuropathy. *Vet Rec.* 2012;171(14):349.
18. Ives E, Freeman PM. A practical approach to common presentations in general practice. In: Freeman PM, Ives E. (eds.) *A Practical Approach to Neurology for the Small Animal Practitioner.* Hoboken, USA: Wiley Blackwell; 2020. p.133–328.
19. Kitshoff AM, Van Goethem B, Stegen L, et al. Laryngeal paralysis in dogs: an update on recent knowledge. *J S Afr Vet Assoc.* 2013;84(1):E1-E9.
20. Menchetti M, Gandini G, Bravaccini B, et al. Clinical, Electrodiagnostic Findings and Quality of Life of Dogs and Cats with Brachial Plexus Injury. *Vet Sci.* 2020;7(3):101.
21. Kerwin SC, Taylor AR. Neurologic Causes of Thoracic Limb Lameness. *Vet Clin North Am Small Anim Pract.* 2021;51(2):357–364.
22. Troupel T, Van Caenegem N, Jeandel A, et al. Epidemiological, clinical, and electrophysiological findings in dogs and cats with traumatic brachial plexus injury: A retrospective study of 226 cases. *J Vet Intern Med.* 2021;35(6):2837–2845.
23. Rossmeisl JH, Pancotto TE. Tumors of the nervous system. In: Vail DM, Thamm DH, Liptak JM (eds.) *Withrow & MacEwen's Small Animal Clinical Oncology*, 6th ed. St. Louis, Missouri: Elsevier; 2020.

CHAPTER 37

Neurogenic bladder dysfunction

Federica Balducci
DVM, DECVN

Neurogenic bladder dysfunction (NBD) refers to lower urinary tract disorders caused by injury or disease affecting the central or peripheral nervous system involved in the control of micturition.[1] Micturition is a two-phase process consisting of storage (passive or reflex filling of the bladder) and periodic elimination (reflex and voluntary bladder emptying) of urine based on the coordinated activity of the urinary bladder (the reservoir) and the bladder neck, urethra, and urethral sphincters (the outlet).[2,3,4] Their structural and functional integrity is necessary for normal micturition to occur.

Micturition dysfunctions are frequently encountered in neurological patients; the lesion localization along the nervous system determines the clinical features of the dysfunction itself.

To correctly approach and treat a patient with NBD, a good knowledge of the functional anatomy and neurological pathways of the lower urinary tract (LUT) is essential.

Functional neuroanatomy of the lower urinary tract

The LUT comprises the urinary bladder, the bladder neck, the urethra, and two urethral sphincters: the internal urethral sphincter (IUS, smooth muscle) and the external urethral sphincter (EUS, striated muscle). The sensory and motor innervation of the LUT relies on three pairs of peripheral nerves: the hypogastric nerve, the pelvic nerve, and the pudendal nerve. Their activity is coordinated and controlled by segmental spinal cord reflexes and supraspinal pathways involving the brainstem, the cerebellum, the hypothalamus, and the cerebral cortex (Fig. 37.1).[4,5]

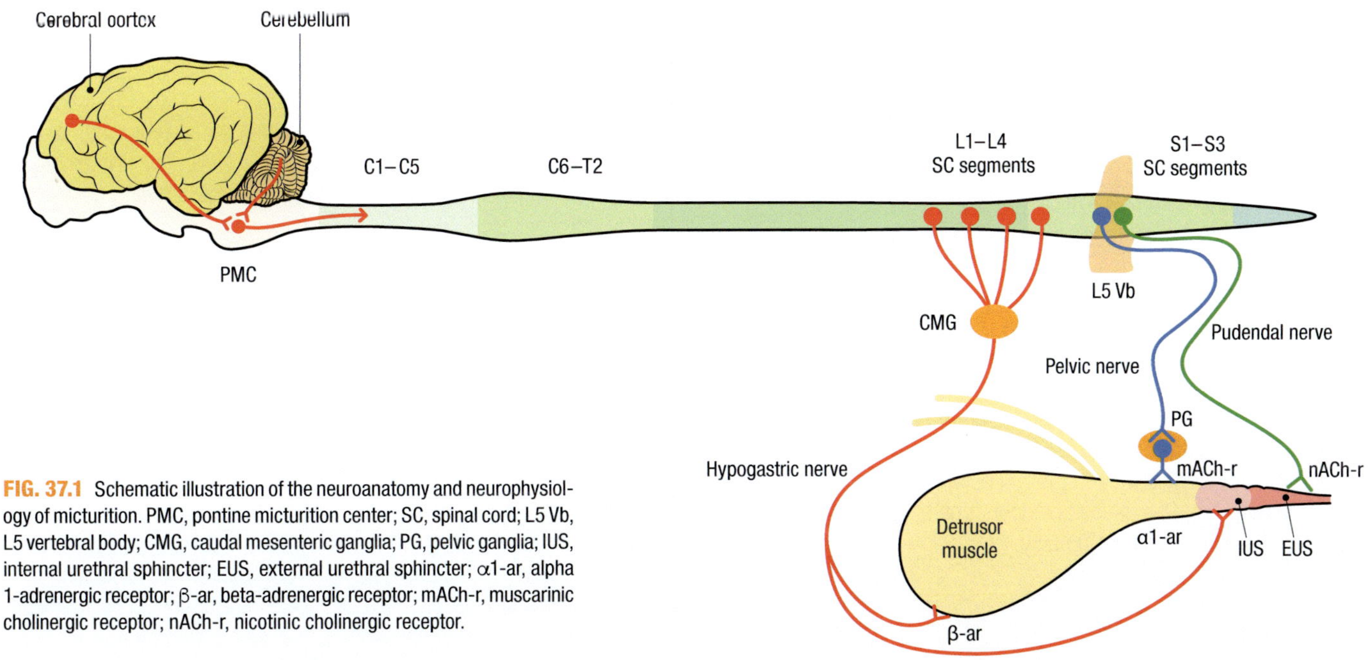

FIG. 37.1 Schematic illustration of the neuroanatomy and neurophysiology of micturition. PMC, pontine micturition center; SC, spinal cord; L5 Vb, L5 vertebral body; CMG, caudal mesenteric ganglia; PG, pelvic ganglia; IUS, internal urethral sphincter; EUS, external urethral sphincter; α1-ar, alpha 1-adrenergic receptor; β-ar, beta-adrenergic receptor; mACh-r, muscarinic cholinergic receptor; nACh-r, nicotinic cholinergic receptor.

Urinary bladder

The urinary bladder musculature (detrusor muscle) is composed of three layers of smooth muscle fibers, connected by tight junctions. The primary function of the urinary bladder is to store urine.

Motor innervation

The detrusor muscle is innervated by:

- The hypogastric nerve (sympathetic nervous system), which emerges from the L1–L4 spinal cord segments. Hypogastric nerve stimulation activates beta-adrenergic receptors in the detrusor muscle, which permits relaxation of this muscle and bladder filling.
- The pelvic nerve (parasympathetic nervous system), which emerges from the S1–S3 spinal cord segments. Pelvic nerve stimulation activates muscarinic cholinergic receptors in the detrusor muscle, producing contraction of this muscle and consequent bladder voiding.[3–6]

Sensory innervation

Sensory innervation in the bladder is supplied by:

- A-delta fibers. Mechanoreceptors responding to bladder distension include the terminal portion of ascending myelinated fibers travelling in the pelvic nerve. These afferent axons start firing when the urinary bladder reaches a certain degree of distension. They ascend the spinal cord, reach the brainstem, and initiate the detrusor reflex (i.e., urine voiding).
- Unmyelinated C-fibers. Nociceptors are free nerve endings within the bladder wall. These afferent fibers travel in the hypogastric nerve. In dogs, this afferent nociceptive pathway is the only one that, after ascending the spinal cord, reaches the cerebral cortex allowing conscious perception of an overdistended and painful bladder.[3–6]

Urethra

From a functional point of view, the bladder neck is considered the proximal part of the urethra. The bladder neck and IUS are made of smooth muscle, whereas the EUS consists of skeletal or striated muscle. The function of the urethra is to prevent urine leakage during bladder filling and allow urine evacuation.

Motor innervation

The urethra is innervated by:

- Descending fibers of the hypogastric nerve, which are responsible for activation of alpha-adrenergic receptors in the bladder neck and IUS. Activation of these receptors produces increased tone and contraction of the urethra, permitting bladder filling.
- Descending fibers of the pudendal nerve (somatic nervous system), which emerges from the S1–S2 spinal cord segments. These fibers are responsible for activation of nicotinic cholinergic receptors in the EUS, which causes contraction of the urethra, thus facilitating bladder filling. The pudendal nerve is under voluntary control. However, it is also the efferent pathway of a reflex activity integrated into the sacral spinal cord and mediated by the pelvic nerve: it produces EUS contraction in response to a sudden bladder stretch, allowing continence when coughing, sneezing, or jumping.[3–6]

Sensory innervation

Sensory innervation of the urethra is provided by:

- Sensory receptors supplied by ascending sensory fibers of the pudendal nerve. These receptors detect stretch, pain, and urine flow.
- Nociceptors supplied by ascending sensory fibers of the hypogastric nerve.[2,6]

Spinal cord and spinal pathways

Motor regions and descending pathways

The motor regions and descending pathways of the spinal cord involved in bladder function include:

- Grey matter, intermediolateral region of the L1–L4 spinal cord segments: preganglionic sympathetic neurons, whose axons travel in the hypogastric nerve.
- Grey matter, intermediolateral region of the S1–S3 spinal cord segments: preganglionic parasympathetic neurons, whose axons enter the pelvic nerve.
- Grey matter, ventral horn of the S1–S2 spinal cord segments (Onuf's nucleus): somatic motoneurons, whose axons travel in the pudendal nerve.
- Descending pontine reticulospinal and bulbospinal tracts (white matter, ventral funiculus). These tracts originate in the reticular formation of the pons (pontine micturition center) and terminate in the grey matter spinal segments, where the lower motoneurons of the hypogastric, pelvic, and pudendal nerves are located (bladder contraction, IUS and EUS relaxation).[5,7]
- Descending corticospinal tract (white matter, lateral funiculus), originating in the frontal cortex area and connecting with the micturition area and, ultimately, the lower motor neurons of the pudendal nerve (S1–S2 spinal cord segments) (voluntary control of micturition).[7]

Sensory regions and ascending pathways

The sensory regions and ascending pathways of the spinal cord involved in bladder function include:

- Grey matter of the dorsal horn of the spinal cord, L1–L4 spinal segments: sensory neurons whose afferent fibers enter the hypogastric nerve, mainly unmyelinated C fibers (nociception from bladder and urethra).[3,7]
- Grey matter of the dorsal horn of the spinal cord, S1–S3 spinal segments: sensory neurons whose afferent fibers enter the pelvic and pudendal nerves, mainly A-delta myelinated fibers (various sensory functions from bladder and urethra).[3,7]
- Ascending spinothalamic tract (white matter lateral funiculus), which originates in the spinal dorsal horn and ends in the thalamus. It carries nociception from the bladder and urethra, allowing conscious perception.[7]
- Ascending spinobulbar tract (white matter), which originates in the dorsal horn of the spinal cord and reaches the pontine micturition center in the brainstem. It carries stretch stimuli from the bladder and participates in the detrusor reflex.[5]
- Ascending spinomesencephalic, spinohypothalamic, and spinoreticular tracts (white matter). They originate in the dorsal horn of the spinal cord and terminate in subthalamic structures.

Brainstem

The micturition center, located in the dorsolateral region of the pons, coordinates bladder filling and voiding through an on–off switching circuit. During urine storage, it receives sensory information on bladder wall distension and maintains concomitant detrusor relaxation and urethral sphincter contraction. During urine voiding, it coordinates simultaneous detrusor contraction and urethral sphincter relaxation.[3,6]

Cerebral cortex and cerebellum

The cerebral cortex receives afferent information from the bladder via the spinothalamic tract and sends efferent axons via the corticospinal tract. Micturition can be voluntarily inhibited by the cerebral cortex (which is the basis of house training) or voluntarily initiated (territorial marking behavior).
The cerebellum inhibits the detrusor reflex.[6]

Storage phase of micturition

Appropriate urine storage requires detrusor muscle relaxation (1) and urethral sphincter contraction (2 and 3) by:

1. Inhibition of the pelvic nerve (muscarinic cholinergic parasympathetic neurons) and stimulation of the hypogastric nerve (beta-adrenergic sympathetic neurons), allowing urine storage by inhibition of detrusor muscle contraction.
2. Stimulation of the hypogastric nerve (alpha-adrenergic sympathetic neurons), allowing urine storage by increasing the tone of the internal sphincter.
3. Stimulation of the pudendal nerve (nicotinic somatic efferent neurons), allowing urine storage by increasing the tone of the external sphincter.

This is a passive phase, mainly regulated by sympathetic thoracolumbar and somatic sacral segmental spinal cord reflexes. The pontine micturition center facilitates involuntary urethral sphincter contraction.[6]
As the urinary bladder reaches its capacity, the stretch receptors start firing and send afferent input to the cerebral cortex and the brainstem micturition center, switching the circuit from the storage to the voiding phase.[6]

Voiding phase of micturition

The phase of urine voiding is controlled by the pontine micturition center and requires coordinated detrusor muscle contraction (1) and urethral sphincter relaxation (2 and 3) by:

1. Stimulation of the pelvic nerve (muscarinic cholinergic parasympathetic neurons), allowing urine voiding by stimulation of detrusor muscle contraction.
2. Inhibition of the hypogastric nerve (alpha-adrenergic sympathetic neurons), allowing urine voiding by decreasing the tone of the IUS.
3. Inhibition of the pudendal nerve (nicotinic somatic efferent neurons), allowing urine voiding by decreasing the tone of the EUS.

In trained dogs, the voiding phase can be controlled by the cerebral cortex. It can inhibit if socially inappropriate, or voluntarily initiate urination.[6]

Etiology

NBD can be caused by any congenital or acquired disease affecting the central and peripheral nervous system pathways controlling micturition. The neurological examination will show other abnormalities related to the neuroanatomical localization, as bladder dysfunction is in most cases associated with other neurological deficits. The most important and common causes of NBD in dogs are spinal cord injuries, in particular intervertebral disc disease (IVDD), trauma, and ischemic myelopathy.[8] In addition, it is essential to remember that urological diseases (urolithiasis, neoplasia, prostatic disease, urethritis, urethral stricture/trauma, bladder displacement/entrapment) or other non-neurogenic conditions affecting the patient's mobility (due to pain or other orthopedic problems) may cause chronic bladder overdistension and consequent detrusor tight junction disruption and bladder atony.[2,3] In the latter cases, the neurological examination, apart from bladder dysfunction, is normal.

Clinical presentation

Clinical features of NBD are strictly dependent on lesion localization and severity.
A complete history should be obtained from the owner regarding any changes in the dog's micturition habits, unsuccessful attempts to urinate or urination while walking, or the presence of urine where the dog sleeps. The onset, duration, and progression of the disease should be recorded.
During the physical examination, the clinician should evaluate the voiding modality, stream size, duration of micturition, urine color and smell, and residual urine volume (normal value in dogs: 0.2–0.4 mL/kg). For this purpose, videos from the owner may be very useful. Palpation of the abdomen, external genitalia, and rectum should be performed to assess for the presence of masses or any abnormalities and to evaluate bladder tone and size.
Finally, a comprehensive neurological examination is essential to correctly localize the lesion and determine if the NBD is caused by a lower motor neuron (LMN) or upper motor neuron disorder (UMN) (Fig. 37.2).[2,3,6]

Lower motor neuron bladder dysfunction

- **Lesion localization:** sacral spinal cord segments (important to remember that the S1–S3 spinal cord segments are located within the L5 vertebral body); sacral nerves within the vertebral canal (cauda equina region); pelvic/lumbosacral plexus within the pelvic canal.
- **Effects:** loss of detrusor muscle function and urethral sphincter tone. The conscious perception of a painful bladder is still present due to the intact function of the L1–L4 spinal cord segments and hypogastric nerve.
- **Clinical features:** urinary incontinence with constant leakage of urine; the patient is frequently soiled with urine. On palpation, the bladder may be distended and is difficult to appreciate and flaccid. Manual bladder expression is easy; however, it is quite difficult to achieve complete bladder emptying.
- **Other possible associated neurological deficits:** decreased/absent perineal reflex, reduced/absent anal sphincter sensation, tail paresis/paralysis, and reduced/absent nociception. Gait, proprioception, and spinal reflexes may be abnormal in the pelvic limbs. Possible lumbosacral pain (Video 37.1).[6]

Upper motor neuron bladder dysfunction

- **Lesion localization:** from the brainstem to the L7 spinal cord segment.
- **Effects**: impairment or abolishment of detrusor reflex due to loss of control over the detrusor muscle, loss of bladder fullness sensation, and urethral sphincter hypertonus.
- **Clinical features:** urinary retention and/or urinary overflow (mainly related to increased abdominal pressure), involuntary intermittent urine emission especially in the chronic phase due to detrusor overactivity. On palpation, the overdistended and firm bladder can be easily identified but may be difficult or impossible to be manually expressed.[6]

Usually, the bladder with a UMN lesion is more overdistended compared to an LMN bladder. This is due to the decrease in internal and external sphincter tone in the LMN bladder, which prevents extreme overdistension by allowing urine to leak after a certain bladder pressure has been reached.

- **Other associated neurological deficits:** there is a plethora of possibly associated neurological signs depending on the lesion localization, mainly including different degrees of paresis and proprioceptive ataxia. For this reason, it is extremely unlikely to have a normal neurological examination with a suspected UMN bladder dysfunction.

Forebrain disorders

Forebrain disease (cognitive dysfunction, cerebral neoplasia) can lead to inappropriate micturition, characterized by loss of learned urination habits, house soiling, or urination in unusual places. As for previously described conditions, other neurological signs such as abnormal mentation, seizures, and motor and sensory deficits are commonly seen.[2,3,8]

Complications of neurogenic bladder

A common complication of NBD is lower urinary tract infection (LUTI), which may be subclinical and challenging to clinically detect due to overlapping of the clinical signs (hematuria, incontinence secondary to myelopathy) and lower urinary tract impaired sensation.[9,10] In particular, for chronic NBD, repeated administration of antibiotics due to recurrent LUTI can lead to multidrug-resistant infections.[10]

A less frequent complication is pyelonephritis, with signs of systemic illness such as uremia, anorexia, fever, painful kidney, and sepsis.[10,11]

Signs of non-neurogenic causes of bladder dysfunction

The description of non-neurological causes of bladder dysfunction is beyond the purposes of this chapter. However, the clinician must be aware that non-neurological causes can lead to storage and voiding dysfunction. For example, one of the most common differential diagnoses for urinary incontinence in young dogs is ectopic ureters, which can produce continuous urine leakage.

Conversely, urethral obstructions (due to urolithiasis, neoplasia, prostatic disease, urethral inflammation) can cause urinary retention.

Inflammatory bladder diseases (e.g., cystitis) produce signs such as stranguria, increased frequency of urination, tenesmus, and repeated attempts to urinate.

Clinicopathological findings

Especially in the case of a normal neurological examination, all the other non-neurological causes possibly affecting micturition should be carefully considered, and the diagnostic workup should always include a complete urinalysis and, in selected cases, an abdominal ultrasound and plain and contrast radiographs.

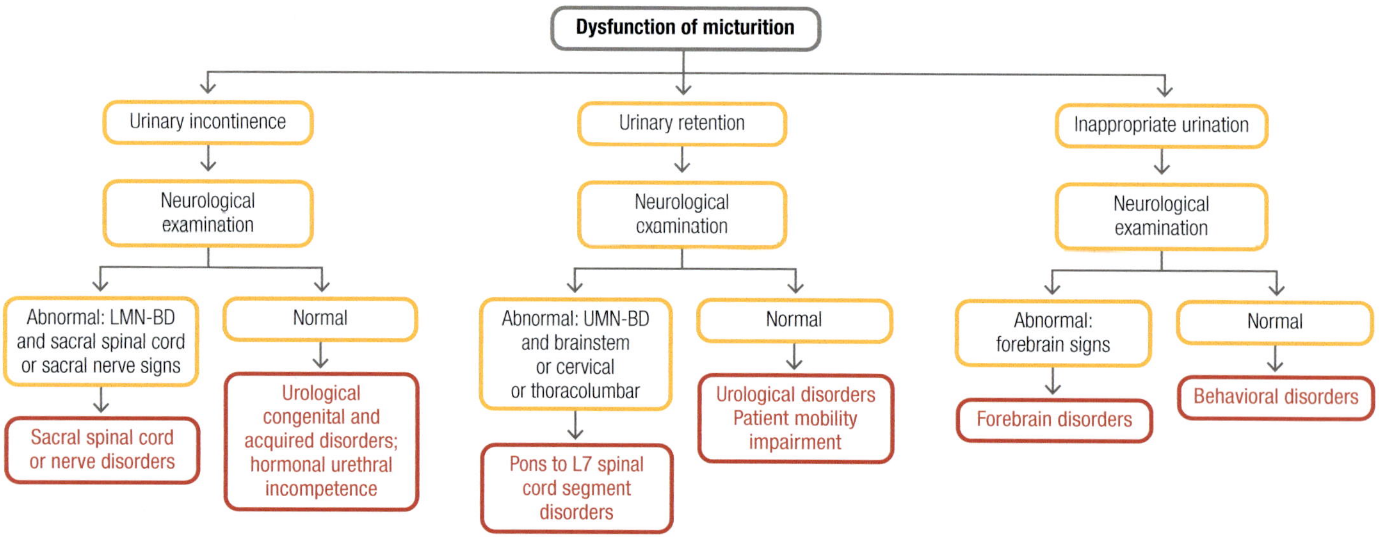

FIG. 37.2 Algorithm for the diagnosis of micturition dysfunction. LMN-BD, lower motor neuron bladder dysfunction; UMN-BD, upper motor neuron bladder dysfunction.

Video 37.1

Five-year-old female Dachshund. Main complaint: unsuccessful attempts to urinate for 24 hours. The neurological examination shows a plegic tail without nociception, absent perineal reflex, dilated anal sphincter, and reduced withdrawal reflex in both pelvic limbs. At palpation, the bladder is flaccid and easy to express manually. Neuroanatomical localization: sacral spinal cord segments/ nerves, pelvic/lumbosacral plexus.

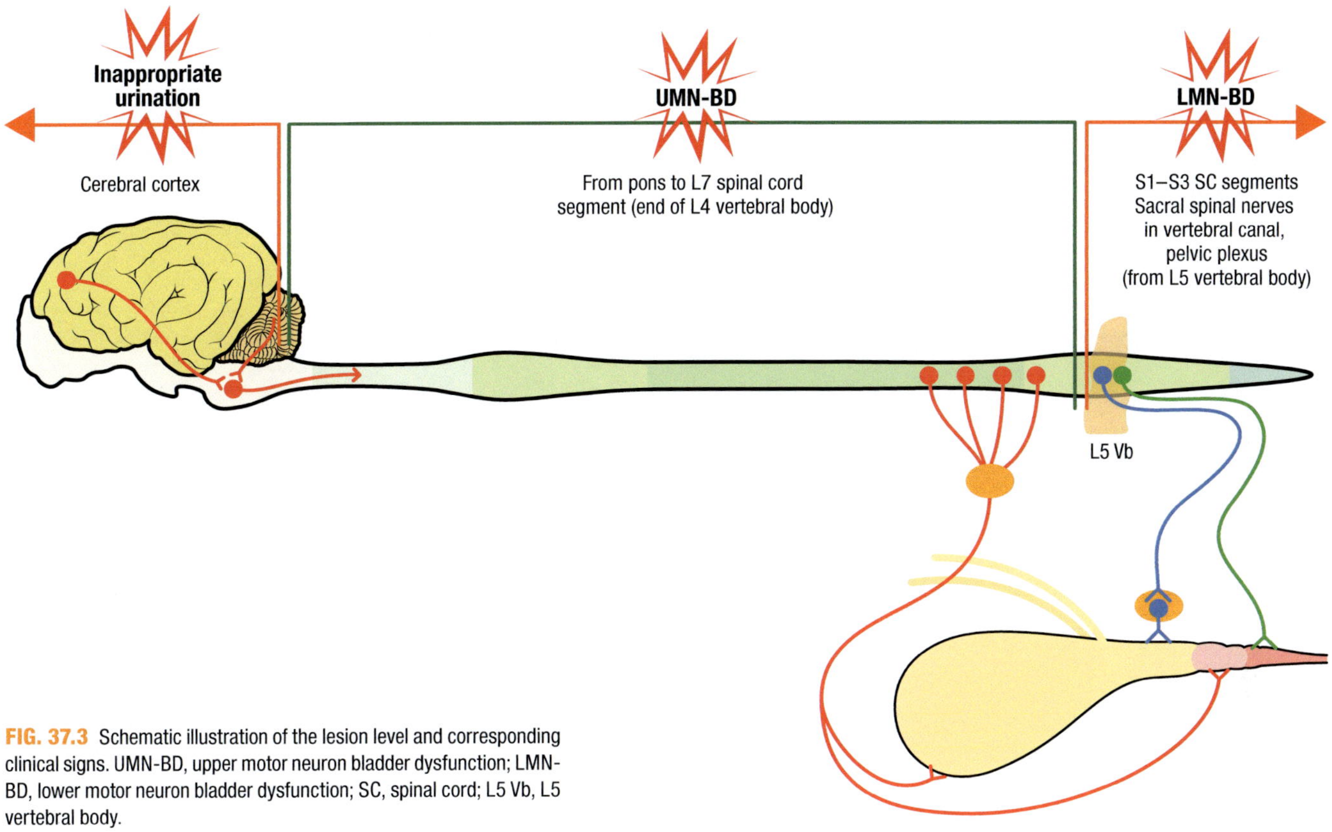

FIG. 37.3 Schematic illustration of the lesion level and corresponding clinical signs. UMN-BD, upper motor neuron bladder dysfunction; LMN-BD, lower motor neuron bladder dysfunction; SC, spinal cord; L5 Vb, L5 vertebral body.

The results of the hematology and complete biochemistry profiles in patients with NBD are typically within normal limits unless there is concurrent pyelonephritis. In such cases, leucocytosis with a left shift, azotemia, and other indicators of renal failure may be observed.[11]

A urinalysis and urine culture may show signs of LUTI, such as pyuria, hematuria, proteinuria, and bacteriuria. Bacteria frequently isolated in urine cultures include *Escherichia coli*, *Enterococcus* spp., *Streptococcus* spp., and *Staphylococcus* spp.[10]

Diagnostic procedures

During NBD, the diagnostic protocol aims to identify the underlying neurological conditions responsible for the clinical signs and is linked to the lesion localization. Survey radiographs of the spine, magnetic resonance imaging (MRI; Fig. 37.4), computed tomography (CT) of the spine or brain, and cerebrospinal fluid analysis may be necessary to reach the diagnosis.

Imaging studies of the urinary tract such as abdominal radiographs (including those taken after administration of an iodine contrast medium) and ultrasonography are particularly useful for:

- Ruling out non-neurological causes of micturition disorders.
- Highlighting non-neurological causes of bladder dysfunction that may occur concurrently with the neurological disease and complicate the diagnosis, especially when the patient shows relevant signs of abnormal micturition not accompanied by equally severe neurological deficits.
- Evaluating the degree of bladder distension and signs of LUTI or pyelonephritis.

Urodynamic studies (cystometry and urethral pressure profiling) and electrophysiological studies may be conducted, although these are infrequently employed in clinical settings. They can aid in providing a neuroanatomical localization and in monitoring neurogenic lower urinary tract dysfunction.[2,3,12]

Treatment

The management of dogs with NBD can be challenging, particularly in chronic cases, as it may extend throughout the patient's entire life, and relies on the following therapeutic options:

- Treatment of the underlying neurological disease.
- Medical treatment of NBD. The choice of medication must be related to the type of dysfunction. For acute UMN bladder dysfunction, since the ability of the detrusor muscle to contract is not decreased, relaxation of the urethral sphincters is the main desired pharmacological action. In the case of chronic UMN bladder dysfunction, the detrusor muscle may become overactive; drugs reducing detrusor contractility may therefore be suggested in addition to those promoting urethral sphincter relaxation, as reported in a recent review.[13] It should be noted that in daily clinical practice, most neurologists treat the chronic UMN bladder only with drugs reducing sphincter tone. For LMN bladder dysfunction, clinicians have very few pharmacological options to treat bladder atony and urethral sphincter incompetence. Several drugs have been used in clinical practice to manage bladder and urethral dysfunction, but clinical data evaluating their efficacy are extremely limited.[12,13] For instance, in one study on 6 normal dogs, administration of bethanechol and oxybutynin did not lead to changes in bladder pressure.[14]

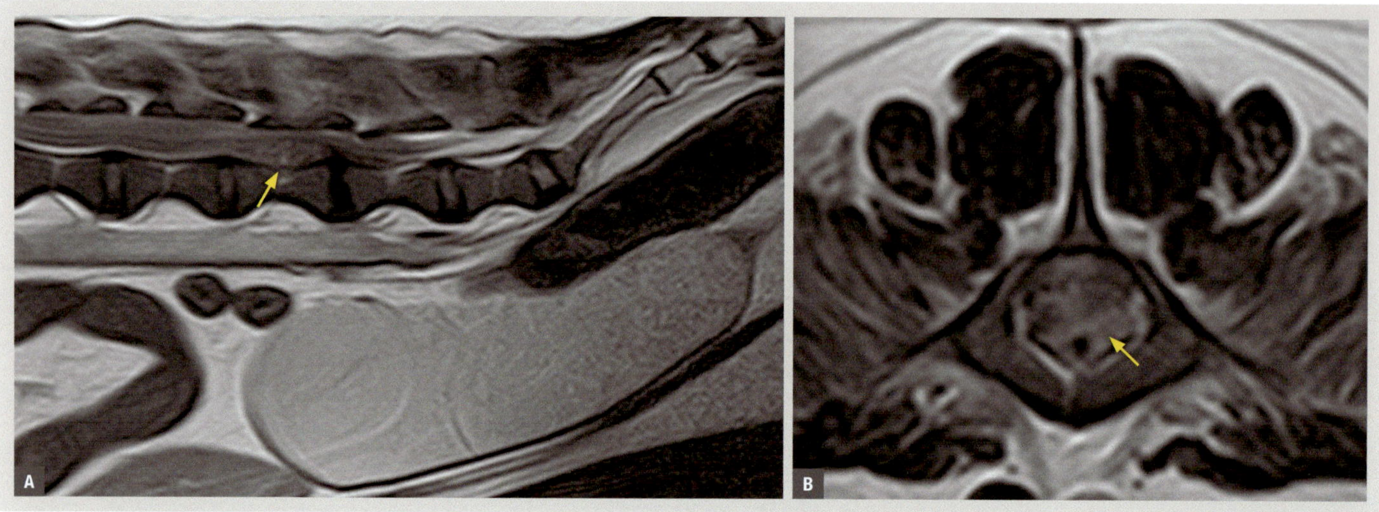

FIG. 37.4 Magnetic resonance images of the lumbosacral spine of the dog featured in Video 37.1. Sagittal T2-weighted (A) and transverse T2-weighted images (B) showing severe spinal cord compression at the level of L5 vertebral body, specifically of the S1–S3 spinal cord segments, caused by an L5–L6 intervertebral disc extrusion (arrows).

Suggested pharmacological agents, their mechanisms of action, functions, dosages, and side effects are summarized in Table 37.1.

- Medical treatment of LUTI. It is strongly recommended to choose the antibiotic treatment based on the urine culture results to minimize the risk of multidrug-resistance infections. Urine acidifiers (ammonium chloride) and urine antiseptics (nitrofurantoin, methanamine hippurate, and methanamine mandelate) may reduce bacterial colonization and aid in preventing LUTI.[13]
- Bladder management and patient care. In the presence of an NBD, it is mandatory to avoid overdistension to prevent detrusor atony. In the acute phase of NBD, there are three methods to empty the bladder: manual expression, intermittent aseptic catheterization, and placement of an indwelling catheter. Each of them has its pros and cons. Manual expression is simple, noninvasive, quick, and economic, but it could be challenging, dangerous, or impossible in some patients. Moreover, it is unlikely to completely empty the bladder, leaving a potentially large residual urine volume in some dogs. Catheterization, either intermittent or permanent, is simple but requires trained staff and allows complete bladder emptying. These methods are less cost-effective, require hospitalization, especially in the case of indwelling catheterization, and are invasive. The risk of developing a LUTI seems to be related more to the duration of bladder management than to the bladder emptying method.[13]

  In patients with chronic NBD, bladder management is typically undertaken by the owner through manual expression, possibly facilitated by drug medical treatment, and only in a few cases through repeated intermittent catheterization.[13]

  The bladder should be emptied at least every 8 hours or sooner if, after palpation, it appears overdistended. It is essential to keep the patient as clean and dry as possible to prevent gut pathogen exposure and urine and fecal scald.[13]
- Surgical treatment. A sacral spinal root stimulator was implanted via sacral dorsal laminectomy in 9 paraplegic dogs unable to urinate following severe thoracolumbar spinal cord injury. This treatment was successful in 8 out of 9 dogs, enabling bladder emptying of over 90% without significant side effects.[15]

Prognosis

The prognosis depends on the etiology, treatability, and severity of the underlying neurological disorders. In general, LMN bladder has a poor prognosis. Acute UMN bladder has a more guarded prognosis than chronic UMN bladder. Most of the data on micturition recovery comes from studies on spinal cord injury caused by IVDD or ischemic myelopathy. In dogs with deep pain perception, recovery of micturition is typically associated with improvement in motor function. This pattern also holds true for dogs without deep pain perception. When they recover motor function, they usually recover the ability to urinate. However, approximately 30% of these dogs will still experience some urinary deficits, such as being unable to hold urine for long periods or experiencing involuntary urination when excited.[13]

TABLE 37.1 Pharmacological agents commonly used in the treatment of neurogenic bladder dysfunction.

Function	Agents	Mechanism of action	Dosage	Adverse effects
Increasing detrusor contractility	Bethanechol	Parasympathomimetic	5–25 mg/kg PO every 8 h	Vomiting, diarrhea, salivation, bradycardia
Decreasing detrusor contractility	Oxybutynin	Muscarinic receptor antagonist	0.5 mg/kg PO every 8–12 h	Reduced gastrointestinal motility, dry mouth, tachycardia
	Mirabegron	Beta-3 adrenergic receptor agonist	<0.3 mg/kg PO every 24 h	Tachycardia, arrythmias, erythema, vomiting, destruction of the zygomatic salivary gland
Increasing urethral resistance	Phenylpropanolamine	Beta-sympathomimetic	1.5 mg/kg PO every 8 h	Hypertension, urine retention
Decreasing urethral resistance	Phenoxybenzamine	Nonspecific, smooth muscle relaxation, alpha-antagonist	0.25–1 mg/kg PO every 8–24 h for 5 days minimum	Hypotension, tachycardia, gastrointestinal upset
	Prasozin	Smooth muscle relaxation, alpha-1 adrenergic receptor antagonist	1 mg/kg PO every 8–12 h in dogs under 15 kg; 2 mg/kg PO every 8–12 h in dogs above 15 kg	Hypotension, salivation, sedation
	Tamsulosin	Smooth muscle relaxation, alpha-1 adrenergic receptor antagonist with high uroselectivity	10–30 µg/kg PO every 12–24 h	Hypotension
	Diazepam	Skeletal muscle relaxation via central effect, benzodiazepine	0.25–1 mg/kg PO every 12–24 h	Sedation, paradoxical excitation
	Dantrolene	Skeletal muscle relaxation, calcium release inhibitor	1–5 mg/kg PO every 8 h	Rare. Weakness, hepatoxicity, vomiting, hypotension
	Baclofen	Skeletal muscle relaxation via direct effect	12 mg/kg PO every 8 h	Weakness, gastrointestinal upset, pruritus

Source: Adapted from Dewey and Da Costa.[6] and Granger et al.[13] PO, orally.

KEY POINTS

- Neurogenic bladder dysfunctions (NBDs) are frequently encountered in dogs with neurological disease, particularly those affected by spinal cord injury.
- Clinical signs of NBD depend on the neuroanatomical localization of the lesion and are usually associated with other neurological deficits, including gait and tail abnormalities.
- In dogs with micturition disorders and a normal neurological examination, it is essential to rule out non-neurogenic disease before undertaking advanced neurological diagnostic procedures.
- Diagnosis of NBD relies on an appropriate diagnostic protocol based on the neuroanatomical localization of the lesion.
- The treatment and prognosis of NBD depend on the etiology, severity, and chronicity of the underlying neurological disease.
- Patients with NBD are at high risk of developing lower urinary tract infections (LUTIs). Frequent urinalyses and urine cultures are necessary to diagnose and correctly treat LUTIs.
- The bladder must be kept small: bladder management, which consists in emptying the bladder at least every 8 hours, is crucial to avoid overdistension and reduce the risk of LUTI. In chronic cases, bladder management may last for the patient's entire life.

References

1. Lane IF. Disorders of micturition. In: Osborne CA, Pineo DR (eds.). *Canine and Feline Nephrology and Urology*, 2nd ed. Baltimore: Williams and Wilkins; 1995. p. 693.
2. Coates JR. Tail, anal and bladder dysfunction. In: Platt S, Olby N (eds.). *BSAVA Manual of Canine and Feline Neurology*, 4th ed. London; 2014. pp. 381–387.
3. Lorenz MD, Coates JR, Kent M. *Handbook of Veterinary Neurology*, 5th ed. Elsevier; 2011. pp. 58–73.
4. De Groat WC, Griffiths D, Yoshimura N. Neural control of the lower urinary tract. *Compr Physiol.* 2015 Jan;5(1):327–396.
5. Gernone F, Uva A, Maiolini A, Zatelli A. A review of the neural control of micturition in dogs and cats: neuroanatomy, neurophysiology and neuroplasticity. *Vet Res Commun.* 2022 Dec;46(4):991–998.
6. Dewey CW, da Costa RC. Neurology and Neuropharmacology of Normal and Abnormal Urination. In: Dewey CW, da Costa RC (eds.). *Practical Guide to Canine and Feline Neurology*, 3rd ed. Ames, USA: Wiley-Blackwell; 2016. pp. 437–444.
7. Uemura EE. *Fundamentals of Canine Neuroanatomy and Neurophysiology.* Ames, USA: Wiley-Blackwell; 2015. pp. 383–410.
8. Gernone F, Uva A, Cavalera MA, Zatelli A. Neurogenic Bladder in Dogs, Cats and Humans: A Comparative Review of Neurological Diseases. *Animals (Basel).* 2022 Nov 22;12(23):3233.
9. Olby NJ, MacKillop E, Cerda-Gonzalez S, et al. Prevalence of urinary tract infection in dogs after surgery for thoracolumbar intervertebral disc extrusion. *J Vet Intern Med.* 2010 Sep-Oct;24(5):1106–1011.
10. Cook L, Byron J, Moore S. Urological Sequelae to Acute Spinal Cord Injury in Pet Dogs: A Natural Disease Model of Neuropathic Bladder Dysfunction. *Top Spinal Cord Inj Rehabil.* 2019 Summer;25(3):205–213.
11. Pressler B, Bartges JW. Urinary Tract Infections. In: Ettinger SJ, Feldman EC (eds.). *Textbook of Veterinary Internal Medicine*, 7th ed. Elsevier; 2010. pp. 2036–2047.
12. Hu HZ, Granger N, Jeffery ND. Pathophysiology, Clinical Importance, and Management of Neurogenic Lower Urinary Tract Dysfunction Caused by Suprasacral Spinal Cord Injury. *J Vet Intern Med.* 2016 Sep;30(5):1575–1588.
13. Granger N, Olby NJ, Nout-Lomas YS. Canine Spinal Cord Injury Consortium (CANSORT-SCI). Bladder and Bowel Management in Dogs With Spinal Cord Injury. *Front Vet Sci.* 2020 Nov 11;7:583342.
14. Noël S, Massart L, Hamaide A. Urodynamic investigation by telemetry in Beagle dogs: validation and effects of oral administration of current urological drugs: a pilot study. *BMC Vet Res.* 2013 Oct 8;9:197.
15. Granger N, Chew D, Fairhurst P, et al. Use of an Implanted Sacral Nerve Stimulator to Restore Urine Voiding in Chronically Paraplegic Dogs. *J Vet Inter Med.* 2013 Jan-Feb;27(1):99–105.

CHAPTER 38

Neuropathic pain and neuroanalgesia

Louise Clark
BVMS, Cert VA, DECVAA, MSc (Clinical Management of Pain), FRCVS

Pain terminology

Readers can refer to the website of the International Association for the Study of Pain (IASP) for definitions of the most common pain-related terms.

Pain definitions

Pain is commonly classified into three categories by cause: nociceptive, neuropathic, and nociplastic. Nociceptive pain is caused by the activation of peripheral nociceptors by a noxious stimulus. This stimulus may be thermal (heat/cold), mechanical, or chemical. Neuropathic pain is caused by an injury or lesion of the nervous system. Nociplastic pain is a relatively newly recognized third category of pain. Pain of this nature is generated by a dysfunction of the central nervous system that serves to distort the processing of normal sensory stimuli. Clinical pain is often a mixture of all these "types" of pain. This chapter concentrates on neuropathic pain, its clinical impact, and its management.

Pain can be considered as a warning about tissue damage; specific receptors and fiber systems that extend from the periphery to the brain communicate this "threat". When the normal pathways are damaged, the immediate consequence is loss or reduction of function, including pain. Sometimes, a condition termed neuropathic pain develops, which has been defined by the International Association for the Study of Pain (IASP) as "pain caused by a lesion or disease of the somatosensory nervous system".[1] The lesion needs to affect the somatosensory system; lesions or diseases outside this system (e.g., in the cerebellum) do not qualify as neuropathic. Terms previously used for pain following injury to the nervous system, such as nerve injury pain, neuralgia, deafferentation pain, neurogenic pain, and central pain, have now been superseded by the term neuropathic pain, to avoid any postulated mechanism or a specific anatomical location of the lesion. When lesions of the nervous system occur peripherally or centrally, they may cause sensory loss in the innervation territory of damaged nerves or in the anatomical area that corresponds to a spinal or brain territory that has been damaged. Therefore, an important distinguishing feature in most cases of neuropathic pain is the paradoxical combination of sensory loss and pain, either with or without sensory hypersensitivity phenomena. Neuropathic pain is associated with a large group of conditions with variable anatomical locations and etiologies.[2]

Mechanisms of neuropathic pain

Neuropathic pain patients show multiple changes in the peripheral nervous system, spinal cord, and brain. Endogenous pain modulation systems may have reduced functionality. The mechanisms involved are incredibly complex and are still being elucidated. The following is simplified for the purposes of aiding understanding and clinical management.

Peripheral nervous system in neuropathic pain

Ectopic activity in primary afferent fibers can have a role in the pathophysiology of neuropathic pain following peripheral nerve injury. For example, patients with a traumatic peripheral nerve injury show a complete loss of ipsilateral spontaneous and evoked pain when treated with a peripheral nerve block (with lidocaine, which blocks voltage-gated sodium channels). If an afferent fiber is disconnected from the periphery due to an injury or a lesion, there will be sensory loss. However, the remnants of the fibers at the injury site can generate ectopic activity (e.g., neuroma C-fiber afferents), resulting in pain from a "numb" area. The remaining intact fibers are hyperexcitable, so-called irritable nociceptors. As a result, the patient can experience ongoing pain, numbness, and evoked pain.[3] Current evidence suggests that the contributions of different types of afferent fibers are state- and context-dependent and vary between disorders.

Contributions of spinal cord circuits to neuropathic pain

Sensory afferents from the periphery terminate at synapses with second-order neurons in the dorsal horn of the spinal cord. Low-threshold (touch) afferents generally terminate and synapse in lamina III and laminae anatomically deep to this, whilst nociceptive afferents synapse in the superficial dorsal horn. Fibers carrying touch information not only synapse in the deeper laminae of the spinal cord but also branch and project directly to nuclei in the brainstem via the dorsal columns. In this way, touch information can reach higher centers directly without synapsing via the spinal cord. Under normal conditions, touch and pain processing areas are spatially segregated in the spinal dorsal horn. Each of these areas contain second-order neurons that act as the next link in the pathways and convey touch and pain information to the brain. Sensory afferent inputs can trigger a prolonged but reversible increase in the excitability and synaptic efficacy of neurons in central nociceptive pathways; this phenomenon is known as central sensitization. Central sensitization manifests as pain hypersensitivity, particularly dynamic mechanical allodynia, secondary punctate or pressure hyperalgesia, aftersensations, and enhanced temporal summation. Allodynia (mechanical or cold allodynia) is one of the features of neuropathic pain in people that is very unpleasant and challenging to manage. It is likely that structural reorganization (plasticity) of synapses, cells, and circuits takes place in pathophysiological states and contributes to the chronic nature of pain.[4]

A desegregation of touch and pain may arise at the level of spinal processing through multiple distinct but not mutually exclusive mechanisms. These include structural remodeling of circuits to enable physical links between nociceptive and non-nociceptive neurons or disinhibition of existing physical links, for which there is currently more evidence.[4] Abnormal neuroimmune interaction is a major contributor to the pathophysiology of neuropathic pain. In summary, these complex mechanisms increase the "gain" of the system resulting in states of facilitation, potentiation, or amplification.

Central pain modulation mechanisms

Some patients with neuropathic pain are moderately affected, whereas others experience debilitating pain. Patients show a large variability in the response to distinct pharmacological and nonpharmacological treatments. A factor involved might be the way that the pain message is modulated in the central nervous system via the descending pain modulatory system (DPMS).[3] This is a complex top-down system in which cognitive, emotional, or autonomic factors can regulate nociceptive processing in a facilitatory or inhibitory manner, thereby heightening or reducing the ultimate pain experience. Descending neurons project from the rostroventral medulla and locus cœruleus to the dorsal horn. The DPMS is influenced by both sensory and affective brain circuits. Pain may be facilitated or inhibited according not only to the degree of injury but also to the emotional status of the individual. Plasticity within the DPMS is a key factor in the transition from acute to chronic pain. Most human patients with neuropathic pain express a pronociceptive pain modulation profile, with augmented pain messages in the central nervous system. The clinical relevance of this in veterinary neuropathic pain patients is currently unknown.

Diagnosis

A comparative approach

In human practice, neuropathic pain presentation is dominated by patient report, i.e., symptoms, and the associated clinical signs are limited. Different scales and questionnaires have been developed to attempt to discriminate between neuropathic and non-neuropathic pain states. No studies have provided a robust, reliable classification of symptoms and signs, and so a hierarchical system has been developed based on grading of evidence for the presence of neuropathic pain, where neuropathic pain is divided into three classes: possible, probable, and definite neuropathic pain (Fig. 38.1). This is based on neurological history, distribution of pain, the presence and location of sensory signs, and finally a confirmatory test.[5]

Clinical presentation in people

It is useful to understand how neuropathic pain presents in people to aid our diagnosis in veterinary patients. Most human patients complain of ongoing or intermittent spontaneous pain. The descriptors used include burning, shooting, pricking, pins and needles, squeezing, or freezing pain. There may be intermittent electric shock–like pain paroxysms, either alone or in addition to an ongoing pain. There may be abnormal sensations, which includes dysesthesias and paresthesia; both may occur spontaneously or be evoked. Evoked types of pain may occur in addition to spontaneous pain and rarely as the only pain manifestation. Usually, this is touch-evoked or cold-evoked pain. On examination, allodynia and hyperalgesia to mechanical or thermal stimuli can be found in addition to sensory loss. There may be aftersensations, which is pain continuing after a stimulation has ceased, and referral of (painful or nonpainful) sensations to denervated areas elicited by stimulation of adjacent body areas.[6] A poor association between self-reported evoked pain and gain on Quantitative Sensory Testing (QST) is well-known, and discrepancy is also documented between bedside examination findings and QST. The tests are inadequate to capture allodynia, and the symptoms sometimes occur intermittently and therefore may not be present at examination. Spontaneous pain often occurs without any evoked pain, and evoked pain may rarely occur without any spontaneous pain. This suggests that evoked and spontaneous pain are caused by different mechanisms, or alternatively, by overlapping mechanisms, but preservation or loss of specific afferent fibers determines the presence or absence of evoked pain.[6]

Diagnosis in veterinary patients

Given the lack of verbal report from veterinary patients, careful history taking is important to identify any behaviors that might indicate the presence of neuropathic pain. These include decreased general activity level and enthusiasm for engaging in activity, reluctance to climb or descend stairs, diminished jumping behavior, difficulty rising, trouble getting into and out of the car, and changes in body posture or appetite. Some of these behavior changes might also be present due to nociceptive or nociplastic pain secondary to musculoskeletal disease (e.g., chronic osteoarthritis), and this must be considered.

Owners may notice reluctance of their dog to being restrained, a new dislike of being held, increasing objection to nail trims and/or venipuncture, and a gradual decrease in the dog's interaction with them. Some dogs are described as increasingly grouchy/self-defensive; this may impact interaction with other dogs including avoidance behavior. Obvious clinical signs include a change in response to palpation or even touch, vocalization in the absence of an overtly painful stimulus, phantom scratching, excessive licking or self-mutilation, and persistent lameness/diminished weight bearing on a limb. An animal that spontaneously rubs its mouth, reacts to (runs from/vocalizes in response to) an invisible stimulus, or exhibits spontaneous panniculus may have neuropathic pain. It should also be suspected when a patient is refractory to conventional analgesic therapy[7] and has shown clinical signs of allodynia and/or hyperalgesia; however, hypoalgesia may also be present depending on the lesion and disease. Box 38.1 lists some conditions that may include neuropathic pain as part of their presentation.

In a veterinary context, QST evaluates the transmission of information related to thermal, mechanical, and chemical stimuli from the periphery

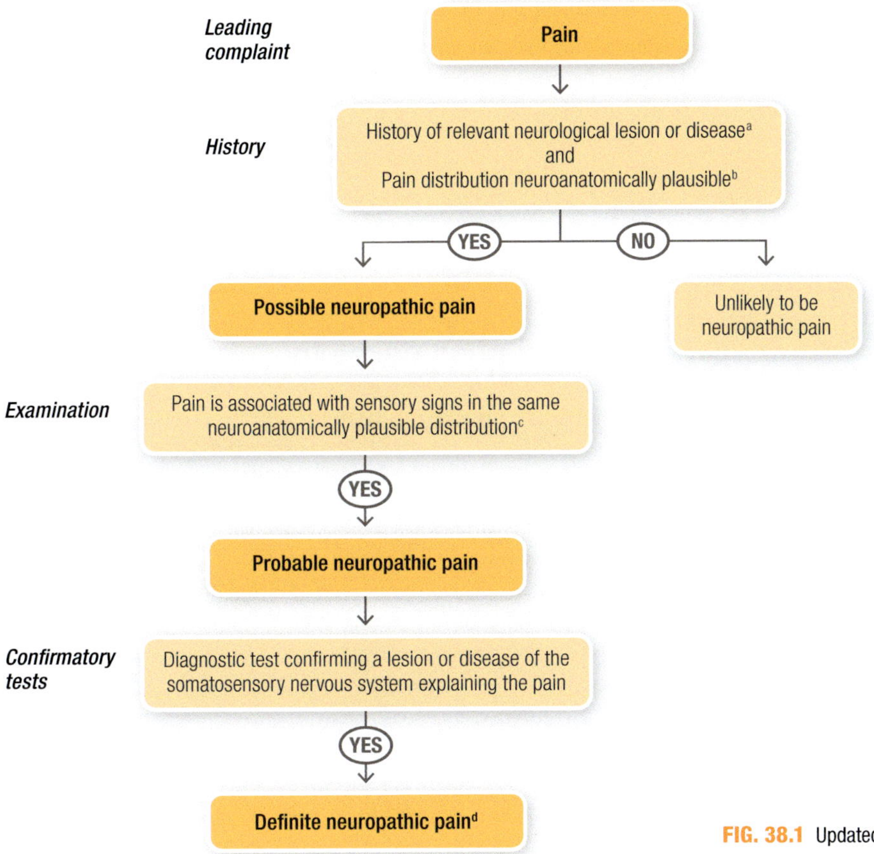

[a] History, including pain descriptors, the presence of nonpainful sensory symptoms, and aggravating and alleviating factors suggestive of pain being related to a neurological lesion and not other causes such as inflammation or non-neural tissue damage. The suspected lesion or disease is reported to be associated with neuropathic pain, including a temporal and spatial relationship representative of the condition; includes paroxysmal pain in trigeminal neuralgia.

[b] The pain distribution reported by the patient is consistent with the suspected lesion or disease.

[c] The area of sensory changes may extend beyond, be within, or overlap with the area of pain. Sensory loss is generally required but touch-evoked or thermal allodynia may be the only finding at bedside examination. In some cases, sensory signs may be difficult to demonstrate although the nature of the lesion or disease is confirmed; for these cases, the level "probable" continues to be appropriate, if a diagnostic test confirms the lesion or disease of the somatosensory nervous system.

[d] The term "definite" in this context means "probable neuropathic pain with confirmatory tests" because the location and nature of the lesion or disease have been confirmed to be able to explain the pain. "Definite" neuropathic pain is a pain that is fully compatible with neuropathic pain, but it does not necessarily establish causality.[5]

FIG. 38.1 Updated grading system for neuropathic pain. Source: Finnerup NB et al.[5]

to the somatosensory cortex. It uses calibrated devices to induce a noxious stimulus against the skin of the animal until a behavioral reaction is observed, at which the end point is objectively recorded (e.g., Newtons, grams, seconds). Quantification of sensory sensitivity allows comparison of animals with and without disease, as well as assessment of treatment efficacy. QST has shown that dogs with thoracolumbar disc herniation showed increased pain facilitation and/or decreased pain inhibition when compared with healthy individuals. QST could provide useful clinical information when incorporated into the physical/neurological examination in the future but also has demonstrable limitations in people (see above). Behavioral changes associated with chronic pain may develop gradually, may be subtle, and may only be detected by someone familiar with the animal. Numerous pain scoring instruments are available to evaluate chronic pain or health-related quality of life (HRQoL) in dogs; however, only a few have been validated and none has specifically been validated in the context of known neuropathic pain. Pain assessment is considered in greater detail in the recent guidelines for the recognition, assessment, and treatment of pain by the World Small Animal Veterinary Association (WSAVA).[7]

Box 38.1 Conditions that may include neuropathic pain as part of their presentation.

- Chiari-like malformation/syringomyelia.
- Radiculopathy caused by chronic cervical or lumbosacral disc disease.
- Diabetic or another painful polyneuropathy.
- Spinal cord injury, e.g., caused by intervertebral disc herniation.
- Central poststroke pain (CPSP) can occur after a cerebrovascular accident. It is characterized by pain and sensory abnormalities in the body parts that correspond to the brain territory injured by the cerebrovascular lesion.
- Persistent postsurgical pain (avoidable), e.g., following cosmetic procedures, which are illegal in many countries.
- Persistent postsurgical pain, e.g., following amputation or thoracotomy.
- Osteoarthritis may present with pain that has neuropathic features; it may be better termed nociplastic pain.

Management of neuropathic pain

Overview of management strategies

The first step in the management of neuropathic pain is identification, whenever possible, of the underlying disease affecting the somatosensory system. This chapter does not consider nociceptive pain, and the likelihood of mixed pain contributing to the clinical presentation should be considered. Strategies for managing nociceptive pain have been reviewed extensively in the recent *WSAVA guidelines for the recognition, assessment and treatment of pain*.[7] Pharmacological therapy should be used rationally, according to the type (mechanism) of pain and based on evidence of efficacy. This may need to be combination therapy because different types and sources of pain can exist simultaneously.

Nonpharmacological interventions may help a return to more normal function. They include weight reduction and avoiding injury from environmental hazards (e.g., using nonslip flooring). Other modalities directed at addressing neuropathic pain include the use of heat and cold therapy, acupuncture, stretching, massage, and exercise. All these modalities need further research. In patients with acute or chronic neuropathic pain with severe clinical signs of hyperalgesia and allodynia, hospitalization might be required to apply neuromodifying techniques (e.g., local anesthetic blocks) and/or administration of intravenous analgesics.[7] Neuropathic pain is difficult to treat and can have a large impact on HRQoL. Ethically, euthanasia should always be considered in cases in which pain cannot be effectively managed.

Practical approach to cases with suspected neuropathic pain

There is limited evidence to support a particular approach to the management of neuropathic pain in veterinary patients. This is a suggested approach based on the available evidence and clinical experience:

- Nonpharmacological interventions should always be considered as part of management as their risk–benefit profile is favorable despite limited evidence of efficacy.
- When severe pain is present, hospitalization and the use of local anesthetic techniques or intravenous options should be considered.[7]
- The Neuropathic Pain Special Interest group (NeuPSIG) of the International Association for the Study of Pain (IASP) has published recommendations for the pharmacological treatment of neuropathic pain in people.[6] Drugs with a moderate to high quality of evidence and strong recommendation are tricyclic antidepressants (TCAs), gabapentin, pregabalin, and serotonin noradrenaline reuptake inhibitors (SNRI: duloxetine and venlafaxine), and these are recommended as first-line drugs. Drugs with a weak recommendation included capsaicin 8% patches, lidocaine patches, and subcutaneous injections of botulinum toxin type A for peripheral neuropathic pain only.[6]
- Oral therapy is the mainstay of the management of neuropathic pain in veterinary patients. Topical approaches such a lidocaine patches, capsaicin patches, and botulinum toxin have been used, but little species-specific evidence exists to support their use as first-line therapeutics.
- Based on the above literature and limited veterinary evidence, initial management with gabapentin or pregabalin would be a rational approach[9] with TCAs as an alternate or potentially additional option.
- This should be as part of multimodal drug therapy, when pain relief with veterinary licensed analgesics is inadequate, and central sensitization or neuropathic pain are thought to be involved.
- Clients should be informed about the uncertainty of a beneficial effect.
- Treatment should include careful monitoring of efficacy and adverse effects.
- Regular assessment and reviews are needed.
- If clinical signs of pain or adverse effects persist despite treatment with gabapentin or pregabalin in the suggested dosage range, after 2 to 3 months, the drug should be withdrawn while introducing an alternative.
- Making more than one change at a time will make it difficult to assess efficacy.

There is a reported risk of rebound seizures with acute withdrawal of gabapentinoids in people, but this is not well documented in canine patients. Sedation and ataxia appear to be the most consistently reported adverse effects with both gabapentin and pregabalin in dogs. Increased appetite and weight gain and diarrhea have also been reported. It is possible that adverse effects such as sedation and ataxia may be interpreted as a worsening of the clinical signs. There may be additive effects with other central nervous system depressants such as sedatives, antidepressants, anesthetics, and opioids (e.g., tramadol). The initial sedation and ataxia may be avoided by gradually increasing the dose over a few days or weeks to the recommended doses or until a clinically relevant effect is obtained.

Practical pharmacology

Gabapentin and pregabalin

Gabapentin and pregabalin are structural analogues of the neurotransmitter gamma-aminobutyric acid (GABA) but are inactive at GABA receptors. They bind to, and inhibit, voltage-gated calcium channels in the central nervous system. Their mode of action is complex, impacting the release of various neurotransmitters including glutamate and noradrenaline. Over several weeks, this leads to a reduction in dorsal horn sensitization; clinically, this corresponds to a reduction in allodynia and hyperalgesia. Gabapentin also binds to the N-methyl-D-aspartate (NMDA) receptor and reduces NMDA-receptor hyperactivity. Both drugs may restore deficiencies in the DPMS. Gabapentin and pregabalin may also be useful for controlling anxiety, but this is beyond the scope of this chapter.

Gabapentin is readily absorbed when given by mouth to dogs. Gabapentin should not be administered within 2 hours of oral antacids as these will hinder absorption. Efficacy in humans is associated with 2 μg/mL plasma concentrations, but the effective concentrations are unknown in the dog. Data suggest 10–20 mg/kg every 8 hours would maintain 2 μg/mL plasma concentrations in dogs. Metabolism of gabapentin is partially by N-methylation (hepatic) in dogs. The drug is thought to be excreted mainly via the kidneys, with an elimination half-life of around 2 to 4 hours in dogs.

The absorption characteristics of pregabalin in dogs are unknown. In humans, metabolism is minimal, with 98% of the drug excreted via the kidneys; the renal route is also thought to be the main elimination route in dogs. Pregabalin is more potent and longer acting than gabapentin in dogs. The elimination half-life is around 7 hours in dogs.

There is a lack of good quality evidence for the efficacy of both gabapentin and pregabalin in dogs with chronic pain. The reference list includes several clinical trials that document the use of gabapentinoids, particularly in Chiari-like malformation/syringomyelia.[10,11,12] There are also several case reports and case series that suggest efficacy, but given the lack of a control group, cannot demonstrate it.[13] This literature should be read critically. Gabapentin and pregabalin are antihyperalgesic, not "analgesic"; they do not affect normal nociceptive pain. They may not be effective in the absence of central sensitization so should not be used as a primary analgesic.

Legal requirements for ordering, storing, and prescribing gabapentin and pregabalin may vary from country to country. They can be abused by people; for example, in the UK, gabapentin and pregabalin are schedule 3 controlled drugs. Gabapentin has become familiar to many veterinarians in practice and so is commonly chosen over pregabalin. However, the need for less frequent dosing due to pregabalin's longer duration of action may be more convenient for many clients.[9]

Tricyclic antidepressants

The effects of TCAs on neuropathic pain are distinct from their antidepressant effects. TCAs including amitriptyline are considered a first-line therapy for neuropathic pain in humans. They exert analgesic effects in several ways, including inhibiting reuptake of serotonin and norepinephrine, antagonism of voltage-gated sodium channels, and antagonism of NMDA receptors. There is limited clinical evidence for use in dogs thus far.[14]

Amantadine

Amantadine is an NDMA antagonist that increases the rate of channel closure following activation of the NMDA complex. It is a weak dopamine agonist and glutamate antagonist that is not widely used in the treatment of neuropathic pain in people. It may decrease central sensitization. Originally an antiviral and antiparkinsonian drug, it may be withdrawn from veterinary use because of its role as an antiviral agent in people and reservation for human use.

Tramadol

Opioids may exacerbate chronic neuropathic pain via neuroinflammation and glial amplification. They are no longer widely advocated for use in people. Tramadol is a weak OP3 (μ) receptor agonist that also inhibits reuptake of noradrenaline and 5-HT. Some individuals do not produce significant quantities of the active metabolite O-desmethyl tramadol. In chronic pain, it is presumed that it is the effects on the descending inhibitory pathways that may be beneficial, and the opioid-like effects may promote sedation, hyperalgesia, and dysphoria. Behavioral changes without analgesic benefit can occur. Careful assessment and discussion with the owners is necessary. It is hard to recommend it in dogs considering the current evidence.[15] In some countries, tramadol is a controlled drug, in others, it is available over the counter, which may impact the frequency of its use. Information relating to ketamine and memantine can be found in Table 38.1.

TABLE 38.1 Pharmacological management of neuropathic pain.

Drug	Dose PO unless specified	Frequency	Comments
Gabapentin	10–20 mg/kg*	Every 8 h	■ Potential accumulation in renal dysfunction. Start with a low dose and gradually titrate upwards ■ * Increasing dose gradually at start of treatment might avoid sedation and ataxia ■ Half-life (2–4 hours) suggests 8-hourly dosing is more likely than 12-hourly dosing to produce a sustained effect
Pregabalin	3‡–4 mg/kg	Every 12 h	■ ‡ Some recommend starting 1 to 2 mg/kg every 12 hours, increasing by 1 mg/kg per week according to effect; 2 mg/kg every 12 hours may be effective
Amitriptyline	1–4 mg/kg	Every 12–24 h	■ Urinary retention reported anecdotally ■ **Do not administer with other serotoninergic drugs**
Amantadine	2–5 mg/kg	Every 12–24 h	■ RCT showing efficacy in dogs with osteoarthritis alongside NSAID ■ Higher doses reported (>10 mg/kg) ■ No withdrawal period required ■ Minimum recommended duration before reassessment is 21 days ■ Long duration therapy may be necessary ■ Usually well tolerated. Agitation, vomiting, flatulence, or diarrhea (which may be watery), possible particularly after first few doses ■ If patient vomits after administration on an empty stomach, try giving with a small meal or treat ■ Use with caution when given with amantadine: anticholinergic drugs, CNS stimulants (includes selegiline), trimethoprim/sulfonamide, thiazide diuretics or urinary acidifiers
Memantine	Dosing 0.3–0.8 mg/kg	Once (or twice) daily	■ Similar mechanism of action to amantadine ■ Much cheaper ■ Less data, information and dosing extrapolated from behavioral medicine ■ Use in chronic pain remains anecdotal ■ Lower incidence of vomiting
Ketamine	0.2–0.5 mg/kg IV then 2–10 μg/kg/min	CRI up to 72 hours, watch for dysphoria at higher doses in prolonged infusions – taper doses	■ Ketamine is not a recognized antineuropathic agent but is often used for the management of refractory chronic pain ■ Ketamine can be used in dogs already receiving other NMDA antagonists (amantadine, memantine) and adverse effects from this are rarely seen ■ Ketamine continuous rate infusions for pain breakthrough where admission to hospital is required ■ Can be used at higher doses during sedation/anesthesia
Tramadol	NOT recommended		■ Do not administer with other serotoninergic drugs

PO, orally; IV, intravenously; CS, subcutaneously; CRI, constant rate infusion; RCT, randomized controlled trial; NSAID, nonsteroidal anti-inflammatory drug; CNS, central nervous system; NMDA, N-methyl-D-aspartate.

Other options

Other drugs may have efficacy against neuropathic pain in specific circumstances. These drugs include:

- Botulinum toxin
- Cannabidiol
- Capsaicin patch
- Lidocaine patch
- Duloxetine
- Lamotrigine
- Levetiracetam
- Oxcarbazepine
- Topiramate
- Venlafaxine

However, the evidence to support their efficacy is often limited in people and very poor in veterinary species, and they are not widely used. Discussion about their use is beyond the limited scope of this chapter.

KEY POINTS

- Neuropathic pain is "pain caused by a lesion or disease of the somatosensory nervous system".
- Terms previously used for pain following injury to the nervous system, including nerve injury pain, neuralgia, deafferentation pain, neurogenic pain, and central pain have now been superseded.
- Neuropathic pain is associated with a large group of conditions with variable anatomical locations and etiology.
- Diagnosis is based on the patient's neurological history, distribution of pain, the presence and location of sensory signs, and a confirmatory (usually imaging) test.
- In people, descriptors used include burning, shooting, pricking, pins and needles, squeezing, or freezing pain. There may be abnormal sensations, which includes dysesthesias and paresthesia; both may occur spontaneously or evoked. Evoked types of pain may occur in addition to spontaneous pain and rarely alone.
- Careful history taking and observation of behavioral changes guides a suspicion of neuropathic pain in veterinary patients.
- Human patients show a large variability in response to distinct pharmacological and nonpharmacological treatments. Pain may be facilitated or inhibited in a manner corresponding to the emotional status of the individual.
- There is weak evidence that gabapentin and pregabalin have antihyperalgesic effects in cats and dogs. Typical adverse effects are dose-related sedation (which might be transient) and ataxia.
- Neuropathic pain is difficult to treat, recommendations are often based on the human literature and an inadequate body of evidence from veterinary medicine. Neuropathic pain can have a negative impact on quality of life and ethically, euthanasia should be considered in cases when pain cannot be effectively managed.

References

1. International Association for the Study of Pain. *Terminology.* International Association for the Study of Pain Website. Retrieved 17th August 2023 from: https://www.iasp-pain.org/resources/terminology/.
2. Scholz J, Finnerup NB, Attal N, et al. Classification Committee of the Neuropathic Pain Special Interest Group (NeuPSIG). The IASP classification of chronic pain for ICD-11: chronic neuropathic pain. *Pain.* 2019;160: 53–59.
3. Colloca L, Ludman T, Bouhassira D, et al. Neuropathic pain. *Nat Rev Dis Primers.* 2017 Feb 16; 3:17002.
4. Kuner R, Flor H, Structural plasticity and reorganisation in chronic pain. *Nat Rev Neurosci.* 2017, 18(1):20–30. Erratum in: *Nat Rev Neurosci.* 2017 Feb;18(2):158. Erratum in: *Nat Rev Neurosci.* 2017 Jan 20;18(2):113.
5. Finnerup NB, Haroutounian S, Kamerman P et al. Neuropathic pain: an updated grading system for research and clinical practice. *Pain.* 2016;157:1599–1606.
6. Finnerup NB, Kuner R, Jensen TS. Neuropathic Pain: From Mechanisms to Treatment. *Physiol Rev.* 2021 Jan 1;101(1):259–301.
7. Monteiro BP, Lascelles BDX, Murrell J, et al, 2022 WSAVA guidelines for the recognition, assessment and treatment of pain. *J Small Anim Pract.* 2023;64:177–254.
8. Moore SA. Managing Neuropathic Pain in Dogs. *Front Vet Sci.* 2016 Feb 22;3:12.
9. Covey-Crump G. *Gabapentin and pregabalin in the management of chronic pain in cats and dogs.* Veterinary Prescriber. Retrieved January 2024 from: https://members.veterinaryprescriber.org/app/cpd/module/gabapentin-and-pregabalin-in-the-management-of-chronic-pain-in-cats-and-dogs.
10. Plessas IN, Volk HA, Rusbridge C, et al. Comparison of gabapentin versus topiramate on clinically affected dogs with chiari-like malformation and syringomyelia. *Vet Rec.* 2015 Sep 19;177(11):288.
11. Sanchis-Mora S, Chang, YM, Abeyesinghe SM, et al. Pregabalin for the treatment of syringomyelia-associated neuropathic pain in dogs: a randomised, placebo-controlled, double-masked clinical trial. *Vet J.* 2019 Aug;250:55–62.
12. Thoefner MS, Skovgaard LT, McEvoy FJ, et al. Pregabalin alleviates clinical signs of syringomyelia-related central neuropathic pain in Cavalier King Charles spaniel dogs: a randomized controlled trial. *Vet Anaesth Analg.* 2020 Mar;47(2):238–248.
13. Schmierer PA, Tunsmeyer J, Tipold A, et al. Randomized controlled trial of pregabalin for analgesia after surgical treatment of intervertebral disc disease in dogs. *Vet Surg.* 2020 Jul;49(5):905–913.
14. Norkus C, Rankin D, KuKanich B. Pharmacokinetics of intravenous and oral amitriptyline and its active metabolite nortriptyline in Greyhound dogs. *Vet Anaesth Analg.* 2015 Nov;42(6):580–589.
15. Donati PA, Tarragona L, Franco JVA, et al. Efficacy of tramadol for postoperative pain management in dogs: systematic review and meta-analysis. *Vet Anaesth Analg.* 2021;48(3):283–296.

Index

O

P